ALZHEIMER'S DISEASE

ALZHEIMER'S DISEASE

Barry Reisberg, M.D., Editor

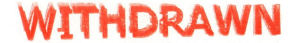

THE FREE PRESS
A Division of Macmillan, Inc.
NEW YORK

Collier Macmillan Publishers
LONDON

The Free Press
A Division of Macmillan, Inc.
866 Third Avenue, New York, N.Y. 10022

Collier Macmillan Canada, Inc.

Printed in the United States of America

printing number

4 5 6 7 8 9 10

Library of Congress Cataloging in Publication Data

Main entry under title:

Alzheimer's disease.

  Includes bibliographical references and index.
  1. Alzheimer's disease.   I. Reisberg, Barry.
[DNLM: 1. Dementia, Presenile. WM 220 A4786]
RC523.A395   1983   616.89′83   83–48030
ISBN 0–02–926230–5

CONTENTS

v

CONTRIBUTORS

BALL, MELVYN J., M.D., F.R.C.P.(C), Professor of Neuropathology, Departments of Pathology, Clinical Neurological Sciences, and Psychiatry, University of Western Ontario; Director, University of Western Ontario Dementia Study; Director, Neuropathology Research Laboratory, University Hospital, London, Ontario, Canada.

BARTUS, RAYMOND T., Ph.D., Director, Geriatric Research Program, and Group Leader/Behavioral Neuroscience, Department of CNS Research, Medical Research Division, American Cyanamid Company, Pearl River, N.Y.; Adjunct Professor, Department of Psychiatry, New York University School of Medicine, New York, N.Y.

BEER, BERNARD, Ph.D., Director, Department of CNS Research, Medical Research Division, American Cyanamid Company, Pearl River, N.Y.; Adjunct Full Professor, City University of New York; Adjunct Full Professor, Department of Psychiatry, New York University School of Medicine, New York, N.Y.

BOLLER, FRANÇOIS, M.D., Ph.D., Associate Professor of Neurology and Psychiatry, University of Pittsburgh School of Medicine, Pittsburgh, Pa.

BOWEN, DAVID M., Ph.D., Reader in Neurochemistry, Institute of Neurology, London, England.

BRANCONNIER, ROLAND J., M.A., Research Director, Geriatric Psychopharmacology, Institute for Psychopharmacologic Research, Brookline, Mass.; Ph.D. candidate in Pharmacology, Boston University; Research Consultant on the Pharmacology of Aging, Laboratory of Neuropsychology, Tufts Medical School; Associate Member, Boston University Gerontology Center, Boston, Mass.

BRINKMAN, SAMUEL, Ph.D., Veterans Administration Medical Center, Allen Park, Mich.; Department of Psychiatry and Neurology, Wayne State University, Detroit, Mich.

BRODY, HAROLD, Ph.D., M.D., Professor and Chairman, Department of Anatomical Sciences, State University of New York, Buffalo, N.Y.

BROWN, PAUL WHEELER, M.D., Medical Director, Laboratory of Central Nervous System Studies, NINCDS, National Institutes of Health, Bethesda, Md.

BRUN, ARNE, M.D., Professor and Chairman, Department of Neuropathology, Institute of Pathology, University of Lund, Lund, Sweden.

BUSSE, EWALD W., M.D., Associate Provost and Dean Emeritus, and J. P. Gibbons Professor of Psychiatry, Duke University Medical Center, Durham, N.C.

BUTLER, ROBERT N., M.D., Professor and Chairman, Department of Geriatrics, Mount Sinai School of Medicine, New York, N.Y.

CARLSSON, ARVID, M.L., M.D. (M.D., Ph.D.), Professor of Pharmacology, University of Göteberg, Göteberg, Sweden.

COHEN, DONNA, Ph.D., Associate Professor of Psychiatry, Medicine, and Neuroscience, and Head, Division of Aging and Geriatric Psychiatry, Montefiore Medical Center and Albert Einstein College of Medicine, Bronx, N.Y.

COHEN, GENE D., M.D., Chief, Center for Studies of the Mental Health of the Aging, National Institute of Mental Health, Rockville, Md.

COPPEL, DAVID, Ph.D., Postdoctoral Fellow, Department of Psychiatry and Behavioral Medicine, University of Washington School of Medicine, Seattle, Wash.

CROOK, THOMAS, Ph.D., Chief, Drug and Alcohol Program, Center for Studies of the Mental Health of the Aging, National Institute of Mental Health, Rockville, Md.

DAVIS, JOHN M., M.D., Gilman Professor of Psychiatry, University of Illinois; Director, Illinois Department of Mental Health, Chicago, Ill.

DAVIS, KENNETH L., M.D., Director, Schizophrenia Biological Research Center, Bronx Veterans Administration Medical Center; Chief, Department of Psychiatry, Veterans Administration Medical Center, Bronx, N.Y.; Associate Professor of Psychiatry and Assistant Professor, Pharmacology, Mount Sinai School of Medicine, New York, N.Y.

DAVISON, ALAN N., B.Pharm., B.Sc., Ph.D., D.Sc., F.R.C. Pathology, Professor of Neurochemistry, Institute of Neurology, The National Hospital for Nervous Diseases, London, England; first president (now vice-president) of the Alzheimer's Disease Society.

DEAN, REGINALD L., III, M.A., Research Scientist, Department of CNS Research, Medical Research Division, American Cyanamid Company, Pearl River, N.Y.

DE LEON, MONY J., Ed.D., Geriatric Study and Treatment Program, Department of Psychiatry, New York University Medical Center, New York, N.Y.

DEVITT, DONALD R., Institute for Psychopharmacologic Research, Brookline, Mass.

DRACHMAN, DAVID A., M.D., Professor and Chairman, Department of Neurology, University of Massachusetts Medical School, Worcester, Mass.

DYSKEN, MAURICE W., M.D., Associate Professor of Psychiatry and Pharmacology, University of Illinois; Research Associate, Illinois State Psychiatric Institute, Chicago, Ill.

EBERT, MICHAEL H., M.D., Section on Experimental Therapeutics and Laboratory of Clinical Science, National Institute of Mental Health, Bethesda, Md.

EISDORFER, CARL, Ph.D., M.D., President, Montefiore Medical Center, Bronx, N.Y.

EMR, MARIAN, Public Affairs Specialist, National Institute on Aging, National Institutes of Health, Bethesda, Md.

EPSTEIN, RACHEAL, Laboratory of Psychology and Psychopathology, National Institute of Mental Health, Bethesda, Md.

ETIENNE, PIERRE, M.D., F.R.C.P.(C), Assistant Professor, Department of Psychiatry, McGill University, Montreal, Canada; Psychiatrist, Department of Geriatrics, and Coordinator of Research in Biological Psychiatry, Douglas Hospital Research Centre, Verdun, Quebec, Canada.

FERRIS, STEVEN H., Ph.D., Geriatric Study and Treatment Program, Department of Psychiatry, New York University Medical Center, New York, N.Y.

FISCHMAN, HARLOW K., Ph.D., Associate Research Scientist, and Head, Cell Genetics Laboratory, New York State Psychiatric Institute; Research Associate, Department of Human Genetics and Development, Columbia University, College of Physicians and Surgeons, New York, N.Y.

FOLSOM, JAMES C., M.D., Director, ICD—International Center for the Disabled; Associate Clinical Professor of Psychiatry, New York University Medical Center School of Medicine, New York, N.Y.

FORTOUL, TERESA, M.D., Postdoctoral Fellow, Department of Pathology, University of California at Los Angeles, Los Angeles, Calif.

FOVALL, PENELOPE, M.A., Ph.D. candidate, Committee on Human Development, University of Chicago, Chicago, Ill.

FRIEDMAN, EITAN, Ph.D., Associate Professor of Psychiatry and Pharmacology, New York University School of Medicine, New York, N.Y.

FULD, PAULA ALTMAN, Ph.D., Associate Professor of Neurology (Psychology), Albert Einstein College of Medicine; Chief, Clinical Neuropsychology, Bronx Municipal Hospital Center.

GAJDUSEK, D. CARLETON, M.D., National Institute of Neurological and Communicative Disorders and Stroke, National Institutes of Health, Bethesda, Md.

GEORGE, AJAX E., M.D., Department of Radiology, New York University Medical Center, New York, N.Y.

GERSHON, SAMUEL, M.D., D.P.M., F.A.P.A., F.R.C. Psychiatry, Department of Psychiatry, Wayne State University, Detroit, Mich.

GIBBS, CLARENCE J., Jr., Ph.D., National Institute of Neurological and Communicative Disorders and Stroke, National Institutes of Health, Bethesda, Md.

GOTTFRIES, CARL-GERHARD, M.D., Ph.D., Professor and Chairman, Department of Psychiatry and Neurochemistry, University of Göteborg; Head Physician, St. Jörgen's Hospital, Hisings-Backa, Sweden.

GREENWALD, BLAINE, M.D., Instructor, Department of Psychiatry, Mount Sinai School of Medicine; Clinical/Research Fellow in Geriatric Psychiatry, Bronx Veterans Administration Medical Center/Mount Sinai School of Medicine, New York, N.Y.

HACHINSKI, VLADIMIR C., M.D., F.R.C.P.(C), Professor of Neurology, Department of Clinical Neurological Sciences, University of Western Ontario, London, Ontario, Canada.

HAYCOX, JAMES A., M.D., Director of Psychiatry, The Burke Rehabilitation Center, White Plains, N.Y.

INGVAR, DAVID H., M.D., Ph.D., Professor and Chairman, Department of Clinical Neuropathology, University Hospital, Lund, Sweden.

IQBAL, KHALID, Ph.D., Head, Chemical Neuropathology Laboratory, and Associate Professor of Neurology, Institute for Basic Research in Developmental Disabilities, Staten Island, N.Y.

JOHN, E. ROY, Ph.D., Brain Research Laboratories, Department of Psychiatry, New York University Medical Center, New York, N.Y.

KAYE, WALTER H., M.D., Section on Experimental Therapeutics and Laboratory of Clinical Science, National Institute of Mental Health, Bethesda, Md.

LERER, BARBARA, Ph.D., Postdoctoral Fellow and Research Scientist, Department of Psychiatry, New York University Medical Center, New York, N.Y.

LIEBERMAN, ABRAHAM N., M.D., Professor of Neurology, New York University School of Medicine, New York, N.Y.

MANN, DAVID M. A., M.D., Lecturer, Department of Neuropathology, The University of Manchester, Manchester, England.

MATSUYAMA, HARUO, M.D., Director General, Saitama National Hospital; Professor of Pathology, Keio University School of Medicine, Japan.

MATSUYAMA, STEVEN S., Ph.D., Veterans Administration Medical Center, and Department of Psychiatry and Biobehavioral Sciences, University of California at Los Angeles, Los Angeles, Calif.

MERVIS, RONALD, Ph.D., Assistant Professor of Neuropathology; Research Coordinator, Office of Geriatrics and Gerontology; and Head, Brain Aging and Neuronal Plasticity Research Group, The Ohio State University College of Medicine, Columbus, Ohio.

MEYER, JOHN STIRLING, M.D., C.M., Chief, Cerebrovascular Research, Veterans Administration Medical Center; Professor of Neurology, Baylor College of Medicine, Houston, Texas.

MICHALEWSKI, HENRY J., Ph.D., Department of Neurology, California College of Medicine, University of California at Irvine, Irvine, Calif.

MONT, FRANCISCO GOMEZ, M.D., Informatics Unit, Mexican Institute of Psychiatry; Co-editor, *Salud Mental,* official journal of the Mexican Institute of Psychiatry; Coordinator, Digital Brain Image Processing Project in collaboration with the Mexican Institute of Psychiatry, the Scientific Center of IBM in Mexico City, New York University, and Brookhaven National Laboratories.

MORTIMER, JAMES A., Ph.D., Associate Director, Geriatric Research, Education, and Clinical Center, Veterans Administration Medical Center; Assistant Professor, Department of Neurology, University of Minnesota Medical School, Minneapolis, Minn.

NANDY, KALIDAS, M.D., Ph.D., Associate Director, Geriatric Research, Education, and Clinical Center, ENR Veterans Hospital, Bedford, Mass.; Professor of Anatomy and Neurology, Boston University Medical Center, Boston, Mass.

ORAM, JULIAN J., M.B., B.S., D(Obs) R.C.O.G., M.R.C.P. (UK), Consultant Physician in Geriatric Medicine, St. George's Hospital, London, England.

PATTERSON, JULIE V., Ph.D., Andrus Gerontology Center, University of Southern California, Los Angeles, Calif.

PERL, DANIEL P., M.D., Professor of Pathology (Neuropathology), University of Vermont College of Medicine, Burlington, Vt.

PERRY, ELAINE K., Ph.D., Research Associate, Department of Neuropathology and MRC Neuroendocrinology Unit, Newcastle General Hospital, Newcastle-upon-Tyne, England.

PERRY, ROBERT H., M.R.C.P., M.R.C. Pathology, Clinical Scientist, MRC Neuroendocrinology Unit, and Honorary Consultant Neuropathologist, Newcastle General Hospital, Newcastle-upon-Tyne, England.

POMARA, NUNZIO, M.D., Department of Psychiatry, Wayne State University School of Medicine, Detroit, Mich.

PRICHEP, LESLIE, Ph.D., Clinical Assistant Professor of Psychiatry, New York University Medical Center, New York, N.Y.

PRIEN, ROBERT F., M.D., Ph.D., Psychopharmacology Research Branch, National Institute of Mental Health, Rockville, Md.

REISBERG, BARRY, M.D., Geriatric Study and Treatment Program, Department of Psychiatry, New York University Medical Center, New York, N.Y.

ROSENBERG, GORDON S., Department of Psychiatry, Veterans Administration Hospital, Bronx, N.Y.

SALAZAR, ANDRÉS M., M.D., F.A.A.N., Colonel in U.S. Army Medical Corps.; 1979–1981: Guest Worker, Laboratory for Central Nervous System Studies, National Institutes of Health, Bethesda, Md.; currently Director, Vietnam Head Injury Study, Walter Reed Army Medical Center, Washington, D.C.

SCHEIBEL, ARNOLD B., M.D., M.S., Professor of Anatomy and Psychiatry, and Member, Brain Research Institute, University of California Center for the Health Sciences, Los Angeles, Calif.; Consultant to Veterans Administration Hospitals, Wadsworth and Brentwood, Calif.

SCHNECK, MICHAEL K., M.D., Clinical Instructor, Department of Psychiatry, New York University School of Medicine, New York, N.Y.

SIMS, N.R., Ph.D., Assistant Professor of Neurochemistry, Institute of Neurology, London, England.

SITARAM, NATRAJ, M.D., Associate Professor of Psychiatry, Wayne State University, Detroit, Mich.

STEINBERG, GERTRUDE, M.A., Family Consultant and Social Researcher in Gerontology, Geriatric Study and Treatment Program, Department of Psychiatry, New York University Medical Center, New York, N.Y.

THOMPSON, LARRY W., Ph.D., Veterans Administration Medical Center, Palo Alto Division, Palo Alto, Calif.

TORACK, RICHARD M., M.D., Professor of Pathology, Washington University School of Medicine, St. Louis, Mo.

WALFORD, ROY L., M.D., Professor of Pathology, University of California at Los Angeles, Los Angeles, Calif.

WEINGARTNER, HERBERT, Ph.D., Chief, Cognitive Studies Unit, National Institute of Mental Health, Bethesda, Md.

WELLS, CHARLES E., M.D., Department of Psychiatry and Neurology, School of Medicine, Vanderbilt University, Nashville, Tenn.

WISNIEWSKI, HENRYK M., M.D., Ph.D., Director, Institute for Basic Research in Developmental Disabilities, Staten Island, N.Y.; Professor of Pathology (Neuropathology), Downstate Medical Center, New York, N.Y.

WISNIEWSKI, KRYSTYNA E., M.D., Ph.D., Associate Director of Clinical Diagnostic Services, Head of Pediatric Neuropathology Laboratory, and Pediatric Neurologist, Institute for Basic Research in Developmental Disabilities, Staten Island, N.Y.

YESAVAGE, JEROME A., M.D., Assistant Professor of Psychiatry, Stanford University Medical School, Stanford, Calif.; Chief, Psychiatric Intensive Care Unit, Veterans Administration Medical Center, Palo Alto, Calif.

PREFACE

Barry Reisberg

Truth must dazzle gradually—lest it blind.
—Emily Dickinson

ALZHEIMER'S DISEASE (AD) has been called "the disease of the century" (1). The medical and social dimensions of this affliction are staggering; surveys indicate that it is the major cause for institutionalization among the more than one million persons in nursing homes in the United States alone (2). (There are, in fact, many more patients in American nursing homes than in all acute and chronic care U.S. hospitals combined, making these numbers even more dramatic.) This nursing home population, however, represents only a fraction of the total AD burden. Thousands of persons with this disease are confined in state institutions and veterans' hospitals. Moreover, perhaps a majority of afflicted persons with severe AD continue to be cared for in their homes, by both relatives and home health aides. Thus, probably far more than a million U.S. citizens suffer sufficiently to require continuous supervision and care.

Inability to care for one's self results in decreased life expectancy. AD is now thought to be the fourth greatest cause of mortality in developed nations, after cardiovascular disease, malignancy, and cerebrovascular disease (Chap. 24 and ref. 3). The psychosocial dimensions of the disease include myriad citizens with ever-diminishing awareness of their lives, or their whereabouts; literally millions of others are physically enthralled caring for AD victims, or psychologically torn by the emotional burdens attendant on the illness.

The above medical, psychosocial, and epidemiologic dimensions refer only to severe forms of AD. Mild and moderate forms of this progressive disease result in early occupational retirement and social withdrawal for millions more throughout the world.

Despite the profound medical and psychosocial impact of this terrible illness, which gradually deprives sufferers of their "minds," the medical and lay communities have largely neglected its study, treatment, and care. The medical community's neglect is best gauged by reference to standard texts.

The clinical condition was described accurately by Esquirol in an 1838 text (4) and the neuropathologic entity was described accurately by Alois Alzheimer in 1907 (5). The medical and epidemiologic aspects have been apparent since Tomlinson, Blessed, and Roth's pioneering investigations, published by 1970 (6, 7). Nevertheless, a standardized American textbook of medicine in 1982 devoted only one of its 2,354 pages to AD, which it accurately describes as "*a major public health problem* . . . approximately 5% of the population at 65 and up to 20% of the population over 80 are affected" (8) (emphasis added). Neglect in specialty textbooks, specifically psychiatry and neurology, has been equally egregious (9, 10).

Laypeople have been no less guilty in removing this illness from public discourse. In literature, Sophocles (11) immortalized the illness in the fifth century B.C. and Shakespeare (12) reinforced these earlier descriptions for laypeople from Elizabethan times to the present. However, the current unabridged dictionary of the English language (13) contains no entry which distinguishes this illness from the general physical symptoms of aging. Naturally, absence of such a specific word or words for the disorder has contributed to removing the ubiquitous AD scourge from conscious public awareness.

The above will assist students, physicians, and other scientists and health professionals in gaining a perspective on why this volume represents possibly the first effort on the part of the medical and scientific communities to formulate, for a general medical audience, a specific and comprehensive textbook of Alzheimer's disease. Clearly, the information contained herein did not spring fully formed from the minds of the scientific community. Rather, it represents a compilation of active research and investigative results from worldwide tests primarily during the past 15 to 20 years.

This volume doesn't by any means represent the only attempt on the part of the scientific community to organize its ever increasing understanding of Alzheimer's disease; there have been many texts resulting from meetings which summarize scientific progress in the field (14–18), volumes directed primarily toward the scientific research community.

At the other end of the informational spectrum, an introductory text describing current concepts of senile dementia and AD has also recently been published (19). None of these compendiums or introductory works, however, has been specifically designed as a comprehensive and up-to-date text to serve medical students, practicing physicians, and other health professionals. The contributors to this volume, most of whom are world-renowned experts in AD and related disciplines, recognize the need for such a text. Thus, more than three-fourths of the internationally recognized experts initially invited to contribute to this volume found themselves eager to participate in this important, somewhat historic, undertaking. The result is a volume in which many world-famous experts in AD and related disciplines are represented. A measure of the eminence of these investigators is the large proportion of the reference citations made to the text's own contributors.

It is hoped that this volume will represent a milestone for the medical community's understanding of Alzheimer's disease in other important ways. It is hoped that this volume will demonstrate to the medical community the profound advances in our understanding of this acknowledged major public health problem in a very short time. Ignorance of AD should not, hereafter, justify undertreatment of this disease process in more general textbooks. Also, it is hoped that presenting the enormous recent advances in the field will stimulate other medical investigators to further discoveries in this important but still largely unexplored illness. The real hope is that this volume will immediately enable clinicians to better serve Alzheimer's patients and their families.

REFERENCES

1. Thomas L: On the problem of dementia. *Discover* 1981; 2:34.
2. National Center for Health Statistics: The projection of the population of the United States, 1975–2050, in *Census Bureau Current Population Report Series 601*. Government Printing Office, 1975, p 25.

3. Katzman R: The prevalence and malignancy of Alzheimer's disease: a major killer (editorial). *Arch Neurol* 1976; 33:217–218.

4. Esquirol JED: *Des maladies mentales.* Paris, Balliere, 1838.

5. Alzheimer A: Uber eine Eigenartige Erkrankung der Hirnrinde. *Allg Z Psychiatrie Psychisch–Gerichtlich Med* 1907; 64:146–148.

6. Tomlinson BE, Blessed G, Roth M: Observations on the brains of nondemented old people. *J Neurol Sci* 1968; 7:331–356.

7. Tomlinson BE, Blessed G, Roth M: Observations on the brains of demented old people. *J Neurol Sci* 1970; 11:205–242.

8. McHugh PR: Alzheimer's disease, in Wyngaarden JB, Smith LH (eds): *Cecil's Textbook of Medicine,* ed 16. Philadelphia, Saunders, 1982, pp 1981–1982.

9. Freedman AM, Kaplan HI, Saddock, BJ: *Comprehensive Textbook of Psychiatry,* ed 2. Baltimore, Williams and Wilkins, 1975, pp 1086–1087.

10. Merritt HH: *A Textbook of Neurology,* ed 5. Philadelphia, Lea and Febiger, 1973, pp 442–445.

11. Boura CM: *Sophoclean Tragedy.* London, Oxford University Press, 1964, p 351.

12. Shakespeare W: *King Lear.* London, Stationer's Register, Nov 26, 1607.

13. *Webster's New Twentieth Century Dictionary,* unabridged, ed 2. Cleveland, Collins–World Publishing Co., 1975, p 1651.

14. Nandy K, Sherwin I (eds): *The Aging Brain and Senile Dementia.* New York, Plenum, 1977.

15. Katzman R, Terry RD, Bick KL (eds): *Aging NY* 1978; 7.

16. Amaducci L, Davison AN, Antuono P (eds): *Aging NY* 1980; 13.

17. Miller NE, Cohen GD (eds): *Aging NY* 1981; 15.

18. Corkin S, Davis KL, Growdon JH, et al: *Aging NY* 1982; 19.

19. Reisberg B. *Brain Failure: An Introduction to Current Concepts of Senility.* New York, Free Press, 1981.

SECTION I
INTRODUCTION

1 An Overview of Current Concepts of Alzheimer's Disease, Senile Dementia, and Age-Associated Cognitive Decline

Barry Reisberg

THE GROWTH OF THE HUMAN POPULATION has been accelerating since the mid-1700s. Until 1900, however, there appears to have been no noticeable decrease in mortality of those over 45 years of age. Since 1900, the percentage of what we term elderly persons has begun to rise dramatically (1). In the United States in 1900, for example, 4% of the population had attained 65 years of age. But by 1980, fully 10.3% of the U.S. population had been estimated to be 65 or more. This demographic trend can be expected to continue in the United States and other developed nations (2). Current demographic projections indicate increased percentages of the elderly in developed nations throughout the remainder of this century, and afterward as well. Similar trends are evidently emerging in the developing nations thanks to a spectrum of interacting social forces.

A sizeable number of these individuals and their families will derive little enrichment from this extension of their lives because of the cognitive impairment which frequently accompanies the aging process.

Until very recently, age-associated cognitive decline has been a neglected medical entity. But with the rise of the aged in our midst, knowledge regarding this common syndrome has been accumulating very rapidly over the past several years, knowledge which is currently being translated into improved strategies for the management of the disorder. Keeping pace, pharmacologic treatments are being investigated based on our increased understanding of the underlying pathophysiology. These interventions and investigations are considerably aided by our freshly acquired understanding of the presentation and differential diagnosis of age-related cognitive impairment.

TERMINOLOGY AND NOSOLOGY OF SENILE DEMENTIA

Although it is possible to describe a clinical syndrome of progressive cognitive decline and to describe the pathophysiologic concomitants, several currently unresolved scientific and epistemologic issues confound attempts to further define the disorder.

The earliest clinically observable symptoms of age-associated cognitive decline are commonly referred to as the syndrome of "benign senescent forgetfulness" (BSF) (3). This terminology is acceptable so long as one recognizes the probability that 5–15% of so-called benign cases may show further deterioration over time. Furthermore, the designation BSF may ultimately prove to be even more inexact in that it removes these BSF-designated persons from the pathophysiologic continuum of progressive change, from normal aging to Alzheimer's disease, within which their symptomatology probably occurs. For these reasons, "forgetfulness phase" has also been proposed for this condition (4), which term avoids the implication of an invariably benign course of the symptomatology. Also, "forgetfulness phase" emphasizes the continuity of this syndrome with both normal aging and with more severe symptomatology such as dementia.

For more severely impaired patients, American psychiatrists have adopted the term "primary degenerative dementia" (PDD) (5, 6). American neurologists and other physicians and investigators throughout the world refer frequently to this same condition as "senile dementia of the Alzheimer type" (SDAT). Neuropathologists and others, alternatively, employ the term "Alzheimer's disease" (AD). Sometimes the abbreviated term "senile dementia" (SD) is used to mean either senile dementia of the Alzheimer type or Alzheimer's disease; however, "senile dementia" may also refer to a broader class of dementias occurring in the aged including, but not limited to, SDAT (or AD). Finally, the distinction is sometimes made between "presenile dementia," or "presenile dementia of the Alzheimer type," and senile dementia, or SDAT; the former has an onset prior to age 65 and the latter has an onset at or after age 65. Each of these terms has certain advantages and disadvantages.

"Primary degenerative dementia" (PDD) was adopted to describe the characteristic clinical syndrome, frequently observed in elderly persons, of progressive cognitive impairment, the onset and course of which are very gradual, generally extending over a period of years. PDD does not imply causative factors or specific pathophysiologic concomitants which, at present, have not been conclusively demonstrated to invariably accompany the clinical syndrome. This terminology is useful to clinicians who can apply this diagnosis to the characteristic clinical syndrome they observe in their living patient, without having to defer a final diagnosis until brain biopsy results or an autopsy report become available. In using the term "Alzheimer's disease," for example, to describe an identical clinical picture, physicians frequently feel obliged to tentatively diagnose the disorder, pending the "definitive" diagnosis from such a brain biopsy or autopsy. Clearly, in a clinical setting this is rarely feasible. The terminology PDD can also be of value to investigators seeking to learn more about the nature of the basic disease process underlying the clinical syndrome. Conversely, although most patients with classical PDD symptoms are also found to have classical Alzheimer-type neuropathologic brain findings, not all patients with classical PDD invariably show these brain changes. Reasons for this absence of total concordance are a matter of active research investigation. Given the lack of complete concordance, however, it is useful for investigators to define the clinical syndrome independently of the neuropathologic syndrome.

"Senile dementia" has been and remains a somewhat ambiguous term. In some cases it refers to dementia that becomes manifest at age 60, or 65, or above; it is also used currently to describe the clinical syndrome regardless of age of onset (7). Furthermore, expanding outward in meaning, senile dementia occasionally embraces a broader class of dementias, including, for example, multi-infarct dementia, which is prognostically, clinically, and pathophysiologically a distinct entity. This terminology is further confounded by the definitions adopted by the World Health Organization and incorporated into the International Classification of Diseases (8). In that system, the disorder falls within two possible categories: "senile dementia, simple type" or "presenile dementia." The former occurs "usually after the age of 65" and excludes "mild memory disturbances, not amounting to dementia, associated with senile brain disease." The latter refers to "dementia occurring, usually before the age of 65, in patients with the relatively rare forms of diffuse or lobar atrophy." This classification has been repeatedly rejected by subsequent forums because of current conceptualizations of the disorder (7, 9).

SDAT is a more circumscribed term than "senile dementia"; it clearly excludes multi-infarct dementia. The diagnosis SDAT is frequently used, however, to describe a clinical syndrome identical in all respects to PDD. When used in this fashion, SDAT has the possible disadvantage of strongly implying the presence of Alzheimer-type neuropathologic changes, which, as stated, have not been demonstrated as an invariable concomitant of the clinical syndrome (10).

Furthermore, the term SDAT strongly implies a dichotomy between progressive age-associated cognitive decline occurring in the "senium" (i.e., after age 65) and that occurring in the "presenium" (i.e., before age 65). This dichotomy is probably archaic: current knowledge does not indicate major differences in the syndrome, either clinically, neuropathologically, or physiologically, reflective in any way upon the age of onset. This age of onset dichotomy developed as a result of historical accident: in the latter part of the nineteenth century, and in the first half of this century, physicians distinguished dementia occurring prior to age 65 from "normal aging." They did not, however, so distinguish dementia after age 65. Hence, until recently, "Alzheimer's disease" referred to a condition occurring primarily in the presenium. Thus, the artificial and unsupported distinction between senile dementia and presenile dementia. Current knowledge would not indicate the value of this distinction except in very specific instances and, hence, it would probably advance our understanding of the illness process if the presenile–senile dichotomy, and terminology implying this dichotomy, were for the present eschewed.

For the reasons stated, in most cases the term "presenile dementia" should likewise be avoided. Like "senile dementia," the term "presenile dementia" is sometimes used to refer to a broad class of dementias. Specifically, "presenile dementia" interchangeably refers to both dementia of the Alzheimer type as well as Pick's dementia, when these conditions become clinically manifest prior to age 65.

The word "dementia" itself means "generalized cognitive and intellectual deterioration." This term describes a clinical syndrome that can be produced at any age by numerous causes including head trauma, brain tumor, nutritional disturbances, encephalitis, heavy-metal poisoning, anoxia, Alzheimer's disease, and the like.

Finally, the term "Alzheimer's disease" is generally used at present to refer to the classical clinical syndrome, with dementia of gradual onset and course accompanied by neuropathologic changes of the Alzheimer type, including neurofibrillary tangles, senile plaques, and granulovacuolar degeneration. Alzheimer's disease, as defined, may thus become manifest either before or after 65 years of age.

TERMINOLOGY TO BE EMPLOYED IN THIS VOLUME

Because of the current confusion with respect to multiple definitions of key terms denoting the disease entities and clinical syndromes in this field, it is necessary to adopt a consistent, if occasionally arbitrary, usage for this volume. This has been done in a manner consistent with the usage preferred by the majority of the contributors and one hopes, also in a manner consistent with the advancement of scientific knowledge and general understanding of the disease process.

"Alzheimer's disease" (AD) will be used throughout this volume to denote the syndrome of age-associated cognitive decline of gradual onset and course, accompanied by Alzheimer-type neuropathologic brain changes. No distinction with respect to age of onset is implied in our usage of the term "Alzheimer's disease," unless specifically stated.

"Senile dementia" will be used to refer to dementia, with onset late in life, generally after age 65, the origin of which may be Alzheimer's disease, multi-infarct dementia, or, possibly, other pathology.

"Presenile dementia" will refer to the dementia syndrome, with age of onset prior to age 65, which is due to various underlying pathologic processes including, but not limited to, Alzheimer's disease (AD).

"Primary degenerative dementia" will be used occasionally to refer to the clinical syndrome of age-associated cognitive decline of gradual onset and course, consistent with, but not invariably associated with, Alzheimer-type neuropathologic brain changes.

CLINICAL CHARACTERISTICS AND INCIDENCE OF AGE-ASSOCIATED COGNITIVE DECLINE AND PRIMARY DEGENERATIVE DEMENTIA

Many aged individuals have neither demonstrable nor subjective cognitive impairment. Others, perhaps constituting a majority of the aged, suffer varying degrees of impairment which are best conceptualized within three broad clinical phases, although seven distinct clinical stages are potentially distinguishable (4, 11). The condition is sufficiently widespread such that professionals will readily recognize the clinical syndromes constituting each of these phases, both from experiences with elderly patients as well as from life experience with family members, colleagues, and personal contacts.

The earliest phase of the process has been termed the "forgetfulness phase." In this phase the deficit is primarily subjective, although it may be objectified utilizing detailed psychometric testing (12). The individual, and frequently the spouse as well, recognizes increased difficulty recalling names of places and objects which had formerly been familiar. Intimates also notice an increased tendency on the patient's part to forget where objects have been placed. The forgetfulness phase individual remains as capable of functioning in social and employment situations as formerly. Nevertheless, the subjective symptomatology is accompanied by an increased sense of concern both on the part of the patient and spouse, as well as heightened irritability and a slight feeling of shame on the part of the patient. Along with these considerations, there is also a mutually identifiable mild increase in strain on the family relationship. Although the onset of these symptoms is met with a sense of appropriate concern, there is no sense of helplessness on the part of the patient or relevant intimates (13).

The precise incidence of forgetfulness phase symptomatology in elderly persons is unknown at present. These symptoms do appear, however, to be quite common. In one pilot survey, it was estimated that over 80% of elderly, community-residing men, with "normal" mood and cognitive function, had memory complaints of varying severity and duration (14). Although forgetfulness phase symptomatology is widespread, there is accumulating evidence that persons with this disorder are distinct behaviorally (12, 15), emotionally (13), and physiologically (16) from persons of the same age who do not suffer from complaints of cognitive decline. Kral (3, 15) proposed the term "benign senescent forgetfulness" to designate this disorder. Implicit in Kral's nomenclature is the hypothesis that the great majority of persons with these symptoms do not suffer any further decline in cognitive capacities. Results from one laboratory support this hypothesis (17). Investigators followed

16 community-residing persons (mean age 68.7 ± 4.05 years) with subjective and psychometrically verified cognitive symptomatology as described above, for a mean interval of 27.2 ± 3.7 months. At the time of follow-up it was found that none of the individuals had measurably worsened cognitively, and all continued alive and well and community-residing.

Analogous results were reported previously by Kral (3) in a somewhat older patient group. He followed 94 subjects with a mean age of 80.5 years. Of this group, 40 subjects had clinically preserved memory function and 20 had senescent forgetfulness over a 4-year observation period. Kral found no significant difference in the death rate between the subjects with preserved memory and those with senescent forgetfulness. However, both groups survived significantly longer than the 34 subjects from the more severely impaired cohort. Furthermore, over the 4-year observation period only one of Kral's 20 senescent forgetfulness patients became more severely cognitively impaired and required subsequent institutionalization.

In a minority of individuals, forgetfulness symptomatology does presage a more overt phase of cognitive deterioration, which has been termed the "confusional phase."

This phase begins at the point at which cognitive deficit becomes identifiable in the course of a detailed clinical interview. Individuals in this phase can no longer function as well in demanding employment or social situations as formerly. The deficit in recalling names becomes more manifest, such that familiar clients and students' names are not easily recalled. The increased deficit in recovering "lost" objects results in the loss or temporary unaccessibility of valuables. Other cognitive deficits also become notable, particularly deficits in the recall of recent events and activities in which the patient had participated. Deficits in the recall of personal history and past events also occur, but are more difficult to demonstrate clinically. Concentration deficits, however, are frequently readily elicited, utilizing such common clinical assessment devices as serial subtractions. Deficits in daily functioning also become manifest in this phase. The earliest clear-cut symptom recalled by family members is sometimes an episode in which the patient had gotten hopelessly lost when traveling to a location which should have been reached without undue difficulty. As deficits become more manifest, confusional phase patients become even less capable of managing their financial affairs.

A sense of helplessness on the part of both patients and those closest to them develops in this phase. Their sense of helplessness appears to replace the slight irritability, shame, and increased familial strain which had accompanied the onset of symptomatology in the earlier phase. Persons in the confusional phase also develop what psychiatrists term a flattening of affect. That is to say, persons in this phase become noticeably less responsive emotionally than heretofore. In part, this results from increased feelings of impotence. At the same time, this decreased emotional responsivity is also a product of the confused patient's lessened ability to process or make sense of incoming stimuli. The adaptive response to these decremental abilities is a partial withdrawal from stimulus input and a lower level of cognitive and emotional responsiveness to ambient events.

Surveys have indicated that the incidence of confusional phase symptomatology (also referred to as "mild to moderate dementia") in northern European populations is 10–12% of all persons aged 65 and greater (18, 19). Looking at these figures, we might estimate that in the United States, approximately 3 million persons presently suffer from confusional phase symptomatology. Although the natural history of confusional phase symptomatology has not been extensively studied, in most patients these symptoms do appear to herald more malignant symptomatology, with further decline, institutionalization, and not infrequently, death within the subsequent 2–5-year period. Of 11 patients (mean age: 72.8 ± 6.0 years) with marked confusional phase symptomatology followed over a period of 27.5

± 5.2 months, 2 were deceased and 1 was institutionalized by the time of follow-up (17). Of the remaining 8 individuals, all continued to function in a community setting. Of these 8, half evidenced significant decline over the follow-up period, while half were not markedly worse in either cognition or functional capacity.

The "dementia phase" can be defined as beginning at the point at which, left on their own, patients can no longer survive. Difficulties in functioning and in carrying out daily basic activities of living are the hallmarks of this phase of cognitive impairment. Early in this phase patients frequently have difficulty in choosing the proper clothing. At this point, individuals become severely circumscribed in movements and activities. Travel, even to familiar neighborhood locations, becomes difficult if not impossible. Financial affairs are taken over by intimates, caretakers, or other family members. Memory worsens to the extent that patients have difficulty recalling the name of the current president, the year, their address, or their current location. Patients also forget the names of schools attended, plus towns and cities in which they have lived.

As the dementia phase progresses, deficits develop in all cognitive and functional areas. The ability to cut one's own food is lost and, ultimately, the capacity to manipulate silverware completely disappears. Patients lose the urge or talent to wash and bathe themselves and must often be coerced to cleanse themselves, even when they are adequately assisted. Patients become incontinent and, finally, require guidance in toileting themselves. They become unsteady in their movements and, eventually, lose psychomotor abilities to the extent that they can no longer ambulate. All memories (recent and remote) and cognitive capacities gradually disappear. Patients forget the name of the spouse upon whom they are entirely dependent for survival and, subsequently, cannot even recognize their own name. In short, all identity is lost. The previous profession of a lifetime is entirely forgotten along with all events from one's past. Calculating and concentrating ability is lost to the extent to which individuals cannot count from one to five consecutively. Ultimately, all ability to speak is lost; patients can only stare blankly and grunt.

Loss of one's cognitive and intellectual capacities is too overwhelming a deficit for conscious contemplation. Consequently, individuals in the dementia phase deny much of their deficit. For instance, a patient may explain that he cannot recall the current president's name because he "doesn't follow politics," or his residence of 20 years because "I've only recently moved." Emotional difficulties, which become manifest in this phase, are also frequently denied. The onset of symptomatology in this phase is met by an acute sense of shame, replaced shortly by irritability and agitation as the condition progresses. Psychiatric manifestations (with suspiciousness, overt paranoia, delusions, and visual or other hallucinatory experiences) frequently occur in middle to late dementia phase patients. These symptoms make caring for the patient particularly difficult, and force even the most heroically concerned family to confront the need for institutionalization.

Estimates have indicated that dementia phase cognitive deficit occurs in approximately 5% of persons aged 65 and older (18, 19). Hence, more than 1 million Americans are probably afflicted with this condition. Government studies indicate that chronic cognitive deficits, probably synonymous in most cases with the condition which we are describing, occur in 58% of the more than 1 million Americans in nursing homes (20). Many such patients are housed in other institutional facilities such as state mental hospitals and veterans' hospitals. More than half of the patients aged 65 or more in state and county mental hospitals carry diagnoses compatible with chronic cognitive decline. Despite these dramatic statistics, it is thought that at least half of all patients in the dementia phase remain within the community where they are assisted by their spouses, siblings, children, or others.

The dementia symptoms described are associated with a sharp decrease in life expectancy (3, 21–24). In one study, the mean survival period was 2.6 years for men and 2.3 years for women, in comparison with 8.7 years and 10.9 years, respectively, for age-matched, nondemented controls (25). Of six community-residing individuals with early dementia phase symptomatology (mean age: 74.2 ± 4.7 years) followed for a mean interval of 23.2 ± 5.8 months, one was deceased by follow-up, two were institutionalized at follow-up, and three remained community-residing and performed only slightly worse, not significantly worse, on a brief Mental Status Questionnaire assessment (17, 26).

PATHOPHYSIOLOGIC CONCOMITANTS OF PROGRESSIVE COGNITIVE DECLINE IN ALZHEIMER'S DISEASE

Intra-individual longitudinal studies of the pathophysiologic concomitants of progressive, age-associated cognitive decline have not yet been reported. Nevertheless, cross-sectional, interindividual studies have revealed a broad spectrum of neuropathologic and neurophysiologic concomitants. These include changes in macroscopic and microscopic brain morphology, neurochemical alterations, changes in cerebral electrophysiology, alterations in cerebral blood flow and metabolism, and neuroimmunologic alterations.

Although changes in brain weight have been observed to accompany the aging process in humans (27–30), such changes have not been notably more numerous in persons who have died with progressive dementia than in decedent age-matched controls (31, 32). Nevertheless, pathologic examination of the brains of persons with severe progressive dementia has frequently revealed evidence of gross brain atrophy. In a classic study, gross cortical atrophy was observed in 9 of 16 cases with severe dementia (32); these degenerative changes were particularly prominent in the parietal, temporal, and frontal lobes of the cortex. Ventricular dilatation to a slight or moderate degree was also observed. Primary motor and sensory areas, such as the precentral and postcentral gyri and the occipital lobe, tended to be relatively preserved.

Recently developed *in vivo* techniques for the assessment of cerebral morphology have confirmed and extended these pathologic observations. Computerized tomographic (CT) studies have revealed significant relationships between cognitive impairment in elderly outpatients, and dilation of both the lateral (33–37) and third ventricles (35). Relationships between progressive cortical atrophy assessed on CT, and progressive cognitive decline, are also significant (35, 36).

The observed changes in gross brain morphology are not readily accounted for by neuronal cellular loss. Although an age-related decrement in neuronal cellular numbers per unit of brain volume has been reported (38, 39), such findings have not been consistently demonstrated with progressive dementia (40). Changes in the neuropil, notably dendritic loss and decreased dendritic arborization (41, 42), as well as changes in the supportive tissue, including increased cortical astrosytosis (43–45), are probably more important constituents of the observed macroscopic brain changes than neuronal cellular loss. Nevertheless, increased neuronal destruction in particular brain regions has been noted with progressive dementia (46, 47).

Microscopic and ultrastructural brain changes have been strongly implicated as concomitants of progressive dementia. The most notable such changes are neuritic plaques, paired helical filaments (PHFs) of the Alzheimer type, and granulovacuolar bodies. Together these micropathologic changes are referred to as "Alzheimer-type brain changes."

"Neuritic plaques," also known as "senile plaques" SPs, are found chiefly in the cerebral cortex, although they have been observed in deeper brain structures (48, 49). Increased concentration of these elements in the cortex has been correlated with the magnitude of cognitive deterioration (32, 50). Neuritic plaques consist of a central core of homogeneous protein material known as amyloid, surrounded by degenerative cellular fragments. The fragments include axonal and dendritic processes, PHFs, lysosomes, and degenerating mitochondria (51, 52). SPs have been found to occur more frequently with aging in humans (53), as well as in other mammals (54, 55). Increased frequency of neuritic plaques in the neocortex has been correlated with "minor features of intellectual decline" (53[p. 49]). Accordingly, confusional or even forgetfulness phase symptomatology may be related to these phenomena. Nevertheless, neuritic plaques are a nonspecific phenomenon found in association with human dementias of diverse etiology. For example, neuritic plaques are observed in kuru and Creutzfeldt–Jakob disease of presumed viral etiology (56–58); in dialysis dementia, a condition in which aluminum toxicity has been implicated (59); and in middle-aged persons with Down's syndrome, a condition in which chromosomal aberrations have clearly been pathogenetically implicated (60).

"Paired helical filaments" (PHFs), also known as "Alzheimer-type neurofibrillary tangles," are found both in the cerebral cortex and in the hippocampus, with the posterior half of the hippocampus more severely affected than the anterior half (61). Additionally, proliferation of PHFs in these areas has been associated with the presence of dementia (32) and the degree of dementia symptomatology (50). Increased appearance of PHFs in the hippocampus in particular, and to a lesser extent in the neocortex, has been strongly related to human aging (53). Not surprisingly, the appearance of PHFs in quantity, particularly in the hippocampus, may be associated with the progression of cognitive impairment in the aged.

Kidd (62) first suggested that the "dense bundles" observed through the light microscope are actually composed of filaments in a double helical configuration. Terry and associates (51) described the ultrastructure of these PHFs as consisting of twisted linear structures with a half period of 80 nm, and a maximum width of 24 nm. Unlike the neuritic plaques, these PHFs appear to occur only in human tissue. As with neuritic plaques, PHFs have been observed in middle-aged persons with Down's syndrome (60). PHFs also occur with greater than normal frequency in the brains of persons with parkinsonian syndromes, including the parkinsonian dementia of Guam and idiopathic parkinsonism (63), as well as in the brains of persons with dementia pugilistica (64). Hakim and Mathieson (65) recently explained the observed association of PHFs with idiopathic parkinsonism by demonstrating that Alzheimer-type pathologic changes in general occur more frequently in association with idiopathic parkinsonism. Furthermore, these Alzheimer-type pathologic changes appear to be related to the tenfold increase in dementia symptomatology in aged persons with Parkinson's disease (66). Finally, while the extrapyramidal symptoms associated with Parkinson's disease do not occur in most persons with confusional phase symptomatology, a statistically significant increase in these symptoms has been observed in patients with these early manifestations of cognitive impairment (67). It follows, then, that Alzheimer-type neuropathology and parkinsonian pathology may often be interrelated.

Granulovacuolar bodies have also been found to be present in large numbers in the hippocampus of patients with age-associated dementia (68). Such lesions have been related to age-associated brain changes *per se,* as well as to age-associated dementia (53). Finally, the occurrence and localization of granulovacuolar bodies in the hippocampus appear to be very closely matched to the occurrence and localization of PHFs in the hippocampus

(53, 69). In both cases, the posterior part of the hippocampus is primarily involved, and the distribution in subareas of the hippocampus is noticeably similar. A common cytotoxic mechanism has accordingly been postulated to underlie both lesions (70).

The most consistently found neurochemical concomitants of the dementia process are changes in the cerebral cholinergic neurotransmitter system. Specifically, there is a decided decrease in the level of choline acetyltransferase (CAT) activity in the brains of those who died with severe dementia as compared with the levels observed in age-matched controls (71–75). The CAT enzyme catalyzes the synthesis of acetylcholine from its precursors acetyl-coenzyme A (acetyl-CoA) and choline. The reduction in CAT levels are also correlated with the concentration of SPs (75). It has not yet been established from these studies whether reduced CAT is an earlier or later change in the disease process.

Decreased activity of the acetylcholine-degradating enzyme, acetylcholinesterase, has also been reported as present in brain specimens of persons with progressive dementia (71, 75, 76). As with CAT activity, there is also an age-related decrement in acetylcholinesterase activity in persons with progressive dementia. Persons with progressive dementia show a much greater decrement in such activity than can be accounted for by age. The extent to which these neurochemical processes parallel age-associated cognitive decline, however, is not certain at present. With respect to Alzheimer-type neuropathologic changes in Down's syndrome, it is noteworthy that analogous cholinergic changes have also been observed in Down's patients (77).

Changes in the level of acetylcholine itself in patients with progressive dementia have recently been reported. Richter and associates (78) directly demonstrated a decrease in measured acetylcholine levels in the temporal cortex of patients with progressive dementia as compared with normal elderly; postsynaptic receptor cholinergic changes do not appear as notable. With one exception (79), all studies have found no change in muscarinic receptor concentrations in AD when compared to control autopsy cases (74, 80, 81). The nicotinic receptor system has not yet been extensively studied.

Other neurochemical systems have also been reported altered in progressive dementia. However, noncholinergic neurotransmitter systems appear to be affected to a lesser extent (81). The most frequently reported noncholinergic neurochemical changes have been those suggestive of decreased dopaminergic activity, particularly as reflected by decreased concentrations of the dopaminergic metabolite homovanillic acid (HVA) in the cerebral spinal fluid (CSF) of persons with progressive dementia (82, 83). Recent work has suggested that patients with low HVA concentrations, although generally indistinguishable clinically from other dementia patients, may be neurochemically and neuropathologically distinct, in that they may not show cholinergic deficits or Alzheimer-type neuropathology (10). The relationship between their proposed subtype and parkinsonian pathology requires further investigation. Decrements in noradrenergic activity have also been reported in patients with progressive dementia (84, 85).

Electrophysiologic changes associated with aging and dementia have been investigated for more than a quarter century. In "senile psychoses," Mundy-Castle and co-workers (86) found diffuse slowing of theta and delta frequencies accompanied by a reduction in beta activity. Analogous findings have frequently been observed accompanying aging in ostensibly normal subjects. Numerous reports support the general conclusion that aged subjects tend to show slowing of the alpha rhythm and a diffuse increase of activity in the delta and theta bands in various head regions (87–91).

Weiner and Schuster (92) found a strong positive relationship between the severity of EEG involvement and the degree of dementia. McAdam and Robinson (93) reported a strong correspondence between the extent of intellectual impairment and EEG abnormalities. On the other hand, other early studies failed to find strong correlations between EEG findings and the extent of intellectual impairment in the early stages of dementia (94–96), while one study even supported the conclusion that the EEG of patients with senile dementia is usually within the range considered normal in old age (96). However, more recent investigations, utilizing modern diagnostic criteria, have supported a relationship between an increase in electrophysiologic slow wave activity and progressive age-associated cognitive decline, even in the early stages (97–100).

Cerebral blood flow studies have usually traced progressive declines throughout the life span from childhood to senescence (101, 102). There is some evidence that severe dementia is accompanied by further decrements in regional cerebral blood flow (103, 104), although these findings have not been entirely consistent (102). These changes in cerebral blood flow, if they indeed occur, may be secondary to a decrease in brain metabolism. One study did not show a reduction in cerebral blood flow and oxygen utilization in normal aging, but did present a significant decrease in these parameters in senile dementia as compared to young and age-matched control subjects (105). Whole brain glucose utilization was found to decline in normal aging, with a more precipitous decline in senile dementia. This study, which utilized the Kety–Schmidt technique (106), provided only whole brain measurements. Positron emission tomographic (PET) techniques, in conjunction with an F^{18}-2-deoxy-D-glucose tracer, now make it possible to evaluate changes in cerebral metabolism accompanying progressive dementia *in vivo* at various brain levels. Preliminary investigations have revealed significant relationships between progressive cognitive decrement, even in the early stages, and decreases in cerebral metabolism (107, 108). It is conceivable that these metabolic changes may account for not only the observed CBF changes, but also the cholinergic deficit. Acetyl-CoA is normally derived from glucose in the brain, and the cholinergic system has been shown to be acutely sensitive to cerebral anoxia (109). On the other hand, the metabolic CBF and cholinergic changes may all be secondary to primary neuronal degeneration.

Immunologic studies have revealed increments in circulating autogenous antibody levels against neuronal tissues in normal aging (110). Increased levels greater than accounted for by age have been observed in severe dementia (110). A recent investigation has revealed that, controlling for age, the increments in circulating autogenous antineuronal antibodies are significantly correlated with the evolution of progressive cognitive decline, even in the very earliest stages (16). These findings, which revealed significant increments in circulating antibody levels in forgetfulness phase subjects, in comparison with age-matched unimpaired persons, and further significant increments in early confusional phase subjects, in comparison with levels in the forgetfulness phase group, provide evidence for physiologic concomitants of even the earliest manifestations of age-associated cognitive decline.

It is important to emphasize that the pathophysiologic correlations just described do enhance our understanding of the disease process. Nevertheless, they do not necessarily provide evidence of a direct, causal relationship between the variables. They seem to point, however, to a pathophysiologic syndrome of change accompanying the behavioral syndrome of progressive cognitive decline.

DIAGNOSIS AND DIFFERENTIAL DIAGNOSIS OF ALZHEIMER'S DISEASE

Age-associated cognitive decline consistent with a diagnosis of AD is a clinical and pathophysiologic syndrome; diagnosis depends upon the clinician's careful exclusion of other possible etiologic factors (111, 112). The latter include (1) toxic causes (e.g., alcohol abuse, heavy-metal poisoning, poisoning secondary to inhalation or ingestion of various organic industrial compounds or organicides); (2) nutritional causes (e.g., pellagra, vitamin B_{12} deficiency, chronic malabsorption syndrome); (3) infectious causes (e.g., encephalitis, syphilis, tuberculosis, fungal infections); (4) endocrinological causes (e.g., myxedema, pituitary insufficiency); (5) neoplastic causes (e.g., primary or metastatic cerebral masses); (6) traumatic causes (e.g., subdural hematoma, cerebral hemorrhage or laceration; (7) circulatory disturbances (e.g., cerebral aneurism, normal pressure hydrocephalus); and others. Many of these secondary dementias can be reversed if identified and treated early.

Wells (113) suggested the following ancillary tests to rule out most reversible causes of cognitive deterioration and dementia: serum enzymes and electrolytes, complete blood cell count, urinalysis, chest x-ray, serological test for syphilis, serum thyroxine or serum-free thyroxine, vitamin B and folate levels, and computed tomography (CT). An electroencephalogram may also be of diagnostic utility. Naturally, every effort should be made to rule out reversible causes of cognitive decline.

After ruling out the above secondary causes of cognitive deterioration, the vast majority of cases among the elderly still remain. Of this caseload, a significant minority are cases in which multiple infarctions are either the sole cause of cognitive deterioration or a major contributor (114). These instances of multi-infarct dementia (MID) need to be differentiated from the syndrome of age-associated cognitive decline of Alzheimer's etiology.

In age-associated cognitive decline consistent with Alzheimer's etiology, there is an insidious onset and a progressive deterioration of cognitive functioning, generally in the absence of any focal neurologic pathology. An increased incidence with age, extending at least to the ninth decade, is common. In MID, onset may be abrupt and the course of the illness generally intermittent and fluctuating, punctuated by episodes of more severe cognitive deficit. There appears to be a stepwise deterioration accompanied by focal neurological signs. Emotional lability, particularly depression, is more usual with MID. Most frequent between the ages of 40 and 60, MID is more frequently seen in men, with hypertension and other stroke risk factors playing major roles. MID often, in fact, develops after a succession of strokes. The mixed-type dementia, which shows both Alzheimer-type changes and diffuse cerebral softening on pathologic examination, presents with a mixed clinical picture as well.

Another significant minority, of patients with cognitive decline of undetermined etiology, will be found to have a functional psychiatric disturbance. Depression, masking as cognitive disturbance, is a not uncommon finding among elderly patients, and can be particularly difficult to differentiate from age-associated cognitive decline. In its mild form, depression can cause symptomatology very similar to that described as accompanying the forgetfulness phase. Specifically, mild depression is accompanied by increased anxiety with a resultant decrease in concentration and cognitive performance. Furthermore, both mildly depressed patients and forgetfulness phase patients report negative self-assessments of their cognitive abilities (13, 115). Additionally, moderate depression can be difficult to distinguish from confusional phase symptomatology: both are accompanied by a flattening of affect and withdrawal. However, moderately depressed patients' complaints of memory disturbance appear to be out of proportion to the magnitude of objectively assessed impairment (116–118). Conversely, confusional phase patients begin to deny the magnitude and extent of objectively observed cognitive disabilities. Finally, severe depression and dementia phase symptomatology can present similar clinical pictures. Both can manifest withdrawal, dysphoria, lack of insight, and associated psychotic symptomatology. At all stages the ultimate differentiation between primary depression and primary cognitive disturbance is based upon the associated symptomatology. True depressive affective disorder is accompanied by a spectrum of vegetative and dysphoric symptoms not often observed in association with primary cognitive disturbance (5). These include sleep and appetite disturbance, as well as feelings of hopelessness and sadness. Furthermore, the onset of depressive affective disorder may be relatively abrupt and the course of illness fluctuates more than in persons with primary cognitive disturbance.

Other functional psychiatric conditions may also be misconstrued with primary cognitive dysfunction. Among these conditions, the residual symptomatology in individuals with a longstanding history of schizophrenia may be particularly difficult to differentiate from true dementia. As with affective disorder, the differences in onset, clinical history, and associated symptomatology are useful in arriving at a proper diagnosis.

TREATMENT APPROACHES TO, AND MANAGEMENT OF, ALZHEIMER'S DISEASE

Dramatically effective pharmacologic treatments for age-associated cognitive decline do not currently exist (119). Our evolving understanding of the pathophysiologic concomitants of the disorder has produced a series of promising treatment rationales which have thus far not resulted in hoped-for pharmacologic treatments (120–125).

The cerebral metabolic enhancers (including the cerebral vasodilators) are the most widely utilized pharmacologic agents in the treatment of age-associated cognitive decline. Many of these compounds have demonstrated small, statistically significant improvements in diverse symptomatology including, but not limited to, cognition over a period of several weeks to several months. Most of these agents have not yet been extensively studied in well-diagnosed, homogeneous patient populations, hence the mood and cognitive effects of the cerebral metabolic enhancers have not been well differentiated (126).

Choline precursors have recently been extensively investigated in the treatment of age-associated cognitive decline. Given alone, for periods of several weeks to months, these precursors have failed to produce therapeutic effects (122–125), although the possibility remains that longer periods of administration (127), or the combination of these cholinergic precursors with other compounds (128) may prove of use.

Dementia phase symptomatology very often includes an increase in agitation as well as an increased incidence of paranoia and other psychotic disturbances. Neuroleptic agents are frequently necessary to assist the family or institution control the patient's misbehavior. Such agents should be prescribed, of course, with great caution; the alterations in cerebral neurochemistry associated with cognitive decline make such patients particularly sensitive to substances which manipulate neurotransmitter status. Hence, such patients are acutely sensitive to even low dosages of neuroleptics.

Psychotherapeutic and environmental interventions are currently among the most crucial in the treatment of age-associated cognitive decline. Although forgetfulness phase patients can benefit from cognitive, mnemonic, and other learning strategies (124), more severely impaired patients do not clearly benefit from such interventions (130). In the confusional and dementia phases, the denial of cognitive deficit that occurs protects patients against much of the psychic pain and trauma that would otherwise accompany the loss of their intellectual capabilities. Denial operates decidedly less forcefully, in the spouses of these patients (13). The latter are forced to devote their lives and their resources to the care of a person who, as the illness progresses, will no longer recognize them, and who immediately forgets whatever kindness or assistance has been shown to them. Even in the confusional phase patient, the spouse is confronted with the destruction of their former lifestyle, marriage, friendships, and other social interrelationships.

Under these circumstances, psychotherapeutic intervention on behalf of the spouse has been found to be of great importance. Although for some spouses individual or family therapy may be useful, for the majority, supportive group therapy has been found to be of particular value (131). Recent work has indicated that such therapy becomes increasingly important as the illness progresses and should ideally extend for a period of years (132).

During the dementia phase the physician can be a valuable resource to both family and patient. In this phase the physician will often be called upon to assist in managing the patient's frequently manifest agitation, aggression, or psychosis. The physician can also assist in identifying and ameliorating the aggressive and hostile reactions evoked in the spouse. At an appropriate time, the physician should recommend that the family consider institutionalization. Assistance should also extend to counseling regarding nursing home placement; and, during and after placement, the physician should attempt to alleviate the profound feelings of guilt which spouses so often feel after the decision to institutionalize the patient.

References

1. McKeown T: *The Modern Rise of Population.* New York, Academic, 1976.
2. US Department of Health, Education and Welfare, Public Health Service, National Institutes of Health: *Changes: Research on Aging and the Aged,* NIH publication no. 78–85. Government Printing Office, 1978, p 8.
3. Kral VA: Benign senescent forgetfulness. *Aging NY* 1978; 7:47–51.
4. Reisberg B: *Brain Failure: An Introduction to Current Concepts of Senility.* New York, Free Press, 1981, pp 81–122.
5. American Psychiatric Association: *Diagnostic and Statistical Manual of Mental Disorders,* ed 3. Washington, DC, American Psychiatric Association, 1980.
6. Lipowski ZJ: Organic mental disorders: their history and classification with special reference to DSM-III. *Aging NY* 1981; 15:37–45.
7. Terry RD: Aging, senile dementia, and Alzheimer's disease. *Aging NY* 1978; 7:11–14.
8. World Health Organization: *Manual of the International Statistical Classification of Diseases, Injuries and Causes of Death,* 9th rev. World Health Organization, Geneva, 1977, vol 1.
9. Clayton PJ, Martin R: Classification of late life organic states and the DSM-III. *Aging NY* 1981; 15:47–54.
10. Bowen DM, Sims NR, Benton JS, et al: Treatment of Alzheimer's disease: a cautionary note. *N Engl J Med* 1981; 305:1016.
11. Reisberg B, Ferris SH, de Leon MJ, et al: The Global Deterioration Scale (GDS): an instrument for the assessment of primary degenerative dementia (PDD). *Am J Psychiatry* 1982; 139:1136–1139.
12. Reisberg B, Ferris SH, Schneck MK, et al: The relationship between psychiatric assessments and cognitive test measures in mild to moderately cognitively impaired elderly. *Psychopharmacol Bull* 1981; 17:99–101.
13. Reisberg B, Gordon B, McCarthy M, et al: Insight and denial accompanying progressive cognitive decline in the aged, in Melnick VS, Dubler N (eds): *Senile Dementia of the Alzheimer's Type: Ethical and Legal Issues Related to Informed Consent.* Government Printing Office, in press.
14. Sluss TK, Rabins P, Gruenberg EM, et al: Memory complaints in community residing men, abstracted. *Gerontologist* 1980; 20:(pt II)5, 201.
15. Kral VA: Senescent forgetfulness: benign and malignant. *Can Med Assoc J* 1962; 86:257–260.

16. Nandy K, Reisberg B, Ferris SH, et al: Brain reactive antibodies and progressive cognitive decline in the aged, abstracted. *J Am Aging Assoc* 1981; 4:3.

17. Reisberg B, Shulman E, Ferris SH, et al: Clinical assessments of age-associated cognitive decline and primary degenerative dementia: prognostic concomitants. *Psychopharmacol Bull* 1983, in press.

18. Katzman R: The prevalence and malignancy of Alzheimer's disease. *Arch Neurol* 1976; 33:217–218.

19. Terry RD: Dementia: a brief and selective review. *Arch Neurol* 1976; 33:1–4.

20. US Department of Health, Education and Welfare: *Vital and Health Statistics,* series 13, no 29, HEW publication no 78–1780. Hyattsville, National Center for Health Resources, 1977.

21. Kay DWK, Norris V, Post F: Prognosis in psychiatric disorders of the elderly: an attempt to define indications of early death and early recovery. *J Ment Sci* 1956; 102:129–140.

22. Larsson T, Sjögren T, Jacobson G: Senile dementia. *Acta Psychiatr Scand Suppl* 1963; 39(suppl 162):3–259.

23. Epstein L, Simon A, Mock R: Clinical neuropathologic correlates in senile and cerebral arteriosclerotic psychoses, in Hansen P (ed): *Old Age with a Future.* Philadelphia, Davis, 1964, pp 272–275.

24. Peck A, Wolloch L, Rodstein M: Mortality of the aged with chronic brain syndrome. *J Am Geriatr Soc* 1973; 21:264–270.

25. Kay DWK, Beamish P, Roth M: Old age mental disorders in Newcastle upon Tyne. *Br J Psychiatry* 1964; 110:146–148.

26. Kahn RL, Goldfarb AL, Pollack KM, et al: Brief objective measures for the determination of mental status in the aged. *Am J Psychiatry* 1960; 117:326–328.

27. Critchley M: The neurology of old age. *Lancet* 1931; i:1119.

28. Corsellis JAN: *Mental Illness and the Aging Brain.* New York, Oxford University Press, 1962.

29. Howell TH: Organ weights in nonagenarians. *J Am Geriatr Soc* 1978; 26:385–390.

30. Howell TH: Brain weights in octogenarians. *J Am Geriatr Soc* 1981; 29:450–452.

31. Tomlinson BE, Blessed G, Roth M: Observations on the brains of nondemented old people. *J Neurol Sci* 1968; 7:331–336.

32. Tomlinson BE, Blessed G, Roth M: Observations on the brains of demented old people. *J Neurol Sci* 1970; 11:205–242.

33. Roberts MA, Caird FL, Grossat KW, et al: Computerized tomography in the diagnosis of cerebral atrophy. *J Neurol Neurosurg Psychiatry* 1976; 39:905–915.

34. de Leon MJ, Ferris SH, Blau I, et al: Correlations between computerized tomographic changes and behavioral deficits in senile dementia. *Lancet* 1979; ii:859.

35. de Leon MJ, Ferris SH, George AE, et al: Computerized tomography evaluations of brain–behavior relationships in senile dementia of the Alzheimer's type. *Neurobiol Aging* 1980; 1:69–79.

36. Mersky H, Ball MJ, Blume WT, et al: Relationships between psychological measurements and cerebral organic changes in Alzheimer's disease. *Can J Neurol Sci* 1980; 7:45–49.

37. Jacoby RJ, Levy R: Computed tomography and the elderly: II. Senile dementia: diagnosis and functional impairment. *Br J Psychiatry* 1980; 136:256–269.

38. Brody H: Organization of the cerebral cortex: III. A study of aging in the human cerebral cortex. *J Comp Neurol* 1955; 102:511–556.

39. Henderson G, Tomlinson BE, Gibson PH: Cell counts in human cerebral cortex in normal adults throughout life using an image analyzing computer. *J Neurol Sci* 1980; 46:113–136.

40. Terry RD, Fitzgerald L, Peck A, et al: Cortical cell counts in senile dementia. *J Neuropathol Exp Neurol* 1977; 36:633.

41. Scheibel ME, Scheibel AB: Structural changes in the aging brain. *Aging NY* 1975; 1:11–37.

42. Buell SJ, Coleman PD: Quantitative evidence for selective dendritic growth in normal human aging but not in senile dementia. *Brain Res* 1981; 214:23–41.

43. Fischer O: Die presbyaphrene Demenz, deren anatomsiche Grundlage, und klinische Abgrenzung. *Ztschr Ges Neurol Psychiat* 1910; 3:371–471.

44. Von Braunmuhl A: Alterserkrankung des Zentralnervensystems. Senile Involution. Senile Demenz. Alzheimersche Krankheit, in Lubarsch O, Henke F, Rossle K, et al (eds): *Handbuch der Speziellen pathologischen Anatomie.* Berlin, Springer, 1957, vol 13, pp 337–539.

45. Schechter R, Yen S-HC, Terry RD: Fibrous astrocytes in senile dementia of the Alzheimer type. *J Neuropathol Exp Neurol* 1981; 40:95–101.

46. Bondareff W, Mountjoy CQ, Roth M: Selective loss of neurones of origin of adrenergic projection to cerebral cortex (nucleus locus coeruleus) in senile dementia. *Lancet* 1981; i:783–784.

47. Whitehouse PJ, Price DL, Clark AW, et al: Alzheimer disease: evidence for selective loss of cholinergic neurons in the nucleus basalis. *Ann Neurol* 1981; 10:122–126.

48. Fuller S: A study of the miliary plaques found in brains of the aged. *Am J Insanity* 1911; 68:147–217.

49. Wisniewski HM, Terry RD: Reexamination of the pathogenesis of the senile plaque. *Prog Neuropathol* 1973; 2:1–26.

50. Farmer PM, Peck A, Terry RD: Correlations among neuritic plaques, neurofibrillary tangles, and the severity of senile dementia. *J Neuropathol Exp Neurol* 1976; 35:367.

51. Terry RD, Gonatas NK, Weiss M: Ultrastructural studies in Alzheimer's presenile dementia. *Am J Pathol* 1964; 44:269–297.

52. Gonatas NK, Anderson A, Evangelista I. The contribution of altered synapses in the senile plaque: an electron microscopic study of Alzheimer's dementia. *J Neuropathol Exp Neurol* 1967; 26:25–39.

53. Tomlinson BE: Morphological changes and dementia in old age, in Smith WL, Kinsbourne M (eds): *Aging and Dementia.* New York, Spectrum, 1977, pp 25–56.

54. Wisniewski HM, Johnson AB, Raine CS, et al: Senile plaques and cerebral amyloidosis in aged dogs: a histochemical and ultrastructural study. *Lab Invest* 1970; 23:287–296.

55. Wisniewski HM, Ghetti B, Terry RD: Neuritic (senile) plaques and filamentous changes in aged Rhesus monkeys. *J Neuropathol Exp Neurol* 1973; 32:556–584.

56. Chou SM, Martin JD: Kuru plaques in a case of Creutzfeldt–Jacob disease. *Acta Neuropathol* 1971; 17:150–155.

57. Hirano A, Ghatak N, Johnson A, et al: Argentophilic plaques in Creutzfeldt–Jacob disease. *Arch Neurol* 1972; 26:530–542.

58. Traub R, Gajdusek DC, Gibbs CJ: Transmissible virus dementia: the relation of transmissible spongiform encephalopathy to Creutzfeldt–Jacob disease, in Smith WL, Kinsbourne M (eds): *Aging and Dementia.* New York, Spectrum, 1977, pp 91–146.

59. Brun A, Victor M: Senile plaques and tangles in dialysis dementia. *Acta Pathol Microbiol Scand A* 1981; 89:193–198.

60. Wisniewski K, Howe J, Williams GV, et al: Precocious aging and dementia in patients with Down's syndrome. *Biol Psychiatry* 1978; 18:619–627.

61. Ball MJ: Neuronal loss, neurofibrillary tangles, and granulovacuolar degeneration in the hippocampus with aging and dementia: a quantitative study. *Acta Neuropathol* 1977; 37:111–118.

62. Kidd M: Paired helical filaments in electron microscopy in Alzheimer's disease. Nature 1963; 197:192–193.

63. Wisniewski H, Terry RD, Hirano A: Neurofibrillary pathology. *J Neuropathol Exp Neurol* 1970; 29:163–176.

64. Corsellis JAN: Posttraumatic dementia. *Aging NY* 1978; 7:125–133.

65. Hakim AM, Mathieson G: Dementia in Parkinson's disease: neuropathologic study. *Neurology* 1979; 29:1209–1214.

66. Lieberman A, Dziatolowski M, Kupersmith M, et al: Dementia in Parkinson's disease. *Ann Neurol* 1979; 6:355–359.

67. Pomara N, Reisberg B, Albers S, et al: Extrapyramidal symptoms in patients with primary degenerative dementia. *J Clin Psychopharmacol* 1981; 1:398–400.

68. Woodward JS: Clinicopathologic significance of granulovacuolar degeneration in Alzheimer's disease. *J Neuropathol Exp Neurol* 1962; 21:85–91.

69. Ball MJ, Lo P: Granulovacuolar degeneration in the aging brain and in dementia. *J Neuropathol Exp Neurol* 1977; 36:474–487.

70. Ball MJ: Topographic distribution of neurofibrillary tangles and granulovacuolar degeneration in hippocampal cortex of aging and demented patients: a quantitative study. *Acta Neuropathol* 1978; 42:73–80.

71. Davies P, Maloney AJF: Selective loss of central cholinergic neurons in Alzheimer's disease. *Lancet* 1976; ii:1403.

72. Perry EK, Gibson PH, Blessed G, et al: Neurotransmitter enzyme abnormalities in senile dementia: choline acetyltransferase and glutamic acid decarboxylase activities in necrotic brain tissue. *J Neurol Sci* 1977; 34:247–265.

73. Spillane JA, White P, Goodhardt MJ, et al: Selective vulnerability of neurons in organic dementia. *Nature* 1977; 266:558–559.

74. White P, Hiley CR, Goodhardt MJ, et al: Neocortical cholinergic neurons in elderly people. *Lancet* 1977; i:668–671.

75. Perry EK, Perry RH; The cholinergic system in Alzheimer's disease, in Roberts RJ (ed): *Biochemistry of Dementia.* New York, Wiley, 1980, pp 135–183.

76. Pope A, Hess HH, Lewin E: Microchemical pathology of the cerebral cortex in presenile dementias. *Trans Am Neurol Assoc* 1964; 89:15–16.

77. Yates CM, Simpson J, Maloney AFJ, et al: Alzheimer-like cholinergic deficiency in Down syndrome. *Lancet* 1980; ii:979.

78. Richter TD, Perry EK, Tomlinson BE: Acetylcholine and choline levels in postmortem human brain tissue: preliminary observations in Alzheimer's disease. *Life Sci* 1980; 26:1683–1689.

79. Reisine TD, Yamamura HI, Bird ED, et al: Pre- and postsynaptic neurochemical alterations in Alzheimer's disease. *Brain Res* 1978; 159:477–480.

80. Davies P: Studies on the neurochemistry of central cholinergic systems in Alzheimer's disease. *Aging NY* 1978; 7:453–459.

81. Bowen DM, White P, Spillane JA, et al: Accelerated ageing or selective neuronal loss as an important cause of dementia? *Lancet* 1979; i:11–14.

82. Yates CM, Allison Y, Simpson J, et al: Dopamine in Alzheimer's disease and senile dementia. *Lancet* 1979; ii:851–852.

83. Gottfries CG: Amine metabolism in normal aging and in dementia disorders, in Roberts RJ (ed): *Biochemistry of Dementia.* New York, Wiley, 1980, pp 213–234.

84. Mann DMA, Lincoln J, Yates CM, et al: Changes in the monoamine containing neurons of the human CNS in senile dementia. *Br J Psychiatry* 1980; 136:533–541.

85. Yates CM, Ritchie IM, Simpson J, et al: Noradrenaline in Alzheimer-type dementia and Down's syndrome. *Lancet* 1981; ii:39–40.

86. Mundy-Castle AC, Hurst LA, Beerstrecher DM: The EEG in senile psychoses. *Electroencephalogr Clin Neurophysiol* 1954; 6:245–252.

87. Davis PA: The electroencephalogram in old age. *Dis Nerv Syst* 1941;2:77.

88. Mundy-Castle AC: Theta and delta rhythm in EEG of normal adults. *Electroencephalogr Clin Neurophysiol* 1951; 3:477–486.

89. Obrist WD: The electroencphalogram of normal aged adults. *Electroencephalogr Clin Neurophysiol* 1954; 6:235–249.

90. Busse EW, Barnes RH, Friedman EL, et al. Psychological functioning of aged individuals with normal and abnormal electroencephalograms: I. A study of nonhospitalized community volunteers. *J Nerv Ment Dis* 1956; 124:135–141.

91. Obrist WD, Busse EW: Temporal lobe abnormalities in normal senescence. *American EEG Society Colloquium* 1960; 12:249–251.

92. Weiner H, Schuster DB: The electroencephalogram in dementia: some preliminary observations and correlations. *Electroencephalogr Clin Neurophysiol* 1956; 8:479–488.

93. McAdam W, Robinson RA: Senile intellectual deterioration and the electroencephalogram: a quantitative correlation. *Br J Psychiatry* 1956; 102:819.

94. Romano J, Engel GI: Delerium; Electroencephalographic data. *Arch Neurol Psychiat* 1944; 51:356–377.

95. Greenblatt M, Levin S, Atwell C: Comparative value of electroencephalogram and abstraction tests in diagnosis of brain damage. *J Nerv Ment Dis* 1945; 102:383–391.

96. Short MJ, Muisella L, Wilson WP: Correlation of affect and EEG in senile psychosis. *J Gerontol* 1968; 23:324–327.

97. Roberts MA, McGeorge AP, Caird FL: Electroencephalography and computerized tomography in vascular and nonvascular dementia in old age. *J Neurol Neurosurg Psychiatry* 1978; 41:903–906.

98. Kaszniak AW, Garren DL, Fox JH: Cerebral atrophy, EEG slowing, age, education, and cognitive functioning in suspected dementia. *Neurology* 1979; 29:1273–1279.

99. Mersky H, Ball MJ, Blume WT, et al: Relationships between psychological measurements and cerebral organic changes in Alzheimer's disease. *Can J Neurol Sci* 1980; 7:45–49.

100. Johannesson G, Hagberg B, Gustafson L, et al: EEG and cognitive impairment in presenile dementia. *Acta Neurol Scand* 1979; 59:225–240.

101. Sokoloff L: Cerebral blood flow and metabolism in the differentiation of dementia: general considerations. *Aging NY* 1978; 7:197–202.

102. McAlpine CJ, Rowan JO, Matheson MS, et al: Cerebral blood flow and intelligence rating in persons over 90 years old. *Age Ageing* 1981; 10:247–253.

103. Ingvar DH, Brun A, Hagberg B, et al: Regional cerebral blood flow in the dominant hemisphere in confirmed cases of Alzheimer's disease, Pick's disease, and multi-infarct dementia: relationship to clinical symptomatology and neuropathological findings. *Aging NY* 1978; 7:203–205.

104. Yamaguchi F, Meyer JS, Yamamoto M, et al: Noninvasive regional cerebral blood flow measurements in dementia. *Arch Neurol* 1980; 37:410–418.

105. Birren JE, Butler RN, Greenhouse SW: *Human Aging: A Biological and Behavioral Study.* Government Printing Office, 1963.

106. Kety SS, Schmidt CF: The nitrous oxide method for the quantitative determination of cerebral blood flow in man: theory, procedure, and normal values. *J Clin Invest* 1948; 27:476–483.

107. Ferris SH, de Leon MJ, Wolf AP, et al: Positron emission tomography in the study of aging and senile dementia. *Neurobiol Aging* 1980; 1:127–131.

108. Ferris SH, de Leon MJ, Christman D, et al: Positron emission tomography (PET) studies of regional brain metabolism in elderly patients, in Jansson B, Perris C, Struwe G (eds): *Biological Psychiatry 1981.* Amsterdam, Elsevier North-Holland, 1981, pp 280–283.

109. Gibson GF, Shimada M, Blass JP. Alterations in acetylcholine synthesis and cyclic nucleotides in mild cerebral hypoxia. *J Neurochem* 1978; 31:757–760.

110. Nandy K: Brain-reactive antibodies in aging and senile dementia. *Aging NY* 1978; 7:503–512.

111. Roth M: Diagnosis of senile and related forms of dementia. *Aging NY* 1978; 7:82.

112. Reisberg B, Ferris SH: Diagnosis and assessment of the older patient. *Hosp Community Psychiatry* 1982; 33:104–110.

113. Wells CE: Management of dementia, in Katzman R (ed): *Congenital and Acquired Cognitive Disorders.* New York, Raven, 1979, pp 281–292.

114. Hachinski VC, Lassen NA, Marshall J: Multi-infarct dementia: a cause of mental deterioration in the elderly. *Lancet* 1974; ii:207–210.

115. Friedman AS: Minimal effects of severe depression on cognitive functioning. *Abnorm Soc Psychol* 1964; 69:237–243.

116. Neville HJ, Folstein MF: Performance on three cognitive tasks by patients with dementia, depression, or Korsakov's syndrome. *Gerontology* 1979; 25:285–290.

117. Sternberg DE, Jarvik ME: Memory functions in depression. *Arch Gen Psychiatry* 1976; 33:219–224.

118. Reisberg B, Ferris SH, Georgotas A, et al: Relationship between cognition and mood in geriatric depression. *Psychopharmacol Bull* 1982; 18:191–193.

119. Reisberg B, Ferris SH, Gershon S: An overview of pharmacologic treatment of cognitive decline in the aged. *Am J Psychiatry* 1981; 138:593–600.

120. Raskin AS, Gershon S, Crook T, et al: The effects of hyperbaric and normobaric oxygen on cognitive impairment in the elderly. *Arch Gen Psychiatry* 1978; 35:50–56.

121. Ferris SH, Sathananthan G, Gershon S, et al: Cognitive impairment in the elderly: effects of deanol. *J Am Geriatr Soc* 1977; 25:241–244.

122. Ferris SH, Sathananthan G, Reisberg B, et al: Long-term choline treatment of memory-impaired elderly patients. *Science* 1979; 205:1039–1040.

123. Thal LJ, Rosen W, Sharpless NS, et al: Choline chloride fails to improve cognition in Alzheimer's disease. *Neurobiol Aging* 1981; 2:205–208.

124. Wurtman RJ, Growden JH, Corkin S, et al: International Study Group on the Pharmacology of Memory Disorders Associated with Aging, meeting report. *Neurobiol Aging* 1981; 2:149–151.

125. Bartus RT, Dean RL, Beer B, et al: The cholinergic hypothesis of geriatric memory dysfunction. *Science* 1982; 217:408–417.

126. Reisberg B: Empirical studies in senile dementia with meta-enhancers and agents that alter blood flow and oxygen utilization, in Crook T, Gershon S (eds): *Strategies for the Development of an Effective Treatment for Senile Dementia.* New Canaan, Powley, 1981, pp 189–206.

127. Mervis R, Bartus RT: Dietary choline increases dendritic spine population in aging mouse neocortex, abstracted. *Soc Neurosci* 1981; 7:370.

128. Friedman E, Sherman KA, Ferris SH, et al: Clinical response to choline plus piracetam in senile dementia: relation to red-cell choline levels. *N Engl J Med* 1981; 304:1490–1491.

129. Zarit SH, Cole KD, Guider RL: Memory training strategies and subjective complaints of memory in the aged. *Gerontologist* 1981; 21:158–164.

130. Zepelin H, Wolfe CS, Kleinplatz F: Evaluation of a yearlong reality orientation program. *J Gerontol* 1981; 36:70–77.

131. Barnes RF, Raskind MA, Scott M, et al: Problems of families caring for Alzheimer patients: use of a support group. *J Am Geriatr Soc* 1981; 29:80–85.

132. Steinberg G, Shulman E: A long-term counseling program for family members of cognitively impaired aged, abstracted. *Gerontologist* (special issue) 1981; 21:286.

SECTION II
SENILE DEMENTIA AND ALZHEIMER'S DISEASE:
Background and
Historical Factors

2 The Early History of Senile Dementia

RICHARD M. TORACK

THE HISTORY OF ALZHEIMER'S DISEASE (AD) and senile dementia usually begins in 1906 with the presentation of a case report of dementia in a middle-aged woman, by Alois Alzheimer. The ensuing argument for a presenile dementia as a distinct nosological entity is now regarded as invalid, and AD has joined senile dementia under the all-encompassing cognomen of "Alzheimer's disease and senile dementia of the Alzheimer type" (SDAT). The recognition of a singular identity has a profound effect on history because, as senile dementia, it certainly existed before Alzheimer. Indeed one would presume that this mental catastrophe has always existed, particularly in aged populations. Therefore, a history that ends rather than begins with Alzheimer might be more appropriate.

Unfortunately, the premise that senile dementia has frequently accompanied aging has not been readily apparent in the medical literature. The term "demence" was coined by Pinel (1797) and before that time, terms like "fatuity" and "dotage" appear with regularity but lack precisely the same meaning. The major problem has been to separate senile dementia from normal aging, and this does not appear to have been less difficult 2,000 years ago than it is today.

GRECO-ROMAN CONCEPTS OF SENILITY

The earliest indication of senile mental deficiency is found in Solon's law regarding the making of wills. About 500 B.C. the Grecian lawgiver revised the usual practice of dividing an inheritance within the family and provided an opportunity to designate extrafamilial heirs. Solon qualified this new privilege, however, by adding "provided his judgment was not influenced by physical pain, violence, drugs, old age or the persuasion of a woman" (1 [p. 232]). Solon also effected extensive land reform so the Greeks, at this time, became largely agrarian, with most of the population being landowners. The elderly, senior members of a stable family unit, were generally regarded with considerable esteem. In Plato's *Republic*, the government is run by the elderly because of their greater experience and proven loyalty. Nonetheless, Plato also recognized senile dementia when he avowed that "the commission of certain crimes (sacrilege, treachery, treason) is excusable in a state of madness or when affected by disease or under the influence of extreme old age or in a fit of childish wantonness" (2 [p. 18]). Although incompetent behavior was recognized in the elderly, Hippocrates did not include it among his mental disorders, which probably means that senile dementia was considered a routine part of the aging process.

The social situation was quite different in Rome about 40 B.C. Republican Rome was rapidly changing, in its most chaotic era, on the threshold of empire. In such circumstances, the elderly were generally vilified. About this time, Horace wrote a letter (Ars Poetica) in which he described the characteristics of old men as "desire for gain, miserliness, lack of energy, quarrelsomeness, praise of the good old days and a condemnation of the younger generation" (3[p. 250]). Little wonder that Cicero was motivated to write an essay in defense of old people. "As wantonness and licentiousness are faults of the young rather than of the old, yet not of all young men but only of the depraved, so the senile folly called dotage is characteristic not of all old men but only of the frivolous" (4[p. 126]). *De senectute* is probably the most widely quoted composition about geriatrics, but it didn't help Cicero, killed by Mark Antony a year later.

Two hundred years later, Rome was an entirely different state under the philosopher-emperors Trajan, Hadrian, and Marcus Aurelius. In this setting, Galen achieved the apex of Greek medicine, especially with his description of the pulmonary circulation. Galen also added "morosis" (dementia) to the list of mental diseases and included old age as one of the situations in which it occurred. Morosis is defined as "some in whom the knowledge of letters and other arts are totally obliterated; indeed they can't even remember their own names. . . . Even now it is seen, that on account of extreme debility in old age, some are afflicted with similar symptoms" (5[pp. 200–201]). Galen also said, "Old age is the driest time of life which follows that what already has been said, because it is indeed the coldest" (6[p. 582]). Galenism migrated to the Arabian world, where his idea was preserved by physicians such as the eminent Maimonides, who described dementia thus: "Sometimes mental confusion and forgetfulness occur purely from senility or extreme weakness" (7[p. 131]).

MEDIEVAL MEDICINE

Unfortunately, Galen was not translated wholly into Latin until the fourteenth century, by which time the mind had become "located" in the heart or diaphragm. Melancholia became heart sickness and mania became phrensy. The terms really did not matter because mental illness was believed to represent witchcraft. In this heroic age, survival from disease or battle was unusual and viewed with suspicion. Consider this damning description of an old man by an unknown author in the fourteenth century:

> His nese ofte droppes, his hand stynkes
> His eres waxes deef and hard to here
> His mouth slavers, his tethe rotes
> His wyttes fayles and he ofte dotes.   (8[p. 263])

Dotage has been considered an equivalent of senile dementia, but in this work the definition is almost obscured by all the other afflictions.

In contrast to these morose definitions, those of Roger Bacon read like science fiction. This celebrated monk is most renowned for his scientific writings, but early in his life (1240?) he apparently studied medicine in Paris. Assigned a thesis on the prolongation of life, his research included the Arabian masters of Galenism: Avicenna, Rhazes, and Haly Regalis. His gleanings included the following:

In the posterior part [of the brain] occurs oblivion and memory concerning which Haly Regalis speaks in his first theoretical treatise, saying that old age is the home of forgetfulness.

An injury to the reasoning faculty happens in the middle part of the brain. Memory is not necessarily impeded. An injury to the imagination occurs in the anterior part of the brain. Memory and judgment are not affected. (8)

Bacon was obviously paraphrasing Arabian Galenism, but the important fact was that no one in Europe had said or written anything like that for 1,000 years and would not do so for another 600 years.

Following Bacon we must return to literary descriptions. In the prologue of Norfolk Reeve, Chaucer gave his thoughts on aging: "With old folk, save dotage, is namore [there is nothing but senility]" (9[p. 108]). In 1595, a humanist cleric in Rome, emulating Cicero, wrote in an essay on aging, "There is not much left of that acumen of mind which some call judgment, imagination, power of reasoning and memory" (10). The masterpiece, of course belongs to Shakespeare in his portrayal of King Lear.

> Does any here know me? This is not Lear.
> Does Lear walk thus? speak thus? Where are his eyes?
> Either his notion weakens, or his discernings
> are lethargied. Ha! waking? Tis not so.
> Who is it that can tell me who I am? (11)

Finally the medical profession began to comment. In 1584, Schenck von Grafenberg observed, "We find Francesco Barbaro totally devoid of any knowledge of Greek in extreme old age, even though he had once been most learned in this subject" (12[p. 153]). In 1599, Du Laurens, a physician to the court of Henry IV of France, wrote a discourse on old age in which he noted, "All the actions of the bodie and minde are weakened and growne feeble, the senses are dull, the memorie lost and the judgement failing so that they become as they were in their infancie" (13[pp. 174–175]). Perhaps the most remarkable evaluation of senile dementia is found in a case report of Salmon, a London practitioner: "For tho Sir John was not mad, or distracted like a man in Bedlam, yet he was so depraved in his intellect that he was become not only a perfect child in understanding but also foolish withall" (14[p. 260]). However, the general lack of public interest in the dementia complex is epitomized by the eminent Boerhaave (1668–1738), who wrote a six-volume textbook in which he made only this comment about the symptoms of aging: "Little by little the mind itself reaches a puerile debility, and finally senility" (15[p. 333]).

By this time, autopsies were being performed for the first time since the 4th century B.C. and many misconceptions of Galenism were being corrected. Unfortunately, the majority of mental disorders do not have an evident anatomical correlate but that did not really deter the anatomists. According to Galen, old meant cold and dry, so the brain must change accordingly. In 1656, Fernel described the brain in "amentia," to which class he assigned the aged. "Of these disorders the cause is an intemperate coldness throughout the brain which renders all its functions torpid and inactive" (16[p. 68]). The Sepulchretum of Bonet was considered to be the authority when it was published in 1679. In this work Bonet describes 23 cases of lapses of reason and memory; "The brain is seen to be pressed by an excess of humidity or cold, the texture of the brain being too solid and crumbling" (17[p. 254]). Boerhaave added, "The brains of the elderly upon examination with a knife are more hard and are more suitable for anatomical demonstrations" (15). The usually observant Haller (1708–1777) wrote, "In madness the brain is dry, hard and friable" (18[p. 572]).

Only the great Morgagni (1682–1771) was purely objective: "I do not lay so much stress upon this hardness, I would have you know that in some persons whose minds had not been disordered, I did not find the cerebrum less hard" (19[p. 161]). The medical profession did not appear to have added much since Galen.

THE MENTAL REVOLUTION

Between 1793 and 1813 the clinical recognition of senile dementia evolved so rapidly that nothing basic has been added since. The first ripple was recognition as a medical entity by Cullen: "Imbecility of judgment, by which men either do not perceive the relation of things or forget them due to diminished perception and memory when oppressed with age [senile dementia]" (20[p. 119]). Another astounding recognition occurred in 1793, 3,000 miles across the sea, from the brilliant Benjamin Rush.

> It would be sufficiently humbling to human nature if our bodies exhibited in old age the marks only of a second childhood; but human weakness descends still lower. I met with an instance of a woman between 80 and 90 who exhibited the marks of a second infancy, by such a total decay of her mental faculties as to lose all consciousness in discharging her alvine and urinary excretions. In this state of the body, a disposition to sleep succeeds the wakefulness of the first stages of old age. (21[p. 311]).

The next chapter in this trilogy occurred in Paris. In 1797, Pinel threw the shackles off the inmates at Bicetre; some of these inmates were senile dements. Pinel coined the term "demence" to indicate that condition in which "there is no judgment either true or false. The ideas appear to be insulated and to rise one after the other without connection, the faculty of association being destroyed" (22[p. 164]). It was, however, Esquirol working with Pinel who really defined senile dementia. "Senile dementia is established slowly. It commences with enfeeblement of memory, particularly the memory of recent impressions. The sensations are feeble; the attention, at first fatiguing, at length becomes impossible; the will is uncertain and without impulsion; the movements are slow and impractical" (23[p. 261]). This 1838 description by Esquirol essentially completed the clinical characterization so that in little more than 40 years, more definition occurred than in the previous two millennia.

Despite the nosological achievement, the anatomical abnormality continued unrecognized. The surprising aspect of the brain changes was the absence of atrophy even in the description of such an astute observer as Morgagni. In 1795, the eminent English pathologist Baillie did make mention of ventricular dilatation: "The brain is sometimes found to be considerably firmer than in a healthy state. Under such circumstances the ventricles are sometimes found enlarged in size and full of water" (24[p. 255]). Yet even in this circumstance the term "atrophy" was not used. In his textbook of 1835, the great clinico-pathologist Abercrombie did not even mention senile dementia.

The first definitive description of atrophy appears to be that of Wilks in 1864. Although Wilks described atrophy due to chronic alcoholism and CNS syphilis, he definitely included senile dementia as another cause. "Should it be the body of an old man where such wasted brain is found, I know that he has long been decrepit; that he has tottered in his walk and that he has been sinking mentally into the stage of second childhood" (25[p. 385]). The atrophy itself was very clear. "Instead of the sulci meeting, they are widely separated and their intervals filled with serum and which, on being removed with the pia mater, the full depth of the sulci can be seen" (25[p. 383]).

After Wilks, atrophy becomes a constant feature in the pathology of dementia. For Clouston, thus, "The next notable appearance [after focal softening] observed was marked atrophy of the whole brain or of considerable portions of its convolutional surface" (26[p. 649]). For Maudsley, in discussing chronic insanity: "Many of the more advanced cases exhibit a degree of atrophy of the brain" (27[p. 506]). For Alzheimer the degeneration became foci of ischemia due to arteriosclerosis which caused neuronal loss and replacement gliosis, thereby explaining both the atrophy and the firmness. The story ends with Redlich's description of a senile plaque in 1898.

CONCLUSION

The definition of senile dementia was essentially completed by 1910. Neurofibrillary tangles and granulovacuolar degeneration described by Alzheimer and Simchowicz in 1906 and 1910, respectively, were the major morphological additions. However, the essential question was not resolved then, and it remains unsolved today. In senile mental impairment the seventh stage of life as described by Shakespeare or is it a true age-related disease? The difference may determine whether national medical insurance pays the bill and, perhaps also, the likelihood of our finding effective treatments for the condition.

REFERENCES

1. Plutarch: *Lives,* North T (trans). New York, AMS Press, 1967.
2. Plato: *The Laws,* EB (trans). Manchester, University Press, 1921, book IX.
3. Coffman GR: Old age from Horace to Chaucer: some literary affinities and adventures of an idea. *Speculum* 1934; 9.
4. Cicero: *De senectute,* quoted in Tibbitts E (ed): *Aging in the Modern World.* Ann Arbor, University of Michigan Press, 1957.
5. Galen: De symptomatum differentiis liber, cap VII, in Kuhn K (ed): *Opera Omnia,* vol 7. Leipzig, Knobloch, 1821–1833.
6. Galen: De temperamentis, lib. II, cap II, in Kuhn K (ed): *Opera Omnia,* vol. I. Leipzig, Knobloch, 1821–1833.
7. *Maimonides: The Medical Aphorisms of Moses Maimonides,* Rosner F, Muntner S (trans). New York, Yeshiva University Press, 1970.
8. Bacon R: *De retardatione accidentium senectutis.* Hants, Gregg, 1966, pp. 18–27.
9. Chaucer G: *Canterbury Tales,* Nicolson JU (trans). Garden City, NY, Garden City Publishing, 1934.
10. Stern K, Cassirer T: A gerontological treatise of the Renaissance. *Am J Psychiatry* 1946; 102:770–773.
11. Shakespeare W: *The Tragedy of King Lear,* Brooke T, Phelps WL (eds). New Haven, Yale University Press, 1947.
12. Schenck von Grafenberg J: *Observationes medicae de capite humano,* obs cxviii. Basel, Froben, 1584.
13. Du Laurens A: *A Discourse of the Preservation of Sight: Of Melancholike Diseases; of Rheumes and of Old Age,* Surphlet R (trans). London, The Shakespeare Association, 1938.
14. Hunter R, Macalpine I: *Three Hundred Years of Psychiatry, 1535–1860.* London, Oxford University Press, 1963.

15. Boerhaave H: *Praelectiones academicae,* von Haller A (ed), vol 3. Venice, 1751.

16. Fernel J: *Universa medicina,* lib III, cap III. Utrecht, à Ziyll & van Ackersdijck, 1656.

17. Bonet T: *Sepulchretum sive anatomia practica,* lib I, sec X, obs I, vol 1. Lyons, Cramer & Perachon, 1700.

18. von Haller A: *Elementa physiologiae corporis humani,* lib XVII, sec I, vol 5. Lausanne, 1763.

19. Morgagni GB: *The Seats and Causes of Diseases Investigated by Anatomy,* Alexander B (trans), bk I, letter viii, art 18, vol 1. Mount Kisco, NY, Futura Publishing Co, 1980.

20. Cullen W: *A Synopsis of Medical Nosology.* Philadelphia, Hall, 1793.

21. Rush B: An account of the state of mind and body in old age, in *Medical Inquiries and Observations,* vol 2. Philadelphia, Dobson, 1793.

22. Pinel P: *A Treatise on Insanity,* Davis D (trans). Washington, DC, University Publications of America, 1977.

23. Esquirol JED: *Des maladies mentales,* vol 2. New York, Arno, 1976.

24. Baillie M: *The Morbid Anatomy of Some of the Most Important Parts of the Human Body,* American ed 2. Oceanside, NY, Dabor, 1977.

25. Wilks S: Clinical notes on atrophy of the brain. *J Ment Sci* 1864; 10.

26. Clouston TS: *Unsoundness of Mind.* New York, Dutton, 1911.

27. Maudsley H: *The Pathology of Mind.* New York, Appleton, 1880.

3 Historical Views and Evolution of Concepts

GENE D. COHEN

CONCEPTS ABOUT SENILE DEMENTIA IN GENERAL have varied and evolved for more than 2,500 years; views on Alzheimer's disease (AD) in particular have developed largely since the start of the 20th century. Moreover, the relationship between AD and senile dementia has often been blurred—as much by semantics as by concepts. Indeed, confusion has accompanied the gamut of considerations about senile dementia and AD, whether the focus has been nomenclature, epidemiology, etiology, diagnosis, clinical course, treatment, prognosis, or prevention. This confusion has historically affected clinical practice, research, and societal response to these disorders.

Some preliminary comments on terminology are in order. The word "senility" adds to the misunderstanding about senile dementia. According to the dictionary, senility is "the quality or state of being senile"—senile in turn is defined as "of, relating to, exhibiting, or characteristic of old age," and especially "exhibiting a loss of mental faculties associated with old age" (1). From these definitions it can easily be inferred that the "loss of mental faculties associated with old age" is "characteristic of old age."

There is unfortunately a long history of both the scientific community's and the lay public's making this circular inference. Dramatic new ideas challenging the perceptions of cognitive dysfunction as a likely or inevitable concomitant of later life and as a normal part of aging represent for the most part a relatively recent phenomenon (2, 3). Growing awareness of the large cohort of elderly individuals moving into advanced old age without measurable decline in intellectual function forces the issue (4). One questions physiological and psychological changes in later life to ask whether they reflect developmental events or clinical disorders.

Encouragingly, with regard to memory, which is usually of central concern in discussions of "senility" and senile dementia, what appears to be change or decline in the elderly may in fact not be. Older people are often accused, or accuse themselves, of memory changes that are not taking place. If a young person misplaces keys or wallet, forgets the name of a neighbor, or calls one sibling by another's name, nobody gives it a second thought. But the same forgetfulness for people in their seventies may raise unjustifiable concern. On the other hand, serious memory difficulties, or noticeable mental decline, should not be dismissed. These symptoms demand differential diagnosis, a search for cause, and a plan for treatment.

Historical Notes

How has mental decline in the form of senile dementia been looked at over the ages? A monumental step in the general understanding of diseases was, of course, taken by Hippocrates in the fourth century B.C. Referred to as the "Father of Medicine," Hippocrates was the first to attempt to explain diseases in terms of natural, as opposed to supernatural, causes (5). In the first century A.D., Aurelius Cornelius Celsus, a Roman writer on medical subjects, introduced the terms "delirium" and "dementia" in his work *De medicina* (5–7). Since then, the term "dementia" has been current for two millennia. During the first and second centuries A.D., two other Roman writers, Aretaeus of Cappadocia and Galen, significantly advanced the understanding of organic factors in mental dysfunction. Aretaeus divided diseases into acute and chronic categories, with the latter containing what would later be called senile dementia. Galen distinguished between primary and secondary brain disease in producing mental disorders, a dichotomy reflected in present day research pursuits for the etiology of AD.

It was then not until the nineteenth century that the term "senile dementia" was first used by Esquirol, Pinel's most outstanding student. After intensive study of physical, psychological, and moral factors in the treatment of mental disorders, Esquirol differentiated three types of dementia—acute, chronic, and senile (6). Acute dementia could be caused by fever or hemorrhage; chronic dementia by such factors as drunkenness, masturbation, epilepsy, or mania; senile dementia by advanced age. It was also around this time, 1837, that the English psychiatrist, James Prichard, described four stages in the progression of dementia: "(1) impairment of recent memory, (2) loss of reason, (3) incomprehension, (4) loss of instinctive action" (6). What should be kept in mind, however, is that reference to dementia up until the twentieth century often did not distinguish between organic and "functional" disorders. The use of the term "dementia praecox" to describe schizophrenia illustrates the point. Even today, the connotation of dementia remains in flux, with the turn-of-the-century specification of irreversibility in its definition no longer an essential feature (8).

Other nineteenth-century notes include the continued use of the rotating, or gyrating, chair by Benjamin Rush, the founder of American psychiatry. Rush believed that congested blood in the brain led to mental illness and that this condition could be ameliorated by rotary movement (5). A century later, a not unrelated theory about inadequate oxygenation of brain tissue leading to senile dementia led to the use of a similarly formidable apparatus—the hyperbaric oxygen chamber—similarly unsuccessful.

In 1898 the term "presenile dementia" was introduced by Binswanger (6). Then in 1906, the German physician Alois Alzheimer described in a patient, aged 51 years, a disease with a characteristic set of clinical and neuropathological findings (9). This disease, given Alzheimer's name, was subsequently designated a presenile dementia. But by the 1970s "Alzheimer's disease" (AD) became commonly used to label senile as well as presenile dementia of unknown etiology; very similar if not identical clinical and neuropathological pictures in both patient age groups was the reason cited.

The role of transmissible agents slowly inducing brain disease and dementia was discovered with the advent of the twentieth century. Fritz Schaudinn, in 1905, discovered the spirochete causing syphilis, and Nideyo Noguchi demonstrated the "spirocheta pallida" organism in the brains of patients suffering from general paresis (5). But it was not until 1965, through the work of D. Carleton Gajdusek, that:

kuru became the first heredofamilial chronic degenerative disease of the CNS of man demonstrated to be a virus-induced slow infection with incubation periods measured in years and with a progressive accumulated pathology restricted to the gray matter of the brain and spinal cord leading to death (10,11).

Subsequently, a similar "slow virus" infection was established by Gajdusek (11) as the cause of Creutzfeldt–Jakob disease, a disorder whose clinical picture can mimic that of AD.

The nineteenth century also witnessed, in the work of Kraepelin, the postulate that brain injury could be due to an unknown metabolite which he called an "autotoxin" (5). In the next century the autoimmunity hypothesis was advanced to explain a number of diseases, including AD.

With the twentieth century came a resurgence of scientific curiosity about the influence of chemistry on function, rivaling the interest in humoral relationships that captured clinical imaginations like that of Alcmaeon of Crotona around 500 B.C. (5). Variations, excesses, and deficits of chemicals in the brain ranging from acetylcholine to aluminum are being currently explored as causes of AD.

PRESENT VIEWS

NOMENCLATURE AND CLINICAL PICTURE

More recently, senile dementia has been considered an organic mental disorder or an organic brain syndrome of unknown cause, characterized by a progressive loss of intellectual function. And at present, senile dementia is increasingly referred to as AD or senile dementia of the Alzheimer type (SDAT). As mentioned earlier, AD was referred to traditionally as a presenile dementia; presenile in general referred to the under-65 age group, and senile to those 65 and older. But because histopathological brain changes of those with senile dementia appear to be essentially indistinguishable from those with presenile dementia of the Alzheimer type, the differentiation is commonly dropped, and AD has come to be used in both instances.

In the third edition of the *Diagnostic and Statistical Manual of Mental Disorders* (DSM III) (8) of the American Psychiatric Association, senile dementia is referred to as "primary degenerative dementia." If the disorder occurs at age 65 or older, as is usually the case, it is classified as "primary degenerative dementia, senile onset"; if it occurs prior to age 65, it is classified as "primary degenerative dementia, presenile onset." During the progression of the disorder significant accompanying or secondary symptoms may develop that are addressed in the DSM-III classification. Specifically, depression or delusions may occur, and in more serious cases delirium may be seen. Hence, in DSM-III primary degenerative dementia is described in terms of four subtypes—presenting with either delirium, delusions, or depression, or as "uncomplicated."

DIAGNOSIS AND DIFFERENTIAL DIAGNOSIS

The DSM-III diagnostic criteria for primary degenerative dementia are threefold:

1. Dementia
2. Insidious onset with uniformly progressive deteriorating course

3. Exclusion of all other specific causes of dementia by the history, physical examination, laboratory tests, psychometric, and other special studies

Proper diagnosis is obviously an important issue among both clinicians and researchers, since various other forms of dementia (other organic brain syndromes) can masquerade as senile dementia of the Alzheimer type. Not all forms of dementia or organic brain syndrome are progressive or irreversible, and initially many of these other disorders may be misdiagnosed as AD. Therefore, the differential diagnostic workup seeks to rule out a range of reversible or nonprogressive brain syndromes of diverse origins, including those attributable to trauma, infection, metabolic disturbances, drug side effects, toxic products, circulatory problems, cerebrovascular disorders, tumors, and a variety of neurological diseases. Moreover, a severe form of depression referred to as "pseudodementia" can manifest signs and symptoms that, at first, may be indistinguishable from those of AD. The ready danger of misdiagnosis should be apparent (12).

EPIDEMIOLOGY AND GENETICS

Epidemiologic and genetic factors represent areas of widespread popular misconception as well as of growing research activity. Rather than AD being a likelihood of later life, the percentage of the more than 25 million people in the United States over age 65 who manifest the disease is closer to 6%. Of course, 6% is still a significant number—more than a million older persons in the United States. The prevalence increases with advancing age, especially after age 75. For reasons that are not clear, the disorder appears to be more common in women than in men. Heredity also appears to be of some importance since the probability of a first degree relative developing AD has been found by some investigators to be four times greater than in the general population, where the risk is well below 1% (2).

ETIOLOGY

Leading hypotheses of the causes of AD now under study include

1. Neurotransmitter or other neurochemical deficits or imbalances (particularly acetylcholine and neuropeptides)
2. Selective brain cell death or injury induced by viral or other transmissible agents in the environment
3. Excessive accumulation in the brain of aluminum or other toxins
4. Genetic factors (defects or predispositions)
5. An autoimmune process (e.g., antibrain antibodies related to aging) (9)

TREATMENT

Two critical junctures crossed in the approach to treatment for AD were (1) recognition of AD as a disease demanding treatment as opposed to a routine part of normal aging, and (2) realization that in developing interventions for a major disorder or disability the concept of care can be as important as that of cure. Consequently, several areas need to be considered with regard to treatment for senile dementia. These include treatment for the disease itself; intervention to assist the individual with adjustment and psychological reaction to the illness; approaches to alleviating excess disability that can accompany the disorder; attention to what can be done to improve conditions in the victim's immediate environment to reduce stress and increase coping capacity; and support for the patient's family (3).

OUTLOOK

AD remains a devastating disorder of unknown cause, but the outlook for breakthroughs in the understanding and treatment of the disease is more optimistic than formerly.

REFERENCES

1. *Webster's New Collegiate Dictionary.* Springfield, Merriam, 1979.
2. Katzman R, Terry RD, Bick KL (eds): *Aging NY* 1978; 7.
3. Miller NE, Cohen GD (eds): *Aging NY* 1981; 15.
4. Reisberg B: *Brain Failure: An Introduction to Current Concepts of Senility.* New York, Free Press, 1981.
5. Alexander FG, Selesnick ST: *The History of Psychiatry.* New York, Harper & Row, 1966.
6. Lipowski ZJ: Organic mental disorders: introduction and review of syndromes, in Kaplan HI, Freedman AM, Sadock BJ (eds): *Comprehensive Textbook of Psychiatry.* Baltimore, Williams & Wilkins, 1980, Vol 2, pp 1359–1392.
7. Lipowski ZJ: Organic mental disorders: their history and classification, with special reference to DSM-III. *Aging NY* 1981; 15:37–45.
8. American Psychiatric Association: *Diagnostic and Statistical Manual of Mental Disorders,* ed 3. Washington, DC, American Psychiatric Association, 1980.
9. *Alzheimer's Disease: A Scientific Guide for Health Practitioners,* NIH publication no. 81–2251. Bethesda, 1980.
10. Gajdusek DC, Gibbs CJ, Jr.: Slow, latent, and temperate virus infections of the central nervous system. *Res Publ Assoc Rev Nerv Ment Dis* 1968; 44:254–280.
11. Gibbs CJ, Gajdusek DC: Subacute spongiform virus encephalopathies: the transmissible virus dementias. *Aging NY* 1978; 7:559–575.
12. Cohen GD: Senile dementia of the Alzheimer type (SDAT): nature of the disorder, in Crook T, Gershon S (eds): *Strategies for the Development of an Effective Treatment for Senile Dementia.* New Canaan, Powley, 1981.

SECTION III

PATHOLOGICAL FEATURES OF ALZHEIMER'S DISEASE AND THE NORMAL AGING BRAIN

4 An Overview of Light and Electron Microscopic Changes

ARNE BRUN

IN VIEW OF ITS ENORMOUS social-medical impact, Alzheimer's disease (AD) has been the subject of numerous treatises and congresses. The reader is referred for further information to refs. 1–12. Macroscopically, the brain may appear normal in early cases of AD. When more advanced, the disease causes a widespread atrophy of the hemispheres. In extreme cases the generalized atrophy results in a reduction of brain weight to 800 g or less, a loss of 400–500 g compared with the normal age-matched weight. This loss of substance is due to a reduction of gray and white matter, white matter atrophy presumably being a secondary and late event. Though generalized, the atrophy is more marked in certain areas of the brain. As a consequence the gyri are narrowed and the sulci widened. The temporal lobe, especially its basal, medial limbic portion (hippocampus and amygdaloid nucleus) and the post–central parietal region, are particularly involved, as well as, to a somewhat lesser extent, the frontal lobes (Fig. 4–1). On the other hand, primary projection areas such as the sensorimotor cortex and calcarine gyrus are largely preserved (2, 3, 8–11, 13). Regional accentuations in late-onset AD are similar to those seen in AD with onset in the presenium, though somewhat less pronounced (14).

The subarachnoid space is widened secondary to the brain atrophy, and the meninges are thickened by fibrosis. In AD, the arteries at the base of the brain usually show little arteriosclerosis, and frank infarctions of the brain are rare. Among older victims, however, vascular lesions more often complicate the picture.

Sectioning of the brain reveals slight to moderate widening of the ventricles, especially of the temporal and parietal-occipital horns. The white matter is usually unremarkable in the early stages of the disease process, but in more advanced cases is contracted, yellowed, and rubbery. Some pallor of the substantia nigra can be seen, but other parts of the brain stem, cerebellum, and spinal cord are usually unaltered. Changes due to other diseases are more frequent in older individuals with AD.

Microscopically, the changes are usually confined to the cerebral cortex, the limbic gray matter, and, to some extent, the mesencephalon. The cerebellum and basal ganglia are rarely affected and changes have not been noted in the spinal cord. In milder cases the gray matter may appear virtually normal using conventional stains, but special techniques (silver impregnation) bring out numerous senile or neuritic plaques (SPs) and neurofibrillary tangles (NFTs). These changes are classical and compulsory for the pathologic diagnosis of AD. They are most likely present during a long subclinical phase, and in early cases

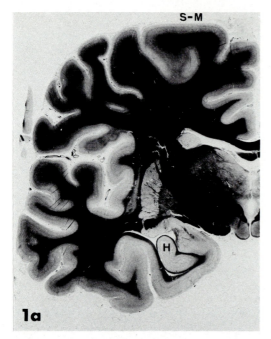

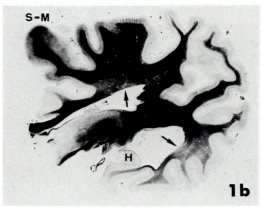

Figure 4–1. Frontal brain sections from patients of the same age: (a) normal and (b) Alzheimer's disease. Normal myelin is stained black. Note atrophy of the gray and white matter, particularly of lower temporal lobe including the hippocampus (H) and a paling of the white matter here as well as above the lateral ventricle (*arrows*). The sensorimotor gyrus (S-M), however, is preserved.

constitute the only microscopic changes. This basic picture is supplemented in more advanced stages by neuronal loss, gliosis, spongiosis, and blurring of cortical cytoarchitecture. In routinely stained sections these latter alterations are the major, striking pathology in the cortex.

Senile plaques are spherical, 5–200-μm lesions, classically consisting of a central amyloid core surrounded by a halo, and more peripherally by a corona composed of argyrophilic (silver-positive) rods and granules, microglial cells, and astrocytes (Fig. 4–2). When viewed under the electron microscope, the rods and granules appear to be made of axonal terminals and preterminals, indicating involvement of synaptic structures. The terminals contain lipid granules, dense bodies, abnormal mitochondria, and paired helical filaments (PHFs) of the type described later in the discussion of NFTs. The SPs can thus be visualized not only with silver staining but with methods which can demonstrate amyloid contained in the core or acid phosphatase contained within microglial cells. The classical form of senile plaques presumably develop from immature forms consisting of a few neurites and wisps of amyloid.

Eventually, the plaques develop into solid amyloid spheres and may finally dissolve or become unidentifiable. Some SPs are associated with vessels from which amyloid appears to leak out into the brain substance (15). SPs tend to accumulate in the depths of sulci and dominate in the superficial cortical layers, although they can, especially in advanced cases, be found diffusely and in all layers (Fig. 4–3). They are common in amygdaloid and hippocampal structures, and also appear in the striate body and anterior septal areas. They are seen occasionally in mesencephalic gray substance but only rarely in the cerebellar cortex and never in the spinal cord.

Neurofibrillary tangles (NFTs) are silver-positive, hairlike hooks or loops in the cyto-

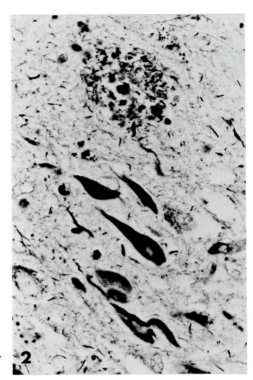

Figure 4–2. Senile plaque (*top*) and several neurofibrillary tangles (*lower half of picture*).

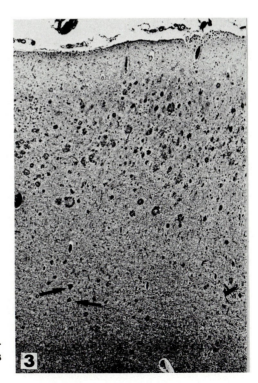

Figure 4–3. Cerebral cortex with numerous senile plaques, mostly in layers III–V, and tangles in neurons below (*arrows*).

plasm of neurons (Fig. 4–2). Electron microscopically, NFTs consist of bundles or masses of 10-nm filaments which are either single and straight or, more usually, paired. The paired filaments are wound about each other in a helical fashion with a periodicity of 80 nm, and are usually designated "paired helical filaments" (PHFs) (16–20) (Fig. 4–4). PHFs presumably take on a β-pleated sheet arrangement as they react histochemically similarly to amyloid. The PHFs composing neurofibrillary tangles have the same structure as PHFs seen in neurites in SPs. Tangles are seen primarily in the pericaryon, but can be detected even at distant synaptic communication points and in the axons, presumably under transport from the cell body to its peripheral ramifications (21).

Granulovacuolar degeneration is usually restricted to the hippocampal formation. As the name implies, it consists of a 1-μm argyrophilic core (granule) in a vacuole measuring 3–5 μm in diameter. The core is electron-dense and the vacuole is membrane-bound (22). This type of degeneration is seen in the cytoplasm of pyramidal neurons, in which RNA is often reduced. Affected neurons often appear to be in stages of terminal degeneration (23). When severe, this change may contribute to the production of dementia (24).

The Hirano body (25) is another discrete type of change seen primarily in the hippocampus. Light microscopically, these bodies appear as eosinophilic rods, 15–30 μm, which under the electron microscope are seen to have a crystalline structure. Their nature and importance are, however, unknown.

Accumulations of lipofuscin in neuronal cytoplasm can be particularly prominent in cases of dementia, but are also seen in other clinical settings. Lipofuscin appears to be a pigmented cellular waste product stored in lysosome-derived vacuoles. The effects of lipofuscin accumulation are unclear. In addition, some neurons, so-called inflated cells, may become swollen with silver-positive inclusions which do not resemble NFTs. Neuronal shrinking or sclerosis can also be seen (2).

Figure 4–4. Electron microscopic view of neurofibrillary tangles composed of paired helical filaments (*arrow*) sweeping along the nuclear membrane in (a) ($\times$ 9,600). Helical twists shown in (b) ($\times$ 80,000).

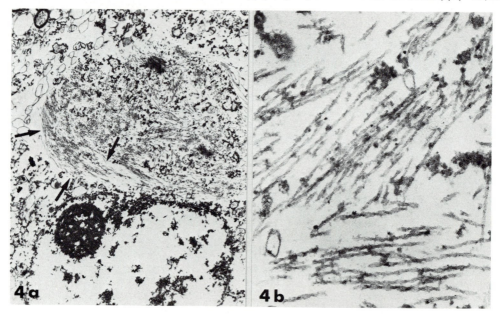

During the development of the neuronal changes described above, the nerve cell extensions become atrophic with loss of dendritic spines and whole dendrites. Attempts at regeneration of dendrites may occur but the main net result is a deafferentation which is probably of considerable functional significance (13, 26, 27).

It thus appears likely that degenerating neurons have a reduced functional capacity even before the final stages of degeneration and neuronal disappearance. This might limit the usefulness of neuronal quantification. Drop-out has also been difficult to ascertain since neurons decrease somewhat with increasing age in the absence of dementia (4–6). Some authors (12, 21, 28–30) in studies of certain brain regions of AD cases found no neuronal drop-out in excess of that which could be expected for the subject's age. Other studies, however, have found in AD, a nearly 60% reduction in neurons and even higher neuronal drop-out in areas of accentuated atrophy, especially in post–central parietal areas and the posterior cingulate gyrus (10, 31, 32).

Spongiosis and gliosis of the cortex are likely results of the neuronal changes and drop-out described above, and represent a progression of the degeneration from the basic stage where only SPs and NFTs are seen. Spongiosis is a loosening of the basic structure of the cortex due to the appearance of minute cavities or vacuoles in the neuropil (Fig. 4–5). These vacuoles may be the result of loss of neurons and their extensions and the swelling of astrocytic processes. Spongiosis is usually first seen in superficial cortical layers, but with disease advancement, spreads to deeper cortical strata. In these deeper layers it is never so marked, possibly because of an attempt at tissue repair at these levels consisting of an increase in the number and size of cortical fibrous astrocytes (33).

Figure 4–5. Cerebral cortex, layers I–IV, with spongiosis mainly of lamina II.

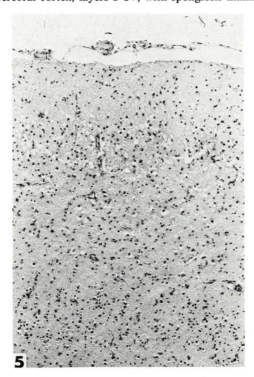

Astrocytic gliosis also helps for a time to maintain the volume of the cortex, which, in the long run, becomes increasingly shrunken. Gliosis is easiest to detect in the outer molecular layer, but is seen to some extent in all cortical layers. In advanced cases the glial fibrils form rounded nests similar to SPs in routinely stained sections (Fig. 4–6). Glial cells and fibrils also give rise to a thickening of membranes along vessels, the ventricular lining, and subpial limiting membrane. At these sites there also appear a large number of pial blue hyaline granules called "brain sand" or "corpora amylacea."

The white matter of the brain appears initially unaltered but may later show some myelin loss. This may at least in part be secondary to the neuronal degeneration which would result in the disappearance of myelinated axons passing through the white matter. In AD, myelin loss is most obvious in the temporal lobe (Fig. 4–1(b)) (10). Arteriolar sclerosis may contribute to white matter alteration with an incomplete noncavitating infarction, especially in AD with late (senile) onset (SDAT) (14) where frank infarctions due to atheromatosis are also more common.

In most cases of AD, the artery and capillary walls in both meninges and cortex show segmental deposits of amyloid (cerebral amyloid angiopathy). Cerebral amyloidosis, manifested by amyloid deposits in SPs and vessels, is almost never associated with amyloid deposits in the viscera. Its presence may point to an immunologic or autoimmune factor in the etiology or pathogenesis of the disease process. The amyloid seen at the various sites does not appear to be of the same type, although it has not yet been well characterized.

Figure 4–6. Cerebral cortex with gliosis: Many enlarged fibrillary astrocytes (*arrows*) and rounded glial nests (*top half of picture*).

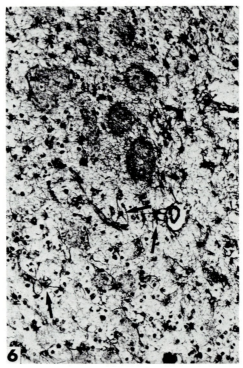

Advancing degeneration results in a progressive loss of internal cortical structure. Its lamination becomes blurred or obliterated and becomes in the end a narrow ribbon with homogeneous cellularity. The changes leading to cortical atrophy tend to proceed from superficial toward deeper cortical layers where only few well-preserved neurons can be seen at the late stages (Figs. 4–7(a)–(c)). In early onset AD, the most degenerated areas may lose up to 50% of their width (10, 32); in AD with late onset, a less pronounced atrophy is noted (28).

The degenerative process is not, however, uniformly severe in all regions. It is most severe in the hippocampus and amygdaloid nucleus, followed, in order of decreasing severity, by the inferior temporal (Brodmann area 20, 21) and post–central parietal areas (Brodmann 7b, 19, 39), the posterior cingulate gyrus (Brodmann 23), and the frontal lobes anterior to the precentral gyrus. On the other hand, the anterior cingulate gyrus (Brodmann 24), the sensorimotor region (Brodmann 4–7a), and the calcarine areas (Brodmann 17) are relatively spared until late in the disease (Figs. 4–8(a) and (b)).

This regional variation may be inconspicuous in the earliest stages but becomes more obvious with disease advancement. The amygdaloid nuclei and hippocampal structures, however, are always affected early. In very advanced cases such regional differences tend to even out. The concept of regional accentuations is supported by the focality of symptoms and signs and the pattern of cerebral blood flow reduction (7–9, 33–36). Obviously, an area selected at random for histologic examination may not be representative of the true state of the disease. A complete picture can be obtained only after extensive pathologic study and consideration of the clinical parameters. The number of SPs is also reported to parallel the severity of dementia (37) except in late stages when SPs appear to dissolve or become unidentifiable (10).

Other causes of dementia can usually be distinguished from AD. The changes of multi-infarct dementia are asymmetrical, whereas those of AD are predictable and usually symmetrical in both hemispheres (see Chap. 25). In Pick's disease the atrophy is most striking in the frontal lobes including the inferior motor area and the anterior portion of the temporal

Figure 4–7. Cerebral cortex (a) preserved, (b) with moderate and (c) severe degeneration. Note distinct lamination and normal cellular density in (a), blurring of lamination in superior half of (b) (*above arrow*), and obliterated structural organization at all depths in (c).

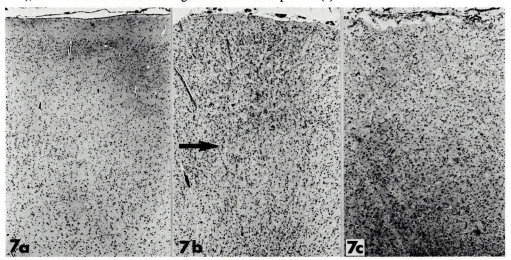

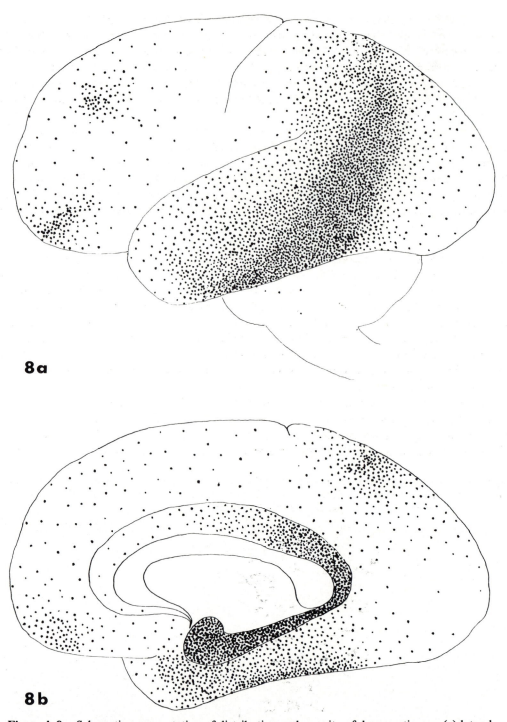

8a

8b

Figure 4–8. Schematic representation of distribution and severity of degeneration on (a) lateral and (b) medial aspect of the brain in an average Alzheimer case. The darker the area, the more pronounced the degeneration. White areas are spared, with only basic change discernible.

lobes, with sparing of the posterior cingulate gyrus and parietal lobes. This pattern is nearly the converse of AD, although the amygdaloid nucleus and hippocampus are involved.

In conclusion, we might state that AD is a generalized corticolimbic disease with regional accentuations, particularly in younger cases. The regional accentuations of the degenerative process in part determine the symptomatology. These are due to neuronal changes with altered metabolism. The pattern of degeneration is consequently mirrored by reductions of both glucose utilization as seen with positron emission tomography (PET) (38) and regional cerebral blood flow (rCBF) using xenon 133, injected (35, 37) or inhaled (36, 39). Cerebral atrophy may also be seen on computed tomography (CT) and correlated with the dementia (40). Finally, cholinergic neuronal transmission in particular is deficient (41) probably due mainly to degeneration of septal and hypothalamic (nucleus basalis Meynert) nuclei where the acetylcholine is produced. With the aid of these methods, which thus reflect the distribution and severity of the pathologic changes, diagnosis and differential diagnosis can be made *in vivo*.

REFERENCES

1. Bowen DM, Spillane JA, Curzon G, et al: Accelerated aging or selective neuronal loss as an important cause of dementia. *Lancet* 1979; i:11–14.

2. Braunmühl A: Alterskrankungen des Zentralnervensystems. Senile involution. Senile demenz. Alzheimersche Krankheit, in Lubarsch O, Henke F, Rössle R (eds): *Handbuch der speziellen pathologischen Anatomie und Histologie*. Berlin, Springer, vol 13, 1937, pp 337–539.

3. Brion S: Démences par atrophie cérébrale primitive. Le concours médical 15–I–88–3, Dossier EPU, 1966, no 31, pp 313–324.

4. Brody H: Organization of the cerebral cortex: III. A study of aging in the human cerebral cortex. *J Comp Neurol* 1955; 102:511–556.

5. Brody H: An examination of cerebral cortex and brainstem aging. *Aging NY* 1976; 3:177–181.

6. Brody H: Cell counts in cerebral cortex and brain stem. *Aging NY* 1978; 7:345.

7. Brun A, Gustafson L, Ingvar DH: Neuropathological findings related to neuropsychiatric symptoms and regional cerebral blood flow in presenile dementia. *Proceedings of the Seventh International Neuropathology*. Amsterdam, Excerpta Medica, 1975, pp 101–105.

8. Brun A, Gustafson L: Distribution of cerebral degeneration in Alzheimer's disease: a clinicopathological study. *Arch Psychiatr Nervenkr* 1976; 223:15–33.

9. Brun A, Gustafson L: Limbic lobe involvement in presenile dementia. *Arch Psychiatr Nervenkr* 1978; 226:79–93.

10. Brun A, Englund E: The pattern of degeneration in Alzheimer's disease: neuronal loss and histopathological grading. *Histopathology* 1981; 5:549–564.

11. Brun A: Alzheimer's disease and its clinical implications, in Platt D (ed): *Geriatrics*. New York, Springer, 1982, vol 1, pp 343–390.

12. Terry RD: Morphological changes in Alzheimer's disease–senile dementia: ultrastructural changes and quantitative studies, in Katzman R (ed): *Congenital and Acquired Cognitive Disorders*. Association for Research in Nervous and Mental Disease, vol 57. New York, Raven, 1979, pp 99–105.

13. Mehraein P, Yamada M, Tarnowska-Dziduszko E: Quantitative study on dendrites and dendritic spines in Alzheimer's disease and senile dementia. *Adv Neurol* 1975; 12:453–458.

14. Englund B, Brun A: Senile dementia: structural basis for etiological and therapeutic considerations, in Perris C (ed): *Proceedings of the Eighth International Congress of Biological Psychiatry.* Amsterdam, Elsevier North-Holland, 1982, pp 951–956.

15. Morel F, Wildi E: General and cellular pathochemistry of senile and presenile alterations of the brain. *Proceedings of the First International Congress of Neuropathology,* vol 2, pp 347–374.

16. Kidd M: Paired helical filaments in electron microscopy of Alzheimer's disease. *Nature* 1963; 197:192–193.

17. Terry RD: The fine structure of neurofibrillary tangles in Alzheimer's disease. *J Neuropathol Exp Neurol* 1963; 22:629–634.

18. Terry RD, Gonatas NK, Weiss M: Ultrastructural studies in Alzheimer's presenile dementia. *Am J Pathol* 1964; 44:269–281.

19. Wisniewski HM, Terry RD: Neuropathology of the aging brain. *Aging NY* 1976; 3:265–280.

20. Yagishita S, Itoh Y, Wang NA: Reappraisal of the fine structure of Alzheimer's neurofibrillary tangles. *Acta Neuropathol* 1981; 54:239–246.

21. Terry RD: Ultrastructural alterations in senile dementia. *Aging NY* 1978; 7:375–382.

22. Ellis WG, McCulloch JR, Corley CL: Presenile dementia in Down's syndrome: ultrastructural identity with Alzheimer's disease. *Neurology* 1974; 24:101–106.

23. Mann DMA: Granulovacuolar degeneration in pyramidal cells of the hippocampus. *Acta Neuropathol* 1978; 42:149–151.

24. Woodard JS: Clinico-pathological significance of granulovacuolar degeneration in Alzheimer's disease. *J Neuropathol Exp Neurol* 1962; 21:85–91.

25. Hirano A, Malamud N, Elizan TS, et al: Amyotrophic lateral sclerosis and parkinsonism-dementia complex on Guam. *Arch Neurol* 1966; 15:35–51.

26. Buell SJ, Coleman PD: Dendritic growth in the aged human brain and failure to grow in senile dementia. *Science* 1979; 206:854–856.

27. Scheibel AB: Dendritic changes in senile and presenile dementia, in Katzman R (ed): *Congenital and Acquired Cognitive Disorders,* vol 57. Association for Research in Nerves and Mental Disease, New York, Raven, 1979, pp 107–124.

28. Terry RD, Fitzgerald C, Peck A, et al: Cortical cell counts in senile dementia. *J Neuropathol Exp Neurol* 1977; 36:316–323.

29. Terry RD: Senile dementia. *Fed Proc* 1978; 37:2837–2840.

30. Tomlinson BE, Henderson G: Some quantitative cerebral findings in normal and demented old people. *Aging NY* 1976; 3:183–204.

31. Colon EJ: The cerebral cortex in presenile dementia: a quantitative analysis. *Acta Neuropathol* 1973; 23:281–290.

32. Shefer VF: Absolute number of neurons and thickness of the cerebral cortex during aging, senile and vascular dementia, and Pick's and Alzheimer's diseases. *Zh Zevropatol Psikhiatr* 1972; 72:1024–1029.

33. Gustafson L, Brun A, Ingvar DH: Presenile dementia: clinical symptoms, pathoanatomical findings, and cerebral blood flow, in Meyer JS, Lechner H, Reivich M (eds): *Cerebral Vascular Disease.* Amsterdam, Excerpta Medica, 1977, pp 5–9.

34. Hagberg B, Ingvar DH: Cognitive reduction in presenile dementia related to regional abnormalities of the cerebral blood flow. *Br J Psychiatry* 1976; 128:209–222.

35. Ingvar DH, Gustafson L: Regional cerebral blood flow in organic dementia with early onset. *Acta Neurol Scand Suppl* 1970; 46(suppl 43): 42–73.

36. Risberg J: Regional cerebral blood flow measurements by 133 Xe-inhalation: methodology and applications in neuropsychology and psychiatry. *Brain Lang* 1980; 9:9–34.

37. Ingvar DH, Brun A, Hagberg B, et al: Regional cerebral blood flow in the dominant hemisphere in confirmed cases of Alzheimer's disease, Pick's disease, and multiinfarct dementia: relationship to clinical symptomatology and neuropathological findings. *Aging NY* 1978; 7:203–211.

38. Ferris, SH, de Leon MJ, Wolf AP, et al: Positron emission tomography in the study of aging and senile dementia. *Neurobiol Aging* 1981; 2:127–131.

39. Gustafson L, Risberg J, Silverskiöld P: Regional cerebral blood flow in organic dementia and affective disorders. *Adv Biol Psychiatry* 1981; 6:109–116.

40. de Leon MJ, Ferris SH, George AE, et al: Computed tomography evaluations of brain–behavior relationships in senile dementia of the Alzheimer's type. *Neurobiol Aging* 1981; 2:66–78.

41. Corkin, S: Acetylcholine, aging, and Alzheimer's disease: implications for treatment. *Trends Neurosci* 1981:287–290.

5 Neurofibrillary Tangles

KHALID IQBAL
HENRYK M. WISNIEWSKI

TOPOGRAPHY, LIGHT, AND ELECTRON MICROSCOPY

Neurofibrillary tangles are the hallmark lesion of the Alzheimer brain, and are commonly referred to as "Alzheimer neurofibrillary tangles" (NFTs) or "Alzheimer neurofibrillary changes." They are stained intensely with silver-impregnation techniques (Fig. 5–1), producing green birefringence in polarized light after staining with Congo red (Fig. 5–2). Such neurofibrillary tangles are found primarily in the cerebral cortex, especially in the hippocampal pyramidal cells of Sommers sector and small pyramidal neurons in the outer laminae of the frontotemporal cortex. They have not been seen in cerebellum, spinal cord, peripheral nervous system, or extraneuronal tissues.

Ultrastructurally, the Alzheimer neurofibrillary tangles are composed of bundles of paired filaments: each filament of the pair is 10–13 nm in diameter, helically wound around

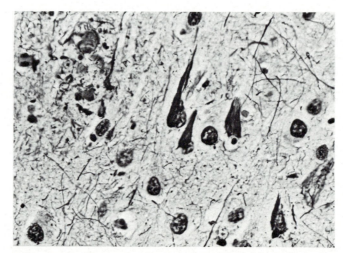

Figure 5–1. Light micrograph of a Bodian-stained section of an Alzheimer hippocampus and parahippocampal area. The NFTs and the neurites of an adjacent neuritic plaque (*upper left corner*) can be easily visualized because of silver impregnation. × 360. *Courtesy Dr. Inge Grundke-Iqbal.*

each other at regular intervals of 80 nm (Fig. 5–3) (1, 2). These paired helical filaments (PHFs) are morphologically unlike any of the normal neurofibers (i.e., neurotubules, neurofilaments, and microfilaments) (Fig. 5–4, Table 5–1).

In addition to the neurofibrillary tangles, the PHFs are found in bundles in the degenerated neurites of the senile (neuritic) plaques (SPs) and less frequently as individual fibers in myelinated axons. The number of both the tangles and the plaques correlates strongly with the degree of dementia (3). It should be noted, however, that plaques and tangles might not be interdependent, since in some Alzheimer cases there are numerous NFTs and very few SPs, and vice versa. Both these lesions are important on their own, therefore, and understanding their pathogenetic mechanisms will enhance our understanding of cerebral aging (4).

In neurons undergoing neurofibrillary changes, PHFs seem to become gradually more densely packed and take over a large proportion of the cell space, displacing cytoplasmic organelles. It remains unclear whether accumulations of such PHFs lead to cell death; whether the affected cells can recover is also unknown. Maintenance of synaptic contact has been observed in situations where presynaptic and postsynaptic processes are filled with PHFs, suggesting that a certain degree of function persists in these affected synapses.

Neurofibrillary Changes: Type and Distribution

Although the neurofibrillary tangles of PHFs are most commonly associated with AD, they are found in small numbers in the brain tissue of normal aged humans, and in great abundance in Guam parkinsonism dementia complex, dementia pugilistica, postencephalitic parkinsonism, and adults with Down's syndrome. This lesion has also been observed in small numbers in several cases of subacute sclerosing panencephalitis (SSPE), in rare cases of Hallervorden–Spatz disease, and in juvenile neurovisceral lipid storage disease (Table 5–2) (for reviews see refs. 5, 6). The accumulation of PHFs is thus associated with normal

Figure 5–2. Alzheimer NFTs in hippocampus (a) stained with Congo red and (b) the same field in polarized light showing the tangles becoming birefringent. × 360. *Courtesy Dr. Inge Grundke-Iqbal.*

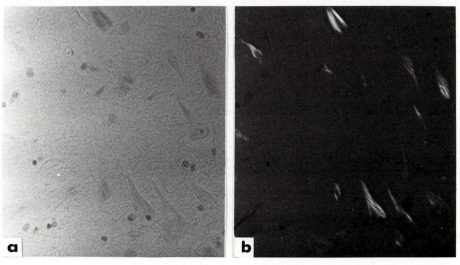

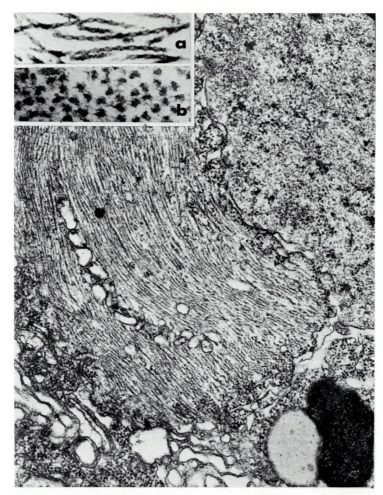

Figure 5–3. Electron micrograph of an NFT from a case of Alzheimer dementia. Bundles of paired helical filaments (PHFs) in the neuronal cytoplasm can be seen. The neuronal nucleus is at the upper right. × 43,500. *Reproduced with permission of Plenum Publishing Corp. from K. Iqbal et al., "Neurofibrillary Pathology: An Update," in The Aging Brain and Senile Dementia, edited by K. Nandy and I. Sherwin, 1977.* Insets: high magnification of PHFs in (a) longitudinal section, × 80,000; and (b) transverse section, × 125,000.

aging, viral infection, chromosomal disorders, and metabolic abnormalities. PHFs of the Alzheimer type, however, have never been observed in any aged animal species nor have they been produced experimentally in animals.

The neurofibrillary changes in human disorders are not always of the Alzheimer type (i.e., made up of PHFs). For instance, in progressive supranuclear palsy, also called Steele–Richardson–Olszewski syndrome, some of the same neurons which contain tangles composed of PHFs in the Alzheimer brain have neurofibrillary tangles composed of 15-nm straight filaments (7). These tangles of 15-nm filaments in progressive supranuclear palsy are sometimes admixed with PHFs (8). In sporadic motor neuron disease, vincristine neuropathy, and infantile neuroaxonal dystrophy in humans, the neurofibrillary changes are of the 10-nm intermediate-filament type. The 10-nm intermediate-filament type neurofibrillary changes

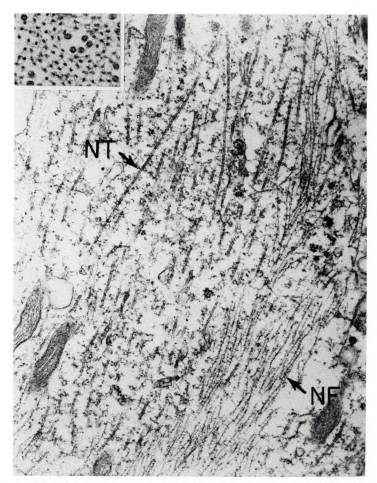

Figure 5-4. Electron micrograph showing neurofilaments (NFs) in a normal neuronal process. X 95,000. NT = neurotubules. *Reproduced with permission of Plenum Publishing Corp. from K. Iqbal et al., "Neurofibrillary Pathology: An Update," in The Aging Brain and Senile Dementia, edited by K. Nandy and I. Sherwin, 1977. Inset:* neurofilaments and neurotubules in a transverse section. X 110,000.

have also been experimentally induced (in animals) with aluminum; mitotic spindle inhibitors such as colchicine, vinblastine, and podophyllotoxin; various nitrates; and acrylamide (for reviews see refs. 5, 6). The aluminum-induced filamentous accumulation is apparently specific to the nervous system, while in the case of the mitotic spindle inhibitors, similar changes occur in a wide range of cell types.

BIOCHEMISTRY OF PHFs

PHFs are stable in both fresh and frozen autopsy tissue and are not in aqueous buffer in the absence of detergents or denaturants. They can be isolated in high purity from autopsied tissue by a combination of sucrose-density-gradient centrifugation and detergent treatment (9). The protein composition of isolated PHFs is different from neurotubules, neurofilaments,

TABLE 5–1
Comparison of Alzheimer's PHFs with Normal Neurofibers

| Characteristic | Neurofiber | | | |
	PHF	Microtubule	Neurofilament	Microfilament
Morphology				
Longitudinal section	Linear, narrowed every 80 nm	Linear, sidearms	Linear, sidearms	Linear —[a]
Cross-section diameter	22 nm–10 nm	24 nm	10 nm	5 nm
Wall	Circular or arciform	Circular	Circular	Circular
Stain				
Argentophilia	+	—	+	—
Congophilia	+	—	—	—
Solubility				
Long formalin	Stable	Soluble	Stable	Stable
Direct osmic acid	Stable	Soluble	Stable	Stable
Glutaraldehyde	Stable	Stable	Stable	Stable
Major proteins	45–62 k	Tubulin: α, 56 k and β, 53 k	Neurofilament triplet 70, 160, and 210 k	Actin: 45 k
Associated proteins	Not identified	Tau: 65–70 k MAPS: 250–350 k	50 k in CNS	

[a] + = takes stain; — = no stain.

and microfilaments (see Table 5–1). Immunochemically, PHFs do not crossreact with microtubules, neurofilaments, or 10-nm filaments induced with aluminum or colchicine. Polypeptides immunochemically crossreactive to PHFs, however, have been observed in normal young human and animal brains (10–13).

It has not yet been determined if PHFs share molecular characteristics with conventional protein species in the brain, or if these crossreactive antigens are secondarily deposited on the tangles in affected neurons, and are not the polypeptides from which the PHFs are primarily polymerized. PHFs might be the product of derepression of previously repressed genes. Alternatively—and most probably—no new proteins are synthesized, but posttranscriptional modifications take place in the affected neurons leading to the formation of PHFs. Such biochemical events might be initiated in the neuron by a variety of insults to the CNS including the interaction of some transmissable agent with host cell proteins. The nature of these biochemical changes leading to the formation of PHFs is, again, not understood.

One of these biochemical changes might be a shift toward the β-pleated conformation of the proteins involved in the formation of PHFs (14, 15). Though there is no evidence for a biochemical relationship between plaque core amyloid and neurofibrillary tangles, both PHF and amyloid fibers are congophilic, producing characteristic green birefringence in polarized light. The optical properties of Congo red–stained fibrillar proteins are believed to depend on the β-pleated sheet formation; this property is shared under appropriate conditions by a number of chemically unrelated proteins (16). Therefore PHFs, although chemically

TABLE 5–2
Condition and Type of Neurofibrillary Changes

Condition	PHFs	10-nm Filament	References
Human			
Aged persons	+	—	1
Alzheimer's dementia	+	—	2–4
Guam parkinsonism dementia	+	—	5,6
Dementia pugilistica	+	—	7,8
Down's syndrome	+	—	9–11
Postencephalitic parkinsonism	+	—	12–13
Subacute sclerosing panencephalitis (SSPE)	+	—	14–16
Hallervorden–Spatz disease	+	—	17
Progressive supranuclear palsy (PSP)	+[a]	+, 15 nm	18,19
Sporadic motor neuron disease	—	+	20–22
Vincristine neuropathy	—	+	23,24
Infantile neuroaxonal dystrophy	—	+	13
Animal			
Aged Rhesus monkey	[b]	—	25
Aged Wobbler mouse	[b]	—	[c]
Chronic alcohol-treated rat	[b]	—	26
Whip spider	[b]	—	27
Aluminum encephalomyelopathy		+	28,29
Spindle inhibitor encephalopathy		+	30,31
Lathyrogenic encephalopathy (IDPN)		+	32,33
Vitamin E deficiency		+	34
Copper deficiency		+	35
Retrograde and Wallerian degeneration		+	36,37

[a] Neurofibrillary tangles of 15-nm filaments are frequently admixed with various amounts of PHFs.
[b] PHFs found in these conditions have different dimensions from that of Alzheimer dementia.
[c] H. M. Wisniewski, personal communication.

REFERENCES TO TABLE 5–2

1. Matsuyama H, Nakamura S: Senile changes in the brain in the Japanese: incidence of Alzheimer's neurofibrillary change and senile plaques. *Aging NY* 1978; 7:287–298.

2. Terry RD: The fine structure of neurofibrillary tangles in Alzheimer's disease. *J Neuropathol Exp Neurol* 1963; 22:629–642.

3. Terry RD, Gonatas NK, Weiss M: Ultrastructural studies in Alzheimer's presenile dementia. *Am J Pathol* 1964; 44:269–297.

4. Kidd M: Alzheimer's disease: an electron microscopical study. *Brain* 1964; 87:307–320.

5. Hirano A, Malamud N, Elizan TS, et al: Amyotrophic lateral sclerosis and parkinsonism-dementia complex on Guam. *Arch Neurol* 1966; 15:35–51.

6. Hirano A, Dembitzer HM, Kurland LT: The fine structure of some intraganglion alterations. *J Neuropathol Exp Neurol* 1968; 27:167–182.

7. Corsellis JAN, Brierley JB: Observations on the pathology of insidious dementia following head injury. *J Ment Sci* 1959; 105:714–720.

8. Wisniewski HM, Narang HK, Terry RD: Neurofibrillary tangles of paired helical filaments. *J Neurol Sci* 1976; 27:173–181.

9. Olson MI, Shaw Ch-M: Presenile dementia and Alzheimer's disease in mongolism. *Brain* 1969; 92:147–156.

10. Ohara PT: Electron microscopical study of the brain in Down's syndrome. *Brain* 1972; 95:681–684.

11. Schochet SS Jr, Lampert DW, McCormick WF: Neurofibrillary tangles in patients with Down's syndrome: a light and electron microscopic study. *Acta Neuropathol* 1973; 23:342–346.

12. Hirano A: Neurofibrillary changes in conditions related to Alzheimer's disease, in Wolstenholme GEW, O'Connor M (eds): *Alzheimer's Disease and Related Conditions.* London, Churchill, 1970, pp 185–207.

13. Wisniewski H, Terry RD, Hirano A: Neurofibrillary pathology. *J Neuropathol Exp Neurol* 1970; 39:163–176.

14. Malamud N, Haymaker W, Pinkerton H: Inclusion encephalitis with a clinicopathologic report of three cases. *Am J Pathol* 1950; 26:133–153.

15. Corsellis JAN: Subacute sclerosing leucoencephalitis: a clinical and pathologic report of two cases. *J Ment Sci* 1951; 97:570–583.

16. Mandybur TI, Nagpaul AS, Pappas Z, et al: Alzheimer neurofibrillary change in subacute sclerosing panencephalitis. *J Neuropathol Exp Neurol* 1976; 35:300.

17. Wisniewski K, Jervis GA, Moretz RC, et al: Alzheimer neurofibrillary tangles in disease other than senile and presenile dementia. *Ann Neurol* 1979; 5:288–294.

18. Tellez-Nagel I, Wisniewski HM: Ultrastructure of neurofibrillary tangles in Steele–Richardson–Olszewski Syndrome. *Arch Neurol* 1973; 29:324–327.

19. Ghatak NR, Nochlin D, Hadfield MG: Neurofibrillary pathology in progressive supranuclear palsy. *Acta Neuropathol* 1980; 52:73–76.

20. Rewcastle NB, Ball MJ: Electron microscopic structure of the "inclusion bodies" in Pick's disease. *Neurology* 1968; 18:1205–1213.

21. Schochet SS Jr, Hartman JM, Ladewig PP et al: Intraneuronal conglomerates in sporadic motor neuron disease: a light and electron microscopic study. *Arch Neurol* 1969; 20:548–553.

22. Hughes JT, Jerone D: Ultrastructure of anterior horn motor neurons in the Hirano–Kurland–Sayre type of combined neurological system degeneration. *J Neurol Sci* 1971; 13:389–399.

23. Schochet SS Jr, Lampert PW, Earle KM: Neuronal changes induced by intrathecal vincristine sulfate. *J Neuropathol Exp Neurol* 1968; 27:645–658.

24. Shelanski, ML, Wisniewski HM: Neurofibrillary degeneration induced by vincristine therapy. *Arch Neurol* 1969; 20:199–206.

25. Wisniewski HM, Ghetti B, Terry RD: Neuritic (senile) plaques and filamentous changes in aged rhesus monkeys. *J Neuropathol Exp Neurol* 1973; 32:566–584.

26. Volk B: Paired helical filaments in rat spinal ganglia following chronic alcohol administration: an electron microscopic investigation. *Neuropathol Appl Neurobiol* 1980; 6:143–153.

27. Foelix RF, Hauser M: Helically twisted filaments in giant neurons of a whip spider. *J Cell Biol* 1979; 19:303–306.

28. Klatzo I, Wisniewski H, Streicher E: Experimental production of neurofibrillary degeneration: I. Light microscopic observations. *J Neuropathol Exp Neurol* 1965; 24:187–199.

29. Terry RD, Peña C: Experimental production of neurofibrillary degeneration: II. Electron microscopy, phosphatase histochemistry, and electron probe analysis. *J Neuropathol Exp Neurol* 1965; 24:200–210.

30. Wisniewski HM, Shelanski ML, Terry RD: Effects of mitotic spindle inhibitors on neurotubules and neurofilaments in anterior horn cells. *J Cell Biol* 1968; 38:224–229.

31. Wisniewski H, Terry RD: Experimental colchicine encephalopathy: I. Induction of neurofibrillary degeneration. *Lab Invest* 1967; 17:577–587.

REFERENCES TO TABLE 5–2 (CONTINUED)

32. Chou SM, Hartmann H: Electron microscopy of focal neuroaxonal lesions produced by B-B-iminodipropionitrile (IDPN) in rats. *Acta Neuropathol* 1965; 4:590–603.
33. Diezel PB, Ule G: Histochemische Untersuchungen an den "ghost cells" beim experimentellen Neurolathyrismus. *Acta Neuropathol* 1963; 3:150–163.
34. Lampert P, Blumberg JM, Pentschew A: An electron microscopic study of dystrophic axons in the gracile and cuneate nuclei of vitamin-E-deficient rats: axonal dystrophy in vitamin-E deficiency. *J Neuropathol Exp Neurol* 1964; 27:60–77.
35. Cancilla PA, Barlow RM: Structural changes of the central nervous system in swayback (enzootic ataxia) of lambs: II. Electron microscopy of the lower motor neuron. *Acta Neuropathol* 1966; 6:251–259.
36. Guillery RW: Some electron microscopical observations of degenerative changes in central nervous synapses. *Prog Brain Res* 1965; 14:57–76.
37. Walberg F, Mugnaini E: Distinction of degenerating fibers and boutons of cerebellar and peripheral origin in the deiters' nucleus of the same animal. *Brain Res* 1969; 14:67–75.

they might unrelated to amyloid, are most likely composed of β-pleated protein fibrils. Furthermore, PHFs are insoluble under physiological conditions and are resistant to proteolytic digestion (9), a characteristic of β-pleated fibrils. This property might lead *in situ* to the accumulation of fibrils made from such proteins, which is indeed the case with the neurofibrillary tangles.

ACKNOWLEDGMENTS

We are very grateful to Dr. Inge Grundke-Iqbal for supplying us with Figures 5–1 and 5–2 and for critical reading of the manuscript as well as helpful suggestions. Studies reviewed from our own laboratory were made possible with technical assistance from Tanweer A. Zaidi and Christopher H. Thompson. Richard Weed helped with photography and Adele Monaco with secretarial tasks. Our laboratory was supported in part by an Over-Recovery Project Award from The Research Foundation for Mental Hygiene and from NIH grants NS 17487 and NS/HD 16971.

REFERENCES

1. Kidd M: Paired helical filaments in electron microscopy of Alzheimer's disease. *Nature* 1963; 197:192–193.
2. Wisniewski HM, Narang HK, Terry RD: Neurofibrillary tangles of paired helical filaments. *J Neurol Sci* 1976; 27:173–181.
3. Tomlinson BE, Blessed G, Roth M: Observations on the brains of demented old people. *J Neurol Sci* 1970; 11:204–242.
4. Wisniewski HM, Iqbal K: Aging of the brain and dementia. *Trends Neurosci* 1980; 3:226–228.
5. Iqbal K, Wisniewski HM, Grundke-Iqbal I, et al: Neurofibrillary pathology: an update, in Nandy K, Sherwin I (eds): *The Aging Brain and Senile Dementia*. New York, Plenum, 1977, pp 209–227.

6. Wisniewski K, Jervis GA, Moretz RC, et al: Alzheimer neurofibrillary tangles in diseases other than senile and presenile dementia. *Ann Neurol* 1979; 5:288–294.

7. Tellez-Nagel I, Wisniewski HM: Ultrastructure of neurofibrillary tangles in Steele–Richardson–Olszewski syndrome. *Arch Neurol* 1973; 29:324–327.

8. Ghatak NR, Nochlin D, Hadfield MG: Neurofibrillary pathology in progressive supranuclear palsy. *Acta Neuropathol* 1980;52:73–76.

9. Iqbal K, Grundke-Iqbal I, Merz PA, et al: Alzheimer neurofibrillary tangle: morphology and biochemistry. *J Exp Brain Res Suppl* 1982; suppl 5:10–14.

10. Grundke-Iqbal I, Johnson AB, Wisniewski HM, et al: Evidence that Alzheimer neurofibrillary tangles originate from neurotubules. *Lancet* 1979; i:578–580.

11. Iqbal K, Grundke-Iqbal I, Johnson AB, et al: Neurofibrous proteins in aging and dementia. *Aging NY* 1980; 13:39–48.

12. Ishii T, Haga S, Tobutake S: Presence of neurofilament protein in Alzheimer's neurofibrillary tangles (ANF): an immunofluorescent study. *Acta Neuropathol* 1979; 48:105–112.

13. Gambetti P, Velasco ME, Dahl D, et al: Neurofibrillary tangles in Alzheimer disease: an immunohistochemical study. *Aging NY* 1980; 13:55–63.

14. Glenner GG, Eanes ED, Bladen HA, et al: β-pleated sheet fibrils: a comparison of native amyloid with synthetic protein fibrils. *J Histochem Cytochem* 1974; 22:1141–1158.

15. Wisniewski HM: Morphology of the aging brain and dementia—human and animal, in Singhal SK, Sinclair NR, Stiller CR (eds): *Aging and Immunity*. Amsterdam, Elsevier North-Holland, 1979, pp 185–194.

16. Glenner GG: Amyloid deposits and amyloidosis, the β-fibrilloses. *N Engl J Med* 1980; 302:1283–1292.

6 Neuritic (Senile) and Amyloid Plaques

Henryk M. Wisniewski

Neuritic (senile) plaques and neurofibrillary changes (1) are the most conspicuous pathological changes found in people with Alzheimer's disease (AD). Morphological (light and electron microscopy) studies of neuritic plaques have revealed that the plaque consists of three elements: dystrophic and degenerating neuronal processes, reactive non-neuronal cells (microglia, phagocytes), and amyloid (2, 3). It is the particular arrangement of two of the three components of the neuritic plaque that determines its type.

The first type is made up of darkly stained rods and dots in Bodian-stained slides, and wisps of amyloid between the normal and abnormal neuronal and astrocytic processes (as seen in polarized light after Congo red staining, or with the aid of the electron microscope). This type is called a "primitive plaque." Plaques with a central core of amyloid surrounded by degenerating and dystrophic neurites are called "typical" or "classical plaques." Plaques made up almost exclusively of amyloid material are called "amyloid plaques" (Figs. 6–1 to 6–3).

Primitive and classical plaques are most commonly found in AD and normal aged people as well as in animals. Amyloid plaques are common in kuru, some cases of Creutzfeldt–Jakob disease (CJD), Gerstmann Straussler syndrome, and scrapie-infected mice (Chap. 39; 4–6).

In AD, primitive and classical plaques are particularly numerous in the cortex (especially the third layer of the frontotemporal cortex) and the hippocampal formation. Some of the plaques are closely associated with small vessels. Amyloid plaques of kuru and CJD are, for the most part, limited to the cerebellar cortex. Neuritic (primitive and classical) and amyloid plaques can be seen with a variety of routine stains, such as hematoxylin and eosin, PAS, Congo red, thioflavin S, and silver impregnation.

Ultrastructural studies of the neuritic and amyloid plaques from AD and other diseases revealed that the amyloid fibers are made of a pair of helically wound filaments. The diameter of the individual filaments making the amyloid fibers, and the periodicity, are not the same in all types of amyloid (7). In AD, amyloid paired filaments measure 4–6 nm, each filament measuring 2–3 nm, with a twist every 30–40 nm.

Between the wisps of amyloid fibers in the primitive plaques or around the amyloid core of the classical plaques, there are aggregates of neuronal processes filled with mitochondria, electron dense bodies, smooth membranes, neurofilaments, and paired helical filaments (PHFs), the latter structures present only in humans.

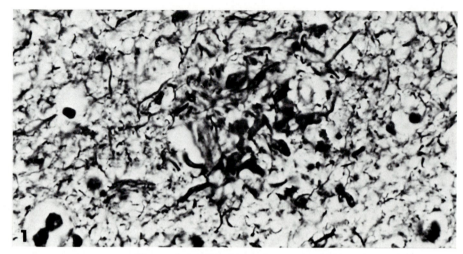

Figure 6–1. Primitive plaque. × 1,152.

Between the dystrophic neurites there are also many other neuronal processes showing Wallerian-like degeneration. Microglia, astrocytes, and their processes, for instance, always accompany these lesions. And while the origin of the protein(s) forming the amyloid fibers is not known, immunocytochemical studies have revealed the presence of gammaglobulin light chains and other blood proteins in the amyloid core of the classical plaque (8, 9). There are also studies showing the presence of neurofilament polypeptides in the amyloid of neuritic plaques (8). Nonetheless, the relationship of these proteins to the amyloid fibers must be viewed with caution, since our recent studies of AD and scrapie-infected brains have shown that (1) blood–brain barrier (BBB) permeability is increased in these diseases and (2) amyloid fibers have a tendency to bind various proteins such as horseradish peroxidase (HRP). Thus the observation that a given protein is associated with amyloid deposits does not mean that it is part of structural protein(s) composing the amyloid fibers.

Recently, the following two hypotheses were put forward to explain the presence of amyloid deposits in AD and related diseases:

Externalized neurofilament (NF) proteins, liberated from degenerate neurites, combine

Figure 6–2. Classical plaque. × 1,152.

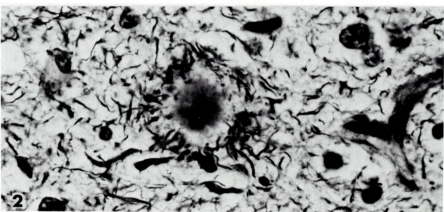

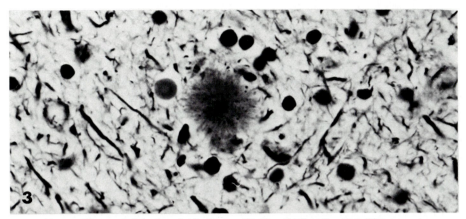

Figure 6–3. Amyloid plaque; Bodian PAS stain. × 1,152.

with glycoproteins and local glycosaminoglycans in the extracellular space to form amyloid (8). In other words, the amyloid fibers are made of heterologous proteins assembled in the extracellular space in a manner similar to the *in vitro* creation of amyloid fibrils from Bence–Jones proteins in multiple myeloma (10). Authors of the first hypothesis see the neuronal pathology as a main source of amyloid protein and are of the opinion that the focus for future pathogenic investigations should be on chronic, intrinsic causes of neuronal degeneration or on extrinsic insults whose targets are specific central nervous system neurons.

According to the second hypothesis, the plaque or vascular amyloid is also produced locally, but the brain's reticuloendothelial system (RES), the microglia and pericytes, are the producers or processors of the amyloidogenic protein(s) (11). Wisniewski and co-workers (11) postulated that as a result of stimulation by a virus or other antigen(s), the brain RES (microglia and pericytes) starts to produce amyloid protein (or proteins) and form amyloid deposits in a manner similar to that observed by Teilum (12,13) in experimental amyloidosis.

According to Teilum, first the reticuloendothelial cells must be stimulated by an antigen to start the synthesis of amyloidogenic protein(s). The proteins are then postulated to polymerize into amyloid fibers. Stiller and Katenkamp (14), studying the pathogenesis of senile cardiac amyloidosis, concluded that perhaps as a result of an aging process or chronic inflammation, the RES cells start to produce abnormal mucopolysaccharides which then form the amyloid fibers. In scrapie-infected mice, CJD, and kuru, the infectious agent is probably responsible for the abnormal local protein synthesis by the central nervous system's RES.

As indicated above, at this point the composition of the amyloid fibers in AD, CJD, and scrapie is not known, although recently it was shown that amyloid deposits are formed at the site of injection of the scrapie agent (11). One can therefore hypothesize that, altered by the infectious agent, local RES cells are the producers of the amyloidogenic protein(s). Since the microglia and pericytes also act as phagocytes, it is possible that the plaque amyloid is not made of homologous protein, but represents a heterogeneous mosaic of proteins (e.g., neurofilament peptides, glia and serum proteins) from a variety of cell types. These proteins, however, do not appear (as suggested by Powers and co-workers) (8) assembled spontaneously in the extracellular space, but are processed, probably inadequately, by the local RES and then combined into β-pleated filaments by the microglia and pericytes acting as "processor cells" in a manner similar to the phagocytes in systemic amyloidosis (15, 16). If the central nervous system's RES proves to be essential for amyloidogenic protein(s) production, then attention should be focused not on the causes leading to externalization of neuronal proteins but on the etiology of how the RES produces the amyloidogenic protein(s).

It is not clear why the dystrophic changes of neurites so prominent in AD—and aged dogs and monkeys—are so minimal in kuru, scrapie, and CJD. One can hypothesize that in the case of AD and affected aged animals, the amyloidogenic stimulus (possibly a CJD-like agent) also alters neurites directly. Alternatively, it is possible that the amyloidogenic protein(s) are more neurotoxic in AD than in the other conditions.

From a study of AD, Larsson and colleagues (17) concluded that their findings were compatible with the effects of an autosomal-dominant gene with reduced penetrance. Other data (5, 6) show that neuritic and amyloid plaque formation in scrapie-infected mice is also under genetic control. From this and the above-discussed morphological similarities between human and animal plaques, it is likely that scrapie and AD plaques reflect the outcome of a common pathogenetic pathway.

ACKNOWLEDGMENT

The author wishes to express his gratitude to Judy Shek for preparation of the histological material, Richard Weed for his excellent assistance in photography, Patricia and George Merz for their critical reading and editorial comments, and Marjorie Agoglia for her superb secretarial assistance.

REFERENCES

1. Wisniewski HM, Iqbal K: Ageing of the brain and dementia. *Trends Neurosci* 1980; 3:226–228.
2. Wisniewski HM, Terry RD: An experimental approach to the morphogenesis of neurofibrillary degeneration and the argyrophilic plaque, in Wolstenholme GEW, O'Conner M (eds): *Alzheimer's Disease and Related Conditions.* London, Churchill, 1970, pp 223–248.
3. Wisniewski HM, Terry RD: Neuropathology of the aging brain, in Terry RD, Gershon S (eds): *Neurobiology of Aging.* New York, Raven, 1976, pp 265–280.
4. Masters CL, Gajdusek DC, Gibbs CJ: Creutzfeldt–Jakob disease virus isolations from the Gerstmann–Straussler syndrome, with an analysis of the various forms of amyloid plaque deposition in the virus-induced spongiform encephalopathies. *Brain* 1981; 104:559–588.
5. Wisniewski HM, Bruce ME, Fraser H: Infectious etiology of neuritic (senile) plaques in mice. *Science* 1975; 190:1108–1110.
6. Bruce ME, Dickinson AG, Fraser H: Cerebral amyloidosis in scrapie in the mouse: effect of agent strain and mouse genotype. *Neuropathol Appl Neurobiol* 1976; 2:471–478.
7. Merz PA, Somerville RA, Wisniewski HM: Abnormal fibrils in scrapie and senile dementia of the Alzheimer type. Read before the Symposium on Non-Conventional Viruses and Effects on the Central Nervous System, November 5–7, 1981, Paris.
8. Powers JM, Schlaepfer WW, Willingham MC, et al: An immunoperoxidase study of senile cerebral amyloidosis with pathogenetic considerations. *J Neuropathol Exp Neurol* 1981; 40:592–612.
9. Wisniewski HM, Kozlowski PB: Evidence for blood–brain barrier changes in senile dementia of the Alzheimer type (SDAT). *Ann NY Acad Sci* 1982; 396:119–129.
10. Glenner GG, Ein D, Eanes ED, et al: Creation of "amyloid" fibrils from Bence–Jones proteins *in vitro. Science* 1971; 174:712–714.

11. Wisniewski HM, Moretz RC, Lossinsky AS: Evidence for induction of localized amyloid deposits and neuritic plaques by an infectious agent. *Ann Neurol* 1981; 10:517–522.

12. Teilum G: Pathogenesis of amyloidosis: the two-phase cellular theory of local secretion. *Acta Pathol Microbiol Scand* 1964; 61:21–45.

13. Teilum G: Origin of amyloidosis from PAS-positive reticuloendothelial cells *in situ* and basic factors in pathogenesis, in Mandema E, Ruinen L, Scholten JH, et al (eds): *Proceedings of the Symposium on Amyloidosis.* Amsterdam, Excerpta Medica, 1968, pp 37–41.

14. Stiller D, Katenkamp D: Histochemistry of amyloid: general considerations, light microscopical, and ultrastructural examinations. *Exp Pathol* 1975; suppl 1, pp 1–116.

15. Glenner GG: Amyloid deposits and amyloidosis. *N Engl J Med* 1980; 302:1283–1292.

16. Scheinberg MA, Cathcart ES: New concepts in the pathogenesis of primary and secondary amyloid disease. *Clin Exp Immunol* 1978; 33:185–190.

17. Larsson T, Sjögren T, Jacobson G: Senile dementia. *Acta Psychiatr Scand Suppl* 1963; 39(suppl 167):1–259.

7 Granulovacuolar Degeneration

MELVYN J. BALL

The fascinating nerve cell lesion known as "granulovacuolar degeneration" was probably originally described by Simchowicz (1), who first noted this striking abnormality in the pyramidal neurons of the hippocampus in cases of severe Alzheimer's disease (AD). Although passing allusion to its relationship with organic dementia was subsequently made (2), the first comprehensive investigation of its occurrence in a wide variety of mental disorders was published in 1962, when Woodard (3) reviewed one hippocampal section from 200 unselected autopsies. More recent surveys include those by Tomlinson and Kitchener (4) and by Ball and Lo (5).

DESCRIPTIVE ANALYSIS

LIGHT-MICROSCOPIC FEATURES

Granulovacuolar degeneration, occurring in the cytoplasm of cerebral cortical neurons, consists of one or more unstained, spherical vacuoles (holes), 3–5 μ in diameter; in the center of each is an argyrophilic (silver-staining), hematoxylinophilic granule (dot), 0.5–1.5 μ wide (Fig. 7–1). Granulovacuolar change is almost never found anywhere but in the large, pyramidal neurons of the hippocampus (6). Some reduction of the stainable Nissl material (cytoplasmic ribonucleic acid) may be observed near the granulovacuole(s) if but few are present in the perikaryon, but when many (sometimes up to 20) vacuoles are present in one paraffin section, the afflicted neuron may appear bulging and edematous.

Granulovacuoles are well demonstrated by hematoxylin-eosin (H and E) stains and by silver-impregnation techniques such as Bielschowsky's or Bodian's. Yet a plethora of histochemical approaches applied to fresh frozen-sectioned tissue, fixed paraffin-processed, and fixed frozen-sectioned material has not appreciably elucidated the nature of the lesions (7, 8). The granules are negative for staining with periodic acid-Schiff (for carbohydrate moieties), Alcian blue (for acid mucopolysaccharides), or Congo red (for amyloid); show a slight affinity for Luxol fast blue (for phospholipids); and are less intensely argyrophilic than the neurofibrillary tangles (NFTs) of Alzheimer or the neuritic (senile) plaques (SPs) that frequently accompany granulovacuolar degeneration.

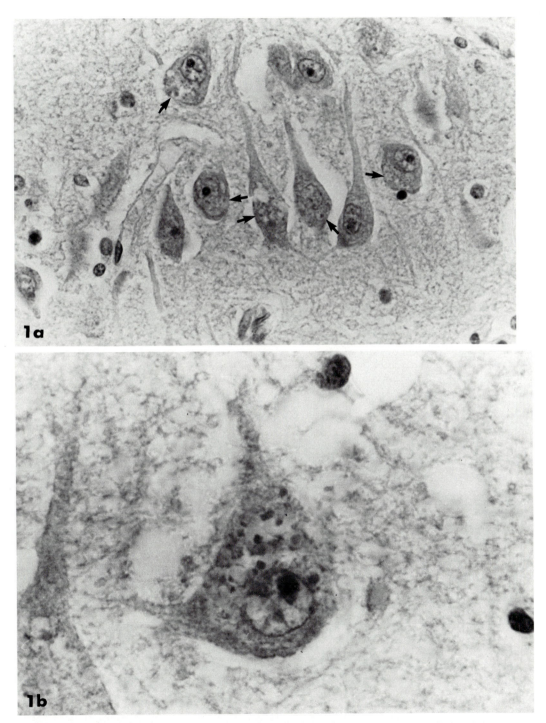

Figure 7–1. (a) Hippocampal pyramidal neurons; those with arrows contain granulovacuoles in their cytoplasm (hematoxylin-eosin, × 400). (b) Granulovacuolar degeneration of Simchowicz in cytoplasm of a hippocampal neuron (H-E, × 1,000).

ULTRASTRUCTURAL FEATURES

Electron microscopy has merely confirmed the apt name for this lesion (Fig. 7–2). Granulovacuoles appear in the cytoplasm each as an empty (electron-lucent) vacuole, probably membrane-bound (9), containing a central or eccentrically located core of dense, osmiophilic, amorphous granular material. This granule itself is between 650 and 1,000 nm in diameter, with no obvious internal structure (10).

The same structural features of granulovacuolar degeneration (GVD) have also been noted in brains of patients with Pick's disease (11), dementia accompanying idiopathic parkinsonism (12), Guam parkinsonism dementia (13), tuberous sclerosis (14), and progressive supranuclear palsy (15). The lesion is, however, unfortunately difficult to identify on electron micrographs of autopsy material (16). In any case, its ultrastructure has not materially advanced our understanding of its pathogenesis.

QUANTITATIVE ANALYSIS

Much more helpful in advancing our understanding of the pathogenesis of AD have been studies of the occurrence and severity of GVD in normal brains of various ages compared with patients afflicted with AD (3, 4, 17, 18). In one laboratory, such a morphometric

Figure 7–2. Electron micrograph of granulovacuoles (GV) in cytoplasm of a pyramidal neuron of the hippocampus. Nucleus = N. Arrows indicate limiting membrane of vacuoles; note electron-dense granular material within each vacuole (formalin-fixed, Spurr, uranyl nitrate – lead citrate, × 7,740).

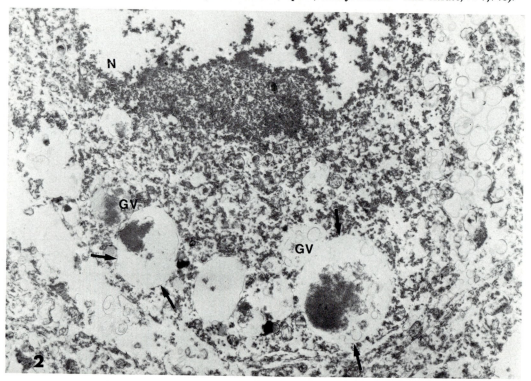

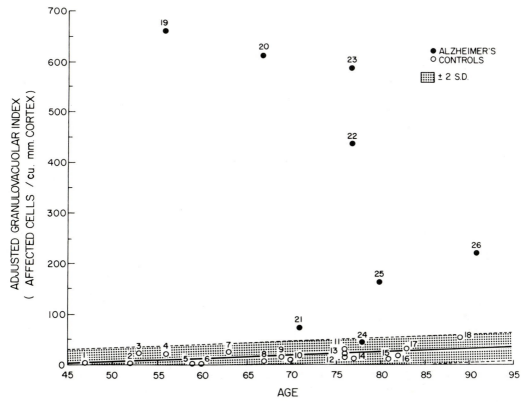

Figure 7–3. Number of hippocampal neurons with granulovacuolar degeneration per mm³ of cortex, at different ages. Best linear regression for controls (*white circles*) shows significant correlation (coefficient $r = 0.59$, $P < .01$). Adjusted Granulovacuolar Index of brains with AD (*black circles*) exceeds that of controls at any age.

approach has been further refined and expanded in a series of 26 subjects: 18 normal controls (aged 47 to 89), and 8 degenerated patients dying from AD, both senile and presenile in onset (5).

The entire hippocampal formation was serially sectioned, and the degree of GVD assessed with a semi-automated sampling stage microscope in 33,811 fields. Whether expressed as the number of (nucleolated) neurons showing GVD per unit volume of temporal cortex (Fig. 7–3) or as the percentage involvement of total hippocampal neurons counted (Fig. 7–4), the severity of GVD, which increases slightly with normal aging, exceeds that of age-matched controls by many times in the brains of people with AD. As with NFTs, the posterior half of each hippocampus seems considerably more susceptible to this augmented GVD in demented cases—a factor of some interest if Penfield and Matthieson (19) are correct that our more remote memories are "processed" in a more posterior portion of the hippocampal formation than recent ones.

Moreover, I (20) have shown that the augmented GVD of AD occurs within a severely shrinking population of surviving pyramidal neurons, wherein the nerve cell fall-out may have already involved nearly half the original neuronal population, and may be up to five times more serious than in normal aging alone. The close (negative) correlation observed between intensity of GVD and neuron density (20), as well as the progressive reduction of

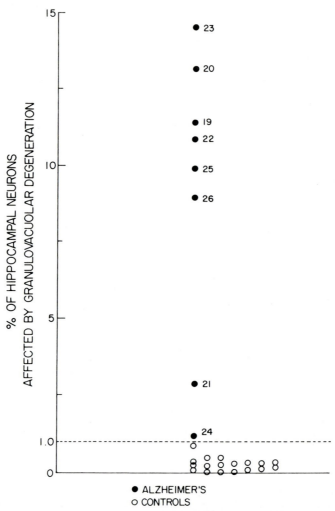

Figure 7–4. Scattergram showing percentage of counted hippocampal neurons affected by GV degeneration. No control brain (*white circles*) exceeds 1% involvement; all brains with AD (*black circles*) do.

cytoplasmic RNA accompanying increasing numbers of granulovacuoles per neuron (21), probably indicate that GVD represents some genuinely deleterious phenomena. This may also be true in Down's syndrome; I have shown a similarly severe GVD and nerve cell loss in brains of adult patients with mongolism (22). These findings accord with the suggestion that GVD represents some type of autophagic (self-digestion) abnormality (23), perhaps lysosomal in nature.

TOPOGRAPHIC CONSIDERATIONS

Because of their predilection for the pyramidal layer of the hippocampus, granulovacuoles have often been noted near Hirano bodies and SPs or even in neurons also showing NFTs (24). Whereas Woodard (3) noted their special prevalence within the ventrolateral quadrant of the hippocampal cortex, Tomlinson and Kitchener (4) felt they were most frequent in Rose's H_1 and H_2 fields.

I (25) have used an XY pen recorder to plot scattergrams of the precise localization of GVD in the mesial temporal cortex, which can be divided into six microanatomical zones. The subiculum and the adjacent H_1 field (Sommer sector of Ammon's horn) are especially predisposed (26). The particular pattern of selective affliction is cytoarchitectonically identical to that seen in normal aged brains (26), as well as in Down's syndrome (27). Such regional predilection hints at a common neurotransmitter substrate, perhaps cholinergic, to account for how it is that only certain groups of these neurons are so predisposed.

FUTURE RESEARCH

Although a sort of vacuolar degeneration has been noted in neuronal perikarya and processes of some aging rats (28), there is no realistically appropriate animal model for GVD, either spontaneous or experimentally induced. Therefore a prospective study has commenced to determine the relationships between GVD (and other neuronal lesions of AD) and several clinical parameters *in vivo,* including specially designed psychometric evaluations of the degree of cognitive function impairment.

Preliminary evidence from our laboratory (MJ Ball, H Merskey, and associates, unpublished data) indicates that tangles, plaques, granulovacuoles, and so on may not in fact correlate equally well with the clinical changes measured. For example, the degree of GVD may have a much higher (positive) relationship with a behavioral rating score than does the extent of NFT formation; the number of cases as yet quantified, however, is too small to permit certainty of this trend.

Nonetheless, it is through such a combined clinicopathological approach that significant advances will be possible in our comprehension of a neuronal lesion which remains unique for the hippocampal cells of the human nervous system.

ACKNOWLEDGMENTS

This work was supported in part by the Ontario Mental Health Foundation. Olive Donaldson prepared the manuscript.

REFERENCES

1. Simchowicz T: Histopathologische Studien über die senile Demenz, in Nissl F, Alzheimer A (eds): *Histologie und Histopathologische Arbeiten über die Grosshirnrinde.* Jena, Fischer, 1911, vol 4, pp 267–444.

2. Malamud N: *Atlas of Neuropathology.* Berkeley, University of California Press, 1957.

3. Woodard JS: Clinicopathological significance of granulovacuolar degeneration in Alzheimer's disease. *J Neuropathol Exp Neurol* 1962; 21:85–91.

4. Tomlinson BE, Kitchener D: Granulovacuolar degeneration of hippocampal pyramidal cells. *J Pathol* 1972; 106:165–185.

5. Ball MJ, Lo P: Granulovacuolar degeneration in the aging brain and in dementia. *J Neuropathol Exp Neurol* 1977; 36:474–487.

6. Tomlinson BE: Discussion, in Wolstenholme GEW, O'Connor M (eds): *Alzheimer's Disease and Related Conditions.* London, Churchill, 1970, p 50.

7. Morel F, Wildi E: General and cellular pathochemistry of senile and presenile alterations of the brain, in *Proceedings of the First International Congress of Neuropathology.* Turin, Rosenberg and Sellier, 1954, vol 2, pp 347–374.

8. Margolis G: Senile cerebral disease: a critical survey of traditional concepts based upon observations with newer technics. *Lab Invest* 1959; 8:335–370.

9. Hirano A, Dembitzer HM, Kurland LT, et al: The fine structure of some intraganglionic alterations. *J Neuropathol Exp Neurol* 1968; 27:167–182.

10. Rewcastle NB, Ball MJ: Electron microscopic structure of the "inclusion bodies" in Pick's disease. *Neurology* 1968; 18:1205–1213.

11. Schochet SS Jr, Lampert PW, Lindenberg R: Fine structure of the Pick and Hirano bodies in a case of Pick's disease. *Acta Neuropathol* 1968; 11:330–337.

12. Kosaka K, Oyanagi S, Matsushita M, et al: Presenile dementia with Alzheimer-, Pick-, and Lewy-body changes. *Acta Neuropathol* 1970; 36:221–233.

13. Hirano A, Malamud N, Elizan JS, et al: Amyotrophic lateral sclerosis and parkinsonism–dementia complex on Guam. *Arch Neurol* 1966; 15:35–51.

14. Hirano A, Tuazon R, Zimmerman HM: Neurofibrillary changes, granulovacuolar bodies, and argentophilic globules observed in tuberous sclerosis. *Acta Neuropathol* 1968; 11:257–261.

15. Steele JC, Richardson JC, Olszewski, J: Progressive supranuclear palsy. *Arch Neurol* 1964; 10:333–359.

16. Gibson PH, Stones M, Tomlinson BE: Senile changes in the human neocortex and hippocampus compared by the use of the electron and light microscopes. *J Neurol Sci* 1976; 27:389–405.

17. Tomlinson BE, Blessed G, Roth M: Observations on the brains of non-demented old people. *J Neurol Sci* 1968; 7:331–356.

18. Tomlinson BE, Blessed G, Roth M: Observations on the brains of demented old people. *J Neurol Sci* 1970; 11:205–242.

19. Penfield W, Mathieson G: Autopsy findings and comments on the role of hippocampus in experiential recall. *Arch Neurol* 1974; 31:145–154.

20. Ball MJ: Neuronal loss, neurofibrillary tangles, and granulovacuolar degeneration in the hippocampus with ageing and dementia. *Acta Neuropathol* 1977; 37:111–118.

21. Mann DMA: Granulovacuolar degeneration in pyramidal cells of the hippocampus. *Acta Neuropathol* 1978; 42:149–151.

22. Ball MJ, Nuttall K: Neurofibrillary tangles, granulovacuolar degeneration, and neuron loss in Down's syndrome: quantitative comparison with Alzheimer dementia. *Ann Neurol* 1980; 7:462–465.

23. Wisniewski HM, Terry RD: Morphology of the aging brain, human and animal. *Prog Brain Res* 1973; 40:167–186.

24. Tomonaga M, Yamanouchi H, Mannen T, et al: On the Hirano bodies observed in the brains of the aged. *Nippon Ronen Igakkai Zasshi* 1975; 12:13–17.

25. Ball MJ: Histotopography of cellular changes in Alzheimer's disease, in Nandy K (ed): *Senile Dementia: A Biomedical Approach.* New York, Elsevier North-Holland, 1978, pp 89–104.

26. Ball MJ: Topographic distribution of neurofibrillary tangles and granulovacuolar degeneration in hippocampal cortex of aging and demented patients: a quantitative study. *Acta Neuropathol* 1978; 42:73–80.

27. Ball MJ, Nuttall K: Topography of neurofibrillary tangles and granulovacuoles in hippocampi of patients with Down's syndrome: quantitative comparison with normal aging and Alzheimer's disease. *Neuropathol Appl Neurobiol* 1981; 7:13–20.

28. De Estable-Puig RF, de Estable-Puig JF: Vacuolar degeneration in neurons of aging rats. *Virchows Arch Cell Pathol* 1975; 17:337–346.

8 Dendritic Changes

ARNOLD B. SCHEIBEL

THE DENDRITIC STRUCTURE OF THE NEURON provides an enormous membrane surface area for the reception of afferent information and for interaction with other neurons. Dendrite patterns vary with cell type and location but, in almost all cases, the dendrite system represents 70–90% of the cell's total surface area (1). No pattern is more familiar than that of the neocortical pyramidal cell, and certainly no cell takes longer to come to full maturity.

In humans, creatures born with a precociously developed cortical dendrite system, full maturation of the basilar ensemble may not occur until the onset of adolescence (Scheibel, unpublished data), and there is evidence that the process of progressive plastic dendritic changes, at least of terminal branchlets, may continue indefinitely (2, 3). The maintenance of so elaborate a protoplasmic system requires considerable outlay of energy, and it is therefore not surprising that some degree of regressive change may eventually characterize all senescent neurons. Routine neuropathological techniques can throw little light on these alterations, and it has been only upon introduction of Golgi-impregnation techniques to the study of aging human and animal tissue (2–10) that such information has become available. The vast majority of studies thus far have been performed on neocortical pyramidal cells of the human and rodent cerebral cortex (2–4, 9, 10), although a few reports are also available on the cerebellum (6), brain stem, and spinal cord (5). Evaluation of dendritic systems in basal ganglia and thalamus are currently in progress (Scheibel, unpublished data).

We shall use the human cerebral cortex as our model and, more specifically, the pyramidal neuron, ignoring the enormous populations of stellate or granule (local circuit) cells, for which there are, to date, insufficient data.

The changes to be described represent steps in a sequence (Fig. 8–1) whose inception and tempo of progression vary from individual to individual. The brain of a 101-year-old patient may in some cases appear remarkably intact, compared with those of some individuals in their fifties and sixties who show advanced changes. Genetic factors are of undoubted, perhaps paramount significance, but emerging evidence increasingly identifies the mental and emotional challenge (environmental enrichment) as an important additional factor in the survivability and vigor of neurons (2, 3).

The appearance of Alzheimer-type dementia, whether of senile or presenile type, accentuates the degree and compresses the timetable of neuronal alterations. An originally robust individual of 50 (presenile type) or 80 (senile type) may thus follow a course that proceeds from a vigorous and productive life to helpless dementia and death in a scant few years. The range of permutations in cellular change is correspondingly great, and the sequence described below will serve as a model, more or less generally applicable no matter what the age of onset, pace, and degree of involvement.

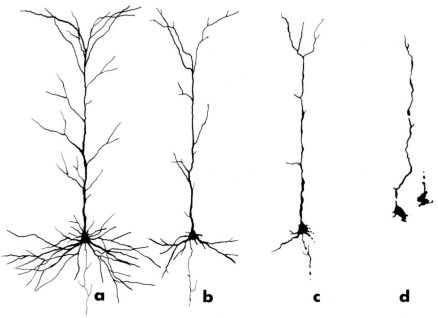

Figure 8–1. Sequence of changes in cortical pyramidal cell during development of Alzheimer's dementia. (a) normal adult pattern; (b) early stages of disease marked by patchy spine loss and thinning out of the dendritic tree, especially horizontally oriented branches; (c) advanced stage with almost complete loss of basilar dendrites; and (d) terminal stage. Drawn from Golgi-stained sections of human prefrontal cortex.

Figure 8–2. Sequence of changes in dendrite spines of cortical pyramidal cell during development of clinical dementia. Dense, regularly spaced spines in (a), become increasingly sparse and pleomorphic, (b) and (c), and finally disappear as dendrite stalk becomes increasingly nodulated. *Above:* greatly enlarged view of representative array of normal spines (NS) and abnormal spines (AS). Drawn from Golgi-stained sections of human prefrontal cortex.

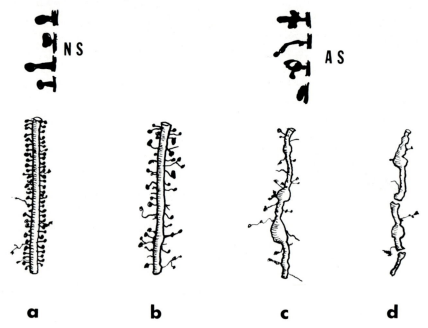

The earliest dendritic changes appear as alterations in the density of spines and in the morphology of the individual spine (Fig. 8–2). There appears to be a progressive thinning out of these small structures which normally cover virtually every part of the mature dendritic tree, except for the proximal 50–200μm of apical shaft and primary basilar dendritic branches. Along with the general decrease in spine density, patchy areas of total spine loss develop along appreciable lengths of dendrite, accompanied by nodulation of the dendrite stalk. Irregular swellings are noted in the dendritic profile—especially at branch points and in the cell body itself. In the case of pyramidal cells, the classic triangular shape is often replaced by an irregular pear-shaped outline, greater in size and more irregular in silhouette than in the healthy mature cell (Fig. 8–3). Along with these alterations is a progressive attrition of the dendritic domain. The basilar dendrite system and the horizontally oriented branches of the apical shaft appear to suffer earliest, starting with distal twigs, and eventually reaching primary branches. The apical shaft itself appears to last the longest, and disappears as the neuron undergoes final pyknotic changes (Figs. 8–1, 8–3). This sequence of age-related structural alterations recapitulates, in reverse order, the development and maturation of the neuron. Electron-microscopic studies indicate that this pattern of neuronal degeneration is accompanied by loss of the normal microtubular endoskeleton, and record its progressive replacement by a coarser system of paired helical filaments (PHFs) (11). Indeed, it is the cohesion of large numbers of these elements which, when stained by reduced silver, form the characteristic NFTs of Alzheimer's.

Figure 8–3. Comparison of Golgi-stained large normal cortical (Betz) pyramidal cell from adult (a) with that of a similar cell in an advanced deteriorative stage (b). Note loss of basilar dendrites and swelling of cell body. Original magnification, × 440.

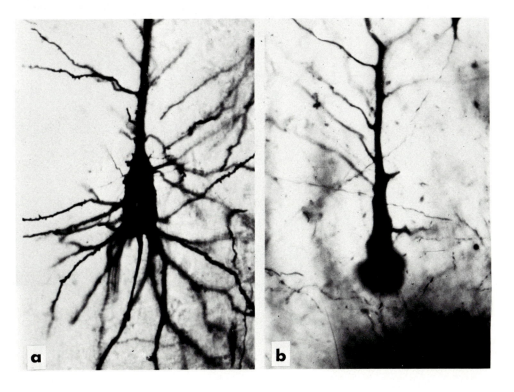

Progressive loss of the complement of spines, and of the dendritic tree, progressively diminishes the amount of membrane surface area available for synaptic afferents. Each neuron thereby receives less information, and the processing capability of the areas involved must consequently diminish. Since changes of this type have already been described in the human cerebral neocortex (9), hippocampus (8), basal ganglia (Scheibel, unpublished data), and cerebellum (6), it is obvious that the individual must eventually reflect such substrate losses in progressive decline of sensorimotor, cognitive, and mnesic functions.

It has recently been shown, both in aged rats (3) and in aged but nondemented humans (2), that the neuron retains some degree of capacity for plastic change and growth. In support of this, animal studies (3) emphasize the importance of environmental challenge or enrichment in stimulating growth response during the senium.

An even more dramatic example of this residual capacity for neural growth has been found in the brains of patients dying of familial presenile dementia of the Alzheimer type. The familial element is stressed since, up to this time, the change to be described has *not* been found in patients with presenile dementia, where a familial history is not present. The change consists of a significant—even explosive—outgrowth of dendritic branches, richly covered with spines, from cells already in late stages of dendritic degeneration (Fig. 8–4). This unexpected and powerful example of vigor in membrane production appears to be more than an isolated phenomenon, and we have seen it in as many as 20–25% of the

Figure 8–4. Cortical pyramidal cell of patient with Alzheimer's presenile dementia of familial type. Darts point to dense clusters of newly sprouting dendrite branches covered with spines. Drawn from Golgi-stained section of prefrontal cortex.

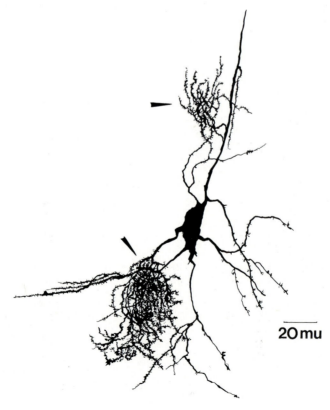

20 mu

cells constituting a microscopic field in the neocortex, hippocampus, or cerebellum. These outbursts of dendrite regeneration may apparently occur anywhere along the cell body or dendrite tree, and do not appear to follow rules of topographic organization characteristic of that cell type. We have therefore provisionally called the phenomenon lawless growth. Electron-microscopic studies will be necessary to determine whether these new dendrites and spines attract presynaptic terminals to their surfaces (10).

The sequence of regressive and destructive alterations in the dendro-spinous structure of the neuron may begin long before significant changes are seen in the cell body. Because of the redundant nature of brain connections, it may well be that early stages of loss in dendritic surface area—and accordingly of synaptic input—produce no obvious change in the individual's mentation or behavior. Once a critical point in the sequence is reached and passed, however, the loss of processing power begins to manifest itself and, in the case of the senile and presenile dementias, will progress until death.

Just as the etiology of AD remains unclear, so is the nature and significance of the histopathological changes described previously and herein. Whether the causative agent is infectious, chemical, or immunologic in nature remains to be determined. Whatever the cause, it is hard to escape the notion that the sequence of regressive changes in dendritic arbors of neurons is fundamental to the development and progression of the catastrophic clinical dementia which is the hallmark of the syndrome.

REFERENCES

1. Atken JT, Bridger JE: Neuron size and neuron population density in the lumbosacral region of the cat's spinal cord. *J Anat* 1961; 95:38–53.

2. Buell S, Coleman P: Dendritic growth in the aged human brain and failure of growth in senile dementia. *Science* 1979; 206:854–856.

3. Connor J, Diamond M, Johnson R: Occipital cortical morphology of the rat: alterations with age and environment. *Exp Neurol* 1980; 68:158–170.

4. Feldman ML: Dendritic changes in aging rat brain: pyramidal cell dendrite length and ultrastructure. *Adv Behav Biol* 1977; 23:23–27.

5. Machado-Salas J, Scheibel ME, Scheibel AB: Neuronal changes in the aging mouse: spinal cord and lower brainstem. *Exp Neurol* 1977; 54:504–512.

6. Mehraein P, Yamada M, and Tarnowska-Dziduszko E: Quantitative study of dendrites and dendritic spines in Alzheimer's disease and senile dementia. *Adv Neurol* 1975; 12:453–458.

7. Scheibel A: Dendritic changes in senile and presenile dementias, in Katzman R (ed): *Congenital and Acquired Cognitive Disorders*. Raven, New York, 1979, pp 107–122.

8. Scheibel ME, Lindsay RD, Tomiyasu U, et al: Progressive dendritic changes in the human limbic system. *Exp Neurol* 1976; 53:420–430.

9. Scheibel M, Scheibel A: Structural changes in the aging brain. *Aging NY* 1975; 1:11–37.

10. Scheibel AB, Tomiyasu U: Dendritic sprouting in Alzheimer's presenile dementia. *Exp Neurol* 1978; 60:1–8.

11. Terry RD: The fine structure of neurofibrillary tangles in Alzheimer's disease. *J Neuropathol Exp Neurol* 1963; 22:629–642.

9 Cell Numbers

Harold Brody

AMONG THE CHANGES associated with increasing age noted within the human CNS, variations of neuronal numbers have attracted an increasing amount of interest. Unfortunately, however, many regions of the brain have not yet been fully examined, so a total picture of the effects of age upon these neuronal populations is still not available. What is clear, however, is that there are observable differences in the degree and rate of cell loss within the CNS.

PREPARATION OF TISSUE

Quantification of neurons depends upon several factors. Since neural tissue is extremely sensitive, precautions must be taken that as little artifact as possible be introduced into the preparation of the specimen tissue used for study. Specimens must be selected from a control cohort without prior history of neurologic disease, to compare them with those who have been diagnosed as Alzheimer patients. Moreover, after death, removal of specimens must be performed as rapidly as possible to prevent artifactual change. In my own studies, a maximum limit of 6 hours has been set between time of death and fixation of the brain, although the majority of specimens are obtained between ½ hour and 4 hours after death. Specimens are perfused with 10% formalin in isotonic saline solution by way of the internal carotid and vertebral arteries, and are then suspended in the fixative solution, whose volume is 5 times the weight of the brain.

SELECTION OF TISSUE TO BE EXAMINED

While the brain stem may be prepared in cross section to identify the nuclear structures to be examined, areas of cerebellar and cerebral cortex must also be carefully identified to provide similar blocks of tissue among the specimens to be examined. In the cerebellar cortex specific landmarks may be identified for orientation, but in the cerebral cortex other precautions are necessary. Since neurons in the cerebral cortex are too great to be completely enumerated, unit areas must be examined. These may be obtained by identifying specific gyri and cutting blocks of tissue perpendicular to the direction of the gyrus.

Further, when a gyrus is of considerable length, it, too, may be subdivided and blocks removed from these smaller sections. This provides a mechanism by which block selection may be more closely duplicated as blocks are removed from other specimens. But, in order to count neurons in the cerebral cortex, one examines the sulcus areas rather than the dome of a gyrus. If the latter were studied, some cells would be counted more than once because the dome is curved and it is necessary to count neurons by columns extending from the pial surface to the underlying white matter.

Tissue blocks, after embedment in paraffin, may be cut at 10 μm and stained with cresyl violet to provide sections of intensely stained nucleoli to contrast with other cell structures still light in color. Since most procedures use the nucleolus as a marker for the neuron, this staining technique facilitates cell counting.

TECHNIQUES

A number of techniques have been developed for estimating cell numbers in the nervous system (for a complete description see ref. 1).

PHOTOGRAPHIC METHOD

A photograph of a section of tissue is produced and cells counted from the print. This technique obviates the possibility of focusing through the entire thickness of the section, and may occasion some difficulty in distinguishing between small neurons and glial cells.

PROJECTION METHOD

A slide may be projected onto a screen and cells counted within predetermined limits.

MICROPHOTOMETRIC METHOD

Light is passed through the specimen tissue onto a photocell of a microphotometer. The current in the photocell may be recorded as a curve, indicating optical density as related to cortical tissue depth.

HOMOGENATE METHOD

Homogenation of brain tissue may produce a suspension of cells. This may be lightly stained with an aniline dye, and a drop of the suspension placed into a hemocytometer. This method appears to have value in estimating total neuronal population in small animal brains, and permits one to distinguish between neurons and glial cells.

DIRECT MICROSCOPIC METHOD

This technique is most commonly used, although it is the most laborious method for counting cells. Nevertheless, it is also the most dependable of all the techniques. Using this method it is possible to differentiate between cell types as well as to determine cell sizes and volume. Cellular structures may also be examined, which may not be possible while using other techniques. Thin sections of tissue are examined under the light microscope with the aid of a micrometer disc that separates the field into small grid squares. Cells can then be counted within these squares; the cell population can be determined by examination of adjacent areas. The cells in a unit area (cerebral cortex) may be counted to compare with similar unit areas from other specimens while in other cases (brain stem nuclei) the entire length of a nucleus may be examined, providing a comprehensive cell count for that structure. This latter technique is incidentally useful in evaluating size changes in nuclear groups during brain maturation.

AUTOMATED TECHNIQUES

Because of the length of time involved in direct methods of counting neurons, many attempts have been made to use automated techniques. One of these was the flying-spot scanner described by Causley and Young (2), and the more recently developed image-analyzing computer system, Quantimet, which transmits an image of a section on a slide through a camera to a television screen and which permits particle counts after the apparatus has been programmed to record specific sizes and shapes. The speed of this apparatus (which can evaluate 8,000 fields in 4 hours) makes this an attractive approach. The problem of cell-type-recognition has not been solved, however, using this system. While automation may very likely be developed to a point of complete dependability, at the present time, the direct microscopic method of counting neurons offers the preferred benefits. Most of the findings reviewed in this section were obtained using this technique.

FINDINGS

CEREBELLUM

The most frequently studied structures in the cerebellum have been Purkinje cells. These cells have been reported to decrease in number with increasing human age (3–8). Corsellis (8) reported a 25% decrease of Purkinje cells in both males and females over a 100-year age span, although the loss was not appreciable until the sixth decade of life. While Purkinje cell decrease has also been reported by Inukai (9) in the rat, Wilcox (10) did *not* find any reportable cell decrease in the aging guinea pig.

CEREBRAL CORTEX

A number of studies have emphasized that certain regions of the cerebral cortex show a significant decrease in neuron number with increasing age while other regions remain stable or demonstrate insignificant changes. I reported significant decreases (11, 12) in the superior temporal gyrus, precentral gyrus, area striata, and superior frontal gyrus; decreases were not significant, however, in the postcentral gyrus or inferior temporal gyrus. Of particular interest were the marked decreases occurring in the granule cells and small pyramidal cells of layers two and four, whose Golgi-type II short-axoned cells are characteristic of associational cells of the human cerebral cortex. These findings have been corroborated by Colon (13) and Shefer (14) using the direct microscopic method of counting, and by Tomlinson (15) with the automatic counting device (Quantimet). In addition, the homogenation technique utilized by Devaney and Johnson (16) demonstrated a 50% loss of all cortical neurons in the macular projection area of the human visual cortex. Johnson and Erner (17), using this same technique, previously described a one-third reduction in the number of nerve cells in the whole brains of Swiss albino mice by 29 months of age. More recently, a study by Terry (18) of cell counts obtained by the automated counting technique in neocortex of individuals with senile dementia of the Alzheimer type demonstrated a small but significant loss of neurons above that seen in normal elderly (human) controls.

OTHER AREAS OF THE CENTRAL NERVOUS SYSTEM

Two structures, the putamen (19) and the substantia nigra (20), which in the human play important roles in the basal ganglia system influencing motor activity, also demonstrate neuronal loss with advancing age.

In the rat, Hsü and Peng (21) reported neuron loss in several hypothalamic areas in aged female rats. These were in the medial preoptic area (MPOA), the anterior hypothalamic area (AHA), and the arcuate nucleus (ARN), but not in the supraoptic (SO), paraventricular (PVN), ventromedial (VMN), and dorsomedial (DMN) nuclei. In a more recent study (22), these findings of neuronal loss could *not* be identified in aged male rats, indicating a correlation with a sex difference in functional changes of the hypothalamic–pituitary–gonadal axis. Sabel and Stein (23) found significant cell loss in the VMN and lateral hypothalamic nuclei, the septum, the corticoamygdaloid nucleus, the substantia nigra, and the reticular formation. These studies of substantial cell changes in the rodent hypothalamus should stimulate similar human studies.

Changes in cell numbers in human brain stem nuclei were not found by Van Buskirk (24) in the facial nucleus; nor by Konigsmark and Murphy (25, 26) in the ventral cochlear nucleus; by Monagle and Brody (27) in the inferior olive; by Vijayashankar and Brody (28) in the abducens nucleus; or by Vijayashankar and Brody (29) in the trochlear nucleus. The only brain stem structure to demonstrate neuronal decrease, in fact, is the locus ceruleus (30). This group of noradrenaline-secreting cells, which projects its processes throughout the CNS, may be involved in the mechanism of paradoxical sleep, in the tonic electrical activation of awakening, in the modulation of cerebellar function, and in reinforcement mechanisms essential in learning.

Peng and Lee (31) commented on regional differences of neuron loss in the aged rat brain to the effect that "the cerebellum is most sensitive to the aging process in respect to neuron loss, while the brain stem is most resistant, and the cerebral hemisphere is in between." This thought confirms similar earlier conclusions by Wright and Spink (32) and by Brody and Vijayashankar (33).

SUMMARY

A review of the data cited in this chapter stresses that areas of the brain vary in the amount and rate of cell loss with increasing age. Although present evidence does not specifically define the mechanism controlling cell loss in postmitotic cell populations, there appears to be some tendency for structures formed earlier in development to maintain a constant neuronal number (brain stem), while more recently developed structures (cerebral cortex) lose cells. Of particular interest is that, even within the cerebral cortex, the more primitive layers (three, five, six) show less neuronal decrease than layers two and four, which develop later. It should be apparent that additional information is needed regarding morphology and quantitative analysis of the aging brain, especially in the large areas not yet examined.

REFERENCES

1. Konigsmark BW: Methods for the counting of neurons, in Ebbessen SOE, Nauta WJ (eds): *Contemporary Research Methods in Neuroanatomy*. Berlin, Springer, 1970, pp 313–340.
2. Causley D, Young JZ: Counting and sizing of particles with flying-spot microscope. *Nature* 1955; 176:453–454.
3. Hodge CF: Changes in ganglion cells from birth to senile death: observations on man and honey bee. *J Physiol* 1894; 17:129–134.
4. Archambault LS: Parenchymatous atrophy of the cerebellum. *J Nerv Ment Dis* 1918; 48:273.
5. Ellis RS: A preliminary quantitative study of Purkinje cells in normal, subnormal, and senescent human cerebella. *J Comp Neurol* 1919; 30:229–252.
6. Ellis RS: Norms for some structural changes in the human cerebellum from birth to old age. *J Comp Neurol* 1920; 32:1–33.
7. Harms JW: Altersscheinungen im Hirn von Affen und Menschen. *Zool Anz* 1927; 74:249–256.
8. Hall TC, Miller AKH, Corsellis JAN: Variations in the human Purkinje cell population according to age and sex. *Neuropathol Appl Neurobiol* 1975; 1:267–292.
9. Inukai T: On the loss of Purkinje cells with advancing age from cerebellar cortex of albino rat. *J Comp Neurol* 1928; 45:1–31.
10. Wilcox HH: Structural changes in the nervous system related to the process of aging, in Birren JE, Imus HA, Windle WF (eds): *The Process of Aging in the Nervous System*. Springfield, Thomas, 1959, pp 16–23.
11. Brody H: Organization of cerebral cortex: III. A study of aging in the human cerebral cortex. *J Comp Neurol* 1955; 102:511–556.
12. Brody H: Structural changes in the aging nervous system, in Blumenthal HT (ed): *Interdisciplinary Topics in Gerontology*. New York, Karger, 1970, vol 7, pp 9–21.
13. Colon EJ: The elderly brain: a quantitative analysis of cerebral cortex in two cases. *Psychiatr Neurol Neurochir* 1972; 75:261–270.
14. Shefer VF: Absolute number of neurons and thickness of cerebral cortex during aging, senile, and vascular dementia and Pick's and Alzheimer's disease. *Neurosci Behav Physiol* 1973; 6:319–324.
15. Tomlinson BE, Henderson G: Some quantitative cerebral findings in normal and demented old people, in Terry RD, Gershon S (eds): *Neurobiology of Aging*. New York, Raven, 1976, pp 183–204.
16. Devaney KO, Johnson HA: Neuron loss in the aging visual cortex of man. *J Gerontol* 1980; 35:836–841.
17. Johnson HA, Erner S: Neuron survival in the aging mouse. *Exp Gerontol* 1972; 7:111–117.
18. Terry RD: Structural changes in senile dementia of the Alzheimer type. *Aging NY* 1980; 13:23–32.
19. Bugiani O, Salvarani S, Mancardi GL: Nerve cell loss with aging in the putamen. *Eur Neurol* 1978; 17:286–291.
20. McGeer PL, McGeer EG, Sazuki JS: Aging extrapyramidal function. *Arch Neurol* 1977; 34:33–35.
21. Hsü HK, Peng MT: Hypothalamic neuron number of old female rats. *Gerontology* 1978; 24:434–440.
22. Peng MT, Hsü HK: No neuron loss from hypothalamic nuclei of old male rats. *Gerontology* 1982; 28:19–22.

23. Sabel BA, Stein DG: Extensive loss of subcortical neurons in the aging rat brain. *Exp Neurol* 1981; 73:507–516.

24. Van Buskirk C: The seventh nerve complex. *J Comp Neurol* 1945; 82:303–333.

25. Konigsmark BW, Murphy EA: Neuronal populations in the human brain. *Nature* 1970; 299:1335.

26. Konigsmark BW, Murphy EA: Volume of ventral cochlear nucleus in man: its relationship to neuronal population and age. *J Neuropathol Exp Neurol* 1972; 31:304–316.

27. Monagle RD, Brody H: The effects of age upon the main nucleus of the inferior olive in the human. *J Comp Neurol* 1974; 155:61–66.

28. Vijayashankar N, Brody H: A study of aging in the human abducens nucleus. *J Comp Neurol* 1977; 173:433–437.

29. Vijayashankar N, Brody H: Aging in the human brain stem: a study of the nucleus of the trochlear nerve. *Acta Anat* 1977; 99:169–172.

30. Vijayashankar N, Brody H: A quantitative study of the pigmented neurons in the nuclei locus coeruleus and subcoeruleus in man as related to aging. *J Neuropathol Exp Neurol* 1979; 38:490–497.

31. Peng MT, Lee LR: Regional differences of neuron loss of rat brain in old age. *Gerontology* 1979; 25:205–311.

32. Wright EA, Spink JM: A study of the loss of nerve cells in the central nervous system in relation to age. *Gerontology* 1959; 3:277–287.

33. Brody H, Vijayashankar N, in Finch CE, Hayflick L (eds): *Handbook of the Biology of Aging.* New York, Van Nostrand Reinhold, 1977, pp 241–261.

SECTION IV
THE NEUROCHEMISTRY OF ALZHEIMER'S DISEASE

10 Chemical-Pathological Changes

David M. Bowen
Alan N. Davison

THE DISEASE DESCRIBED in Alois Alzheimer's 1907 report, "On a Peculiar Disease of the Cerebral Cortex," was soon designated "Alzheimer's disease" by Kraepelin and others (1). Alzheimer described a generally atrophic brain without macroscopic lesions, in which remarkable changes in the neurofibrils appeared. Since these could be stained with other than the usual dyes, he reasoned that a chemical alteration must have taken place. He also concluded that numerous neocortical nerve cells had disappeared entirely and that a refractory substance had been deposited in the cerebral cortex (the "core" of the senile plaque).

The findings of the first systematic examination of the incidence of senile degeneration are described by Corsellis (2). In this study, 80% of the patients who died in a psychiatric hospital over a 4½-year period were first classified using clinical criteria and then examined for pathological brain changes. There was no great difference in the mean age at death between patients in the two main diagnostic groups (functional and organic illnesses), yet the various morphological degenerative changes of old age were clearly more intense in the organic group. This was particularly so for neurofibrillary degeneration. The incidence of depression was much lower in the AD group (6%) than in those with dementia of vascular origin (20%); paranoid symptoms were similar in both groups, about 20% in each being affected. These latter findings illustrate the difficulty of using only clinical criteria to decide whether a patient has a functional or organic brain disorder. This is particularly so in the early stages of paranoid, depressive, and dementing conditions, where identifiable syndromes are necessary if meaningful drug trials are to be carried out. Bergmann (3) reviewed the problem of early diagnosis, and Bowen and associates (4) emphasized the importance of cerebral biopsy in diagnosing presenile AD as well as in detecting neurochemical deficits in individual demented patients. The data of Corsellis (2) indicated that about one-fifth of the patients studied with an organic or neurological disorder had AD. Later work by Tomlinson and associates and by Marsden and Harrison (for a review see ref. 5) demonstrated that AD is the major cause of dementia in both the presenile and senile age range.

BIOCHEMISTRY OF LESIONS DETECTED BY NEUROHISTOLOGY

Electron microscopic studies on biopsy samples of neocortex led Kidd (6) to describe neurofibrillary degeneration as being paired helical filaments (PHFs), and this has been confirmed. Although the PHFs or tangles have been described only in human nerve cells, they occur in the brains of normal elderly subjects, and in conditions such as Down's syndrome, postencephalitic parkinsonism, brain-damaged boxers, and the amyotrophic lateral sclerosis–parkinsonism dementia complex. The protein component of tangles seems to be antigenically related to a fibrous protein that normally occurs in the brain, but the identity of precursors is unclear (Chap. 5). The core of the senile plaque is composed of (or contains) amyloid, possibly derived from immunoglobulin (IgG) and suggesting that immunological factors are involved in pathogenesis (5). Granulovacuoles, confined to the pyramidal cells of the hippocampus, are like senile plaques (SPs) and tangles in that they increase in number with advancing years in nondemented subjects (7). They show a positive reaction to acid phosphatase and other hydrolases (8), which is indicative of a change in neuronal lysosomes. Subcellular fractionation suggests that lysosomes in the neocortex are also affected (9).

GLIAL CELL MARKERS

Cathepsin A activity, which provides insight into the activity of microglia or brain macrophages, appears high in the AD brain; this conforms to the established view that cells of this type occur in the Alzheimer brain (5). It is often assumed that astrocytes greatly increase in number in areas of the brain undergoing degenerative change, although work on the striatum from the brain tissue of Huntington's chorea patients suggests this is not so (10). The relative number of macroglia (astrocytes and oligodendrocytes) in the temporal lobe of the AD brain has been assessed using β-glucuronidase and carbonic anhydrase activities. Glial cells seem to survive better than neurons (11), suggesting that neuronal degeneration precedes changes in glia (12).

CORRELATES OF BRAIN ATROPHY AND NEURON LOSS

With increasing age, from about 25 years, there is a steady loss of wet weight of the brain (13). Thus, the mean weight of the brain in a 25-year-old male is 1,449 g and in that of a female is 1,309 g. At 70–80 years of age, the mean weights are 1,344 g for men (−7.3%) and 1,213 g for women (−7.4%). Shrinkage of the brain is associated with widened sulci and slight enlargement of the ventricles. In AD, the brain is often found to be considerably smaller than in age-matched controls, although the difference is not always large.

From the brain volume measurements (14) it is noteworthy that only in those AD patients dying before 80 years of age does the entire cerebrum undergo atrophy more than do the cerebrums of controls. The hindbrain is little changed. Although total cortical deficit appears to be more than loss of white matter, in the temporal lobe there is considerable reduction in white matter volume. In patients younger than 80 years of age, the temporal lobe was found to be the most atrophic of areas examined, and in very old AD patients the temporal lobe shows selective atrophy. These observations suggest that AD is a disease process particularly affecting the temporal lobes, and that dementia is not simply an exaggeration of normal aging.

Since the temporal lobe is particularly affected in AD, Bowen and associates (11, 12) made a number of biochemical analyses of the whole temporal lobe in control and AD patients of different ages. Most AD patients died in the same hospital as those studied by Corsellis (2). Altogether, 35 biochemical constituents were measured to give indications of possible cellular change which could be correlated with the disease in relation to aging. There was evidence of atrophy (wet weight and total protein loss) of the temporal lobe, and patients below 80 years old were more affected than those over 80. Similarly, other constituents such as those associated with nerve and glial cells, and those representing neurotransmitters (particularly the presynaptic cholinergic system, indicated by loss of choline acetyltransferase activity) were lost more frequently in patients younger than 80 years of age. This study also provided evidence of a distinct disease process which more seriously affects the relatively younger patients. Interestingly, the content of the major metabolite of serotonin (5-hydroxyindole acetate) was more sharply reduced in older patients, although indoleamine-receptive cells (LSD binding) were significantly reduced in only the more severely affected (i.e., younger) group (Chap. 13). Cholinoreceptive and adrenoreceptive cells were unaltered as indicated by binding of quinuclidinyl benzilate and dihydroaloprenolol, respectively, which also indicates a sparing of basal structures (based on measurements of the whole caudate nucleus).

In AD, a 20% shrinkage of the temporal lobe occurs, associated with a loss of about one-third of nerve cell components common to all nerve cells, and a 65% loss of choline acetyltransferase activity (12). If these changes are not attributable to shrinkage of perikarya and dendritic trees, they may reflect reduction in the nerve cell population. If so, this would be consistent with histological findings showing a substantial loss of neocortical neurons (particularly the large ones) (15). Other regions of the brain, however, show either neuronal loss or neurofibrillary degeneration (NFD). These are the substantia innominata, dorsal raphe nucleus, and locus ceruleus, which are thought to project, respectively, cholinergic, serotoninergic, and noradrenergic fibers to the neocortex (16). The major cause of cortical atrophy, therefore, remains unclear.

CHANGES IN OTHER MAJOR BIOCHEMICAL CONSTITUENTS

AMINO ACIDS

Examination of the amino acid composition of brain tissue has proved useful, despite alterations occurring postmortem (e.g., increase in γ-aminobutyric acid concentration). In a study on the hippocampus (17), the only significant change in AD was an increase in the concentration of the basic amino acid arginine. Tarbit and co-workers (17) suggested that the trend toward increasing free amino acids may be related to an elevated rate of proteolysis. Increased brain catheptic activity has been observed in AD (9, 18).

PROTEINS

A reduction in RNA and the volume of the nucleolus was taken to indicate a decline in protein synthesis (19). However, Suzuki and associates (20) reported that protein synthesis is normal in a crude microsomal preparation of cerebral cortex, although it is unclear whether sufficient controls were studied. Studies should be carried out using more sophisticated techniques as has been done in choreic brain tissue (21). Such studies might provide information about neuron-specific synthesis in AD. It is of interest that changes in cerebrospinal fluid–specific proteins have been found in patients with AD compared to those with multi-infarct dementia (22).

GLUCOSE UTILIZATION

This has been measured *in vitro,* with tissue prisms (essentially, preparations of nerve endings) of neocortex removed at diagnostic craniotomy from presenile AD cases (23). Incubations were performed in both 5-mmol and 31-mmol potassium concentrations to measure utilization in simulated resting and stimulated conditions. Glucose ^{14}C was used as the radioactive precursor, and its utilization was measured by trapping the $^{14}CO_2$ evolved. The $^{14}CO_2$ production was apparently increased by 39%. Paradoxically, neurophysiological measurements, such as positron emission tomography using deoxyglucose (Chap. 36), suggest that glucose utilization is decreased in AD; such change detected *in vivo* may be related to alterations in specific neurotransmitter pathways (i.e., the reticular activating system), which could obscure an underlying subcellular change.

SUMMARY

In AD, intrinsic cortical neurons (e.g., γ-aminobutyric acid–containing cells) seem to be preserved (24, 25), while loss of neurons seems to occur in areas of brain which project long axons to the neocortex. However, it is by no means generally accepted that extracortical brain regions play a key role in either the pathogenesis or cognitive and behavioral disturbances of AD. Previously, the substantia innominata was implicated in schizophrenia (26) and was the supposed target in psychosurgery for intractable psychoneurosis (27). Our metabolic study suggested that overall glucose utilization by the tissue prisms may be increased (23). Terry (28) commented that mitochondria surrounding the core of SPs appear to be undergoing a change similar to that caused by a reduced ATP–ADP ratio, so our result may reflect uncoupling of oxidative phosphorylation (23). Further work is needed to determine the full importance of all of these observations and the relationship, if any, to the pattern of cell loss, distribution of senile degeneration, and clinical features of the disease. In AD, however, by analogy with Parkinson's disease (where there is still considerable uncertainty about pathogenesis, and little is known about etiology), transmitter replacement should be considered. Combined therapy aimed at restoring activity of the cholinergic, noradrenergic, and serotinergic systems may even be necessary.

ACKNOWLEDGMENT

Dr. Bowen is grateful to JAN Corsellis for the samples and neurohistology employed in the studies described in refs. 11 and 12.

REFERENCES

1. Torack RH: *The Pathologic Physiology of Dementia.* Berlin, Springer, 1978, pp 5–15.
2. Corsellis JAN: *Mental Illness and the Aging Brain.* Maudsley Monograph, Oxford University Press, 1962, no. 9.
3. Bergmann K: The problem of early diagnosis, in Glen AIM, Whalley LJ (eds): *Alzheimer's Disease: Early Recognition of Potentially Reversible Deficits.* Edinburgh, Livingstone, 1979, pp 68–77.
4. Bowen DM, Sims NR, Benton S, et al: Biochemical changes in cortical brain biopsies from demented patients in relation to morphological findings and pathogenesis. *Aging NY* 1982; 19.

5. Bowen DM: Alzheimer's disease, in Thompson RHS, Davison AN (eds): *The Molecular Basis of Neuropathology.* London, Arnold, 1981, pp 649–665.

6. Kidd M: Paired helical filaments in electron microscopy of Alzheimer's disease. *Nature* 1963; 197:192–193.

7. Ball MJ, Vis CL: Relationship of granulovacuolar degeneration in hippocampal neurons to aging and to dementia in normal-pressure hydrocephalus. *J Gerontol* 1979; 33:815–824.

8. Krigman MR, Feldman RG, Bensch K: Alzheimer's presenile dementia: a histochemical and electron microscopic study. *Lab Invest* 1965; 14:381–396.

9. Bowen DM, Smith CB, Davison AN: Molecular changes in senile dementia. *Brain* 1973; 76:849–856.

10. Lange H, Thorner G, Hopf A, et al: Morphometric studies of the neuropathological changes in choreatic diseases. *J Neurol Sci* 1976; 28:401–425.

11. Bowen DM, Smith CB, White P, et al: Chemical pathology of the organic dementias: II. Quantitative estimation of cellular changes in post-mortem brains. *Brain* 1977; 100:427–453.

12. Bowen DM, White P, Spillane JA, et al: Accelerated ageing or selective neuronal loss as an important cause of dementia? *Lancet* 1979; i:11–14.

13. Dekaban AS, Sadowsky D: Changes in brain weights during the span of human life: relation of brain weights to body heights and body weights. *Ann Neurol* 1978; 4:345–356.

14. Hubbard BM, Anderson JM: A quantitative study of cerebral atrophy in old age and senile dementia. *J Neurol Sci* 1981; 50:135–145.

15. Terry RD, Peck A, DeTeresa R, et al: Some morphometric aspects of the brain in senile dementia of Alzheimer type. *Ann Neurol* 1981; 10:184–192.

16. Bowen DM, Sims NR, Davison AN: Neurochemistry of Alzheimer's disease: an update. *Expl Br Res Suppl* 1982; suppl 5:127–132.

17. Tarbit I, Perry EK, Perry RH, et al: Hippocampal free amino acid in Alzheimer's disease. *J Neurochem* 1980; 35:1246–1250.

18. Pope A, Hess HH, Lewin E: Studies on the microchemical pathology of human cerebral cortex, in Cohen MM, Snider RS (eds): *Morphological and Biochemical Correlates of Neural Activity.* New York, Harper, 1964, pp 98–111.

19. Mann DMA, Sinclair KGA: The quantitative assessment of lipofuscin pigment, cytoplasmic RNA, and nucleolar volume in senile dementia. *Neuropathol Appl Neurobiol* 1978; 4:129–135.

20. Suzuki K, Korey SR, Terry RD: Studies on protein synthesis in brain microsomal system. *J Neurochem* 1964; 11:403–412.

21. Marotta CA, Brown BA, Strocchi P, et al: *In vitro* synthesis of human brain proteins, including tubulin and actin, by purified post-mortem polysomes. *J Neurochem* 1981; 36:966–975.

22. Wikkelsø C, Blomstrand C, Rönnbäck L: Cerebrospinal fluid–specific proteins in multi-infarct and senile dementia. *J Neurol Sci* 1981; 49:293–303.

23. Sims NR, Bowen DM, Davison AN: ^{14}C-acetylcholine synthesis and ^{14}C-carbon dioxide production from U-^{14}C-glucose by tissue prisms from human neocortex. *Biochem J* 1981; 196:867–876.

24. Spillane JA, White P, Goodhardt MJ, et al: Selective vulnerability of neurons in organic dementia. *Nature* 1977; 226:558–559.

25. Emson PC, Lindvall O: Distribution of putative transmitters in the neocortex. *Neuroscience* 1977; 4:1–30.

26. David GB: The pathological anatomy of the schizophrenias, in Richter D (ed): *Schizophrenia: Somatic Aspects.* Oxford, Pergamon, 1957, p 109.

27. Goktepe FO, Young LB, Bridges PK: A further review of the results of stereotatic subcaudate tractotomy. *Br J Psychiatry* 106:270–280.

28. Terry RD: Ultrastructural alterations in senile dementia. *Aging NY* 1978; 7:375–382.

11 Changes in Choline Acetyltransferase and in Acetylcholine Synthesis

N. R. SIMS

DAVID M. BOWEN

OVER THE PAST DECADE there has been a rapid increase in studies aimed at elucidating biochemical changes associated with Alzheimer's disease (AD). These investigations have attempted to identify functions that may be related to the clinical presentation of the disease and which could indicate rational approaches to therapy.

An early finding was of a large reduction in the activity of the enzyme choline acetyltransferase (CAT) in the neocortex of brains obtained at postmortem from AD patients. CAT is the enzyme responsible for synthesis of the neurotransmitter acetylcholine from its immediate precursors, choline and acetyl-CoA (1, 2). Subcellular fractionation of brain tissue indicates that the enzyme is predominately located in the nerve terminals (3), to which it is carried by slow axonal transport, following synthesis in the cell body (4). In the brain, the enzyme distribution is similar to that of both acetylcholine (5) and the high-affinity uptake of choline (6). It is generally accepted as primarily associated with cholinergic neurons, and has been used extensively as a marker for the cholinergic system. Thus, a decreased CAT activity in AD was suggestive of a defect in cholinergic function.

CHOLINE ACETYLTRANSFERASE IN ALZHEIMER'S DISEASE

The dramatic reduction of CAT in AD has been shown in many studies (7–13). These generally indicate a loss of CAT activity to 30–50% of control values in the neocortex, although Davies (12) reported even greater losses of activity. The magnitude of this deficiency relative to other neural components was exhibited in an examination of 43 biochemical parameters in the temporal lobe (7). Table 11–1 selectively reports findings from this examination. CAT activity was reduced to 35% compared with controls, whereas markers indicative of the total neuronal population were present at 60% or more of the control values. CAT was particularly appropriate for investigation in autopsy material as it seems relatively impervious to changes related to postmortem decay and the agonal state, which have confounded the interpretation of findings with some other markers (14–17). Determination of CAT activity in biopsy samples removed from AD patients for diagnostic purposes has confirmed both

TABLE 11–1
Selected Changes in the Whole Temporal Lobe in Alzheimer's Disease

Marker	Possible Indices of:	% Reduction in Comparison with Controls ($P < .01$ in All Cases)
Choline acetyltransferase	Cholinergic neurons	35
2',3'-cyclic nucleotide phosphodiesterase Ganglioside NANA	Number of nerve cells	60–70
Lobe weight Total protein	Atrophy	77–81

Source: Adapted from Bowen and associates (7).

Values were expressed as content per whole temporal lobe to permit estimation of total changes in the tissue.

the absolute values and the magnitude of the deficit observed using autopsy material (7, 18).

The reduction in CAT activity is most marked in those regions in which the characteristic histopathological features of the disease are most prevalent, being even more severely affected in the hippocampus (12, 19) than in the neocortex. Activity in the caudate nucleus, which rarely exhibits pathological changes, is relatively unaffected (7, 15, 19). In the neocortex, a significant correlation has been demonstrated between senile plaque count and CAT activity in AD (20); moreover, a correlation between the enzyme and neurofibrillary tangles (NFTs) was shown in the hippocampus in a mixed population of demented and nondemented individuals (19).

ACETYLCHOLINE SYNTHESIS IN ALZHEIMER'S DISEASE

Interpretation of the reduction in CAT activity in relation to the cholinergic system as a whole is complicated for two reasons. First, the results do not indicate whether changes in CAT activity arise from a reduction in the enzyme in each neuron or from actual loss of the neuron or its nerve terminal. Second, animal studies suggest that the enzyme is not rate-limiting in acetylcholine synthesis (4, 21) and is present in large excess over requirements for normal synthesis. Therefore, synthesis could be relatively unimpaired despite a reduction in CAT activity. Thus, a direct estimate of acetylcholine synthesis has been obtained by examination of the capacity of tissue from neocortical biopsy samples to synthesize acetylcholine ^{14}C using glucose ^{14}C as substrate (18). As Table 11–2 shows, in samples exhibiting the histological features of AD, acetylcholine ^{14}C production was reduced by greater than 50% compared with control tissue (removed to allow access to tumors). By contrast, samples from demented patients which lacked the characteristic histology of AD retained their ability to synthesize acetylcholine. CAT activity showed a similar reduction in the AD group and there was a correlation between this and acetylcholine ^{14}C synthesis. This finding is best interpreted as indicating the loss (functionally, if not necessarily anatomically) of cholinergic nerve endings, such that the two markers were reduced in parallel. Such a loss of functional nerve endings could arise for a number of reasons that are not distinguishable by the present study. Recent evidence indicating that cell body numbers are reduced in the nucleus basalis

TABLE 11–2

CAT Activity and Acetylcholine ^{14}C Synthesis in Biopsy Samples of Demented Patients

| | Control | Dements | |
		with Alzheimer Histology	w/o Alzheimer Histology
CAT activity	7.7 ± 2.9 (24)[a]	3.4 ± 1.7 (15)[c]	9.1 ± 4.5 (5)
Acetylcholine ^{14}C synthesis[b]	7.0 ± 1.4 (31)	3.2 ± 1.2 (17)[c]	6.8 ± 1.9 (6)

Source: Data from Sims and associates (18, 27).

  [a] Values shown are mean ± standard deviation, with the number of cases in parenthesis.
  [b] Measured using tissue prisms incubated in the presence of 31 mmol K$^+$ and 2 mmol choline.
  [c] Significantly different from control ($P < .01$; Wilcoxon rank test).

of Meynert in AD (22) may be relevant, as this region is believed to be the site of a diffuse projection of cholinergic neurons to the neocortex.

RELATIONSHIP OF CHOLINERGIC CHANGE TO CLINICAL PRESENTATION OF AD

Although it is difficult to determine the relevance of the cholinergic change to the clinical symptoms of the disease, two lines of evidence indicate the possibility of a direct involvement. First, Perry and co-workers (20) showed that the neocortical CAT activity in postmortem samples correlated with a mental test score determined within 6 months prior to death for a group of patients with either AD or depression (CAT is not significantly reduced in the neocortex in depression). Second, there is extensive evidence from animal studies that the cholinergic system plays an important role in memory and learning (19). Furthermore, cholinergic drugs have been found to alter memory and other cognitive functions in humans (23–25) and to produce memory changes in healthy young individuals similar to those changes encountered in untreated elderly subjects (26). While neither of these observations alone can be taken as evidence of a cause and effect relationship between cholinergic function and cognitive changes in AD, they are at least consistent with such a possibility.

RELATIONSHIP OF CHOLINERGIC NEUROCHEMISTRY TO NORMAL AGING

As the histological features of AD are also found (to a lesser extent) in the nondemented elderly population, the possibility that the disease is an exacerbation of the normal aging process must be considered. CAT activities in the hippocampus show a significant decline with advanced age (9, 12), but in the neocortex some studies have produced evidence of no significant changes with age (7, 10, 15, 17) while others have shown large decreases (9, 12, 16). The explanation for these discrepancies is as yet unforthcoming. They could be related to the many variables involved in the handling of postmortem material and the selection of samples considered normal on histological and clinical grounds. Two other observations suggest that the cholinergic defect in AD is not related to an aging change. First, synthesis of acetylcholine ^{14}C in the neocortical biopsy samples was not found to change with age in control samples from patients aged 15 to 68 years (27). Second, studies in aging rats and mice, which have provided more consistent results than have human studies, show little evidence of changes in either CAT activity (28–30) or acetylcholine ^{14}C synthesis (31) in the neocortex or the hippocampus, although decreases occur in striatal tissue.

IMPLICATIONS OF CHOLINERGIC NEUROCHEMISTRY FOR THERAPY

Although there are changes in the presynaptic cholinergic function, the postsynaptic muscarinic receptors (i.e., the cholinergic binding sites) appear to be essentially preserved (7, 9, 10, 32). This finding, coupled with successes achieved with dopamine replacement therapy (by administration of a precursor) in parkinsonism, has prompted attempts to enhance acetylcholine concentrations in AD. These approaches to therapy are fully discussed in later chapters, but as yet there are no reports of substantial improvements. This may reflect the difficulties of providing suitable treatments when a large proportion of the cholinergic nerve endings are apparently malfunctioning, when some other neurotransmitters may also be affected (Chap. 13), and when complex mental processes are treatment targets.

SUMMARY

Investigation of CAT activity and acetylcholine ^{14}C synthesis demonstrates a large defect in the cholinergic system probably related to a loss of functional nerve endings. This change is correlated with histological and clinical features of AD and may be relevant to the symptoms.

REFERENCES

1. Nachmansohn D, Machado AL: The formation of acetylcholine: a new enzyme: choline acetylase. *J Neurophysiol* 1943; 6:397–403.
2. Korey SR, de Braganza B, Nachmansohn D: Choline acetylase: V. Esterifications and transacetylations. *J Biol Chem* 1951; 189:705–715.
3. Fonnum F: Topographical and subcellular localisation of choline acetyltransferase in rat hippocampal region. *J Neurochem* 1970; 17:1029–1037.
4. Tucek S: *Acetylcholine Synthesis in Neurons.* London, Chapman and Hall, 1978.
5. Hebb C: Formation, storage, and liberation of acetylcholine, in Koelle GB (ed): *Cholinesterases and Anticholinesterase Agents.* Berlin, Springer, 1963, pp 55–58.
6. Kuhar MJ, Sethy VH, Roth RH, et al: Choline: selective accumulation by central cholinergic neurons. *J Neurochem* 1973; 20:581–593.
7. Bowen DM, White P, Spillane JA, et al: Accelerated ageing or selective neuronal loss as an important cause of dementia? *Lancet* 1979; i:11–14.
8. Davies P, Maloney AJF: Selective loss of central cholinergic neurones in Alzheimer's disease. *Lancet* 1976; ii:1403.
9. Perry EK, Perry RH, Blessed G, et al: Necropsy evidence of central cholinergic defects in senile dementia. *Lancet* 1977; i:189.
10. White P, Hiley CR, Goodhardt MJ, et al: Neocortical cholinergic neurones in elderly people. *Lancet* 1977; i:668–670.

11. Reisine TD, Yamamura HI, Bird ED, et al: Pre- and post-synaptic neurochemical alterations in Alzheimer's disease. *Brain Res* 1978; 159:477–480.

12. Davies P: Neurotransmitter-related enzymes in senile dementia of the Alzheimer type. *Brain Res* 1979; 138:385–392.

13. Rossor M, Fahrenkrug J, Emson P, et al: Reduced cortical choline acetyltransferase activity in senile dementia of Alzheimer type is not accompanied by changes in vasoactive intestinal polypeptide. *Brain Res* 1980; 201:249–253.

14. Bird ED, Iversen LL: Huntington's chorea: postmortem measurement of glutamic acid decarboxylase, choline acetyltransferase, and dopamine in basal ganglia. *Brain* 1974; 97:457–472.

15. Bowen DM, Smith CB, White P, et al: Neurotransmitter related enzymes and indices of hypoxia in senile dementia and other abiotrophies. *Brain* 1976; 99:459–496.

16. McGeer PL, McGeer EG: Enzymes associated with the metabolism of catecholamines, acetylcholine, and GABA in human controls and patients with Parkinson's disease and Huntington's chorea. *J Neurochem* 1976; 26:65–76.

17. Spokes EGS: An analysis of factors influencing measurements of dopamine, noradrenaline, glutamate decarboxylase, and choline acetylase in human post-mortem brain tissue. *Brain* 1979; 102:333–346.

18. Sims NR, Bowen DM, Smith CCT, et al: Glucose metabolism and acetylcholine synthesis in relation to neuronal activity in Alzheimer's disease. *Lancet* 1980; i:333–336.

19. Perry EK, Perry RH: The cholinergic system in Alzheimer's disease, in Roberts PJ (ed): *Biochemistry of Dementia.* New York, Wiley, 1980, pp 135–183.

20. Perry EK, Tomlinson BE, Blessed G, et al: Correlation of cholinergic abnormalities with senile plaques and mental test scores in senile dementia. *Br Med J* 1978; 2:1457–1459.

21. Marchbanks RM, Wonnacott S: Relationship of choline uptake to acetylcholine synthesis and release. *Prog Brain Res* 1978; 49:77–88.

22. Whitehouse PJ, Price DL, Clark AW, et al: Alzheimer's disease: evidence for selective loss of cholinergic neurons in the nucleus basalis. *Ann Neurol* 1981; 10:122–126.

23. Crow TJ, Grove-White IG: An analysis of the learning deficit following hyoscine administration to man. *Br J Pharmacol* 1973; 49:322–327.

24. Drachman DA, Leavitt J: Human memory and the cholinergic system: a relationship to ageing? *Arch Neurol* 1974; 30:113–121.

25. Peterson RC: Scopolamine-induced learning failures in man. *Psychopharmacology* 1977; 52:283–289.

26. Drachman DA: Memory, dementia, and the cholinergic system. *Aging NY* 1978; 7:141–148.

27. Sims NR, Bowen DM, Davison AN: [^{14}C] Acetylcholine synthesis and [^{14}C] carbon dioxide production from [U-^{14}C] glucose by tissue prisms from human neocortex. *Biochem J* 1981; 196:867–876.

28. McGeer EG, Fibiger HC, McGeer PL, et al: Aging and brain enzymes. *Exp Gerontol* 1971; 6:391–396.

29. Meek JL, Bertilson L, Cheney DL, et al: Aging-induced changes in acetylcholine and serotonin content of discrete brain nuclei. *J Gerontol* 1977; 32:517–522.

30. Lai JCK, Leung TKC, Lim L: Brain regional distribution of glutamic acid decarboxylase, choline acetyltransferase, and acetylcholinesterase in the rat: effects of chronic manganese chloride administration after two years. *J Neurochem* 1981; 36:1443–1448.

31. Sims NR, Marek KL, Bowen DM, et al: Production of [^{14}C] acetylcholine and [^{14}C] carbon dioxide from [U-^{14}C] glucose in tissue prisms from aging rat brain. *J Neurochem,* in press.

32. Davies P, Verth AH: Regional distribution of muscarinic acetylcholine receptor in normal and Alzheimer-type dementia brains. *Brain Res* 1978; 138:385–392.

12 Acetylcholinesterase in Alzheimer's Disease

ELAINE K. PERRY
ROBERT H. PERRY

ACETYLCHOLINESTERASE AND THE CHOLINERGIC SYSTEM

The existence of an esterase that hydrolyzes acetylcholine (ACh) was predicted by Dale (1) as long ago as 1914. Many years elapsed before enzymes capable of hydrolyzing ACh, acetylcholinesterase and pseudocholinesterase, were clearly identified in tissues of the central nervous system and other systems (2). Of these enzymes, acetylcholinesterase (AChE) is considered principally responsible for hydrolyzing ACh at the cholinergic synapse. In this respect ACh, as opposed to other choline esters, is the preferred substrate for AChE. Pseudocholinesterase (pseudo-ChE), in contrast, hydrolyzes esters such as butyrylcholine or propionylcholine more efficiently. AChe not only differs from pseudo-ChE in its substrate affinities but it can also be experimentally distinguished by a characteristic substrate inhibition that occurs *in vitro* at high (mmol) acetylcholine concentrations, as well as by the appropriate use of a selective inhibitor of AChE such as BW 284c51 (1:5-bis [4-allyldimethylammonium-phenyl]-pentan-3-one dibromide). In most tissues, including those of the mammalian brain, AChE exists in a variety of molecular (isoenzyme or polymeric) forms; estimates of the molecular weights of these forms vary from under 100,000 to over 600,000 (2).

Although several functions have been attributed to AChE, its principal function is likely to be the rapid degradation of the transmitter, ACh, at the cholinergic synapse. In hydrolyzing ACh, AChE is one of the most active enzymes known: in the excitable eel membrane, for example, 1 g of tissue could theoretically hydrolyze 30 kg of ACh in 1 hour (3). Such a phenomenal capacity is not encountered in the mammalian brain, where cholinergic neurons are interspersed among numerous other neuron types. In brain regions AChE is considered associated predominantly with the cholinergic system, the activities of this enzyme are distributed unevenly in conjunction with cholinergic markers such as choline acetyltransferase, the enzyme that synthesizes ACh. Thus, the highest levels are found in such areas as the caudate nucleus and putamen, and the lowest levels (apart from white matter) in the cerebral cortex (4). In the cortex, although not in certain other brain areas such as the substantia nigra, AChE is apparently confined to the cholinergic system, and is confined mainly in presynaptic axonal processes and their terminal ramifications (5). Afferent cholinergic fibers containing AChE arise from various discrete underlying nuclei (6) and distribute widely throughout different cortical areas and in the various cortical (grey matter) layers. Both anterograde and retrograde axonal transport of AChE have been demonstrated and, in addition, release of the enzyme from the neuron occurs in various tissues including the brain (7).

In pathological conditions, such as in Alzheimer's disease (AD), a reduction of cortical AChE activity may occur in conjunction with several abnormalities. These include an actual degeneration of cholinergic processes, an impairment of axonal transport, or excessive release of the enzyme from terminal processes. Distinguishing between these alternatives in postmortem human brain tissue remains difficult at present.

ALZHEIMER'S DISEASE AND THE CHOLINERGIC SYSTEM

An involvement of the cholinergic system in AD is now well established, and has been described in detail elsewhere (Chap. 11;5). Currently unresolved issues include the precise nature of the cholinergic abnormality; the extent to which it is directly or primarily related to the disease process; and whether, at least in earlier stages, the cholinergic deficit is selective or amenable to treatment. In these respects, investigations relating to the enzyme AChE may be of particular importance. Thus, in areas such as the cortex, in which the enzyme is a reliable cholinergic marker, biochemical and histochemical findings should reflect the state of the cholinergic system. In addition, particular forms of AChE in the blood may possibly reflect alterations in central cholinergic neurons. Therapeutically, selective inhibition of the enzyme resulting in increased ACh levels may ultimately be of some value.

ACETYLCHOLINESTERASE IN ALZHEIMER'S DISEASE

BRAIN BIOCHEMISTRY

The first report relating to AChE in AD actually dates back to 1964, when Pope and associates (8) demonstrated a loss of activity in biopsy brain tissue. Since then, reduced activity in postmortem tissue has been reported, to a greater or lesser extent, by several other groups (9–11). Enzyme loss in the cortex is not generally seen in a variety of other unrelated neurological or psychiatric diseases (5), although it is of interest that in Down's syndrome, in which Alzheimer-type neuropathological changes are present, there is also a significant reduction in cortical AChE (12).

In AD the extent of the AChE reduction is apparently related to the severity of the disease process, assessed either by the degree of senile plaque formation (13) or extent of neurofibrillary tangle (NFTs) formation (5). The reduction in AChE (as judged by measurements of total biochemical activity) is not apparent at earlier stages of the disease process and, in pathologically moderate or severe cases, the loss of AChE is not as extensive as that of choline acetyltransferase, the enzyme that synthesizes ACh. (Fig. 12–1). This may partly reflect the more specific localization of the latter to cholinergic nerve terminals. Interestingly, butyrylcholine esterase appears to increase as AD advances (Fig. 12–1).

The general resemblance between alterations in cortical or hippocampal cholinergic activities in AD and, as far as this has been investigated, cholinergic derangements in similar brain areas of experimental animals following lesions of the afferent fibers to these areas has been discussed elsewhere (5). This similarity raises the possibility that AD may actually be associated with cholinergic fiber degeneration, although other possibilities include a defect in the axonal transport of cholinergic components from subcortical nuclei to cortical brain

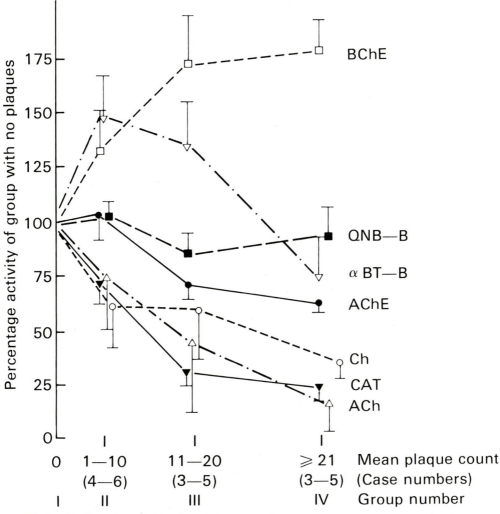

Figure 12–1. Cholinergic activities in relation to senile plaque density. Elderly nondemented and demented (Alzheimer-type) cases have been grouped according to mean cortical plaque counts (per 1.4-mm optical field), as indicated. Results (mean ± SE) expressed as activity in each group as a percentage of activity in group with no plaques. Activities include acetylcholinesterase (AChE), butyryl-choline esterase (BChE), choline acetyltransferase (CAT), acetylcholine (ACh), choline (Ch), QNB- and α-Bungarotoxin–bindings (QNB–B and α-BT–B, respectively) in temporal cortex (Brodmann area 21, except for α-BT–B in hippocampus). Significant differences (where $P < .05$) compared with group with no plaques include AChE (third and fourth groups), CAT (second, third, and fourth groups), ACh (fourth group), Ch (fourth group), and BChE (third and fourth groups). *Results on α-BT–B are unpublished observations of B. T. Volpe and E. K. Perry.*

regions. Further investigations of areas such as the substantia innominata, which appears in the human brain to contain a major cholinergic component (14), may help to distinguish between these alternatives.

Brain Histochemistry

Histochemical studies of AChE in neocortical and archicortical areas have not only confirmed the overall reduction in enzyme activity in AD but have also demonstrated interest-

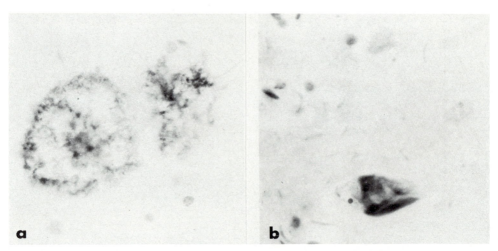

Figure 12–2. Senile plaques (a) and a neurofibrillary tangle (b) stained for acetylcholinesterase (15). Plaques in occipital cortex (× 640) and tangle in hippocampal pyramidal layer (× 800) in an elderly patient with Alzheimer-type dementia. Staining not apparent in sections pre-incubated with AChE inhibitor BW 284c51 (5 × 10⁻⁵M)

ing relationships between the enzyme localization and particular neuropathological features of the disease (15). Thus, in both normal elderly persons and some AD patients, senile plaques (SPs) and neurofibrillary tangles (NFTs) are associated with AChE histochemical activity (Fig. 12–2). In more advanced cases of AD, this staining decreases in conjunction with the loss of staining of the neuropil. The apparently elevated activity around some plaques (Fig. 12–2[a]) raises the question of whether, at some stage in plaque development, axonal proliferation occurs perhaps as part of an "abortive" attempt at regeneration. The staining of NFTs with an enzymatic activity such as AChE (Fig. 12–2[b]) may also be of considerable interest in relation to the etiology and nature of the paired helical filaments (PHFs). Whether the enzyme activity of the tangle is loosely associated with or is an integral part of the PHFs is not yet known, nor is it clear whether this AChE originates in the cholinoceptive pyramidal neuron or from impinging cholinergic terminals.

BLOOD BIOCHEMISTRY

In the absence of consistent evidence that cerebrospinal fluid (CSF) AChE reflects central cholinergic function, investigation of blood cholinergic activities in AD is of considerable interest. Red blood cell AChE is apparently below normal in AD (16, 17), although other evidence of similar reductions in depression (17, 18) suggests this is probably not a specific abnormality. In a recent comparison of plasma (as opposed to red blood cell) AChE in clinically assessed cases of Alzheimer-type dementia and age-matched nondemented cases, a highly significant increase in the mean value is apparent in the suspected cases of AD (Fig. 12–3). Although the overlap between the two groups was considerable, there was no difference between the groups in plasma pseudocholinesterase and the plasma AChE elevation was not apparent in endogenous depression, indicating the relative specificity of this change. Plasma AChE (as opposed to pseudocholinesterase) has received scant attention due partly to difficulties in measuring low levels of AChE against a background of high pseudocholinesterase. Nevertheless, elevated activities of plasma AChE have also been reported in motor

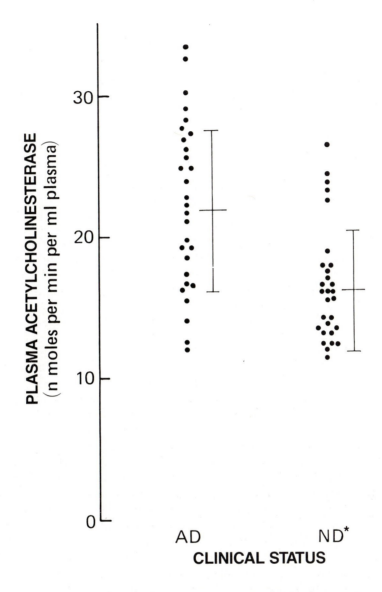

*Nondemented, age-matched controls

Figure 12–3. Acetylcholinesterase activity, estimated by the method of Ellman (19), in plasma of clinically assessed nondemented patients (ND), including normal, depressed, and schizophrenic individuals, and patients with senile dementia of the Alzheimer type (AD). Mean (± S.D.) ages of the two groups were 77.7±5.5 (ND) and 79.4±6.1 (AD). Assays were performed in the presence of 10^{-4}M tetra-isopropylpyrophosphoramide to inhibit pseudocholinesterase activity. The activity here represents the difference between estimations in the presence and absence of the specific AChE inhibitor 10^{-5}M BW 284c51, and is considered entirely due to AChE itself.

neuron disease (20), where degeneration of cholinergic neurons of the spinal cord occurs. In light of these recent findings, it might be postulated that during active degeneration of central cholinergic neurons, a stage which may occur in AD, there could be abnormal release of AChE via the cerebral vasculature into the plasma. Further investigation of plasma AChE is warranted, since the possibility of establishing a diagnostic blood abnormality is worth pursuing in a disease such as AD where early clinical diagnosis is often quite difficult.

SOME FUTURE TRENDS

ENIGMATIC ASPECTS

Among the more interesting of the numerous unresolved issues relating to AChE are the functions and localizations in nervous tissue of the different molecular forms of the enzyme, the possible role of AChE in peptide hydrolysis (21), and the neurophysiological role of AChE release (7). In AD it is now necessary to establish whether particular enzyme forms in the brain are affected, and whether pathological abnormalities occurring in the release of AChE might provide an index of central cholinergic function in such body fluids as the plasma. Of further interest in a degenerative disease like AD is the role of growth promoting agents such as nerve growth factor, which in such tissues as rat pheochromocytoma regulates the AChE activity (22).

THERAPEUTIC POTENTIAL

A role for the cholinergic system in normal memory has been suggested by experimental pharmacological manipulations in man and animals (for a review see ref. 5), and small but significant dose-dependent improvements have been reported in normal individuals following infusion of the reversible AChE inhibitor physostigmine (23). Whether physostigmine provides, at particular dose levels, clinical benefit in AD patients is not yet clear, although in a recent report (24) consistent improvements in memory function were observed during intravenous injections of physostigmine with optimal responses at doses in the region of 0.4 mg; further research is required to determine the usefulness in the treatment of AD of this or other centrally active AChE inhibitors. In the meantime, it is no doubt encouraging to consider that future research into the effects of AChE inhibitors on the human CNS may be directed not, as in the past, toward the development of nerve gases with potential military application but toward designing agents which ameliorate conditions of human confusion or dementia in the elderly.

ACKNOWLEDGMENTS

The work reported here was conducted, in part, in collaboration with B. E. Tomlinson, G. Blessed, I. Wilson, M. Bober, J. Atack, J. A. Richter, B. T. Volpe, and J. McLennan and was financially supported by the Wellcome Trust.

REFERENCES

1. Dale HH: The action of certain esters and ethers of choline and their relation to muscarine. *J Pharmacol Exp Ther* 1914; 6:147–190.

2. Silver A: *The Biology of Cholinesterases.* Amsterdam, North-Holland, 1974.

3. Nachmansohn D: Biochemistry as part of my life. *Annu Rev Biochem* 1972; 41:1–28.

4. McGeer PL, McGeer EG: Enzymes associated with the metabolism of catecholamines, acetylcholine, and GABA in human controls and patients with Parkinson's disease and Huntington's chorea. *J Neurochem* 1976; 26:65–76.

5. Perry EK, Perry RH: The cholinergic system in Alzheimer's disease, in Roberts PJ (ed): *Biochemistry of Dementia.* New York, Wiley, 1980, pp 135–183.

6. Wenk H, Bigl V, Meyer U: Cholinergic projections from magnocellular nuclei of the basal forebrain to cortical areas in rats. *Brain Res* 1980; 2:295–316.

7. Hollunger EG, Niklasson BH: The release and molecular state of mammalian brain acetylcholinesterase. *J Neurochem* 1973; 20:821–836.

8. Pope A, Hess HH, Lewin E: Studies on the microchemical pathology of human cerebral cortex, in Cohen MM, Snider RS (eds): *Morphological and Biochemical Correlates of Neural Activity.* New York, Harper, 1964, pp 98–111.

9. Op Den Velde W, Stam FC: Some cerebral proteins and enzyme systems in Alzheimer's presenile and senile dementia. *J Am Geriatr Soc* 1976; 24:12–16.

10. Davies P, Maloney AJF: Selective loss of cholinergic neurons in Alzheimer's disease. *Lancet* 1976; ii:1403.

11. Perry EK, Perry RH, Blessed G, et al: Changes in brain cholinesterases in senile dementia of the Alzheimer type. *Neuropathol Appl Neurobiol* 1978; 4:273–277.

12. Yates CM, Simpson J, Maloney AFJ, et al: Alzheimer-like cholinergic deficiency in Down's syndrome. *Lancet* 1980; ii:979.

13. Perry EK, Tomlinson BE, Blessed G, et al: Correlation of cholinergic abnormalities with senile plaques and mental test scores in senile dementia. *Br Med J* 1978; 2:1457–1459.

14. Candy JM, Perry RH, Perry EK, et al: Distribution of putative cholinergic cell bodies and various neuropeptides in the substantia innominata of the human brain. *J Anat* 1981; 133:124–125.

15. Perry RH, Blessed G, Perry EK, et al: Histochemical observations on cholinesterase activities in the brains of elderly normal and demented (Alzheimer-type) patients. *Age Aging* 1980; 9:9–16.

16. Chipperfield B, Newman PM, Moyes ICA: Decreased erythrocyte cholinesterase activity in dementia. *Lancet* 1981; i:199.

17. Perry RH, Wilson ID, Bober MJ, et al: Plasma and erythrocyte acetylcholinesterase in senile dementia of Alzheimer type. Lancet 1982; i:174–175.

18. Milstoc M, Teodoru CV, Fieve RR, et al: Cholinesterase activity and the manic-depressive patient. *Dis Nerv Syst* 1975; 36:197–199.

19. Ellman GL, Courtney DK, Andres V, et al: A new rapid calorimetric determination of acetylcholinesterase activity. *Biochem Pharmacol* 1961; 7:88–95.

20. Festoff BW, Fernandez HL: Plasma and red blood cell acetylcholinesterase in amyotrophic lateral sclerosis. *Muscle Nerve* 1981; 4:41–47.

21. Chubb IW, Hodgson AJ, White GH: Acetylcholinesterase hydrolyses substance P. *Neuroscience* 1980; 5:2065–2072.

22. Lucas CA, Czlonkowska A, Kreutzberg GW: Regulation of acetylcholinesterase by nerve growth factor in the pheochromocytoma PC12 cell line. *Neurosci Lett* 1980; 18:333–337.

23. Davis KL, Mohs R, Tinklenberg JR, et al: Physostigmine: improvements of long-term memory processes in normal humans. *Science* 1978; 201:272–273.

24. Christie JE, Shering A, Ferguson J, et al: Physostigmine and arecoline: effects of intravenous infusions in Alzheimer presenile dementia. *Br J Psychiatry* 1981; 138:46–50.

13 Changes in Neurotransmitter Systems in the Aging Brain and in Alzheimer's Disease

ARVID CARLSSON

NEUROTRANSMITTER CHANGES IN THE AGING BRAIN

The brain starts to deteriorate at about age 60. An example of such deterioration is the increase in persons over 60 who become "delirious" when exposed to stressors such as trauma, fever, or environmental changes. A reduction of cerebral blood flow, as well as oxygen and glucose consumption, is also observed after this milestone (1). Signs of cerebral atrophy with increased ventricular size (2) and loss of brain weight, are also evident (3).

Age-related cerebral atrophy, however, is by no means uniform. For example, the cerebral cortex atrophies more than the brain stem. Also, certain neurons demonstrate greater age-dependent changes than others. For example, whereas brain stem nuclei in general show only slight age-related neuronal loss, the cell count shows a significant decrease with age in both the locus ceruleus (4) and the substantia nigra (5), indicating an above-average sensitivity of catecholamine-storing neurons.

Changes with age have also been demonstrated in the catecholamine-synthesizing enzyme tyrosine hydroxylase (TH) (5). Interestingly, the most rapid decline in TH activity occurs before the age of 20. However, there seems to be a continuing age-related decline, a decline that could be related to the decrease in the cell count. The acetylcholine-synthesizing enzyme choline acetyltransferase (CAT) shows a slight but significant age-related drop in the caudate, but no significant decrease in the putamen. Also, the γ-aminobutyric acid (GABA)-synthesizing enzyme shows a slight age-related decrease (5).

With regard to actual transmitter levels, as investigated postmortem, I have shown that dopamine in the caudate shows a significant decrease with age (6). In this study I added the metabolite 3-methoxytyramine to dopamine because I believe, on the basis of animal studies, that virtually all the 3-methoxytyramine found in the brain has been formed postmortem. When rat brain is taken very quickly after death and frozen, the 3-methoxytyramine level is very low indeed. Therefore, if we add up the dopamine and 3-methoxytyramine, we arrive at a total that is probably closer to the actual sum at the time of death. The results with dopamine alone, however, give a very similar picture.

Also, corrected data taking into consideration the decline that occurs with the time interval between death and autopsy did not significantly alter the basic findings. An interesting

100

observation in this study was that the decline in dopamine with age accelerated significantly after about age 60. This is consistent with other neurochemical data and may suggest that some form of signal occurs around the age of 60, accelerating the process of aging.

It was also found that the dopamine level in the putamen decreased with age. However, the age dependence was less pronounced than in the caudate nucleus ($r = -.36$ for the sum of dopamine and 3-methoxytyramine, corrected for postmortem delay, $N = 61$, $P < .01$). In fact, the putamen–caudate ratio of dopamine plus 3-methoxytyramine was found to increase significantly with age ($r = .47$, $N = 61$, $P < .001$).

As shown in Table 13–1, several different brain regions, transmitters, transmitter metabolites, and enzymes have been examined (7). For dopamine (as discussed earlier) there is a significant decline with age, and this is also the case for its metabolite homovanillic acid (HVA) although the latter decline does not reach statistical significance because of the small number of estimations. In several brain regions there is no significant decline in norepinephrine with age, but in the hippocampus, a statistically significant decline was found. A major metabolite of norepinephrine, 3-methoxy-4-hydroxyphenylglycol (MHPG) does not show a significant change with age but tends to show a positive correlation with age in the hippocampus, in contrast to the strong negative correlation for norepinephrine itself in the same region.

A corresponding difference between transmitter and metabolite is seen for 5-hydroxytryptamine (5-HT) where a clear-cut decrease occurs with age in the gyrus cinguli, but the metabolite 5-hydroxyindoleacetic acid (5-HIAA) does not change. In the medulla oblongata the correlation between 5-HT and age is actually positive. The most striking age dependence observed is with monoamine oxidase (MAO), however, only with the B enzyme. There are two monoamine oxidases, the A and the B enzymes. MAO-A generally does not show any change with age. MAO-B, in contrast, shows a dramatic increase with age in all brain parts examined. Choline acetyltransferase (CAT) did not show a significant decrease with age in this particular investigation. About half the published studies have reported decreases in CAT with aging. Probably the decrease in CAT occurs only in certain brain regions. Thus, a heterogeneous picture exists with respect to the age dependence of the neurotransmitters and their metabolites in different brain regions (8).

TABLE 13–1
Age Dependence of Neurotransmitters

	Gyrus Cinguli	Hippo-campus	Caudate	Putamen	Thala-mus	Hypothal-amus	Mesen-cephalon	Medulla Oblongata
Dopamine[a]	—	—	−0.57[b]	−0.36[c]	—	−0.18	−0.51[e]	−0.11
Homovanillic acid	0.33	0.25	−0.43[f]	—	—	0.04	—	—
Norepinephrine	0.12	−0.51[c]	−0.15	—	0.04	−0.18	−0.23	0.14
MHPG	0.07	0.20	0.27	—	—	−0.37	—	—
5-HT	−0.45[d]	−0.23	−0.25	—	−0.32	−0.22	0.19	0.50[c]
5-HIAA	0.11	−0.09	0.10	—	−0.14	−0.13	0.15	0.22
MAO-B	0.85[b]	0.60[c]	0.59[d]	—	—	0.57[d]	—	—
CAT	−0.08	−0.12	0.04	—	—	0.01	—	—

[a] The values for caudate and putamen refer to dopamine plus 3-methoxytyramine.
[b] $P < .001$.
[c] $P < .01$.
[d] $P < .02$.
[e] $P < .05$.
[f] $P < .1$.

Following the observation of an increase with age in MAO-B in both the gyrus cinguli and the caudate nucleus, I conducted an experiment to determine whether I could produce a similar increase by hemitransection of the brain in rats (9). Because of the large number of axons cut in the hemispheres, an extensive neuronal degeneration is induced. Within a couple of weeks following the hemitransection, there was a clear-cut increase in MAO-B activity in the striatum and the cerebral cortex, whereas in the limbic areas this increase, if it existed, did not reach statistical significance. Perhaps the increase in MAO-B with age is related in some way to neuronal degeneration. MAO-A did not change at all in this experiment. Some data suggest that MAO-B occurs more in glia than in neurons, whereas the opposite is true of MAO-A (10). There is also the possibility that MAO-B serves as a biochemical marker of glial cells, and that what we observe here is a sign of gliosis induced by neuronal degeneration.

NEUROTRANSMITTER CHANGES IN ALZHEIMER'S DISEASE

A survey of the literature on transmitters in senile dementia reveals that the conclusions arrived at depend very much on the particular transmitter an investigator studies (11–13). Workers who focus on acetylcholine frequently conclude that this is the transmitter mainly involved in senile dementia, and that the memory disturbance is due to loss of acetylcholine in the hippocampus. Others have suggested that the catecholamines are involved. One could also make a case for 5-HT. Of course, there are also many transmitters that have not yet been analyzed. In Sweden, a group of investigators tried to resolve this problem by measuring as many transmitters and transmitter markers as possible in the same individual (7).

In this collaborative effort we focused mainly on late-onset AD (7). Table 13–2 presents the results. It is apparent that in the caudate nucleus, dopamine, 3-methoxytyramine, and HVA levels are all below normal. Norepinephrine is reduced, but interestingly its metabolite MHPG is significantly above normal, suggesting an increased turnover of norepinephrine. 5-HT is very much reduced, while 5-HIAA is lowered but not significantly reduced. MAO-B, which showed such a sharp rise with age, is increased here, too. Choline acetyltransferase is reduced to about the same extent as the other markers. It happened that material from severe chronic alcoholics was processed in this same analysis, along with the AD cases, and in many respects the changes in alcoholics were found to be similar to those in late-onset AD. We speculate that perhaps in alcoholism the aging process in the brain is accelerated.

Similar changes were also found in the gyrus cinguli, hippocampus, and hypothalamus: i.e., a decrease in norepinephrine but an increase in its metabolite; a decrease in 5-HT with no change in its metabolite; an increase in MAO-B; and a decrease in choline acetyltransferase.

In view of the considerable clinical differences between cases of AD and controls, one wonders whether a similar clear-cut distinction between the two groups can be made, based on the biochemical data. This is not so. For example, choline acetyltransferase in the hippocampus shows a considerable overlap between dementia and control cases, and this is true also of dopamine in the caudate nucleus, as well as the other transmitters studied so far. This overlap between AD patients and normal individuals suggests it is not possible to single out one neurotransmitter as being clearly responsible for AD. Some clear-cut AD patients have values within normal limits when each transmitter is considered separately.

TABLE 13–2
Neurotransmitters in the Caudate Nucleus

	Controls		AD	Alcoholism
	Mean ± S.E.M.		% Control	% Control
	N = 17		N = 15	N = 13
Dopamine, nmole/g	15.8 ±	0.90[d]	54[a]	45[a]
3-methoxytyramine, nmole/g	6.6 ±	0.34[d]	70[b]	43[a]
Homovanillic acid, nmole/g	22.7 ±	1.37	67[b]	86
Norephinephrine, nmole/g	0.16±	0.012	73[c]	65[c]
MHPG, nmole/g	0.10±	0.019	183[c]	164
5-HT, nmole/g	0.51±	0.043	49[a]	30[a]
5-HIAA, nmole/g	1.4 ±	0.11	87	60[b]
MAO-B	3,390 ±	158	115[c]	85
Choline acetyltransferase, pkatal/1	17,172	± 1,879	55[b]	90

Source: Carlsson et al (7).

[a] $P < .001$.
[b] $P < .01$.
[c] $P < .05$.
[d] $N = 54$.

But if one looks at each individual case and takes into account all the different values measured, a distinct separation is obtained between the controls and the AD cases.

Figure 13–1 illustrates how to distinguish AD patients from normals neurochemically. This is a three-dimensional picture where we have entered the values of dopamine, 5-HT, and norepinephrine in each individual case. It can be seen that some of the AD cases are very low in dopamine, 5-HT, and norepinephrine. There is also a group of AD cases moderately low in dopamine, and in some cases also low in norepinephrine and 5-HT. Subjects in this group are separated from the main group where practically all the controls are located. There is only one control among these AD cases, and, in his case, hospital records indicated that during the last two or three years of life the patient had become confused and delirious at night. Thus, the subject may not have been an appropriate control. Among the group of controls, there were a number of dementia cases (six cases in the right part of Fig. 13–1), but all these cases are below the range of the controls with respect to 5-HT levels. Apart from the one (doubtful) control case, there is a clear-cut separation between the senile dementia cases and controls, and these observations considered only three neurotransmitters. If we had also considered the enzyme choline acetyltransferase, the distinction between groups would have been even sharper. Probably the more neurotransmitters taken into account, the more clear-cut the separation in biochemical terms between AD cases and normals. What this suggests is that AD is multifactorial. Different neurotransmitters and different types of neurons are involved to a varying extent. Thus, clinical symptomatology in AD results from the sum of many different neuronal deficiencies.

In a subsequent analysis AD patients were divided into two groups: a younger group that would generally correspond to so-called presenile dementia, and an older group that would correspond to so-called senile dementia. In the younger group, the changes relative to age-matched controls were much more severe than in the older group (Table 13–3).

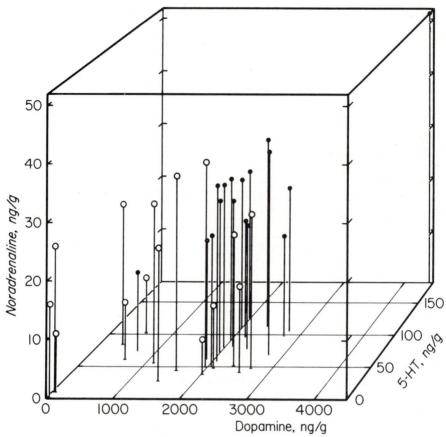

Figure 13–1. Three-dimensional diagram of norepinephrine, dopamine, and 5-HT in the caudate nucleus of AD patients (♀) and controls without known brain pathology (♂).

TABLE 13–3
Neurotransmitters in Two Age Groups of AD Patients
Values expressed in percent of age-matched controls

	Caudate		Hippocampus	
	≤73 yr N = 9	>73 yr N = 5	≤73 yr N = 9	>73 yr N = 4
Choline acetyltransferase	47[a]	96	35[b]	61
Dopamine	62[c]	76	—	—
Norepinephrine	73[c]	82	66[d]	62[d]
5-HT	51[a]	64[b]	21[a]	27[c]
MAO-B	122[d]	108	128[d]	139[b]

Significance versus control:
[a] $P < .001$.
[b] $P < .01$.
[c] $P < .025$.
[d] $P < .05$.

This is true both for the caudate and for the hippocampus. In the older group, a clear-cut reduction of 5-HT, but not of the other transmitters, was seen.

SUMMARY

Postmortem examination of various brain regions in subjects without known brain pathology showed an age-related decrease in the levels of dopamine in the nigrostriatal system, norepinephrine in the hippocampus, and 5-HT in the gyrus cinguli. However, there was an increase of 5-HT in the medulla oblongata, and MAO-B in several brain regions.

In AD, all these monoamines, as well as choline acetyltransferase, were reduced, whereas MAO-B was increased. When all the different transmitters were taken into account, a virtually complete separation between the AD group and the control group was obtained. The data suggest that the process of neuronal aging is exaggerated in senile dementia.

In chronic alcoholics, changes similar to those in senile dementia were observed, suggesting an acceleration of the neuronal aging process in this condition as well.

ACKNOWLEDGMENTS

This chapter is reprinted, with changes by the editor, from a chapter by A. Carlsson in *Strategies for the Development of an Effective Treatment for Senile Dementia,* T. Crook, S. Gershon (eds.), 1981. Reprinted by permission of the publisher, Mark Powley Associates, Inc., New Canaan.

REFERENCES

1. Gottstein U, Held K: Effects of aging on cerebral circulation and metabolism in man. *Acta Neurol Scand Suppl* 1979; 60 (suppl 72).

2. Jacobs L, Kinkel WR, Painter F, et al: Computerized tomography in dementia with special reference to changes in size of normal ventricles during aging and normal pressure hydrocephalus. *Aging NY* 1978; 7.

3. Brody H: Aging of the vertebrate brain, in Rockstein M, Sussman ML (eds): *Development and Aging in the Nervous System.* New York, Academic, 1973.

4. Brody H: An examination of cerebral cortex and brain stem aging. *Aging NY* 1973; 3.

5. McGeer EG: Aging and neurotransmitter metabolism in the human brain. *Aging NY* 1978; 7.

6. Carlsson A, Winblad B: Influence of age and time interval between death and autopsy in dopamine and 3-methoxytyramine levels in human basal ganglia. *J Neural Transm* 1976; 38:271.

7. Carlsson A, Adolfsson R, Aquilonius SM, et al: Biogenic amines in human brain in normal aging, senile dementia, and chronic alcoholism, in Goldstein M, Caine DB, Liberman A, et al (eds): *Ergot Compounds and Brain Function: Neuroendocrine and Neuropsychiatric Aspects.* New York, Raven, 1980.

8. Pradhan SN: Central neurotransmitters and aging. *Life Sci* 1980; 26:1643.

9. Carlsson A, Fowler CJ, Magnusson T, et al: The activities of monoamine oxidase −A and −B, succinate dehydrogenase and acid phosphatase in the rat brain after hemitransection. *Naunyn Schmiedebergs Arch Pharmacol* 1981; 316:51.

10. Student AK, Edwards DJ: Subcellular localization of type A and B monoamine oxidase in rat brain. *Biochem Pharmacol* 1977; 26:2337.
11. Bowen DM, Davison AN: Biochem changes in the cholinergic system of the aging brain and in senile dementia. *Psychol Med* 1980; 10:315.
12. De Boni U, McLachlan DRC: Senile dementia and Alzheimer's disease: a current view. *Life Sci* 1980; 27:1.
13. Gottfries CG: Biochemical aspects of dementia, in van Praag HM, Lader MH, Rafaelsen OJ, et al (eds): *Handbook of Biological Psychiatry.* New York, Dekker, 1980, vol 4.

14 Changes in Protein Synthesis

David M. A. Mann

The brain's capacity for synthesizing proteins is high, comparable to that of liver and pancreatic tissue, where the production of proteins is assumed to be a main function. Much of this synthetic activity is directed toward the production of structural proteins; the 5–6-nm microfilament composed of actin, the 10-nm filament composing the principal cytoskeletal element of the nerve cell, and the 24-nm microtubule composed mainly of tubulin. Production of the latter accounts for 10–25% of the total protein output.

The ultrastructural hallmark of Alzheimer's disease (AD) is the accumulation within nerve cells of the cerebral cortex of paired helically wound filaments (PHFs) (Chap. 5), each strand of which resembles the 10-nm straight filament; these, en masse, constitute the structures commonly termed neurofibrillary tangles (NFTs). Under the light microscope, NFTs are readily demonstrated within the nerve cell body using silver impregnation techniques. However, electron microscopy shows PHFs to be present within the axon, as well as within the abnormal processes forming the neuritic or senile plaque (SP).

PHFs are widely present in the nerve cells of mentally preserved, but aged, individuals (1), and also in some long-surviving patients of all ages with chronic neurological illnesses (2). Yet their presence in concentrations of more than an order of magnitude higher in AD than in normally aged individuals (3, 4), together with a correlation between number of PHFs and degree of dementia (3, 4), implies that the disordering of production or assimilation of structural proteins may be a basic aspect of AD pathogenesis. Histological examination (Fig. 14–1a–d) shows that a progressive degeneration of the nerve cells of the cerebral cortex occurs in AD, (5), characterized by gradual loss of cytoplasmic basophilia and reduction in the size of the nucleus and nucleolus. The latter eventually fragment and disappear. Biochemical analysis (6) reveals a decreased RNA/DNA ratio in the temporal cortex, consistent with widespread diminished protein synthesis capacity (illustrated by the reduced nucleolar volume and cytoplasmic RNA content) in the temporal cortex and other areas in the brains of AD patients (Table 14–1) (5, 7–10). These findings are in accordance with the above cytological observations (Fig. 14–1). Moreover, these changes are not related to autolytic or other events occurring at, around, or following the time of death, nor do they seem to represent a late aspect of the disorder, occurring only in the chronically demented, since similar changes are present in biopsy specimens of the temporal cortex (5) from less affected individuals (Table 14–2).

Separate analysis of PHF- and non-PHF-containing nerve cells from autopsy tissues (10) shows that, as might be expected, protein synthesizing capacity is greatly reduced in the PHF cells (Table 14–3). However, protein production is also decreased, though to a lesser degree, in those nerve cells that do not contain PHFs (Table 14–3). At biopsy (11),

107

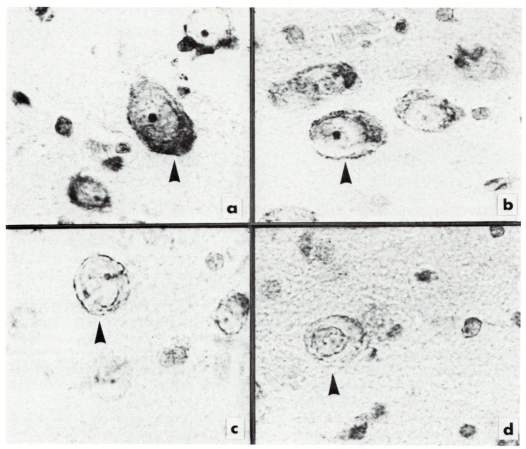

Figure 14–1. Nerve cells of temporal cortex in Alzheimer's disease at biopsy, showing from (a) to (d) a progressive loss of cytoplasmic basophilia, with shrinkage of nucleus and nucleolus, both of which fragment and disappear. Reproduced from Mann et al (5) by permission of the *Journal of Neurology, Neurosurgery and Psychiatry.*

however, protein synthesis is diminished equally in PHF- and non-PHF-containing cells (Table 14–4). These results, therefore, indicate that the ability of nerve cells of the cerebral cortex and of many other areas to produce proteins is altered early in the course of the illness, and may lead to the formation and intracellular accumulation of PHFs. Initially, the PHF material seems to be accommodated within the cell body without metabolic detriment. Eventually, however, when cells are heavy with PHFs, there is further reduction in protein synthesis. This may occur as a result of disruption and displacement of intracellular membranes and organelles, combined with disturbances of transport of substances within the cell body and its processes, affecting feedback mechanisms between the nucleus and cell terminals.

The appearance of PHFs in nerve cells may be a response to changes in protein metabolism within the cell. These changes may be:

1. induced by genetic changes following viral infection or metallic intoxication;
2. the result of a misassembly, or structural alteration, of normal neurofilament proteins;

TABLE 14–1
Widespread Reductions in Nucleolar Volume and Cytoplasmic RNA Content of Nerve Cells, of Types Shown, as Measured in Cases of Alzheimer's Disease and Age-Matched Controls, at Autopsy

Brain Area	Nucleolar Volume (μm³) Control	Nucleolar Volume (μm³) Alzheimer	% Loss from Alzheimer Group	Cytoplasmic RNA Content (Arbitrary Units) Control	Cytoplasmic RNA Content (Arbitrary Units) Alzheimer	% Loss from Alzheimer Group
Temporal cortex (3)	12.6 ± 0.7	7.0 ± 0.5	44.3	29.3 ± 1.5	15.2 ± 1.1	48.1
Temporal cortex (5)	14.5 ± 0.8	8.2 ± 0.5	43.7	31.3 ± 1.7	14.4 ± 1.2	54.0
Frontal cortex	16.0 ± 0.5	12.3 ± 0.9	23.2	26.7 ± 1.6	15.6 ± 0.9	41.6
Parietal cortex	16.1 ± 1.2	12.8 ± 1.2	20.5	20.8 ± 1.9	11.6 ± 0.7	44.3
Insular cortex	10.5 ± 0.7	7.9 ± 0.8	24.8	20.7 ± 1.0	12.6 ± 0.5	39.2
Entorhinal cortex	13.9 ± 0.9	10.6 ± 0.8	23.8	18.7 ± 1.2	10.3 ± 0.5	45.0
Amygdala	35.6 ± 2.1	20.0 ± 1.9	43.8	39.6 ± 1.4	22.7 ± 1.3	42.7
Hippocampus	25.2 ± 0.7	19.5 ± 0.6	22.5	20.6 ± 0.4	14.5 ± 0.6	41.6
Betz cell	65.6 ± 2.4	45.0 ± 1.9	31.4	53.7 ± 0.8	41.7 ± 1.0	22.3
Supraoptic	32.9 ± 2.0	25.1 ± 1.4	23.7	36.9 ± 1.0	26.6 ± 0.8	38.0
Paraventricular	32.7 ± 1.8	20.8 ± 1.2	36.4	35.2 ± 1.0	24.8 ± 0.9	29.5
Thalamus	26.8 ± 1.3	21.5 ± 1.2	19.8	25.8 ± 1.1	22.5 ± 0.8	13.0
Purkinje cell	43.3 ± 1.6	32.5 ± 1.6	25.1	31.6 ± 1.0	22.7 ± 2.6	28.2
Dentate nucleus	27.4 ± 1.2	20.0 ± 1.2	27.0	24.5 ± 1.0	16.3 ± 1.1	30.8
Inferior olives	21.2 ± 0.7	16.0 ± 0.7	24.5	11.2 ± 0.7	8.2 ± 1.2	26.2
Trigeminal	46.2 ± 1.8	37.8 ± 1.6	18.2	39.0 ± 1.6	32.1 ± 0.9	17.9
Facial	48.8 ± 1.9	39.2 ± 2.0	19.7	42.0 ± 1.9	28.2 ± 1.2	32.8
Hypoglossus	40.3 ± 1.5	30.6 ± 0.9	24.1	32.9 ± 1.3	29.2 ± 1.1	11.3

Source: Data reproduced in part with permission from the following journals: from Mann and Sinclair (7) by permission of the *Journal of Neuropathology and Applied Neurobiology;* from Mann, Yates, and Barton (8) by permission of the *Journal of Neurology, Neurosurgery and Psychiatry;* from Mann et al (5) by permission of the *Journal of Neurology, Neurosurgery and Psychiatry;* from Mann et al (9) by permission of *Lancet;* from Mann and Yates (10) by permission of *Mechanisms of Ageing and Development.*

TABLE 14–2
Mean Values of Nuclear Volume, Nucleolar Volume, and Cytoplasmic RNA Content of Pyramidal Cells of Layers 3 and 5 of Temporal Cortex, as Measured in 13 Cases of Alzheimer's Disease and 5 Controls; Tissue from Biopsy

	Nuclear Volume (μm³) Layer 3	Nuclear Volume (μm³) Layer 5	Nucleolar Volume (μm³) Layer 3	Nucleolar Volume (μm³) Layer 5	Cytoplasmic RNA Content (Arbitrary Units) Layer 3	Cytoplasmic RNA Content (Arbitrary Units) Layer 5
Control	1,714.3	2,017.8	17.7	18.1	36.3	37.9
(N = 5)	±71.1	±135.5	±0.5	±0.3	±0.7	±0.6
Alzheimer's disease		1,209.6	12.6	11.8	28.1	28.6
(N = 13)	±67.1	±90.6	±0.6	±0.5	±0.6	±0.7
% loss in Alzheimer's disease	42.5	40.1	28.8	34.8	22.6	24.6
Mean loss	41.3		31.8		23.6	

Source: Data reproduced in part from Mann et al (5) by permission of the *Journal of Neurology, Neurosurgery and Psychiatry.*

TABLE 14–3

Reduced Protein Synthesis Capacity of PHF-Containing and Non-PHF-Containing Nerve Cells, as Measured at Autopsy in 10 Different Areas of Brain in Alzheimer's Disease

Brain Area	Nucleolar Volume (μm³)			% Loss from Alzheimer Group	
	Control	Alzheimer		Non-PHF	PHF
		Non-PHF	PHF		
Frontal cortex	16.0 ± 0.9	12.6 ± 0.9	9.2 ± 0.7	21.3	42.5
Temporal cortex	14.5 ± 0.8	9.8 ± 0.6	8.0 ± 0.6	32.4	44.8
Occipital cortex	4.9 ± 0.3	3.6 ± 0.2	3.0 ± 0.2	26.5	38.8
Parietal cortex	16.1 ± 1.2	13.1 ± 1.0	9.7 ± 0.6	18.6	39.8
Insular cortex	10.5 ± 0.7	8.2 ± 0.7	6.1 ± 0.4	22.9	41.9
Motor cortex	15.9 ± 1.0	13.4 ± 0.8	10.0 ± 0.7	15.7	37.1
Entorhinal cortex	13.9 ± 0.9	10.9 ± 0.8	8.6 ± 0.5	21.6	38.1
Amygdala	35.6 ± 2.1	21.3 ± 1.8	18.6 ± 1.5	40.2	47.8
Hypothalamus	29.3 ± 1.8	22.0 ± 2.1	15.9 ± 1.2	24.9	45.7
Aqueductal grey matter	43.4 ± 2.0	30.8 ± 1.6	21.2 ± 1.4	29.0	51.2

Source: Data reproduced in part from Mann and Yates (10) by permission of *Mechanisms of Ageing and Development.*

3. derived from other protein pools, which undergo a configurational change;
4. the result of a failure of protein degradation leading to partially degraded filaments, forming PHFs.

Current evidence favors the preferential biosynthesis of a new protein following nucleus level alterations. For example, the amount of protein synthesizing euchromatin is reduced (12) and is accompanied at each stage in the degenerative process (see Fig. 14–1) by a greater reduction in nuclear volume than that of nucleolar volume or RNA content (Fig. 14–2) (both of which may be of normal value in the early stages). These findings suggest a selective "switching off" of part of the genome, with preference for production of certain protein species, rather than an overall decline in all cell proteins. In this context, it has recently been noted (13) that the amount of protein of molecular weight 20,000 (P 20) is

TABLE 14–4

Protein Synthesis Capacity Is Reduced Equally in PHF-Containing and Non-PHF-Containing Nerve Cells of Temporal Cortex, Measured in Five Biopsy Cases of Alzheimer's Disease Compared with Five Control Cases

Biopsy Case	Nucleolar Volume (μm³)		% Loss from Alzheimer Cases	
	Non-PHF	PHF	Non-PHF	PHF
Control mean	18.1 ± 0.3	—	—	—
1	10.7 ± 0.3	10.6 ± 0.4	42.1	42.3
2	9.8 ± 0.4	9.7 ± 0.3	47.1	46.3
3	13.4 ± 0.6	13.2 ± 0.6	27.6	28.3
4	11.2 ± 0.5	10.8 ± 0.4	38.4	41.7
5	9.9 ± 0.3	9.8 ± 0.3	46.2	46.9
Mean	11.0 ± 0.7	10.8 ± 0.6	40.4	41.2

Source: Data reproduced in part from Mann et al (11) by permission of the *Journal of Neuropathology and Applied Neurobiology.*

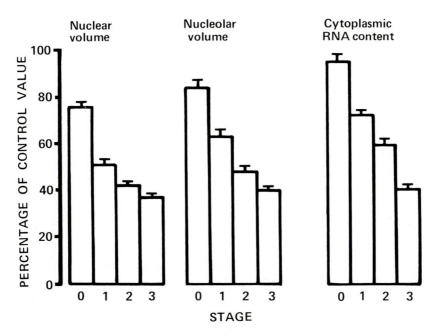

Figure 14–2. Histogram showing values of mean (±S.E.) nuclear and nucleolar volume and cytoplasmic RNA content, of nerve cells of temporal cortex at biopsy, expressed as percentage of control value and classed into stages 0 to 3, according to morphological appearance shown in Figs. 14–1(a) to (d), respectively. Reproduced from Mann et al (5) by permission of the *Journal of Neurology, Neurosurgery and Psychiatry.*

enhanced in neuron-enriched fractions of areas of the cerebral cortex rich in PHFs, but is not so increased in those areas relatively free of PHFs, implying that the P 20 protein may be related to the abnormal filament protein of AD.

RELATIONSHIPS BETWEEN CHANGES IN PROTEIN SYNTHESIS AND OTHER POSSIBLE ORIGINS OF AD

The possibility that these types of changes may be virally induced has long been attractive and, because of its propensity to produce latent infections, particularly of the temporal lobe, herpes simplex virus (HSV) has been thought a likely candidate, a suggestion strengthened by a report of raised HSV antibody in the cerebrospinal fluid (14). Although nucleic acid hybridization techniques (15, 16) have yielded ambiguous results, attempts to locate HSV or other viral genomes in AD brain tissue by immunohistochemical methods (17) have been unsuccessful. Similarly, some histocompatibility studies of HLA antigens (18, 19) have not pointed to any consistent differences in AD patients. Despite these essentially negative findings, however, the report (20) that an extract of AD brain tissue can induce PHFs in cultured nerve cells means an infective etiology remains worthy of consideration.

What is also possible is that the changes in protein production stem from the effects of intoxication of the brain, causing alterations in the functioning of enzymes concerned with DNA synthesis, repair, or transcription, and leading to a cascade of metabolic changes, of which PHFs may be just one facet. These may culminate in cellular dysfunction and, eventually, cell death.

In this respect, there has been some controversy over the past years as to whether aluminum exerts a toxic effect on the nervous system and, if so, whether this is an important factor in the pathogenesis of AD. Since aluminum binds to DNA (21) and can be detected mainly in those nerve cells containing PHFs, (22) the premise is that interference with transcription of genetic information occurs, with the formation of PHFs resulting. Indeed, experimental aluminum encephalopathy causes neurofibrillary degeneration of nerve cells in certain species (21). But although the aluminum is again DNA-bound (23), the induced neurofibrils are structurally dissimilar to PHFs (24). Furthermore, although in AD brain aluminum levels are often increased (25–27), this does not seem to be a result of serum level elevation (28, 29) as in renal dialysis encephalopathy, where both brain (30) and serum (28) levels are elevated. In renal dialysis encephalopathy, brain aluminum is cytoplasm bound (31) and no PHFs are formed. (32)

Thus, while it may well be that, in situations such as renal dialysis, aluminum exerts a direct toxic effect on nerve cell metabolism, it is less certain whether in AD aluminum causes PHFs, or whether its presence is responsible for or even necessary for, the early changes in protein synthesis. Indeed, since elevated levels of other metals are seen in AD (33) and metals other than aluminum are increased in non-AD neurological disorders, (27). it may be that the ability to concentrate metals from their immediate environment is a secondary characteristic of already changed nerve cells. The effects of this concentration may, however, cause still additional tissue or cellular damage that may compound, or even be necessary for, full clinical expression of the condition.

If metal toxins are held to play a vital role in the pathogenic process, one must consider how the toxins accumulate, given that serum concentrations may be within normal limits. The rate of blood flow through, and the permeability of, the cerebral microcirculation are regulated by the noradrenaline-containing neurons of the locus ceruleus (34). These cells, acting in conjunction with those of the hypothalamus and dorsal motor nucleus of the vagus nerve, maintain homeostasis within the CNS (35) by monitoring, via pituitary and parasympathetic contacts, changed conditions at the periphery. In AD there is severe atrophy and loss of the cells of the locus ceruleus and dorsal motor nucleus of the vagus (36) (Table 14–5). There are also decreases in brain noradrenaline (37), its metabolite (38), MHPG, and the noradrenaline-synthesizing enzyme, dopamine β hydroxylase (39). Reduced function occurs in the cells of the hypothalamus (9) (Table 14–1). Loss of noradrenaline cells, together with changes in the functional integrity of their associated pathways, may lead to foci of losses of control over permeability within the microcirculation, which eventually culminate in failure of the blood brain barrier. This process permits accumulation within the brain of metals or other substances with potential toxic effects. Findings of various serum proteins, as well as immunoglobulins, within senile plaques (SPs) near damaged blood vessels in cases of AD, multi-infarct dementia, and aged controls (40) would also support this supposition.

Furthermore, the dementia, or gross mental impairment seen in conditions such as Down's syndrome, dementia pugilistica, Parkinson's disease, or progressive supranuclear palsy, may also be partly due to the loss and degeneration of the locus ceruleus nerve cells occurring in all of these conditions (41), disorders in which neurofibrillary pathology also forms a common aspect. Because of their widespread nerve networks and general regulatory effect, changes in these cells could plausibly lead to global impairment of brain function through extensive alterations in protein synthesis, even leading to PHF formation following secondary intoxication or viral action. Why these particular cell types should be damaged in the first instance is not clear. One explanation may be their predilection (in middle age and later life) to accumulate excessive quantities of melanin pigment (42), a substance known

TABLE 14–5

Mean (±S.E.) Number of Nucleolated Neurons per 20-μm Section and Nucleolar Volume of Nerve Cells of Locus Ceruleus and Vagus Nerve Nucleus in Alzheimer's Disease and in Age-Matched Controls. Also Shown Is Percentage Cell Loss and Reduction in Nucleolar Volume in Alzheimer Group

Cell	Mean Number of Nucleolated Nerve Cells		% Loss from Alzheimer Group
	Control ($N = 21$)	Alzheimer ($N = 19$)	
Locus ceruleus	75.8 ± 3.2	34.3 ± 3.8	54.8
Vagus	7.2 ± 0.3	2.9 ± 0.3	59.5
Cell	Mean Nucleolar Volume (μm³)		% Loss from Alzheimer Group
	Control ($N = 21$)	Alzheimer ($N = 19$)	
Locus ceruleus	69.9 ± 1.0	56.6 ± 1.8	19.0
Vagus	52.6 ± 0.8	39.3 ± 1.4	25.2

Source: Data reproduced from Mann et al (36) by permission of the *Journal of Neurology, Neurosurgery and Psychiatry.*

to be associated with cytotoxic effects. (43) This process may render the neural cells weak and particularly vulnerable, consequently, to "attack" by extraneous agents.

REFERENCES

1. Tomlinson BE, Blessed G, Roth M: Observations on the brains of nondemented old people. *J Neurol Sci* 1968; 7:331–356.

2. Wisniewski K, Jervis GA, Moretz RC, et al: Alzheimer neurofibrillary tangles in diseases other than senile and presenile dementia. *Ann Neurol* 1979; 5:288–294.

3. Tomlinson BE, Blessed G, Roth M: Observations on the brains of demented old people. *J Neurol Sci* 1970; 11:205–242.

4. Ball MJ: Neurofibrillary tangles and the pathogenesis of dementia: a quantitative study. *Neuropathol Appl Neurobiol* 1976; 2:394–410.

5. Mann DMA, Neary D, Yates PO, et al: Alterations in protein synthetic capability of nerve cells in Alzheimer's disease. *J Neurol Neurosurg Psychiatry* 1981; 44:97–102.

6. Bowen DM, Smith CB, White P, et al: Chemical pathology of the organic dementias. *Brain* 1977; 100:427–453.

7. Mann DMA, Sinclair KGA: The quantitative assessment of lipofuscin pigment, cytoplasmic RNA, and nucleolar volume in senile dementia. *Neuropathol Appl Neurobiol* 1978; 4:129–135.

8. Mann DMA, Yates PO, Barton CM: Cytophotometric mapping of neuronal changes in senile dementia. *J Neurol Neurosurg Psychiatry* 1977; 40:299–302.

9. Mann DMA, Yates PO, Bansal DV, et al: Hypothalamus and dementia. *Lancet* 1981; i:393–394.

10. Mann DMA, Yates PO: The relationship between formation of senile plaques and neurofibrillary tangles and changes in nerve cell metabolism in Alzheimer-type dementia. *Mech Ageing Dev* 1981; 17:395–401.

11. Mann DMA, Neary D, Yates PO, et al: Neurofibrillary pathology and protein synthetic capability in nerve cells in Alzheimer's disease. *Neuropathol Appl Neurobiol* 1981; 7:37–47.

12. Crapper DR, Quittkat S, De Boni U: Altered chromatin conformation in Alzheimer's disease. *Brain* 1979; 102:483–495.

13. Selkoe DJ: Altered protein composition of isolated human cortical neurons in Alzheimer's disease. *Ann Neurol* 1980; 8:468–478.

14. Libikova H, Pogady J, Wiedermann V: Search for herpetic antibodies in CSF in senile dementia and mental retardation. *Acta Virol* 1975; 19:493–495.

15. Sequiera LW, Carrasco LH, Curry A, et al: Detection of Herpes simplex viral genome in brain tissue. *Lancet* 1979; ii:609–612.

16. Middleton PJ, Petric M, Kozak M, et al: Herpes simplex viral genome and the senile and presenile dementias of Alzheimer and Pick. *Lancet* 1980; i:1038.

17. Mann DMA, Yates PO, Davies JS, et al: Viruses, parkinsonism, and Alzheimer's disease. *J Neurol Neurosurg Psychiatry* 1981; 44:651.

18. Sulkava R, Koskimies S, Wikstrom J, et al: HLA antigens in Alzheimer's disease. *Tissue Antigens* 1980; 16:191–194.

19. Wilcox CB, Caspary EA, Behan PO: Histocompatibility antigens in Alzheimer's disease. *Eur Neurol* 1981; 20:25–28.

20. De Boni U, Crapper DR: Paired helical filaments of the Alzheimer type in cultured neurons. *Nature* 1978; 271:566–568.

21. Klatzo I, Wisniewski HM, Streicher E: Experimental production of neurofibrillary degeneration. *J Neuropathol Exp Neurol* 1965; 24:187–199.

22. Perl DR, Brody AR: Detection of local accumulations of aluminum (Al) and silicon (Si) within neurofibrillary tangle bearing neurons of Alzheimer's disease. *J Neuropathol Exp Neurol* 1979; 38:335.

23. De Boni U, Scott JW, Crapper DR: Intracellular aluminum binding: a histochemical study. *Histochemistry* 1974; 40:31–37.

24. Terry RD, Pena C: Experimental production of neurofibrillary degeneration. *J Neuropathol Exp Neurol* 1965; 24:200–210.

25. Crapper DR, Krishnan SS, Quittkat S: Aluminum, neurofibrillary degeneration, and Alzheimer's disease. *Brain* 1976; 99:67–80.

26. Trapp GA, Miner GP, Zimmerman RL, et al: Aluminum levels in brain in Alzheimer's disease. *Biol Psychiatry* 1978; 13:709–718.

27. Traub RD, Rains TC, Garruto RM, et al: Brain destruction alone does not elevate brain aluminum. *Neurology* 1981; 31:986–990.

28. Crapper DR, Karlick S, de Boni U: Aluminum and other metals in senile (Alzheimer) dementia. *Aging NY* 1978; 7:471–485.

29. Shore D, Millson M, Holtz JL, et al: Serum aluminum in primary degenerative dementia. *Biol Psychiatry* 1980; 15:971–977.

30. McDermott JR, Smith AI, Ward MK, et al: Brain aluminum concentration in dialysis encephalopathy. *Lancet* 1978; i:901–904.

31. Crapper DR, Quittkat S, Krishnan SS, et al: Intranuclear aluminum content in Alzheimer's disease, dialysis encephalopathy, and experimental aluminum encephalopathy. *Acta Neuropathol* 1980; 50:19–24.

32. Burks JS, Alfrey AC, Huddleston J, et al: A fatal encephalopathy in chronic hemodialysis patients. *Lancet* 1976; i:764–768.

33. Yoshimasu F, Yasui M, Yase Y, et al: Studies on amyotrophic lateral sclerosis by neutron activation analysis. *Folia Psychiatr Neurol Jpn* 1980; 34:75–82.

34. Raichle ME, Hartman BK, Eichling JO, et al: Central noradrenergic regulation of cerebral blood flow and vascular permeability. *Proc Natl Acad Sci USA* 1975; 72:3726–3730.

35. Swanson LW, Hartman BK: Biochemical specificity in central pathways related to peripheral and intracerebral homeostatic function. *Neurosci Lett* 1980; 16:55–60.

36. Mann DMA, Yates PO, Hawkes JS: The noradrenergic system in Alzheimer's and multi-infarct dementias. *J Neurol Neurosurg Psychiatry* 1982; 45:113–119.

37. Mann DMA, Lincoln J, Yates PO, et al: Changes in monoamine containing neurons of the human CNS in senile dementia. *Br J Psychiatry* 1980; 136:533–541.

38. Mann DMA, Lincoln J, Yates PO, et al: Monoamine metabolism in Down's syndrome. *Lancet* 1980; ii:1366–1367.

39. Cross AJ, Crow TJ, Perry EK, et al: Reduced dopamine-β-hydroxylase activity in Alzheimer's disease. *Br Med J* 1981; 1:93–94.

40. Mann DMA, Davies JS, Yates PO, et al: Immunohistochemical staining of senile plaques. *Neuropathol Appl Neurobiol* 1982; 8:55–61.

41. Mann DMA, Yates PO, Hawkes J: Pathology of the human locus ceruleus. *Clin Neuropathol* 1983; 2:1–7.

42. Mann DMA, Yates PO: Lipoprotein pigments: their relationship to aging in the human nervous system: II. The melanin content of pigmented nerve cells. *Brain* 1974; 97:489–498.

43. Graham DG, Tiffany SM, Bell WR: Auto-oxidation versus covalent binding of quinones as the mechanism of toxicity of dopamine, 6-hydroxy-dopamine, and related compounds towards C1300 neuroblastoma cells *in vitro. Mol Pharmacol* 1978; 14:644–653.

15 Pathologic Association of Aluminum in Alzheimer's Disease

Daniel P. Perl

THE CLASSIC TRIAD OF NEUROPATHOLOGIC LESIONS encountered in the brains of individuals with Alzheimer's disease (AD) consists of neurofibrillary tangles (NFTs), senile or neuritic plaques (SPs), and granulovacuolar degeneration (GVD) of Simchowitz. Although the neuropathologic hallmark of AD, NFTs are not confined exclusively to this condition, as NFTs are encountered in association with a wide variety of conditions (1). These include postencephalitic parkinsonism (2, 3), Down's syndrome (4, 5), posttraumatic dementia (dementia pugilistica) (6, 7), amyotrophic lateral sclerosis–parkinsonism dementia complex endemic to the Chamorro people of Guam (8, 9), subacute sclerosing panencephalitis (SSPE) (10), chronic manganese poisoning (11), and lead poisoning (12, 13). While this list embraces diseases related to a wide range of etiologic factors, the formative mechanism for NFTs in each diverse clinical setting remains unknown, and may reflect common underlying pathogenetic mechanisms for this specific neuronal response.

Recently, data have been presented to suggest that aluminum accumulation in the brain may play a role in the pathogenesis of senile dementia; more specifically, in the formation of the NFTs associated with this condition. This concept stems initially from a 1965 report of the experimental induction of neurofibrillary degeneration in rabbits by exposure to aluminum salts (14), accomplished by the inoculation of aluminum phosphate into the rabbit cerebral cortex. Within 14 days, the rabbits exhibited generalized seizures as well as changes in neurons which, by light microscopic criteria, were relatively similar to naturally occurring NFTs.

Aluminum salts other than aluminum phosphate were tried successfully, and it was subsequently learned that the cat and the ferret are also susceptible to this alteration, whereas mice, rats, and the rhesus monkey are resistant to neurofibrillary changes following comparable aluminum exposure (15). Cats exposed to aluminum have shown deficits in short-term retention of newly learned tasks (16) and decreased rates of acquisition of conditioned avoidance responses (16, 17). Repeated subcutaneous injections of aluminum lactate or aluminum tartrate in rabbits have been reported to produce elevated brain aluminum levels with subsequent widespread neurofibrillary degeneration (15). *In vitro* induction of neurofibrillary changes by aluminum salts has also been reported in dorsal root ganglion organ cultures (18) and in mouse neuroblastoma cell cultures (19).

Ultrastructural examination of the aluminum-induced neurofibrillary changes has revealed that the experimental tangles consist of 10-nm straight filaments (20), a diameter comparable to that of the filamentous accumulations seen in the human NFTs of AD; however, the aluminum-induced tangles do not take on the paired helical configuration encountered in human NFTs. Recently, Wisniewski and co-workers (21) described a chronic animal model for aluminum-induced neurofibrillary changes utilizing repeated intracysternal or intraventricular inoculation of aluminum chloride in young rabbits. Although the distribution of lesions and clinical characteristics of the young rabbits were somewhat different from those seen in adult animals exposed to a single injection of an aluminum salt, no significant ultrastructural differences were noted in the tangles characteristic of these relatively long-term studies. Of interest is the finding of fewer NFTs in animals examined at 85 and 100 days following aluminum chloride exposure, suggesting the apparent reversibility of neurofibrillary degeneration in this experimental model.

In 1973, Crapper and co-workers (22, 23) reported the presence of increased aluminum in the brains of four individuals with senile dementia as compared to nondemented controls. Further work attempted to correlate regional brain aluminum concentration with the presence of senile changes in specific brain regions (24). The investigation involved determination of the aluminum concentration of 585 samples derived from the brains of ten autopsied AD patients. The aluminum concentrations ranged from 0.4 to 107.0μg/g of dry weight; 28% of the samples had an aluminum level greater than 4.0μg/g. Five of six cerebral cortical biopsies from AD patients also revealed an elevated aluminum content. (The mean aluminum concentration of seven brains derived from neurologically normal individuals was 1.9 $\pm$ 0.75 μg/g of dry weight.) The investigators concluded that brain aluminum concentrations greater than 4.0μg/g were abnormally high and correlated positively with the presence of senile changes. This level of aluminum accumulation is roughly comparable with those obtained in cats with experimentally induced neurofibrillary degeneration (4.0–6.0μg/g) (23).

Aluminum levels were assayed by atomic absorption spectroscopy. There was considerable regional variation in the aluminum concentration of any particular brain specimen, with the highest amounts present in those areas containing the most prominent senile changes (frontal and temporal cortex of the hippocampus). Because the assay system destroyed tissue, the authors were unable to further localize the aluminum within the samples. Nevertheless, they suggested a correlation between excess aluminum and sampled areas abundant in NFTs; lesser amounts of aluminum were present in areas with only SPs and relatively few NFTs.

Corroborative attempts by others to reproduce these findings have met with varied success. McDermott and associates (25, 26) reported increased brain aluminum concentration with normal human aging but failed to detect a significant difference in brain aluminum content between AD patients and age-matched controls. Trapp and co-workers (27) found brain aluminum levels 1.4 times greater in patients with AD than in age-matched controls; the differences were significant ($P > .05$). All of these studies used atomic absorption spectroscopy, but differing methods of tissue digestion, sample preparation, and assay configuration. Using instrumental neutron activation analysis, Markesbury and co-workers (28) recently reported brain aluminum content for AD and aged controls. They found no significant difference in brain aluminum content between AD patients and controls.

de Boni and co-workers (29) attempted to further localize excess aluminum in the tissues by means of a histochemical procedure employing the fluorescent dye morin. Morin is a dye which combines with aluminum to produce a bright yellow fluorescence when exposed to ultraviolet illumination. Morin stains demonstrated fluorescence in the nuclei of neurons and astroglia in the cerebral cortex and the hippocampal pyramidal neurons of cats with aluminum-induced encephalopathy. Capillary endothelial cells and ependymal cells also showed positive fluorescence. Human senile changes were apparently not examined in this study. Cell fractionation studies of specimens derived from both AD patients and cats and rats exposed intercerebrally to aluminum have revealed excess accumulation of the element within nuclear and chromatin fractions, particularly within the heterochromatin components (30).

Brief mention should be made of the association of aluminum with the progressive encephalopathic syndrome occurring in patients chronically on hemodialysis (31, 32). This condition, referred to as "dialysis dementia," includes dementia, dyspraxia, myoclonus, focal and grand mal seizures, and a characteristic EEG pattern. Studies have shown a dramatic accumulation of aluminum within the grey matter of the cerebral cortex of patients with this condition. Such aluminum accretion in the brain has been related to ingestion of large amounts of aluminum containing phosphate binding gels (33) or to aluminum present in the dialysate solution. (34) These dialysis patients do not show neuropathologic evidence of senile changes despite the high levels of aluminum in the brain. Galle and associates (35), using x-ray microprobe analysis, demonstrated aluminum accumulation within lysosomes of neurons in the cerebral cortex of aluminum exposed rats, as well as in two patients with dialysis dementia (36). Crapper and co-workers (30) reported relatively low aluminum levels within the nuclear fraction of five brains derived from patients with dialysis dementia. Whether this difference in aluminum distribution within the brain is responsible for the absent neurofibrillary tangle formation in these cases remains unknown.

Perl and Brody (37, 38) used scanning electron microscopy (SEM), in conjunction with x-ray spectrometry, to analyze intraneuronal trace element composition. With these sensitive techniques, aluminum accumulations within the nuclear region of neurofibrillary tangle-bearing neurons of the hippocampus were identified from autopsied AD patients. For these studies, frozen tissue sections were stained using a modified Bielschowsky silver-impregnation method prior to their examination in the electron microscope. The backscattered electron-imaging capabilities of the SEM successfully disclosed the NFTs and SPs. In this way, individual neurons could be determined to be tangle-bearing or tangle-free prior to multipoint x-ray energy analysis. In initial studies on three cases of AD, 91.2% of tangle-bearing hippocampal neurons demonstrated a peak corresponding to the $K\alpha$ energy emission of aluminum in any of the four probe sites in the nuclear region of the cell (37, 38). Overall, 38.4% of the nuclear probe sites were positive for aluminum within these cells. In contrast, only 3.8% of the adjacent nontangled neurons from the AD cases emitted a peak for aluminum in the nuclear region. Examination of numerous tangle-free neurons from elderly nondemented subjects failed to show evidence of aluminum emission (5.9% of cells positive).

It is still unclear whether aluminum plays an active role in the pathogenetic sequence leading to NFT formation in AD. The aluminum accumulations demonstrated by SEM–x-ray spectroscopy may reflect nonspecific uptake of the element by a malfunctioning, partially damaged cell. In order to clarify these questions, Perl (39) recently attempted to evaluate the elemental content of NFT-bearing neurons encountered in other clinical settings. The study reported aluminum peaks comparable to those found in AD specimens in the tangle-bearing neurons of a case of Down's syndrome with extensive senile changes. Work has also begun on evaluating the noted tendency toward NFT formation exhibited by the Chamorro natives of Guam (40). The tendency toward NFT formation in the Chamorro population is accompanied by an inordinately high incidence of parkinsonism in association with severe dementia and amyotrophic lateral sclerosis (ALS). Perl and co-workers (40) recently reported preliminary evidence of prominent intraneuronal aluminum accumulation within

NFT-bearing hippocampal neurons of patients manifesting the ALS–parkinsonism dementia complex of Guam. These data tend to support the hypothesis that aluminum plays an active role in the induction of NFTs and that environmental conditions unique to Guam may play a significant role in the neurodegenerative phenomena encountered there.

Aluminum is encountered widely in our environment, primarily in geologic forms, yet it serves no known biologic function (41). This element constitutes approximately 8% of the earth's crust; as such, aluminum is our most abundant metallic element. The selective intraneuronal accumulation of aluminum in association with NFT formation as seen in a number of clinical settings has yet to be explained. Trapp and associates (27) suggested that aluminum may bind with tubulin and thus interfere with the formation of microtubules. An analogy can be made to the induction of 10-nm filamentous accumulations associated with colchicine intoxication and vinca alkaloid poisoning, compounds known to bind with tubulin, and thus prevent its assembly into organized microtubules. It has been suggested that neurofilamentous elements accumulate in the perikaryal cytoplasm due to failure of assembly of essential subunits into neurotubular elements, or to impaired axoplasmic flow related to the neurotubular deficiency. In addition, aluminum is known to bind with DNA and at least at high doses does interfere with the reaggregation of DNA strands following thermal denaturation (42); it is still unclear whether aluminum binding to DNA causes errors in DNA transcription.

REFERENCES

1. Wisniewski K, Jervis GA, Moretz RC, et al: Alzheimer neurofibrillary tangles in diseases other than senile and presenile dementia. *Ann Neurol* 1979; 5:288–294.

2. Hirano A: Neurofibrillary changes in conditions related to Alzheimer's disease, in Wolstenholme GEW, O'Connor M (eds): *Alzheimer's Disease and Related Conditions.* London, Churchill, 1970, pp 185–201.

3. Wisniewski H, Terry RD, Hirano A: Neurofibrillary pathology. *J Neuropathol Exp Neurol* 1970; 29:163–176.

4. Burger PC, Vogel FS: Development of pathologic changes of Alzheimer's disease and senile dementia in patients with Down's syndrome. *Am J Pathol* 1973; 73:457–476.

5. Ellis WG, McColloch JR, Corley CL: Presenile dementia in Down's syndrome: ultrastructural identity with Alzheimer's disease. *Neurology* 1974; 24:101–106.

6. Corsellis JAN, Bruton CJ, Freeman-Browne D: The aftermath of boxing. *Psychol Med* 1973; 3:270–275.

7. Wisniewski HM, Narang HK, et al: Ultrastructural studies of the neuropil and neurofibrillary tangles in Alzheimer's disease and post-traumatic dementia. *J Neuropathol Exp Neurol* 1976; 35:367.

8. Malamud N, Hirano A, Kurland LT: Pathoanatomic changes in amyotrophic lateral sclerosis on Guam: special reference to the occurrence of neurofibrillary changes. *Arch Neurol* 1961; 19:573–578.

9. Hirano A, Malamud N, Kurland LT: Parkinsonism–dementia complex, an endemic disease on the island of Guam: II. pathological features. *Brain* 1961; 84:662–679.

10. Mandybur TI, Nagpaul AS, Pappas Z, et al: Alzheimer neurofibrillary change in subacute sclerosing panencephalitis. *J Neuropathol Exp Neurol* 1976; 35:300.

11. Banta RG, Markesbury WR: Elevated manganese levels associated with dementia and extrapyramidal signs. *Neurology* 1977; 27:213–216.

12. Niklowitz WJ, Mandybur TI: Neurofibrillary change following childhood encephalopathy: case report. *J Neuropathol Exp Neurol* 1975; 34:445–455.

13. Niklowitz WJ: Neurofibrillary changes after acute experimental lead poisoning. *Neurology* 1975; 25:927–934.

14. Klatzo I, Wisniewski H, Streicher E: Experimental production of neurofibrillary degeneration: I. Light microscopic observations. *J Neuropathol Exp Neurol* 1965; 24:187–199.

15. Crapper DR, Karlik S, de Boni U: Aluminum and other metals in senile (Alzheimer) dementia. *Aging NY* 1978; 7:471–489.

16. Crapper DR, Dalton AJ: Alterations in short-term retention, conditioned avoidance-response acquisition, and motivation following aluminum induced neurofibrillary degeneration. *Phys Behav* 1973; 10:925–933.

17. Crapper DR, Dalton AJ: Aluminum induced neurofibrillary degeneration, brain electrical activity, and alterations in acquisition and retention. *Physiology & Behavior* 1973; 10:935–945.

18. Seil FJ, Lampert PW, Klatzo I: Neurofibrillary spheroids induced by aluminum phosphate in dorsal root ganglia neurons *in vitro*. *J Neuropathol Exp Neurol* 1969; 28:74.

19. Miller CA, Levine EM: Effects of aluminum salts on cultured neuroblastoma cells. *J Neurochem* 1974; 22:751–758.

20. Terry RD, Pena C: Experimental production of neurofibrillary degeneration. *J Neuropathol Exp Neurol* 1965; 24:200–210.

21. Wisniewski HM, Sturman JA, Shek JW: Aluminum chloride induced neurofibrillary changes in the developing rabbit: a chronic animal model. *Ann Neurol* 1980; 8:479–490.

22. Crapper DR, Krishnan SS, Dalton AJ: Brain aluminum in Alzheimer's disease and experimental neurofibrillary degeneration. *Trans Am Neurol Assoc* 1973; 98:17–20.

23. Crapper DR, Krishnan SS, Dalton AJ: Brain aluminum distribution in Alzheimer's disease and experimental neurofibrillary degeneration. *Science* 1973; 180:511.

24. Crapper DR, Krishnan SS, Quittkat S: Aluminum neurofibrillary degeneration and Alzheimer's disease. *Brain* 1976; 99:67–80.

25. McDermott JR, Smith AI, Iqbal K, et al: Aluminum and Alzheimer's disease. *Lancet* 1977; ii:710.

26. McDermott JR, Smith AI, Iqbal K, et al: Brain aluminum in aging and Alzheimer's disease. *Neurology* 1979; 29:809–814.

27. Trapp GA, Miner GD, Zimmerman RL, et al: Aluminum levels in the brain in Alzheimer's disease. *Biol Psychol* 1978; 13:709–718.

28. Markesbury WR, Ehmann WD, Hossain TIM, et al: Instrumental neutron activation analysis of brain aluminum in Alzheimer's disease and aging. *Ann Neurol* 1981; 10:511–516.

29. de Boni U, Scott JW, Crapper DR: Intracellular aluminum binding: a histochemical study. *Histochemistry* 1974; 40:31–37.

30. Crapper DR, Quittkat S, Krishnan SS, et al: Intranuclear aluminum content in Alzheimer's disease, dialysis encephalopathy, and experimental aluminum encephalopathy. *Acta Neuropathol* 1980; 50:19–24.

31. Alfrey AC, LeGendre FR, Kaehny WD: The dialysis encephalopathy syndrome: possible aluminum intoxication. *N Engl J Med* 1976; 294:184–188.

32. Burks JS, Huddleston J, Alfrey AC, et al: A fatal encephalopathy in chronic hemodialysis patients. *Lancet* 1976; i:764.

33. Kaehny WD, Hegg AP, Alfrey AC: Gastrointestinal absorption of aluminum from aluminum-containing antacids. *N Engl J Med* 1977; 296:1389–1390.

34. Ward MK, Ellis HA, Feest TG, et al: Osteomalacic dialysis osteodystrophy: evidence for a water-borne etiological agent, probably aluminum. *Lancet* 1978; i:841.

35. Galle P, Berry JP, Duckett S: Electron microprobe ultrastructural localization of aluminum in rat brain. *Acta Neuropathol* 1980; 49:245–247.

36. Galle P, Chatel M, Berry JP, et al: Progressive dialytic encephalopathy. *Nouv Presse Med* 1979; 8:1071.

37. Perl DP, Brody AR: Detection of focal accumulations of aluminum (Al) and silicon (Si) within neurofibrillary tangle-bearing neurons of Alzheimer's disease. *J Neuropathol Exp Neurol* 1979; 38:335.

38. Perl DP, Brody AR: Alzheimer's disease: x-ray spectrometric evidence of aluminum accumulation in neurofibrillary tangle-bearing neurons. *Science* 1980; 208:297–299.

39. Perl DP: SEM–x-ray spectrometric studies of aluminum in neurofibrillary tangle-bearing neurons, in Hirano A, Miyoshi K (eds): *Neuropsychiatric Disorders in the Elderly.* Tokyo, Igaku–shoin, 1983, pp. 52–58.

40. Perl DP, Gajdusek DC, Garruto RM, et al: Intraneuronal aluminum accumulation in amyotrophic lateral sclerosis and parkinsonism dementia of Guam. *Science* 1982; 217:1053–1055.

41. Underwood EJ: *Trace Elements in Human and Animal Nutrition.* New York, Academic, 1977.

42. Karlik SJ, Eichhorn GL, Lewis PN, et al: Interaction of aluminum species with deoxyribonucleic acid. *Biochemistry* 1980; 19:5991–5998.

16 Biochemical Changes in Blood and Cerebrospinal Fluid

CARL-GERHARD GOTTFRIES

SINCE BIOPSIES CANNOT USUALLY be performed directly from the human brain, the investigation of brain material must generally be done postmortem. In the living patient the investigation of cerebrospinal fluid (CSF) can give valid information about the metabolism in brain tissue. It is possible that Alzheimer's disease (AD) is not entirely localized in the CNS; findings in fact indicate that other parts of the body are also involved in this dementing disorder. It may therefore also be of value to study changes in the blood. Findings in the blood may to some extent also reflect the metabolism of the brain. In this chapter blood- and CSF-findings in AD will be discussed.

CHANGES IN BLOOD

CHROMOSOME BANDING PATTERN

AD manifests itself sporadically, although a small number of cases are familial (1, 2). Cytogenetic studies have been performed with lymphocytes and in some investigations a pathological chromosome banding pattern in AD has been reported (3). Alzheimer patients have a higher frequency of acentric fragments than other dementia patients, which to a lesser extent were found in patients with multi-infarct dementia, but not in controls or patients with Down's syndrome (4). Normal chromosome banding patterns have also, however, been reported (5, 6). Further studies are needed before chromosome aberrations can be accepted as an etiological factor in AD (see Chaps. 21 and 22 in this volume).

GLUCOSE METABOLISM

Studies of the metabolism of glucose in patients with AD have shown pathological values. Demented patients have a lower fasting blood sugar and a smaller area under the glucose curve in loading tests, as compared to age-matched controls (7). The metabolism of glucose is dependent upon central neuroendocrine mechanisms, and the pathological findings may indicate disturbed central regulation.

PLATELET MONOAMINE OXIDASE

In postmortem investigations of human brain tissue, the activity of the enzyme MAO-B has been found to increase with age. In patients with AD there is a still higher increase of this enzyme activity. As the blood platelets contain the same type of enzyme, MAO-B, as the brain, the platelets from patients with AD were investigated (8). The platelet MAO-B activity was increased when compared to age-matched controls, which finding may suggest that the disease is associated with a generalized increase in MAO activity, although results from other tissues are necessary to confirm such a view. The finding indicates that biochemical changes in AD patients are not entirely localized to the brain.

SERUM LEVELS OF BIOPTERIN

In AD, levels of serum biopterin have also been investigated (9). The results revealed significantly reduced levels of serum biopterin in patients with AD when compared with normals, and with a group of confusional phase patients. Tetrahydrobiopterin is the essential cofactor in the hydroxylation of tyrosine, tryptophan, and phenylalanine. As there are biochemical findings indicating disturbed neurotransmitter function in the brain, this finding has special importance.

INVESTIGATIONS OF CEREBROSPINAL FLUID (CSF)

Postmortem investigations of human brains from patients with AD have shown disturbances of neurotransmitters and related enzyme activities. There are reports indicating that not only the metabolism of acetylcholine, but also monoamines such as GABA are disturbed. Hence, CSF investigations have focused on studying biochemical variables reflecting the brain metabolism of many neurotransmitter systems.

METABOLISM OF ACETYLCHOLINE

The biochemical evidence for altered cholinergic function in brains from patients with AD is well known (10–12) wherein the activity of choline acetyltransferase (CAT) and acetylcholinesterase (AChE) has been shown to be reduced.

There are methodological difficulties in studying cholinergic brain functions via CSF investigations. The lumbar CSF choline may relate closely to acetylcholine turnover in the brain (13), but the validity of this has been disputed (14). CSF from intracranial sites may be needed to accurately measure biochemical processes in brain tissue (15).

The relationship between the CSF content of acetylcholine occurring at extremely low levels, and the functional state of the central cholinergic system, remains to be determined.

Soininen and associates (16) investigated AChE in CSF from controls as well as patients with AD. There were significantly reduced levels of AChE in the AD patients; patients with severe dementia recorded the lowest activities.

AChE is the predominant cholinesterase in human CSF, while blood contains butyrylcholine esterase. In AD patients, the blood brain barrier is believed to be intact and the finding thus supports reduced AChE activity in brain tissue. The finding may reflect the loss of cholinergic neurons or disturbed cholinergic metabolism in the brain.

Modern biochemical methods capable of measuring small amounts of CSF constituents may perhaps improve the possibility of studying cholinergic brain function via CSF investigations.

METABOLISM OF MONOAMINES

Postmortem investigations of human brains have also revealed disturbances of the metabolism of monoamines in AD patients. The synthesis of dopamine (DA) and noradrenaline (norepinephrine) (NA), and the metabolism of these active neurotransmitters to their end metabolites, homovanillic acid (HVA) and 3-methoxy-4-hydroxy-phenylglycol (MHPG), can be seen in Figure 16–1. The synthesis and the breakdown of 5-hydroxytryptamine (5-HT) to its end metabolite, 5-hydroxyindolacetic acid (5-HIAA), is described in Figure 16–2. In the CSF the acid metabolites HVA and 5-HIAA are measurable; these acid metabolites are transported out from the fluid compartment by an active process. In normal aging it has been reported that there is an increase of these metabolites, perhaps due to reduced active transport from the CSF (17, 18). Methods have also been introduced to measure MHPG in the CSF. On the other hand, the active neurotransmitters DA, NA and 5-HT are not found in the CSF in measurable quantities.

If a patient is given probenecid, the acid metabolite outflow is reduced since probenecid blocks the transport mechanism. Probenecid has been used, therefore, as a loading test. If the accumulation of acid metabolites is studied, information can be obtained about monoamine brain turnover. The probenecid test is, however, far from perfect since the kinetics of CSF probenecid must be carefully monitored. Nevertheless this test is perhaps the only test utilized to study metabolic processes and monoamine function in human CSF (19).

AD patients, diagnosed on the basis of clinical criteria, have reduced levels of HVA and 5-HIAA in their CSF. These findings were first demonstrated in 1969 (20). A relationship could also be shown between the levels of HVA and 5-HIAA in the CSF and the degree of dementia (21–23). Although the reduced levels of HVA and 5-HIAA in CSF in patients with AD could not be confirmed by Mann, there have been other investigations in which the finding has been reproduced (24–28). In some of these investigations a correlation between reduced acid metabolite levels and degree of dementia has also been noted. Of interest is that the strongest relation is seen between the degree of dementia and the HVA level. No changes have been reported to date in MHPG levels in patients with AD (29).

The reduced activity in the monoaminergic neurotransmitters in patients with AD has stimulated treatment trials in which investigators attempt to activate these failing systems. CSF investigations have been used to study the pharmacodynamic effect of such treatment. Argentiero and Tavolato (25) treated AD-patients with brain phospholipids, because animal experiments had shown that these phospholipids did influence the metabolic pathways of cerebral catecholamines. By dint of CSF investigations they were able to demonstrate a significant increase in the levels of HVA and 5-HIAA after prolonged administration of brain phospholipids.

METABOLISM OF γ AMINOBUTYRIC ACID

GABA is considered an inhibitory transmitter in the CNS. The principal synthesizing enzyme is glutamic acid decarboxylase (GAD). Bowen and associates (30) found reduced levels of GAD in brains of AD patients. But this finding was later refuted, and biopsy studies by Spillane and associates (31) could not confirm GAD reductions in patients with

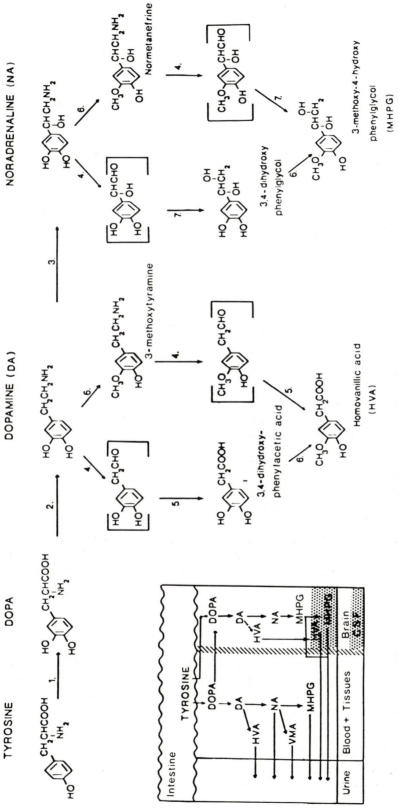

Figure 16-1. Synthesis and breakdown of dopamine and noradrenaline. CSF = cerebrospinal fluid; 1 = tyrosine hydroxylase; 2 = dopadecarboxylase; 3 = dopamine-β-hydroxylase; 4 = monoamine oxidase (MAO); 5 = aldehyde dihydrogenase; 6 = catechol-O-methyltransferase; 7 = aldehyde reductase. Inserted in the figure are the pathways in different tissues. As seen from the figure, those monoamines and monoamine metabolites which are found in urine and blood do not originate from the brain only, but come from other organs as well.

125

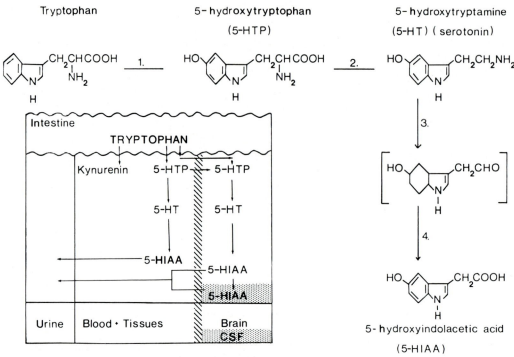

Figure 16–2. Synthesis and breakdown of 5-hydroxytryptamine (5-HT). CSF = cerebrospinal fluid; 1 = tryptophan hydroxylase; 2 = 5-hydroxytryptophan decarboxylase; 3 = monoamine oxidase (MAO); 4 = aldehyde dihydrogenase. Inserted in the figure is the pathway of 5-HT in different tissues. As seen from the figure, the 5-HT and 5-HIAA found in blood and urine do not come only from the brain but from other organs as well.

AD. Levels of GABA in the CSF have been studied by Enna and co-workers (32), in patients with neurological disorders. The patients included three subjects with AD; two of these had low levels of GABA in the CSF. In a study by Manyam and associates (33) GABA levels in the CSF were measured in a clinical group including 12 patients with dementia, 5 of whom were diagnosed as having AD. There were no significant differences between the subgroups of dementia; dementia patients with diverse etiologies had significantly reduced levels of GABA. Thus, a reduction of the GABA levels in the CSF in AD may occur.

PROTEIN PATTERNS IN CSF

CSF has been studied for its protein pattern in numerous degenerative diseases. The majority of CSF proteins are derived from plasma but the CSF also contains specific brain proteins. Accordingly, a separation technique has been introduced (34). In investigations of CSF from patients with senile dementia, characteristic changes in the CSF protein were found which differentiated AD patients from those with multi-infarct dementia (35).

IMMUNOGLOBINS

An interrelationship between the CNS and immune functions has been postulated. Cohen and associates (36) studied the correlation between serum levels of the immunoglobin IgG and IgM fractions with tests measuring intellectual functions, and disclosed a positive relationship. Also, based on the assumption that the etiology of AD may involve an infectious agent, such as a virus, the γ-globulin banding in CSF from patients with presenile dementia has been studied. Such a virus hypothesis became attractive with the discovery that Creutzfeldt–Jakob disease is caused by a slow virus. Using an agarose gel electrophoretic technique, Williams and co-workers (37) studied serum and CSF proteins in patients with presenile-onset dementia. The electrophoretic pattern demonstrated three homogeneous bands in the gamma globulin region in five of eight patients with AD. The bands were not present in the serum. The authors concluded that the bands found in the CSF of the AD patients supported the hypothesis that an infectious agent, or abnormal regulation of the immune system, is significant in the disease etiology.

METABOLISM OF ALUMINUM

Another hypothesis involving exogenous agents as contributors to AD is that of aluminum intoxication (38). At least, aluminum seems to accumulate in the brain of AD patients, indicating that the metabolism of heavy metals may be disturbed (39). Delaney (40) investigated the CSF aluminum level in patients with AD. His sample included 180 male patients with varying diagnoses. Although in most instances no correlation could be identified he noted ten AD patients who showed significantly lowered concentrations of CSF aluminum. This finding, however, contrasts with previous findings of high concentrations of aluminum in brain tissue. Thus pinpointing the relationship between brain tissue aluminum and CSF aluminum requires further study.

BRAIN HYPOXIA

An important and still unanswered question is whether the degenerative changes in brain tissue in AD are due to hypoxia. Both lactic and pyruvic acids diffuse readily into the CSF. It is well established that the lactate concentration and the lactate–pyruvate ratio in the CSF increase in acute hypoxic conditions (41). Lactate and pyruvate values in CSF have also been used to demonstrate brain tissue hypoxia in subacute conditions such as neonatal asphyxia (42). In an investigation by Gottfries and co-workers (23), 15 patients with AD were investigated for their CSF pyruvate and lactate levels. There were small but significant increases in the lactate concentration and lactate–pyruvate ratio, indicating that cellular hypoxia may indeed be present in AD.

SUMMARY

As it is not possible to take brain biopsies from living patients, the investigation of patients with degenerative diseases of the CNS must alternatively be done by examining other tissues such as the CSF and blood.

Investigations using blood tissue have sometimes revealed chromosomal aberrations in the lymphocytes. These findings are of particular interest since hereditary factors do play some role in the etiology of AD. The findings are, however, reported from investigations utilizing small quantities of specimens. Moreover, other investigators have found a normal chromosomal banding pattern in AD.

In AD the activity of MAO-B in brain tissue is increased. The platelets contain the same type of enzyme and it has been found that platelets from patients with AD manifest a higher activity of MAO-B than age-matched controls. This finding, based on limited patient material, has yet to be confirmed, but it provides further evidence that AD is not wholly localized in the brain.

Pathological glucose metabolism has been observed in patients with AD. The glucose loading test shows a flatter curve and a smaller area under the curve when these patients are compared to age-matched controls. Serum biopterin derivatives are found in reduced concentrations in patients with senile dementia. Tetrahydrobiopterin is an essential co-factor in the hydroxylation of tyrosine, tryptophan, and phenylalanine.

Postmortem investigations of brains from patients with AD have revealed reduced activity in some neurotransmitter systems. It appears that both the acetylcholine and the monoamine systems are damaged. It is difficult on the basis of CSF studies, however, to make conclusions about acetylcholine metabolism in the brain. The monoamines, however, can be studied by estimating their end metabolites in CSF. It is fairly well documented that the turnover of DA and 5-HT is reduced in patients with AD. In CSF, this is indicated by reduced levels of HVA and 5-HIAA, and a reduced accumulation of these acid metabolites during probenecid loading. The concentration of these acid metabolites is inversely related to the level of dementia. GABA levels seem to be reduced in the CSF from patients with AD, but investigations as of this time have been limited.

Brain-specific proteins have been studied in the CSF and characteristic patterns have been described in patients with SD. This finding may ultimately be of help in diagnostic work.

By agarose electrophoresis, it has been possible to demonstrate homogeneous bands in the γ-globulin reagent in the CSF of patients with AD. Though based on a small quantity of material, the finding supports the hypothesis that infectious agents, or abnormal regulation of the immune system, may be significant in the etiology of AD.

Increased levels of aluminum have been reported in brain tissue from patients with AD. Investigations of CSF provided the surprising finding that patients with AD have lower aluminum concentrations than controls.

The question whether there is a relative hypoxia in brains from patients with AD has been proposed. Studies of lactate and pyruvate in the CSF could not exclude the possibility of a relative hypoxia in brains from patients with AD.

REFERENCES

1. Zerbin, Rübin E: Hirnatropische Prozesse, in Becker PE (ed): *Humangenetik*. Stuttgart, Thieme, 1967, pp 84–146.

2. Pratt RTC: The genetics of Alzheimer's disease, in Wolstenholme, O'Connor (eds): *Alzheimer's Disease*. London, Churchill, 1970, pp 137–143.

3. Bergener M, Jungklaass FK: Genetische Befunde bei Morbus Alzheimer und seniler Demenz. *Gerontology* 1970; 71–75.

4. Nordenson I, Adolfsson R, Beckman G, et al: Chromosomal abnormality in dementia of Alzheimer type. *Lancet* 1980; i:481–482.

5. Mark J, Brun A: Chromosomal deviations in Alzheimer's disease compared to those in senescence and senile dementia. *Gerontology* 1973; 15:253–258.

6. Brun A, Gustafson L, Mitelman F: Normal chromosome banding pattern in Alzheimer's disease. *Gerontology* 1978; 24:369–372.

7. Adolfsson R, Bucht G, Lithner F, et al: Hypoglycemia in Alzheimer's disease: preliminary report. *Acta Med Scand* 1980; 208:387–388.

8. Adolfsson R, Gottfries CG, Oreland L, et al: Increased activity of brain and platelet monoamine oxidase in dementia of the Alzheimer type. *Life Sci* 1980; 27:1029–1034.

9. Leeming RJ, Blair JA, Melikian V: Biopterin derivatives in senile dementia. *Lancet* 1979; i:215.

10. Davies P, Maloney AJF: Selective loss of central cholinergic neurons in Alzheimer's disease. *Lancet* 1976; ii:1403.

11. Perry EK, Perry RH, Blessed G, et al: Necropsy evidence of central cholinergic deficits in senile dementia. *Lancet* 1977; i:189.

12. Bowen DM, Spillane JA, Curzon G, et al: Accelerated ageing or selective neuronal loss as an important cause of dementia? *Lancet* 1979; i:11–14.

13. Aquilonius SM, Schubert HJ, Sundwall A: Choline in the cerebrospinal fluid as a marker for the release of acetylcholine, in Heilbronn E, Winter A (eds): *Drugs and Cholinergic Mechanisms in the CNS*. Stockholm, Försvarets Forskningsanstalt, 1970, pp 399–410.

14. Schubert J, Jenden DJ: Transport of choline from plasma to cerebrospinal fluid in the rabbit with reference to the regions of choline and to acetylcholine metabolism in brain. *Brain Res* 1975; 84:245–256.

15. Haber B, Grossman RG: Acetylcholine metabolism in intracranial and lumbar cerebrospinal fluid and in blood, in Wood JH (ed): *Neurobiology of Cerebrospinal Fluid*. New York, Plenum, 1980, pp 345–351.

16. Soininen H, Halonen T, Riekkinen PJ: Acetylcholinesterase activities in cerebrospinal fluid of patients with senile dementia of the Alzheimer type. *Acta Neurol Scand* 1981; 64:217–224.

17. Bowers MB, Gerbode FA: Relationship of monoamine metabolites in human cerebrospinal fluid to age. *Nature* 1968; 219:1256–1257.

18. Gottfries CG, Gottfries I, Johansson B, et al: Acid monoamine metabolites in human cerebrospinal fluid and their relations to age and sex. *Neuropharmacology* 1971; 10:665–672.

19. Ebert NH, Kartzinel R, Cowdry RW, et al: Cerebrospinal fluid amine metabolites and probenecid test, in Wood JH (ed): *Neurobiology of Cerebrospinal Fluid*. New York, Plenum, 1980, pp 97–112.

20. Gottfries CG, Gottfries I, Roos BE: Homovanillic acid and 5-hydroxyindoleacetic acid in the cerebrospinal fluid of patients with senile dementia, presenile dementia and parkinsonism. *J Neurochem* 1969; 16:1341–1345.

21. Gottfries CG, Gottfries I, Roos BE: Homovanillic acid and 5-hydroxyindoleacetic acid in cerebrospinal fluid related to rated mental and motor impairment in senile and presenile dementia. *Acta Psychiatr Scand* 1970; 49:257–263.

22. Gottfries CG, Roos BE: Acid monoamine metabolites in cerebrospinal fluid from patients with presenile dementia (Alzheimer's disease). *Acta Psychiatr Scand* 1973; 49:257–263.

23. Gottfries CG, Kjällquist A, Pontén U, et al: Cerebrospinal fluid PH and monoamine and glucolytic metabolites in Alzheimer's disease. *Br J Psychiatry* 1974; 124:280–287.

24. Guard O, Renaud B, Chazot G: Métabolisme cérébral de la dopamine et de la sérotonine au cours des maladies d'Alzheimer et de Pick: étude dynamique par le test au probénecide. *Encephale* 1976; 2:293–303.

25. Argentiero V, Tavolato B: Dopamine (DA) and serotonin metabolic levels in the cerebrospinal fluid (CSF) in Alzheimer's presenile dementia under basic conditions and after stimulation with cerebral cortex phospholipids. *J Neurol* 1980; 224:53–58.

26. Mölsä P: *Dementia: A Clinical Study in the Finnish Population*, thesis. Turku, 1980.

27. Soininen H, MacDonald E, Rekonen M, et al: Homovanillic acid and 5-hydroxyindoleacetic acid levels in cerebrospinal fluid of patients with senile dementia of the Alzheimer type. *Acta Neurol Scand* 1981; 64:101–107.

28. Shimizu T, Fujita M: Monoamine metabolite levels in the cerebrospinal fluid of patients with dementias. *Abstracts of the 12th World Congress of Neurology, Kyoto, Sept 20–25, 1981,* p 80.

29. Mann JJ, Stanley M, Neophytides A, et al: Central amine metabolism in Alzheimer's disease: *in vivo* relationship to cognitive deficit. *Neurobiol Aging* 1981; 2:57–60.

30. Bowen DM, Flack RHA, White P, et al: Brain-decarboxylase activities as indices of pathological change in senile dementia. *Lancet* 1974; i:1247–1249.

31. Spillane JA, White P, Goodhardt MJ, et al: Selective vulnerability of neurones in organic dementia. *Nature* 1977; 266:558–559.

32. Enna SJ, Stern LZ, Wastek GJ, et al. Cerebrospinal fluid γ-aminobutyric acid variations in neurological disorders. *Arch Neurol* 1977; 34:683–685.

33. Manyam NVB, Katz L, Hare TA, et al: Levels of γ-aminobutyric acid in cerebrospinal fluid in various neurologic disorders. *Arch Neurol* 1980; 37:352–355.

34. Wikkelsö C, Blomstrand C, Rönnbäck L: Separation of cerebrospinal fluid–specific proteins: a methodological study (pt 1). *J Neurol Sci* 1980; 44:247–257.

35. Wikkelsö C, Blomstrand C, Rönnbäck L: Cerebrospinal fluid–specific proteins in multiinfarct and senile dementia. *J Neurol Sci* 1981; 49:293–303.

36. Cohen D, Matsuyama SS, Jarvik LF: Immunoglobulin levels and intellectual functioning in the aged: short communication. *Exp Aging Res* 1976; 2:345–348.

37. Williams A, Papadopoulos N, Chase TN: Demonstration of CSF gamma-globulin banding in presenile dementia. *Neurology* 1980; 30:882–884.

38. Crapper DR, Krishnan SS, Dalton AJ: Brain aluminum distribution in Alzheimer's disease and experimental neurofibrillary degeneration. *Science* 1973; 180:511–513.

39. Crapper DR, Quittkat S, Krishnan SS, et al: Intranuclear aluminum content in Alzheimer's disease, dialysis encephalopathy, and experimental aluminum encephalopathy. *Acta Neuropathol* 1980; 50:19–24.

40. Delaney JF: Spinal fluid aluminum levels in patients with Alzheimer's disease. *Ann Neurol* 1979; 5:580–581.

41. Siesjö BK, Nilsson L: The influence of arterial hypoxemia upon labile phosphates and upon extracellular and intracellular lactate and pyruvate concentration in the rat brain. *Scand J Clin Lab Invest* 1971; 27:83–96.

42. Svenningsen NW, Siesjö BK: Cerebrospinal fluid lactate–pyruvate ratio in normal and asphyxiated neonates. *Acta Psychiatr Scand* 1972; 61:117–124.

17 Peptidergic Hormonal Factors

JULIAN J. ORAM

THE SO-CALLED HYPOTHALAMIC-REGULATING HORMONES, thyrotrophin-releasing hormone (TRH), gonadotrophin-releasing hormone (GnRH), and somatostatin, plus an additional hypothalamic neuropeptide, vasopressin, have been implicated in the Alzheimer's disease (AD) pathogenic process. I have used the term "so-called" hypothalamic-regulating hormones in reference to the neuropeptide hormones TRH, GnRH, and somatostatin because until recently it was thought that the ability of certain hypothalamic neurons to secrete peptides reflected a specialization related wholly to the hypothalamic control of the pituitary gland; it is now known that the biosynthesis and release of small peptide messengers is a widespread property of neurons in many other regions of the CNS as well.

Neuropeptides have complex multiple actions ranging from their effects on the pituitary to roles in other areas of the CNS involving synaptic function and behavior. The discovery of these neuropeptides, which are rapidly growing in number and include, for example, substance P and enkephalin, has led to a greatly improved understanding of brain physiology and of the integration of neural and endocrine function. The hypothalamic peptides are small, each containing fewer than 15 amino acid chains, and it is probable that they are synthesized ribosomally in the cell bodies of neurons as part of macromolecular precursors (1). This macromolecule may contain entire sequences of peptides. By enzymic cleavage of this pro-peptide, multiple offspring of different biologically active peptides can be produced.

Neuropeptides have specific effects on behavior; for example, GnRH (also known as luteinizing hormone releasing factor [LHRF]) has been shown to stimulate sexual behavior in rats (2). So GnRH, as well as stimulating the release of luteinizing hormone (LH) from the pituitary to act on gonadal function, also elicits sexual behavior by an alternative pathway.

TRH has been shown to: antagonize the effects of ethanol narcosis in rats (3); potentiate the effects of strychnine in animals; and cause mood changes, namely, euphoria in humans. TRH is also involved in thermoregulation; under cold conditions not only does it cause thyrotrophin to be released from the pituitary, which in turn releases thyroxine, leading to increased metabolic heat, but it also induces thermoregulatory behavior, such as shivering and locomotor activity. Somatostatin has been found in rats to have some behavioral effects which are in many cases directly opposite to those of TRH (4). TRH increases spontaneous motor activity in animals, for example, whereas somatostatin decreases spontaneous motor activity. It is presently believed that TRH may be a CNS stimulant while somatostatin may be a CNS depressant.

While GnRH is confined mainly to the hypothalamus, and TRH is found in large quantities in other areas of the CNS, somatostatin, in addition to being found in substantial

131

quantities in extrahypothalamic neural tissue, is also found outside the CNS. Vasopressin, too, is found in various parts of the brain, although it is mainly found in the supraoptic and paraventricular nuclei of the hypothalamus. Vasopressin is actually stored in the posterior pituitary and has a well-known effect on the distal part of the nephron, causing more water to be reabsorbed, but it has also been shown to have a beneficial effect on memory in animal experiments (5).

The evidence described above represents only a fraction of current knowledge, indicating a wide range of distribution and multiplicity of actions possessed by these hypothalamic neuropeptides. Collectively, their role is of great importance in neuroendocrinology. That neuropeptides are so widely distributed increasingly suggests that cerebrospinal fluid (CSF) acts as a transport medium for these peptides and lends supports to the ependymal transport theory, which suggests that neuropeptides are released into the ventricular system, taken up in luminal processes of the cells of the median eminence from the third ventricle, and then actively transported to the capillary end of the cell, where they are released into the portal vessel complex and transported to the pituitary. Studies by Oliver and associates (6) with respect to TRH and by Onde and co-workers (7) with respect to LHRF have provided convincing evidence of this alternative pathway of hypothalamic peptide control of the pituitary.

Experiments involving deafferentation of the hypothalamus in rats have demonstrated that the content of neuropeptides subsequently declines markedly (8, 9). This suggests either that these neuropeptides arise from cells outside the hypothalamus or that the production of hypothalamic peptides is controlled by cells outside this area.

Clinical experience has shown involvement of the hypothalamus in cases of memory loss, and Reeves and Plum (10) describe a patient with gross obesity and marked short-term memory loss who had an harmartoma affecting the ventromedial nucleus while the remaining hypothalamus was spared. The Wernicke–Korsakoff syndrome (thiamine deficiency), in which there is marked short-term memory loss, is most frequently associated with lesions of the mamillary bodies, but patients with hypothalamic disease also manifest this syndrome. Tumors invading the ventromedian hypothalamus and mamillary bodies lead to short term memory loss; it is likely that both structures are important in short-term memory. Reasons for investigating hypothalamic peptides in AD are threefold:

1. Cerebral peptides have established actions on neuronal function and behavior (including memory).
2. Complex mechanisms of biosynthesis, secretion and disposal provide ample opportunity for genetic and other neurochemical lesions to affect peptidergic systems.
3. Peptidergic systems have marked interactions with aminergic neurons which have previously been implicated in AD.

The precise mechanism of hypothalamic influence on intelligence and memory is unknown, but it is closely tied to the amygdala, hippocampus, limbic system, and mamillary bodies, all of which play a major part in memory, emotion, and behavior. These hypothalamic peptides may bear on memory either through their hypothalamic role or via their widespread distribution and function throughout the cortex as modulators of other neurotransmitters such as acetylcholine. Certainly in the median eminence, for example, in addition to the hypothalamic neuropeptides, there is found dopamine, acetylcholine and gamma aminobutyric acid in reasonable quantities; it is likely that in this region, where there is such a high density of nerve terminals, there is considerable interaction between these neurohormones and neurotransmitters.

TABLE 17–1

Mean (±S.E.M.) Concentrations of Thyrotrophin-Releasing Hormone and Gonadotrophin-Releasing Hormone in Lumbar CSF from Patients with Cerebral Tumors, Disc Lesions, and Idiopathic Senile Dementia[a]

	Thyrotrophin-Releasing Hormone	Gonadotrophin-Releasing Hormone
Cerebral tumors	49 cases: range <10 (3 cases) to 220 pg/ml, mean value 69.7 ± 7.5 pg/ml	42 cases: range <10 (14 cases) to 130 pg/ml, mean value 27.6 ± 4.5 pg/ml
Disc lesions	51 cases: range <10 (3 cases) to 270 pg/ml, mean value 78.3 ± 8.1 pg/ml	49 cases: range <10 (18 cases) to 93 pg/ml, mean value 26.6 ± 3.7 pg/ml
Senile dementia	19 cases: range 14 to 48 pg/ml, mean value 26.5 ± 2.1 pg/ml	All 19 cases: <10 pg/ml, the level of sensitivity of the assay, mean value 5.0 ± 0 pg/ml

[a] Presumably secondary in most cases to Alzheimer's disease.

Oram and associates (11) measured CSF neuropeptides in several clinical groups which included cerebral tumors, spinal disc lesions, senile dementia, and, finally, a group of miscellaneous neurological disorders (cerebrovascular accidents, degenerative disorders, trauma, and meningitis). Measurement, of TRH and GnRH from these clinical groups are shown in Table 17–1, and of somatostatin and vasopressin, in Table 17–2.

The significantly lower levels of CSF, TRH, GnRH, and somatostatin in the groups afflicted with senile dementia, compared with the other clinical groups may indicate a deficit in central peptidergic mechanisms in this disorder (10). If this is the case, however, then even the derangement of peptide-secreting neurons must be selective since CSF levels of vasopressin were found to be normal in the senile dementia group. In a study by Jenkins and co-workers (12) the normal CSF range of vasopressin was shown to lie between 1 and 4 pg/ml.

Interestingly, CSF levels of vasopressin were found to be normal in the dementia group, since a study by Rossor and associates (13) showed reduced levels of vasopressin in five areas of the brains of demented patients when compared with controls. However, these findings were of statistical significance only in the area of the globus pallidus. Additionally, Mann and colleagues (14) showed a significant reduction of vasopressin in the nerve cells of the supraoptic and paraventricular nuclei of the hypothalamus in patients dying from senile dementia.

TABLE 17–2

Mean Concentrations of Somatostatin and Arginine Vasopressin in Lumbar CSF from Patients with Miscellaneous Neurological Disorders and Idiopathic Senile Dementia[a]

	Somatostatin	Mean (±S.E.M.)	Arginine Vasopressin	Mean (±S.D.)
Controls	17 cases: range 10 to 97 pg/ml	48 ± 6.9 pg/ml	12 cases: range 1.4 to 3.6 pg/ml	2.4 ± 0.7 pg/ml
Senile dementia	16 cases: range 10 (6 cases) to 28 pg/ml	12.9 ± 2.0 pg/ml	18 cases: range 1.0 to 3.8 pg/ml	2.6 ± 0.93 pg/ml

[a] Presumably secondary in most cases to Alzheimer's disease.

Studies of somatostatin-like immunoreactivity (SLI) in brain specimens of patients with AD, compared with controls, have revealed even more generalized decreases in many brain regions (15–18). SLI was found to be reduced in 12 AD brain specimens compared with 12 controls in 7 of 9 brain regions examined in one study (15).

Our knowledge of the involvement of hypothalamic neuropeptides in AD is currently in its infancy. But present evidence indicates that these neurohormones may have a significant part to play in unearthing the key to this devastating illness.

REFERENCES

1. Rupnow J, Hinkle PM, Dixon JEA: Macromolecule which gives rise to TRH. *Biochem Biophys Res Commun* 1979; 89:721–728.

2. Pfatt DW: Luteinizing hormone releasing factor (LRH) potentiates lordosis behavior in hypophysectomized ovariectomized female rats. *Science* 1973; 182:1148.

3. Prasad C, Matsui T, Kofsky PA: Antagonism of ethanol narcosis by histidyl-proline-diketopiperazine. *Nature* 1977; 268:142–144.

4. Brown M, Vale W: Central nervous system effect of hypothalamic peptides. *Endocrinology* 1975; 96:1333–1336.

5. De Wied D, Van Wimersma Greidanus TJB, Bohus B, et al: Vasopressin and memory consolidation. *Prog Brain Res* 1976; 45:181–194.

6. Oliver C, Ben-Jonathan N, Mical RS, et al: Transport of thyrotrophin releasing hormone from cerebrospinal fluid to hypophysial portal blood and the release of thyrotrophin. *Endocrinology* 1975; 97:1138–1143.

7. Onde J, Eskay RL, Mical RS, et al: Release of LH by LRF injected into the CSF: a transport role for the median eminence. *Endocrinology* 1973; 93:231–237.

8. Brownstein MJ, Viger RD, Palkovitz M, et al: Effect of hypothalamic deafferentation on thyrotrophin-releasing hormone levels in rat brain. *Proc Natl Acad Sci USA* 1975; 72:4177–4179.

9. Brownstein MJ, Arimura A, Schally AV, et al: The effect of surgical isolation of the hypothalamus on its luteinizing hormone–releasing hormone content. *Endrocrinology* 1976; 98:662–665.

10. Reeves AG, Plum F: Hyperphagia, rage, and dementia accompanying a ventromedial hypothalamic neoplasm. *Arch Neurol* 1969; 20:616–624.

11. Oram JJ, Edwardson J, Millard PH: Investigation of cerebrospinal fluid neuropeptides in idiopathic senile dementia. *Gerontology* 1981; 27:216–223.

12. Jenkins JS, Mather HM, Ang V: Vasopressin in human cerebrospinal fluid. *Endrocrinology* 1980; 50:364–367.

13. Rossor MN, Iversen LL, Mountjoy CQ, et al: Arginine, vasopressin, and choline acetyltransferase in brains of patients with Alzheimer-type senile dementia. *Lancet* 1980; ii:1367–1368.

14. Mann DMA, Yates PO, Bansal DV, et al: Hypothalamus and dementia. *Lancet* 1981; i:393–394.

15. Davies P, Katz DA, Crystal HA: Choline acetyltransferase, somatostatin, and substance P in selected cases of Alzheimer's disease. *Aging NY* 1982; 19:9–14.

16. Davies P, Katzman R, Terry RD: Reduced somatostatin-like immunoreactivity in cerebral cortex from cases of Alzheimer disease and Alzheimer senile dementia. *Nature* 1980; 288:279–280.

17. Davies P, Terry RD: Cortical somatostatin-like immunoreactivity in cases of Alzheimer's disease and senile dementia of the Alzheimer type. *Neurobiol Aging* 1981; 2:9–14.

18. Rossor MN, Emson PC, Mountjoy CQ, et al: Reduced amounts of immunoreactive somatostatin in the temporal cortex in senile dementia of the Alzheimer type. *Neurosci Lett* 1980; 20:373–377.

18 Immunologic Factors

Kalidas Nandy

ALZHEIMER'S DISEASE (AD) AFFLICTS PRIMARILY older people, significantly increasing in incidence with age. Aging is also associated with marked deterioration of the immune system and a significant increase in the incidence of autoimmune diseases (1–3). The age-related decline in immune functions is partly the result of deterioration of thymus derived (T cell) functions, and may also be related to the involution of the thymus (4, 5). It has been reported that thymectomy accelerates the age-related loss of IgG and high-affinity antibody response (5). On the other hand, when spleen cells from old animals were exposed to a young thymus gland or exogenous thymopoietin, the high-affinity antibody response was restored (6). The neuropathological changes in the AD brain include neuronal loss, loss of dendritic spines, and formation of neuritic (senile) plaques (SPs) and neurofibrillary tangles (NFTs), but the underlying pathogenesis of these phenomena is not clearly understood as yet (7). This chapter concerns the various immunologic factors that play a significant role in the neuropathology of aging and AD.

Antibodies against neuronal structures have previously been reported in various neurological diseases such as multiple sclerosis, cerebrovascular accidents, schizophrenia, Huntington's chorea, and systemic lupus erythematosus (8–14). An increased age-related concentration of the γ-globulin fraction of human serum, which binds specifically with neurons in sections of human brain, has also been described (15).

Brain-reactive antibodies (BRAs) have been extensively investigated in my laboratory (16). These have been demonstrated in serum from aging rodents, nonhuman primates, and humans both through indirect immunofluorescence as well as chromium 51 cytotoxicity tests. These antibodies are composed of γ-globulin and are specific to brain tissue, although some cross-reaction with thymic tissue has been observed (17, 18). BRAs begin to appear in serum from C57BL/6 mice at 6–12 months of age and thereafter increase progressively as a function of age (19). When serum from 12-month-old germ-free (Charles River Laboratories) and control female mice was tested for BRAs, no significant difference was noted in the serum levels (20). The study indicated that antibody formation probably resulted from the stimulation of the immune system by an autogenous antigen, rather than an exogenous antigen such as an infectious agent (20). The cytotoxicity of BRAs was studied (21) by injecting the serum intracerebrally in young and old mice. Both antigen–antibody reaction as well as evidence of morphological damage were then noted primarily in the mouse neurons within 7 days. The possible role of the blood–brain barrier in separating the circulating antibodies from the brain tissue was investigated using ^{125}I-labeled γ-globulin injected intraperitoneally into the animals. While a high level of radioactivity was seen in the blood and most organs within 6 hours of administration of the isotope, the maximum levels of radioactivity in the cerebrum were reached in 24 hours. It appeared from this study (16, 22) that the blood–brain barrier largely separates the circulating γ-globulin from the brain tissue. BRA levels have also been studied in the serum of nonhuman female primates, *Macaca nemestrina,* of different ages (4, 10, and 20 years) (23). Antibodies were detected in all age groups and a significant age-related BRA level increase was noted.

Serum levels of BRAs in clinically diagnosed cases of senile dementia, including AD, have been compared with levels in age-matched normal subjects (age range 48–82 years) (24). BRA levels observably increased as a function of age in normal people and were significantly higher in senile dementia patients than in the age-matched controls.

The formation of BRAs in young and old C57BL/6 mice has been followed through various immunological manipulations. A high BRA level, for instance, was attained in young mice following irradiation and transfer of hemopoietic cells from old animals. Antibody levels were significantly reduced in old mice, however, when these animals also had a neonatal thymus graft performed in addition to the injection of hemopoietic tissue from young animals. The age-related thymic involution appears to play an important role in BRA formation, as well as in the immunodysfunction associated with aging.

Since NZB mice have a shorter lifespan and a greater propensity for autoimmune diseases (increased formation of antinuclear, antierythrocytic, and antithymocytic antibodies) than C57BL/6 mice (25) serum BRA levels and learning ability (condition avoidance response) were compared in both strains. While C57BL/6 mice exhibited a gradual but steady decrease in their learning ability with age, NZB mice exhibited a virtual inability to meet the criteria even at the age of 2–4 months. It was apparent that the youngest (2–4 months) NZB mice were worse in their cognitive performance than the oldest (24–25 months) C57BL/6 mice. This NZB learning deficit was due neither to any significant difference in sensitivity to paw shock nor to auditory motor deficits. These NZB mice also showed higher levels of BRA than C57BL/6 at each age group. Although specific neuropathological changes of AD have not been described in NZB mice, the finding of "precocious" BRA formation and the observation that NZB mice behave as if they are "senile" with respect to memory function lead one to hypothesize that these mice may serve as an animal model for an enhanced understanding of the mechanism of senile dementia (37). Scrapie-infected mice have also been suggested (26–29) as an animal model of AD on the basis of parallel formation of amyloid and SPs in the brain (but not NFTs). However, no learning deficits have been described in these animals. Although the precise role of the various immunologic changes, including BRA formation, in the pathogenesis of the specific brain changes in aging and AD is not clear, antibody levels have been correlated with cognitive impairment in recent studies using animals and humans. The high incidence of SPs with an amyloid core in AD patients appears significant, since amyloid-B bears a marked similarity to light chains of immunoglobulin (30–33). It has been suggested that amyloid deposits probably represent antigen-antibody complexes and might induce neuritic degeneration and senile plaque formation (7). The experimental induction of amyloid and SP formation in scrapie-infected mice offers further evidence in favor of immunological factors in these neuropathological changes (29, 34). In addition, Dahl and Bignami (35) observed that rabbit antineurofilamentous serum prepared against antigens isolated from chicken brain or human sciatic nerve reacted strongly with NFTs induced by intracerebral injection of aluminum phosphate in the rabbit. Attempts are under way to prepare antisera to isolated paired helical filaments from AD brains. Subsequently, the induction of neurofibrillary tangle formation in the brains of experimental animals will be attempted (36). It has also been possible to significantly delay the age-related dysfunction of the immune system, including BRA formation, by dietary restriction in experimental animals (38–41). The demonstrated association of HLA-B7 antigen with greater cognitive function loss (39) probably suggests that HLA genes, or genes linked thereto, may influence AD (Chap. 23).

In summary, evidence that immunologic changes play an important role in the neuropathology and cognitive impairment of AD is mounting, and studies of these changes might yield valuable insight into the condition.

REFERENCES

1. Makinodan T: Immunobiology of aging. *J Am Geriatr Soc* 24:249–252.

2. Burch PRJ: *An Inquiry Concerning Growth, Disease and Aging.* Edinburgh, Oliver & Boyd, 1968.

3. Burnet FM: An immunological aspect of aging. *Lancet* 1970; ii:358–360.

4. Kay MMB, Makinodan T: Immunobiology of aging: evaluation of current status. *Clin Immunol Immunopathol* 1976; 6:394–413.

5. Weksler ME, Innes JB, Goldstein G: Immunological studies of aging: IV. The contribution of thymic involution to the immune deficiencies of aging mice. *J Exp Med* 1978; 148:996–1009.

6. Weksler ME: The senescence of the immune system. *Hosp Prac,* October 1981, pp 53–64.

7. Wisniewski HM, Terry RD: Morphology of aging brain, human and animal. *Prog Brain Res,* 1973; 40:167–186.

8. Bluestein HG: Neurocytotoxic antibodies in serum of patients with systematic lupus erythematosus. *Proc Natl Acad Sci USA* 1978; 75:3965–3969.

9. Heath RG, Krupp IM: Schizophrenia as an immunologic disorder. *Arch Gen Psychiatry* 1967; 15:1–9.

10. Motycka A, Jezkova Z: Autoantibodies and brain ishaemia topography. *Cas Lek Cesk* 1975; 114:1455–1457.

11. Skalickova O, Jezkova Z, Jezkova V: Immunological aspects of psychiatric gerontology. *Rev Czech Med* 1962; 8:264–275.

12. Pandey RS, Gupta AL, Chaturvedi UC: Autoimmune model of schizophrenia with special reference to antibrain antibodies. *Biol Psychiatry* 1981; 16:1123–1135.

13. Husby G, Rijn IVE, Zabriskia JB, et al: Antibodies reacting with cytoplasm of subthalamic and caudate nuclei neurons in chorea and acute rheumatic fever. *J Exp Med* 1976; 144:1094–1110.

14. Diederrichsen H, Pyndt IC: Antibodies against neurons in a patient with systematic lupus erythematosus, cerebral palsy and epilepsy. *Brain* 1968; 93:407–412.

15. Ingram CR, Phegan KJ, Blumenthal HT: Significance of an aging-linked neuron binding gamma-globulin fraction of human sera. *J Gerontol* 1974; 20:20–27.

16. Nandy K: Significance of brain-reactive antibodies in serum of aged mice. *J Gerontol* 1975; 30:412–416.

17. Nandy K, Fritz RB, Threat J: Specificity of brain-reactive antibodies in serum in old mice. *J Gerontol* 1975; 30:269–275.

18. Threatt J, Nandy K, Fritz R: Brain-reactive antibodies in serum of old mice demonstrated by immunofluorescence. *J Gerontol* 1971; 26:316–323.

19. Nandy K: Brain-reactive antibodies in mouse serum as a function of age. *J Gerontol* 1972; 27:173–177.

20. Nandy K: Brain-reactive antibodies in serum of germ-free mice. *Mech Ageing Dev* 1972; 1:133–138.

21. Nandy K: Neuronal degeneration in aging and after experimental injury. *Exp Gerontol* 1972; 7:303–311.

22. Nandy K: in Nandy K, Sherwin I (eds): *The Aging Brain and Senile Dementia.* New York, Plenum, 1977, pp 181–196.

23. Nandy K: in Mortimer JA, Shuman LM (eds): *Epidemiology of Senile Dementia.* New York, Oxford University Press, 1981, pp 87–100.

24. Nandy K: *Aging NY* 1978; 7:503–574.

25. Shirai T, Mellors RC: Natural thymocytotoxic autoantibodies and reactive antigen in New Zealand black and other mice. *Proc Nat Acad Sci USA* 1971; 68:1414–1415.

26. Dickinson AG, Fraser H, Bruce M: Animal models for the dementias, in Glen AIM, Whalley LJ (eds): *Alzheimer's Disease: Early Recognition of Potentially Reversible Deficits.* New York, Livingstone, 1979, pp 42–45.

27. Fraser H: The pathology of natural and experimental scrapie, in Kimberlin RH (ed): *Slow Virus Diseases of Animals and Man.* New York, Elsevier North-Holland, 1976, pp 209–241.

28. Fraser H: Neuropathology of scrapie: the precision of the lesions and their diversity, in Prusiner SB, Hadlow WJ (eds): *Slow Transmissible Diseases of the Nervous System.* New York, Academic, 1980, vol 1, pp 387–406.

29. Wisniewski H: Infectious etiology of neuritic (senile) plaques in mice. *Science* 1975; 190:1108–1110.

30. Ishii T, Shimizu S: Identification of components of immunoglobulins in senile plaques by means of fluorescent antibody techniques. *Acta Neuropathol* 1975; 32:157–162.

31. Ishii T, Haga S: Immuno-electron microscopic localization of immunoglobulins in amyloid fibrils of senile plaques. *Acta Neuropathol* 1976; 36:243–249.

32. Glenner GG, Harbough J, Ohms JI, et al: Amyloid protein: the amino-terminal variable fragment of immunoglobulin light chain. *Biochem Biophys Res Commun* 1970; 41:1287–1289.

33. Glenner GG: Current knowledge of amyloid deposits as applied to senile plaques and congophilic angiopathy. *Aging NY* 1978; 7:493–501.

34. Merz PA, Somerville RA, Wisniewski HM, et al: Abnormal fibrils from scrapie-infected brain. *Acta Neuropathol* 1981; 54:64–74.

35. Dahl D, Bignami A: Immunochemical cross-reactivity of normal neurofibrils and aluminum-induced neurofibrillary tangles. *Exp Neurol* 1978; 58:74–80.

36. Iqbal K, Grundke-Iqbal I, Merz PA, et al: Age-associated neurofibrillary changes. *Aging NY* 1982; 20:247–257.

37. Nandy K, Lal H, Bennett M: Brain-reactive antibodies and learning deficits in NZB mice: an animal model of senile dementia. Submitted for publication.

38. Nandy K: Effects of caloric restriction on brain-reactive antibodies in old mice. *Age* 1982; 4:117–121.

39. Nandy K: Effects of dietary restriction on brain-reactive antibodies in aging mice. *Mech Ageing Dev* 1981; 18:97–102.

40. Gerbase-DeLima N, Liu RK, Cheney KE, et al: Immune function and survival in a long-lived mouse strain subjected to undernutrition. *Gerontology* 1975; 21:184–202.

41. Bell RG, Hazell LA: Influence of dietary protein restriction on immune competence: I. Effect on the capacity of cells from lymphoid organs to induce graft vs. host reactions. *J Exp Med* 1975; 141:127–137.

Section V

EPIDEMIOLOGIC AND GENETIC FACTORS IN ALZHEIMER'S DISEASE

19 Alzheimer's Disease and Senile Dementia: Prevalence and Incidence

JAMES A. MORTIMER

JAMES A. MORTIMER

PREVALENCE

Among persons over age 65, the *prevalence* (percentage afflicted at a given time) of severe dementia has been estimated at 1.3–6.2% (Table 19–1). Such a wide range in prevalence estimates could be attributed primarily to differences in diagnostic critera. Reliable estimates for the prevalence of dementia among persons under age 65 are not available, due to the relative infrequency of this condition in the younger population, the absence of uniform reporting procedures, and the difficulty of screening a sufficiently large population for cognitive loss. Heston and Mastri (1), using a death certificate method, estimated that Alzheimer's disease (AD) accounted for 70/100,000 deaths in the state of Minnesota from 1952 to 1961. Assuming an average disease duration of 7 years (1), this suggests that the prevalence could be as high as 0.5% among persons in the 40–70 age range. Many of these cases, however, are likely to have begun after age 60. Hence, severe AD appears to be uncommon in the fifth and sixth decades of life.

In addition to severe dementia, mild forms of senile dementia have been estimated as prevalent in 2.6–20.0% of the elderly (Table 19–1; ref. 2). The difficulty in recognizing mild dementia is evident from the markedly different criteria applied by investigators to identify such cases. Nielson (3), who reported a 15.4% prevalence of mild dementia among persons over age 65, included individuals with depression and delirium in this category; whereas Kay and co-workers (4) used more stringent criteria, and identified only 2.6% of persons in this age group as having mild dementia syndromes. Since AD is progressive, it is conceivable that mild dementia syndromes represent early cases. However, only one-fifth of severe dementia cases identified in a random population of 711 older persons living in Newcastle-upon-Tyne, England, were previously identified as having mild dementia syndromes at the time of a survey performed 2–4 years earlier (5). This suggests that many cases of mild dementia may represent a nonprogressive entity distinct from AD.

Estimates for the proportion of cases with AD among the demented have been based largely upon the study of Tomlinson, Blessed, and Roth (6), who found that approximately 60% of a sample of 50 institutionalized older persons with moderate to severe dementia before death had brain lesions characteristic of AD at autopsy. The fact that the population studied by these investigators was institutionalized may have led to an overestimate of the

TABLE 19–1
Prevalence of Organic Brain Syndromes Among the Aged

Study	Country	Years of Survey	N (65+)	Organic Brain Syndromes (Cases/100)		Type of Prevalence	Type of Sample
				"Severe"	"Mild"		
Essen-Möller et al. (22)	Sweden	1947	443[a]	5.0	10.8	Point	Delimited rural population
Primrose (23)	Scotland	1959–60	222	4.5	—	Period: 1 yr	Delimited rural population
Nielson (3)	Denmark	1961	978	3.1	15.4	Period: 6 mo	Delimited rural population
Kay et al. (24)	England	1960	505	5.6	5.7	Point	Randon urban sample
Åkesson (21)	Sweden	1964	2979	1.3	—	Point	Delimited rural population
Kay et al. (4)	England	1960, 1964	758	6.2	2.6	Point	Randon urban sample living at home
Bollerup (25)	Denmark	1967	626[b]	1.6	5.0	Point	Delimited urban population of 70-year-olds
Broe et al. (19)	Scotland	Not given	808	3.8	4.3	Point	Randon urban sample living at home

Source: Reproduced from Mortimer, Schuman, and French (10) by permission of Oxford University Press.

[a] Age 60 and over.
[b] Age 70 only.

importance of AD relative to other conditions, since cases of nonprogressive intellectual impairment would likely have been excluded. More recent studies in noninstitutionalized populations show that the percentage of persons referred for evaluation of an apparent dementia syndrome, for whom a diagnosis of AD or primary degenerative dementia is made, is lower than the Tomlinson, Blessed, and Roth findings among institutionalized elderly (7, 8).

Using 4.15% as the median prevalence rate of severe dementia among persons over age 65 (Table 19–1), the prediction can safely be made that at any time, approximately 1 million persons in the United States are afflicted with a severe dementia syndrome. If 60% of these million persons have AD, the number of cases of this disease would be comparable to that of Parkinson's disease and would far exceed that of other degenerative neurologic diseases (Table 19–2).

INCIDENCE

Determination of the *incidence* (frequency of occurrence of new cases) of senile dementia requires that a population be followed over time and that occurrence of new cases of the disease be carefully monitored. Few studies of this type have been performed. Kay's (5)

TABLE 19–2
Prevalence of Selected Neurologic Disorders in the United States, 1976

Disease	Prevalent Cases
Alzheimer's disease–senile dementia	600,000
Parkinson's disease	500,000
Multiple sclerosis	250,000
Huntington's disease	10–14,000
Amyotrophic lateral sclerosis	5–10,000

Source: Office of Scientific and Health Reports, National Institute of Communicative Disorders and Stroke (26).

4-year study of the Newcastle population indicated an annual incidence rate of 1.4% for a combination of senile and arteriosclerotic dementia among persons over age 65. Jarvik, Ruth, and Matsuyama (9) reported a somewhat higher incidence (2.7%) for senile dementia for a small sample of 22 persons who averaged 83 years of age at the beginning of the 6-year study period. Computations performed by Mortimer, Schuman, and French (10) on the Baltimore Longitudinal Study data (11) yielded an average annual incidence of slightly more than 1% among persons aged 65 or over in that study. An indirect estimate for the incidence can also be obtained by dividing the prevalence rate by the average disease duration. Using 4% as the prevalence rate, and assuming an average duration of 4 to 7 years (11a), an incidence rate of 0.6% to 1.0% is obtained for severe dementia. Thus, with the exception of the study by Jarvik and associates (9) in which a much older population was followed, there appears to be good agreement that approximately 1% of the elderly population develop senile dementia each year.

AGE-SPECIFIC PREVALENCE AND INCIDENCE

Knowledge of the average incidence and prevalence of senile dementia among persons 65 and over is necessary in planning for general health and social service delivery. However, the changing age composition among the elderly makes it important to know the year-by-year age-specific prevalence and incidence of dementing illness as well. In 1950, those over age 85 accounted for only 4.9% of the population above age 65. By 1976, that percentage had risen to 8.4%; and it is projected to rise further, to 11.5%, by the year 2000 (12).

Fig. 19–1 summarizes findings of three different studies of the age-specific prevalence of senile dementia and related conditions. The marked increase in prevalence with age is especially evident in the fastest growing segment of the older population, those 80 and over. Although there is the temptation to explain this great increase in prevalence with age by a parallel change in incidence, the available data suggest that this explanation may be incorrect. For example, Fig. 19–2 shows age-specific hospitalization and incidence rates for patients with senile dementia, based on the data of Larsson, Sjögren, and Jacobson (13), who identified 657 cases of senile dementia from those persons admitted to Stockholm mental hospitals.

Although these data suggest that the incidence rate of senile dementia levels off at around 75 years of age, the incidence rates at ages 85 and above is based on too few cases

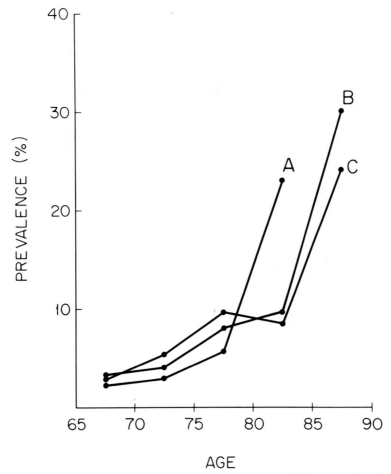

Figure 19–1. Prevalence rates of senile dementia and related conditions: results of three surveys. *Curve A: Kay et al. (4); curve B: Staff of the Mental Health Research Unit, New York State Department of Hygiene (1960); curve C: Nielson (3). Adapted from Gruenberg (27).*

to judge whether this trend continues. Indirect evidence that individuals living into the ninth and tenth decades of life may have a reduced risk of developing the brain lesions characteristic of AD is provided by three independently conducted autopsy studies demonstrating decreased severity of Alzheimer's type neuropathological findings in the tenth decade of life (14–16). Although these findings were obtained from an unselected series of older persons in whom dementia was not confirmed before death, they provide indirect support for a possible survival effect, in which persons living to very old ages may be less likely to have neuropathological manifestations of AD.

Another explanation for the marked increase in prevalence of senile dementia with age is the greater reduction in expected survival duration among persons who develop AD at younger ages, compared with those with later onset. Heston (17) found little difference in the absolute mean duration of survival between patients who developed AD in their forties and fifties and those who developed AD in their sixties and seventies. However,

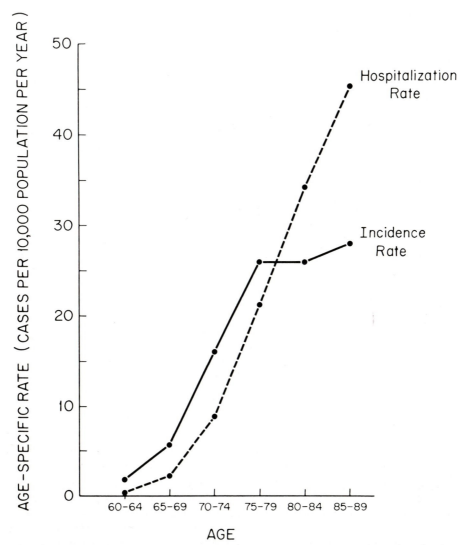

Figure 19–2. Age-specific average annual hospitalization and incidence rates of senile dementia in Stockholm, 1935–1950. Derived from published data of Larsson, Sjögren, and Jacobson (13). *Solid lines:* age-specific average incidence rates of senile dementia as determined from medical records, males and females combined (from Table 40, "Final Assessment"). *Dashed lines:* age-specific average annual first-admission rates to mental hospitals for senile dementia, males and females combined (from Tables 1 and 38). *Reproduced from Mortimer, Schuman, and French (10) by permission of Oxford University Press.*

because older persons have higher mortality rates than younger, the reduction in the *expected* survival time is much greater for persons who develop the disease at an early age than for those who develop it later in life when the chances of dying, regardless of whether one has dementia or not, are considerably higher. The loss of early onset cases through premature death has the effect of reducing the *prevalence* of dementia among persons in their fifties and sixties, thereby accentuating the increase in prevalence seen with age.

CUMULATIVE MORBIDITY RISK

Prevalence rates, while very useful for assessing the impact of a disease upon society, do not necessarily provide good estimates of the risk to individuals of becoming afflicted with the disease during their lifetimes. The *cumulative morbidity risk* or *probability that a person living to a certain age will develop a condition* provides a measure of this risk. As the name implies, this measure is derived by summing the age-specific risk or incidence of the disease for each year of life. Using data from the studies of Larsson and associates (13) and Roth and colleagues (18), Mortimer and associates (10) computed the cumulative risk of severe dementia to be 20% by age 85. A very similar prediction (17% by age 80) was made by Sluss, Gruenberg, and Kramer (11), who employed a life table analysis of data from the Baltimore Longitudinal Study. These figures are consistent with the cumulative risk that would be obtained by multiplying the average annual incidence of senile dementia after age 65 (1%) by the number of years a person is exposed to that risk. That the cumulative morbidity risk is four to five times the prevalence rate is perhaps surprising, but this is a direct consequence of the reduced life expectancy of persons who develop dementing illness. To maintain a prevalence of 4%, new cases must continually occur to replace those that die.

VARIATIONS IN PREVALENCE BY PERSON, PLACE, AND TIME

Little information is available concerning the variations in prevalence of dementia by place, time or personal characteristics (other than age and sex). Kay (5) reported a higher prevalence of senile dementia in females. However, data from other studies (13, 19) do not support a differential prevalence by sex of senile dementia. Despite the lack of agreement on this issue, it is clear that females with senile dementia significantly outnumber males with this condition, because of their increased life expectancy, coupled with the high incidence rates for this condition in the ninth decade of life (Fig. 19–2).

The racial, religious, and ethnic distribution of dementing illness is currently unknown. Kay, Beamish, and Roth (20) found no relationship between social class and the prevalence of senile dementia. Other personal characteristics that have been examined, that do not appear to be associated with the occurrence of senile dementia, include birth order, fertility, and mortality among relatives (13, 21).

Since most prevalence studies have been carried out in northern Europe, little is known regarding geographic variation in the prevalence of dementia. Urban–rural differences in prevalence are not apparent among the studies cited in Table 19–1. Although no change in the incidence of senile dementia over time has been documented, it would be difficult to judge whether one had occurred, given the changes in diagnostic criteria and nosology that have taken place over the past 30 years. Prospective studies utilizing uniform diagnostic criteria are needed to clarify this issue.

SUMMARY

Studies of the prevalence of senile dementia suggest that about 4% of the population over age 65 is afflicted with a severe form of dementing illness at any given time. Although the prevalence of AD among persons under age 65 is unknown, it is likely that the disease is uncommon in this age group, particularly when onset occurs in the fifth and sixth decades of life.

Estimates of the prevalence of mild forms of dementia are unlikely to be reliable, given the difficulty of recognizing this condition. Many mild dementias may represent nonprogressive entities distinct from AD.

Clinicopathological studies suggest that approximately 65% of the elderly patients with dementia may have AD. This percentage may be lower in noninstitutionalized populations of elderly patients who present with cognitive impairment.

Studies of the incidence of senile dementia indicate that approximately 1% of those over age 65 develop this condition each year. A marked increase in prevalence occurs between age 70 and 85. However, the present data suggest that the incidence rate may level off around age 75. The greater reduction in expected survival duration among early onset cases likely contributes to the sharply rising prevalence of senile dementia with age.

The cumulative morbidity risk to the general population of developing severe dementia may reach 15–20% by the age 80.

Little is known regarding the variations in prevalence of senile dementia by place, time, or personal characteristics.

ACKNOWLEDGMENT

The author thanks L. Ronald French for helpful comments during the preparation of this chapter.

REFERENCES

1. Heston LL, Mastri AR: The genetics of Alzheimer's disease: associations with hematologic malignancy and Down's syndrome. *Arch Gen Psychiatry* 1977; 34:976–981.

2. Brody JA: An epidemiologist views senile dementia: facts and fragments. *Am J Epidemiol* 1982; 115:155–162.

3. Nielson J: Geronto-psychiatric period–prevalence investigation in a geographically delimited population. *Acta Psychiatr Scand* 1963; 38:307–330.

4. Kay DWK, Bergmann K, Foster ΕM, et al: Mental illness and hospital usage in the elderly: a random sample followed up. *Comp Psychiatry* 1970; 11:26–35.

5. Kay DWK: Epidemiological aspects of organic brain disease in the aged, in Gaitz CM (ed): *Aging and the Brain.* New York, Plenum, 1972, pp 15–27.

6. Tomlinson BE, Blessed G, Roth M: Observations on the brains of demented old people. *J Neurol Sci* 1970; 11:205–242.

7. Hutton JT: Results of clinical assessment for the dementia syndrome: implications for epidemiologic studies, in Mortimer JA, Schuman LM (eds): *The Epidemiology of Dementia.* New York, Oxford University Press, pp 62–69.

8. Maletta GJ, Pirozzolo FJ, Thompson G, et al: Organic mental disorders in a geriatric outpatient population. *Am J Psychiatry* 1982; 139:521–523.

9. Jarvik LF, Ruth V, Matsuyama SS: Organic brain syndrome and aging: a six-year follow-up of surviving twins. *Arch Gen Psychiatry* 1980; 37:280–286.

10. Mortimer JA, Schuman LM, French LR: Epidemiology of dementing illness, in Mortimer JA, Schuman LM (eds): *The Epidemiology of Dementia.* New York, Oxford University Press, pp 3–23.

11. Sluss TK, Gruenberg EM, Kramer M: The use of longitudinal studies in the investigation of risk factors for senile dementia–Alzheimer type, in Mortimer JA, Schuman LM (eds): *The Epidemiology of Dementia,* New York, Oxford University Press, pp 132–154.

11a. Go RCP, Todorov AB, Elston RC, et al: The malignancy of dementias. *Ann Neurol* 1978; 6:559–561.

12. US Bureau of the Census: Projections of the population of the United States, 1977–2050, in *Current Population Reports,* series P-25, no. 704. US Government Printing Office, 1977.

13. Larsson T, Sjögren T, Jacobson G: Senile dementia: a clinical, sociomedical and genetic study. *Acta Physiol Scand Suppl* 1963; 39 (suppl 167): 1–259.

14. Tomlinson BE, Kitchener D: Granulovacuolar degeneration of hippocampal pyramidal cells. *J Pathol* 1972; 106:165–185.

15. Peress, NS, Kane WC, Aronson SM: Central nervous system findings in a tenth decade autopsy population. *Prog Brain Res* 1978; 40:473–483.

16. Matsuyama H, Nakamura S: Senile changes in the brain in the Japanese: incidence of Alzheimer's neurofibrillary change and senile plaques. *Aging NY* 1978; 7:287–297.

17. Heston LL: Genetic studies of dementia, with emphasis on Parkinson's disease and Alzheimer's neuropathology, in Mortimer JA, Schuman LM (eds): *The Epidemiology of Dementia.* New York, Oxford University Press, 1981, pp 101–114.

18. Roth M: Epidemiological studies. *Aging NY* 1978; 7:337–339.

19. Broe GA, Akhtar AJ, Andrews GR, et al: Neurological disorders in the elderly at home. *J Neurol Neurosurg Psychiatry* 1976; 39:362–366.

20. Kay DWK, Beamish B, Roth M: Old age disorders in Newcastle-upon-Tyne: II. A study of possible social and medical causes. *Br J Psychiatry* 1964b; 110:668–682.

21. Åkesson HO: A population study of senile and arteriosclerotic psychoses. *Hum Hered* 1969; 19:546–566.

22. Essen-Möller E, Larsson H, Uddenberg C, et al: Individual traits and morbidity in a Swedish rural population. *Acta Psychiatr Neurol Scand Suppl* 1956; suppl 100:156.

23. Primrose EJR: *Psychological Illness. A Community Study.* Springfield, Ill, Thomas, 1962.

24. Kay DWK, Beamish P, Roth M: Old age mental disorders in Newcastle-upon-Tyne: I. A study of prevalence. *Br J Psychiatry* 1964a; 110:146–158.

25. Bollerup TR: Prevalence of mental illness among 70-year-olds domiciled in nine Copenhagen suburbs: the Glostrup survey. *Acta Psychiatr Scand* 1975; 51:327–339.

26. Office of Scientific and Health Reports, National Institute of Neurological and Communicative Disorders and Stroke: *Neurological and Communicative Disorders. Estimated Numbers and Cost.* Washington, DC: DHEW publication no. NIH 77–152, 1976.

27. Gruenberg EM: Epidemiology of senile dementia, in Schoenberg BS (ed): *Neurological Epidemiology: Principles and Clinical Applications.* New York, Raven, 1978, pp 437–457.

20 Incidence of Neurofibrillary Change, Senile Plaques, and Granulovacuolar Degeneration in Aged Individuals

HARUO MATSUYAMA

ALZHEIMER'S NEUROFIBRILLARY CHANGE, SENILE PLAQUES, and granulovacuolar degeneration are generally considered the anatomical substrates of Alzheimer's disease (AD). These brain changes are also found to some extent in elderly people who are apparently within normal functional range for their age. The following description concerns the incidence of the above changes in the nondemented population.

ALZHEIMER'S NEUROFIBRILLARY CHANGE

Early Alzheimer-type change is characterized by a progressive increase in argyrophilia (silver staining) and increased thickening and tortuosity of cytoplasmic fibrillary neuronal structures (Fig. 20–1). These changes are, in the cerebrum, almost exclusively confined to the median temporal lobe, and the anterior half of the temporal lobe is more vulnerable (1, 2). In fulminant AD, the entire cerebral cortex is involved, and the posterior half of the hippocampus is also severely affected (1). Within the median temporal lobe, deeper layers of the cortical ribbon in the lateral aspect of the parahippocampal gyrus and the glomerular formation of the same gyrus are most vulnerable (Fig. 20–2). Other than the median temporal lobe, the cingulate gyrus, insula, and other parts of the cortex may also be involved. Among brain stem nuclei, a fairly high incidence of the change in locus ceruleus was reported (2).

Abnormal fibrils persist in tissue as remnants of dead nerve cells (Fig. 20–1). The ratio of cells with residual neurofibrillary changes tends to increase with advanced lesions. For instance, in the case of a 71-year-old woman who died of carcinoma of the cervix, shown in Figure 20–2, the ratio of residual fibrillary structures to intracytoplasmic fibrillary change is 2:1. Ball reported that the later phase of neurofibrillary change was four times more than the early phase, in sections from the median temporal lobe of a case of AD (1).

Figure 20–3 shows incidence of Alzheimer's neurofibrillary change by age, based on

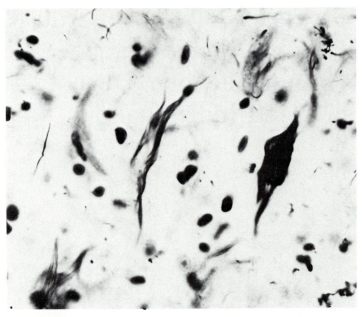

Figure 20–1. Coarse structure of the fibrillary material with dense argyrophilia represents earlier change (*right*). Networks of fine fibrils are identified as remnants of dead neurons. Silver impregnation. × 600.

Figure 20–2. Predilection site of Alzheimer-type neurofibrillary change. Distribution of Alzheimerized cells in the median temporal lobe at the level of the mamillary body.

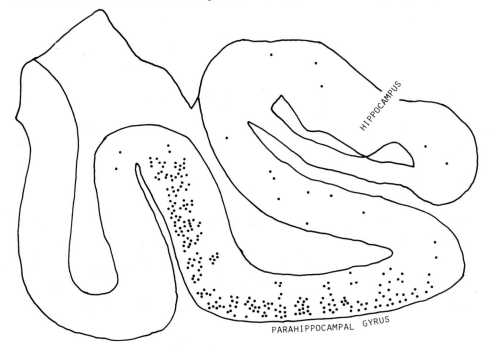

HIPPOCAMPUS

PARAHIPPOCAMPAL GYRUS

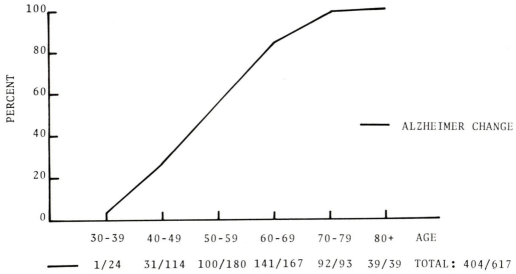

Figure 20–3. Incidence of Alzheimer-type neurofibrillary change by age.

observation of 617 brains obtained from autopsies in Tokyo and suburbs during the period of 1957 to 1972. The incidence of Alzheimer-type neurofibrillary changes increases linearly with age. A comparison of severity of the change in each age group is shown in Figure 20–4. Under age 60 the number of such cells, if any, is usually fewer than ten in a single section. In the six cases examined of age 90+ patients, affected cells actually decreased in number in comparison with the 80–89 year old age group. (See: Incidence of senile plaques in same age group, in Fig. 20–6.)

The incidence of neurofibrillary changes shown in Figure 20–3 is much higher than in reports from other countries (3–5). This may be at least partially due to methodologic

Figure 20–4. Histograms of Alzheimer-type neurofibrillary change by age. N = number of positive cases with Alzheimer-type neurofibrillary change.

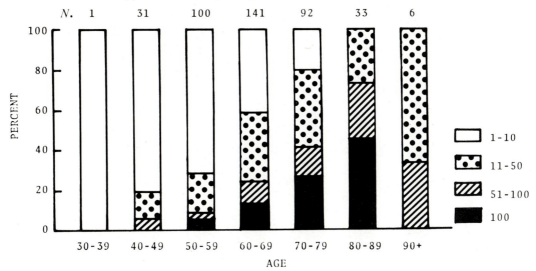

differences. For example, Anderson et al. reported in a study of 69 brains from the Guamanian Chamorro population without known evidence of dementia, parkinsonism, or amyotrophic lateral sclerosis that Alzheimer-type neurofibrillary changes appeared at much earlier ages than previously recognized; 29% of cases at the fourth decade in their study (6).

There is no significant gender difference in the frequency of neurofibrillary change. The incidence also does not appear to be influenced by, or associated with, any systemic condition. If the Alzheimer's neurofibrillary changes are confined to the median temporal lobe, they may be considered one of the "normal" physiological aging changes of the brain, and the number of these cells may be an indicator of gradation in the aging process.

Senile Plaques

Senile plaques (SPs) consist of a central core of amyloid, surrounded by thickened neurites including synaptic endings, both of which show strong argyrophilia (Fig. 20–5). The cerebral cortex is a common site of plaque formation; other subcortical gray matter rarely contains plaques. The distribution in normal aging varies in different regions of the cortex and the density is also irregular; in contrast, in AD it is uniformly heavy throughout the cortex. Figure 20–6 shows the incidence of the SPs by age among the Japanese. The incidence of SPs is much lower than that of Alzheimer-type neurofibrillary changes. The values shown in Figure 20–6 are, however, much lower than those of most reports from European countries (4), although the percentage of cases at different ages with SPs is little higher in comparison with similar Japanese reports which appeared prior to 1954 (7).

Both sexes are, again, equally affected. There is no correlation between the number of cells with Alzheimer-type neurofibrillary changes and the distribution and density of SPs.

Granulovacuolar Degeneration

Granulovacuolar degeneration (GVD) consists of one or more intracytoplasmic vacuoles, each of which contains argyrophilic and hematoxylinophilic granules (Fig. 20–7). The changes

Figure 20–5. Senile plaque. Silver impregnation. × 600.

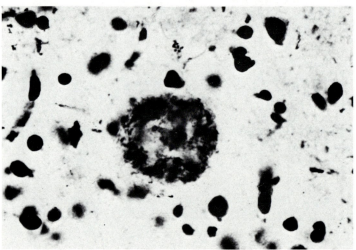

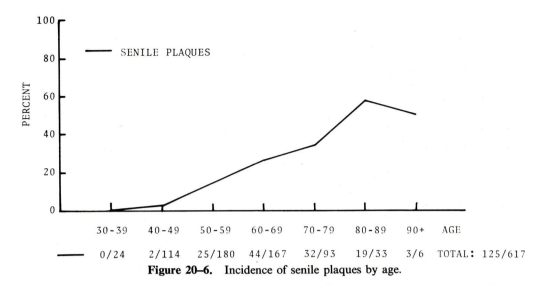

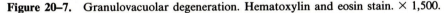

Figure 20–6. Incidence of senile plaques by age.

are almost entirely confined to Ammon's horn and its adjacent area. Outside of these regions, isolated nerve cells are sometimes rarely affected, in the amygdaloid nucleus and in some parts of the cortex. The prevalence is lower than for Alzheimer-type neurofibrillary changes, even though both types of pathologic change may affect an individual cell.

Tomlinson and Kitchner examined the hippocampal neurons in 219 cases taken from an acute-treatment general hospital (8). Granulovacuolar change was rare below the age of 60 years; above 60 years it was found with increasing frequency, and above 80 years was present in approximately 75% of all cases. From the seventh decade, the number of affected cells involved increased, as did the severity of the change in individual cells. Comparative studies agree that the incidence regularly increases above 60 years of age (7, 9).

Figure 20–7. Granulovacuolar degeneration. Hematoxylin and eosin stain. × 1,500.

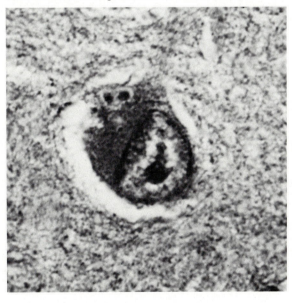

References

1. Ball MJ: Neurofibrillary tangles and the pathogenesis of dementia: a quantitative study. *Neuropath Appl Neurobiol* 1976; 2:395–410.

2. Matsuyama H, Nakamura S: Senile changes in the brain in the Japanese: incidence of Alzheimer's neurofibrillary change and senile plaques. *Aging NY* 1978; 7:287–297.

3. Dayan AD: Quantitative histological studies on the aged human brain: I. Senile plaques and neurofibrillary tangles in normal patients. *Acta Neuropathol* 1970; 16:85–94.

4. Gellerstadt N: Zur Kenntnis der Hirnveränderungen bei der normalen Altersinvolution. *Upsala Läkareförenings Förhandlingar* 1933; 38:194–408.

5. Tomlinson BE, Blessed G, Roth M: Observations on the brains of non-demented old people. *J Neurol Sci* 1968; 7:331–356.

6. Anderson FW, Richardson EP, Okazaki H, et al: Neurofibrillary degeneration on Guam: frequency in Chamorros and non-Chamorros with no known neurological disease. *Brain* 1979; 102:65–77.

7. Inose T: Die Pathologie des Gehirns im Praesenium und Senium. *Yokohama Med Bull* 1954; 5:287–303.

8. Tomlinson BE, Kitchener D: Granulovacuolar degeneration of hippocampal pyramidal cells. *J Pathology* 1972; 106:165–185.

9. Peress NS, Kane WC, Aronson SM: Central nervous system findings in a tenth decade autopsy population. *Prog Brain Res* 1978; 40:473–483.

21 Genetic Factors in Dementia of the Alzheimer Type

Steven S. Matsuyama

Evidence for genetic factors in the etiology of Alzheimer's disease (AD) has come from individual pedigrees, numerous family studies, and a twin study (for a review see ref. 1). Nearly all early genetic investigations distinguished between Alzheimer's disease of early and late onset. For this reason these conditions are reviewed separately.

GENETIC STUDIES

Alzheimer's Disease, Presenile Onset

Genetic factors in the etiology of AD have emerged from a number of pedigree studies (for a review see ref. 2). Caution is indicated, however, in relying on pedigree information as the sole basis of evaluating genetic influence since pedigrees usually come to attention because they contain a strikingly high accumulation of affected individuals.

The first systematic study of AD was performed in Sweden by Sjögren and co-workers (3), who collected a series of 36 index cases with AD, 18 of which had histopathologically verified diagnoses. Geneological data were collected from parish records, and personal visits made to the families of the index cases and to secondary cases. In addition, all individuals suspected of having a mental disorder were evaluated by a psychiatrist. For those who had died prior to the investigation, hospital records were reviewed. From these data, morbidity risks for AD were calculated at 10.7% for the parents and 3.8% for siblings of AD index cases, as compared to the general population AD morbidity risk in Sweden of 0.1%. First-degree relatives had, by deduction, a 38–107 times greater risk. Drawing on their data, the authors proposed a polygenic mode of transmission for AD.

Constantinides and associates (4) reviewed family histories derived from hospital records of individuals with AD admitted to the Bel Air Clinic in Geneva, Switzerland, between 1901 and 1958, and arrived at a 3.3% risk for siblings, and 1.4% for parents. Their data appeared most compatible with an autosomal dominant mode of inheritance with reduced penetrance. While the risk for siblings was similar in both the Swiss and Swedish studies, the risk for parents was much lower in the Swiss. This discrepancy may be due, at least in part, to the fact that Constantinides and associates relied on less extensive hospital records, whereas Sjögren and colleagues (3) carried out probing personal psychiatric interviews.

Heston (5), and Heston and Mastri (6), reported on a retrospective family study of 30 well-documented and histopathologically confirmed AD cases. These cases were collected from a consecutive series of autopsies in Minnesota state psychiatric facilities between 1952 and 1972; all patients had an onset before the age of 65. Relatives of the index cases were then contacted, at least one member of each family was interviewed, and a medical history compiled. Recurrence risks of 23% for parents and 10% for siblings were found, frequencies much higher than those previously reported. This may be because these researchers included both early and late onset cases of AD in their calculations, whereas previous investigators had studied only those cases beginning in the presenium. The data from the Minnesota study was compatible with both an autosomal dominant (low penetrance) and a polygenic model. Heston (5) and Heston and Mastri (6) also reported a marked increase in the frequency of Down's syndrome and myeloproliferative (leukemic) disorders among the families of Alzheimer patients. Aside from this association, it had been known that patients with Down's syndrome, if they survived, developed dementia at relatively early ages (in their thirties or forties), showing characteristic Alzheimer-type brain changes (7, 8), and had an increased risk of leukemia (9). Based on these associations, Heston (5) hypothesized a defect in the spatial organization of microtubules as a common pathological mechanism.

In an expanded study, Heston (10) investigated 86 additional probands with senile dementia and 10 with AD, bringing the total sample to 126 (30 from the original report) (5). Preliminary analysis revealed 67 secondary cases with recurrence risks of $12 \pm 2\%$ for siblings and $19 \pm 4\%$ for parents. The association with Down's syndrome was again found. Furthermore, examination of the distribution of cases by age at onset of the probands revealed that the excess of Down's syndrome cases was seen only among the relatives of the younger probands. By contrast, the initial report of an excess of hematologic malignancies among the relatives of probands, as compared to national rates, was no longer evident with the addition of the relatives of the older probands.

ALZHEIMER'S DISEASE, SENILE ONSET

Evidence for genetic factors in the etiology of senile dementia come from several family studies and one twin study. Family studies date back over 50 years (4, 11–13). Despite the small sample sizes in these early studies, they do give evidence of an increased familial incidence of senile dementia and indicate further that the hereditary factors are specific for senile dementia, as distinct from schizophrenia or other psychoses.

In the monumental study of senile dementia by Larsson and co-workers (14), records from two large mental hospitals in Stockholm were screened for persons diagnosed as senile dementia patients over a 15-year period. These case records were carefully analyzed, and 377 index cases were identified with 3,426 relatives; 2,675 of the relatives were investigated in the community and this effort led to the identification of 55 additional cases of senile dementia. The cases identified among the relatives did not deviate from the index cases with regard to onset, symptoms, or course of the disease. The morbidity risk for senile dementia among first-degree relatives was assessed at 4.3 times that in the general population. Again, there was no increase in the frequencies of other mental disorders. Not a single case of presenile-onset AD or presenile-onset Pick's disease was uncovered among the relatives, suggesting to the authors that senile dementia with onset in the presenium and AD with senile onset are separate entities. From general population figures, however, one would not expect to find any cases of AD with onset in the presenium in so small a sample, and other studies (4, 10) have reported both presenile- and senile-onset AD within the same family. Larsson and associates (14) found no evidence for sex linkage, and sociomedical factors did not appear to influence the morbidity risk for senile dementia.

Åkesson (15) studied an entire population in a well-defined area of islands off the coast of Sweden in an attempt to identify every case of significant dementia (serious enough to warrant more than casual comment). Although prevalence was lower than any previously reported, there was a sharply elevated risk for parents and siblings. In this study of 47 patients with the diagnosis of senile psychosis, nearly 20% of siblings aged 60 or older (23/125) also suffered from senile psychosis, the frequency increasing with age; 15% of the 80 parents who survived past 60 years of age (12/80) were also affected; with again an age-related increase in frequency.

Finally, there is one twin study in the literature (16). In that study, concordance rates were 8.0% for dizygotic twins, and 42.8% for monozygotic twins, with frequencies of 6.5% for siblings and 3.0% for parents.

Taken together, the studies reviewed in this section provide evidence for a significant genetic component in the etiology of AD. Although a number of models have been proposed, the precise mode of inheritance is not yet known and may vary from family to family.

CYTOGENETIC STUDIES FOR CHROMOSOMAL CORRELATES OF DEMENTIA

The search for chromosomal correlates of dementia began in the late 1960s with publications originating from Jarvik's (17, 18) and from Nielsen's laboratory (19, 20).

The subjects of the initial studies by Jarvik and associates (17, 18) were twins who formed part of the first and only prospective gerontological twin study in the United States, organized by Kallmann and associates (21) in the 1940s and maintained to the present time (22, 23). In the follow-up investigation, (18) a subsample of subjects was identified with the clinical diagnosis of chronic organic brain syndrome with onset after age 60. Those individuals for whom there was evidence in favor of multi-infarct dementia were excluded, and the final sample included 14 subjects, 8 women and 6 men, who fit the then current criteria of AD. The women showed a statistically significant increased frequency of chromosome loss, or "hypodiploidy" (21.6%, compared to 12.9% of 15 age-matched women without dementia; $P < .001$). By contrast, the six men with AD showed no significant difference in aneuploidy when compared to the seven age-matched men without evidence of dementia (15.4% hypodiploidy for those with dementia versus 16.5% for those without dementia).

Nielsen (20) examined 30 elderly women (10 with senile dementia, 10 with arteriosclerotic dementia, and 10 controls) and found the highest frequency of hypodiploidy in the senile dementia group, almost twice the level found in the age-matched controls (18.0% versus 10.1%; $P < .001$). The hypodiploidy frequency was similar between the arteriosclerotic dementia group and the controls (9.4% and 10.1%, respectively). As in the previous investigation, no increased frequency of hypodiploid cells was found in men with senile dementia. The sex difference is as yet unexplained but is in accord with numerous studies reporting that aged women have a higher frequency of chromosome loss than young women, but old and young men have about the same frequency (Matsuyama and Jarvik, in preparation).

Ward and co-workers (24) examined the chromosomes of three groups of subjects: 8 sporadic cases of presenile-onset AD, 5 familial cases of presenile-onset AD, and 9 unaffected siblings of the familial AD cases. They detected an increased frequency of chromosome loss in the AD cases, with the familial group exhibiting a higher frequency of loss than the sporadic group. Chromosome loss was significantly elevated in 2 of the 9 unaffected siblings, which led the authors to conclude that these two individuals were at greater risk of developing AD than were the other siblings. Unfortunately, because these investigators did not report the aneuploidy frequency for individuals in their control group, comparisons with individuals in the other three groups are precluded. Furthermore, of the 9 siblings examined, 7 came from a single family not represented among the 5 familial cases but included one family member with another chromosomal abnormality (XYY). Although this individual was not included in the analysis, the two individuals with elevated chromosome loss were among the remaining 6 siblings in this particular family. Thus, the elevated hypo-diploid frequency in a family prone to nondisjunction may be related to other factors aside from AD, and clearly many more families will need to be studied. In another study, a group of Swedish investigators (25), reported a significant increase in the frequency of hypo-diploid cells in 10 dementia patients (5 males and 5 females) compared to 10 sex-matched controls of comparable age (11.3% versus 7.8%, $p < .01$).

The studies described above focused primarily on alterations in chromosome number. Chromosome structure, too, has been examined in patients with early-onset AD. Normal karyotypes were reported in two studies (2, 26), and normal banding patterns in a third (27) Brun and associates (27) studied ten women with dementia of the Alzheimer type, including five familial cases.

Bergener and Jungklaass (28) described the occurrence of chromosomes without visible "centromeres" (acentric fragments) in cells from patients with AD. Unfortunately, the number of patients examined was not stated. Recently, Nordenson and colleagues (25) reported in their previously cited study: compared to ten healthy controls, ten individuals with nonfamilial dementia had a significant increase in the frequency of cells with acentric fragments. Reexamination of the data collected by Jarvik and associates (17, 18, 23) failed to confirm an increased frequency of structural chromosomal abnormalities for twins with AD (29). Neither men nor women showed a significantly increased frequency of chromosomal abnormalities, although the frequency was slightly higher in the dementia group than in the control group (for women 1.66% versus 1.33%; for men 2.50% versus 2.02%; for both sexes combined, the frequencies were 2.05% versus 1.53%, not statistically significant). The sister chromatid exchange (SCE) technique was recently applied to lymphocyte cultures from six women with AD (30) and an elevated frequency of SCEs was reported for the patients compared to controls. Clearly, further research on sister chromatid exchange is needed.

The chromosomal changes reported in the literature suggest the need for further cytogenetic studies. That chromosomal abnormalities may play a role in AD is an assumption strengthened by Heston's (5, 6, 10) report of an increased frequency not only of Alzheimer-type dementia but also of solid lymphoproliferative cancers and Down's syndrome (a chromosomal disorder) among relatives of patients with AD. At the moment, however, chromosomal findings cannot be used to make individual predictions of who is or is not at increased risk of developing AD. There is much overlap within studies and inconsistency from study to study.

Summary

There is evidence for a significant genetic component in the etiology of AD, and Heston and Mastri (5, 6, 10) have provided the first hypothesis concerning a mechanism. The mode of transmission may vary between families, both autosomal dominant with reduced penetrance and polygenic models having been proposed. Genetic markers which could help to identify persons at increased risk have not as yet been detected. The available data do not support using frequency of aneuploidy or any other indicator as predictors of disease, although eventually chromosome changes may be among the laboratory markers that collectively will enable researchers to make individual risk predictions.

ACKNOWLEDGMENTS

I wish to thank Lissy F. Jarvik, M.D., Ph.D., for helpful comments and suggestions during the preparation of this chapter.

REFERENCES

1. Matsuyama SS, Jarvik L: Genetics and mental functioning in senescence, in Birren JE, Sloane RB (eds): *Handbook of Mental Health and Aging.* Englewood Cliffs, Prentice-Hall, 1980, pp 134–148.

2. Feldman RG, Chandler KA, Levy L, et al: Familial Alzheimer's disease. *Neurology* 1963; 13:811–824.

3. Sjögren T, Sjögren H, Lindgren AGH: Morbus Alzheimer und Morbus Pick. *Acta Psychiatr Neurol Scand Suppl* 1952; 82:1–152.

4. Constantinides J, Garrone G, De Ajuriaguerra J: L'hérédité des démences de l'âge avancé. *Encephale* 1962; 51:301–344.

5. Heston LL: Alzheimer's disease, trisomy 21, and myeloproliferative disorders: associations suggesting a genetic diathesis. *Science* 1976; 196:322–323.

6. Heston LL, Mastri AR: The genetics of Alzheimer's disease: associations with hematologic malignancy and Down's syndrome. *Arch Gen Psychiatry* 1977; 34:976–981.

7. Jervis GA: Premature senility in Down's syndrome. *Ann NY Acad Sci* 1970; 171:559–561.

8. Olsen MI, Shaw CM: Presenile dementia and Alzheimer's disease in mongolism. *Brain* 1969; 92:147–156.

9. Ager EA, Schuman LM, Wallace HM, et al: An epidemiological study of childhood leukemia. *J Chronic Dis* 1965; 18:113–132.

10. Heston LL: Genetic studies of dementia, with emphasis on Parkinson's disease and Alzheimer's neuropathology, in Mortimer JA, Schuman LM (eds): *The Epidemiology of Dementia.* New York, Oxford University Press, 1981, pp 101–114.

11. Meggendorfer F: Über familiengeschichtliche Untersuchungen bei arteriosklerotischer und seniler Demenz. *Zentrabl Gesamte Neurol Psychiatr* 1925; 40:359.

12. Weinberger HL: Über die hereditären Beziehungen der seniler Demenz. *Zeitsch Gesamte Neurol Psychiatr* 1926; 106:666–701.

13. Cresseri A: L'ereditarietà della demenza senile. *Boll Soc Ital Biol Sper* 1948; 24:200–201.

14. Larsson T, Sjögren T, Jacobson G: Senile dementia: a clinical, sociomedical and genetic study. *Acta Psychiatr Scand Suppl* 1963; 39 (suppl 167):1–259.

15. Åkesson HO: A population study of senile and arteriosclerotic psychoses. *Hum Hered* 1969;19:546–566.

16. Kallmann FJ: *Heredity in Health and Mental Disorder.* New York, Norton, 1953.

17. Jarvik LF, Kato T: Chromosomes and mental changes in octogenarians: preliminary findings. *Br J Psychiatry* 1969; 115:1193–1194.

18. Jarvik LF, Altshuler KZ, Kato T, et al: Organic brain syndrome and chromosome loss in aged twins. *Dis Nerv Syst* 1971; 32:159–170.

19. Nielsen J: Chromosomes in senile dementia. *Br J Psychiatry* 1968; 114:303–309.

20. Nielsen J: Chromosomes in senile, presenile and arteriosclerotic dementia. *J Gerontol* 1970; 25:312–315.

21. Kallmann FJ, Sander G: Twin studies on senescence. *Am J Psychiatry* 1949; 106:29–36.

22. Jarvik LF, Yen FS, Ful TK, et al: Chromosomes in old age: a six-year longitudinal study. *Hum Genet* 1976; 33:17–22.

23. Jarvik LF, Ruth V, Matsuyama SS: Organic brain syndrome and aging: a six-year follow-up of surviving twins. *Arch Gen Psychiatry* 1980; 37:280–286.

24. Ward BE, Cook RH, Robinson A, et al: Increased aneuploidy in Alzheimer disease. *Am J Med Genet* 1979; 3:137–144.

25. Nordenson I, Adolfsson R, Beckman G, et al: Chromosomal abnormality in dementia of the Alzheimer type. *Lancet* 1980; i:481–482.

26. Mark J, Brun A: Chromosomal deviations in Alzheimer's disease compared to those in senescence and senile dementia. *Gerontol Clin* 1973; 15:253–258.

27. Brun A, Gustafson L, Mitelman F: Normal chromosome banding pattern in Alzheimer disease. *Gerontology* 1978; 24:369–372.

28. Bergener M, Jungklaass FK: Genetische Befunde bei Morbus Alzheimer und seniler Demenz. *Gerontol Clin* 1970; 12:71–75.

29. Matsuyama SS: Chromosomes and dementia of the Alzheimer type. Read before the Mini White House Conference on Aging: Alzheimer's Disease and Related Disorders, Washington, DC, Jan 16, 1981.

30. Fischman HK, Albu P, Reisberg B, et al: Elevation of sister chromatid exchanges in female Alzheimer's disease patients. *Am J Hum Genet* 1980; 32:69A.

22 Chromosomal Factors

Harlow K. Fischman

There is evidence that chromosomes play a role in the etiology or development of Alzheimer's disease (AD). A number of authors have presented data which, although sometimes based on small numbers of patients, and occasionally contradictory, indicate that chromosomal abnormalities are often associated with the disease.

Aneuploidy

Nielsen (1) reported increased "aneuploidy" (abnormal chromosome number) in senile dementia patients over that of age- and sex-matched normal and arteriosclerotic dementia controls (age range 65–89). His results were, however, based on only three females and three males. Mark and Brun (2) reported no increase of aneuploidy in eight Alzheimer patients ranging from 37 to 74 years in age. However, since one of the patients had Down's syndrome and no contemporary controls were used for comparison, it is hard to draw firm conclusions from their observations. Jarvik, Yen, and Goldstein (3) investigated the degree of aneuploidy in 78 institutionalized older women and reported that their average chromosome loss was 15.2% (12/78), compared with 10.1% and 10.6% in young and middle-aged women, respectively. There was some indication that the degree of "hypodiploidy" (chromosome loss) was greater in women diagnosed as having either a moderate or severe degree of organic brain syndrome (16.0%) (13/78) than for those showing mild or no such symptoms (14.4%) (11/78), but the difference was not statistically significant. They speculated that the changes might be due to aging, cognitive decline, or some factor associated with institutionalization.

Ward and associates (4) found increased aneuploidy in five familial and five out of eight sporadic Alzheimer patients. One of the most intriguing aspects of their investigation is the observation that aneuploidy was considerably greater in familial (13.0%) than in sporadic (8.1%) Alzheimer patients. This finding, together with the observation that asymptomatic siblings of patients with familial AD also had an increased aneuploidy over that of controls (5.4% versus 3.2%), indicated genetic loading, and suggested that people at risk for the disease or carrying it may be detectable by cytogenetic means. The data from Ward's investigation are hard to interpret, however, because of the low number of cases, and the observation that the 23 controls did not show the age-related increase in hypodiploidy found by many other investigators in normal females (5–10). Ward and associates' (4) findings were strengthened by the report of Honma and Hasegawa (11), who examined the prevalence of "hyperdiploid" cells (more than the normal number of chromosomes) in five Alzheimer patients and three control subjects. All of the Alzheimer patients had higher numbers of such cells, averaging 2.5% more, with a range of 1.2–4.8%, compared with the controls, who averaged 0.7%, with a range of 0.6–0.8%. Although the number of patients analyzed in this investigation was small, significance may lie in the observation of increased numbers of hyperdiploid cells. Although chromosome loss could be attributed to methodological error, the presence of extra chromosomes is more likely to be of real significance and could be attributed to "nondisjunction" (failure of chromosomes to separate during division).

Nordenson and co-workers (12) also observed a significantly higher frequency of hypodiploid cells in Alzheimer patients (11.3%) than in the controls (7.8%), although there was no significant difference in chromosome breakage (26 breaks per 1,581 cells in Alzheimer patients, compared with 15 breaks per 940 cells in the controls).

In Fischman and associates' investigation (13), the analysis of aneuploidy proved inconclusive, due to the wide range of chromosome loss and gain observed in the cells of both Alzheimer patients (0–20%, S.D. = 7.64%) and their controls (5–18%, S.D. = 6.05%).

Martin, Kellet, and Kahn (14) examined aneuploidy in lymphocyte cultures of 54 hospitalized Alzheimer patients (46 females and 8 males) and 73 aged controls (55 females and 18 females). They reported (unpublished data) that hypodiploidy was higher in both groups than in young controls and was also higher in female (12%) than in male (6%) AD patients. There was, however, no significant difference between the Alzheimer patients and their aged controls. Recently, White and colleagues (15) examined aneuploidy in 7 familial and 5 sporadic AD patients, 12 age- and sex-matched controls, and 19 relatives. They found no increase, on the average, in either aneuploidy or chromosome aberrations in any of these groups. Unfortunately, all metaphases with fewer than 44 or more than 48 chromosomes were excluded from the data, thus throwing some doubt on the conclusions from this otherwise well conceived study.

The results with regard to aneuploidy have therefore been contradictory. Possible explanations of this are: small numbers of AD patients in some of the investigations, methodological and technical differences, and the possibility that the different patient populations (from Scandinavia, England, Colorado, Washington, D.C., and New York) differ in some as yet undefined respect.

Sister Chromatid Exchanges

Another problem in Alzheimer's disease concerns "sister chromatid exchanges" (SCEs). SCEs are microscopically detectable interchanges between the replicated chromatids of metaphase chromosomes, and are believed to be involved in repair of damaged DNA (16). In a number of inherited disorders, such as Bloom's syndrome and Fanconi's anemia, faulty DNA repair mechanisms result in an elevation of SCEs. Exposure to mutagens or carcinogens also results in dose-dependent elevation of SCEs, and when repair-deficient cells are treated with these agents, larger increases in SCEs result.

Sulkava, Rossi, and Knuutila (17) reported no increase in SCEs in four females with AD compared with five controls (all of whom were under medication), in which they analyzed only 18–25 cells per patient. Their data reveal a slight increase in SCEs of the AD patients (10.44 SCEs per cell) over the controls (9.91 SCEs per cell) which could not be shown to be statistically significant, possibly due to the low number of patients and cells analyzed. Fischman and associates (13) analyzed blood cultures from six female Alzheimer outpatients and four age- and sex-matched controls. SCEs were scored on 30–40 second-division metaphases for each subject. The mean SCE level for the Alzheimer patients was 11.40 SCEs per metaphase, whereas that of the controls was 9.12. The difference between the two groups was found to be significant, as shown by the Wilcoxon Rank-Sum Test. Such an increase in SCE level is equivalent to that induced by 1.0×10^{-4} M Benz(a)pyrene, a potent carcinogen, in Chinese hamster ovary (CHO) cells (18). Additionally, it was observed that the only patient belonging to the Alzheimer group, who had an SCE level in the range of that of the controls (9.42), was diagnosed according to the Global Deterioration Scale (GDS) (19) as a mild case (GDS3) whereas the others were considered moderately deteriorated (GDS4 in four cases) or moderately–severely deteriorated (GDS5 in one case). Thus, there is some indication that the increase in SCE level was dependent on the gravity of the disease relatively early in the disease process. Furthermore, the addition of Mitomycin-C, a potent mutagen, to the cultures, increased the SCE level in the Alzheimer patients' cells to 31.63 SCEs per metaphase, while increasing that of the controls to a lesser extent (23.3 SCEs per metaphase).

There has been speculation that AD may be caused by a slow virus (20). In this light, it is interesting to note that Kurvink, Bloomfield, and Cervenka (21), among others, observed an elevation of SCEs in patients with viral diseases. Indeed, Sutherland and associates (22) reported an increase of SCEs in patients with multiple sclerosis, a suspected slow virus disease. Therefore, elevation of SCE level in AD patients may be caused by the presence of a virus. Schneider and co-workers (23) and Zanzoni and co-workers (24) observed that although baseline and mutagen-induced SCE levels do differ for human fibroblasts from individuals of differing age and early and late passages of cell lines, they do not differ in human white blood cells taken from both young and old donors. Thus, age of the subject, which is a factor in aneuploidy, apparently need not be considered when analyzing SCE level. However, a recent report by Schmidt and Sanger (25) is in disagreement. Fischman and colleagues (13) also reported that cell cycle time was considerably longer in both Alzheimer patients (31.7 hours) and aged controls (31.5 hours) than in normal young adults (22.5 hours).

CHROMOSOMAL ALTERATIONS

Bergener and Jungklaass (26) described the presence of large acrocentric marker chromosomes in Alzheimer patients (abnormally shaped, with the centromere closer to one end), but did not mention any loss or gain of chromosomes. This observation had not been confirmed until recently, when Nordenson and associates (12) reported fragments in ten nonfamilial Alzheimer patients (41 fragments per 1581 cells) compared with ten sex-matched controls (1 fragment per 940 cells), a highly significant difference. The fragments were described as varying in size from G- to B-type chromosomes and appearing most often in diploid cells. All of the Alzheimer patients had at least one fragment and seven of the ten patients had two to three fragments in at least one cell each. In most cells with more than one fragment, the fragments were of identical size. Nordenson speculated that the fragments may in reality be chromosomes that have undergone premature centromere division. Fischman and co-workers (13) observed these entities also, although in smaller number, and suspected that at least some of them are prematurely separated X chromosomes.

SUMMARY

Still awaiting clarification is whether chromosome alterations are involved in AD and, if so, to what extent and through what mechanism(s). Results of investigations of aneuploidy have been contradictory. Reports by Martin and associates (14) and by White and associates (15) indicate that hypodiploidy plays no role in the disease. However, Honma and Hosegawa's (11) results suggest that hyperdiploidy requires more extensive investigation. The situation with regard to SCEs is at present controversial, with conflicting reports. An investigation analyzing considerably more patients of the same sex and age range is needed to clarify the situation. Since three investigators (12) have independently reported the presence of chromosome fragments in leucocyte cultures from Alzheimer patients, this phenomenon bears scrutiny, especially because the identity, function and significance of these fragments is in doubt. Finally, observations on the length of the cell cycle and the effects of mutagens on cell cycle time and SCE level ought to be followed up with more comprehensive studies.

References

1. Nielsen J: Chromosomes in senile, presenile, and arteriosclerotic dementia. *J Gerontol* 25:312–315.

2. Mark J, Brun A: Chromosomal deviations in Alzheimer's disease compared to those in senescence and senile dementia. *Gerontology* 1973; 15:253–258.

3. Jarvik LF, Yen FS, Goldstein F: Chromosomes and mental status: a study of women residing in institutions for the elderly. *Arch Gen Psychiatry* 1974; 30:186–190.

4. Ward BE, Cook RH, Robinson A, et al: Increased aneuploidy in Alzheimer's disease. *Am J Med Genet* 1979; 3:137–144.

5. Jacobs PA, Court-Brown WM, Doll R: Distribution of human chromosome counts in relation to age. *Nature* 1961; 191:1178–1180.

6. Jacobs PA, Court-Brown WM: Age and chromosomes. *Nature* 1966; 212:823–824.

7. Galloway SM, Buckton KE: Aneuploidy and aging: chromosome studies on a random sample of the population using G-banding. *Cytogenet Cell Genet* 1978; 20:78–95.

8. Fitzgerald PH, McEwan CM: Total aneuploidy and age-related sex-chromosome aneuploidy in cultured lymphocytes of normal men and women. *Hum Genet* 1977; 39:329–337.

9. Vormittag W: Age dependence of chromosomal findings. *Acta Med Austriaca* 1977; 4:1–6.

10. Jarvik LF, Yen FS, Fu TK, et al: Chromosomes in old age: a six-year longitudinal study. *Hum Genet* 1976; 33:17–22.

11. Honma A, Hasegawa K: Chromosome abnormalities in dementia of the middle age. *Seishin Shinkeigaku Zasshi* 1979; 81:110–113.

12. Nordenson I, Adolfsson R, Beckman G, et al: Chromosomal abnormality in dementia of the Alzheimer type. *Lancet* 1980; i:482–483.

13. Fischman HK, Albu P, Reisberg B, et al: Elevation of sister chromatid exchanges in female Alzheimer's disease patients. *Am J Hum Genet* 1980; 32:A69.

14. Martin JM, Kellett JM, Kahn J: Aneuploidy in cultured human lymphocytes: II. A comparison between senescence and dementia. *Age Ageing* 1981; 10:24–28.

15. White BJ, Crandall C, Boudsmit J, et al: Cytogenetic studies of familial and sporadic Alzheimer's disease. *Am J Med Genet* 1981; 10:77–89.

16. Latt S: Sister chromatid exchanges. *Genetics* 1979; 92(May suppl):85–95.

17. Sulkava R, Rossi L, Knuutila S: No elevated sister chromatid exchange in Alzheimer's disease. *Acta Neurol Scand* 1979; 59:156–159.

18. Takehisa S, Wolff S: Induction of sister chromatid exchanges in Chinese hamster cells by carcinogenic mutagens requiring metabolic activation. *Mutat Res* 1977; 45:263–270.

19. Reisberg B, Ferris SH, Crook T: Signs, symptoms, and course of age-associated cognitive decline. *Aging NY* 1982; 19:177–181.

20. Wisniewski HM: Possible viral etiology of neurofibrillary changes and neuritic plaques. *Aging NY* 1978; 7:555–558.

21. Kurvink K, Bloomfield CD, Cervenka J: Sister chromatid exchange in patients with viral disease. *Exp Cell Res* 1978; 113:450–454.

22. Sutherland GR, Seshadri RS, Black A: Increased sister chromatid exchange in multiple sclerosis. *N Engl J Med* 1980; 303:1126.

23. Schneider EL, Kram E, Nakanishiy, et al: The effect of aging on sister chromatid exchange. *Mech Ageing Dev* 1979; 9:303–311.

24. Zanzoni F, Bauman JWA, Jung EG: Sister chromatid exchange (SCE) in human lymphocytes: effect of UV C irradiation and age. *Arch Dermatol Res* 1979; 265:283–287.

25. Schmidt MA, Sanger, WG: Sister chromatid exchange in aged human lymphocytes. A brief note. *Mech Age and Develop* 1981; 16:67–70.

26. Bergener M, Jungklaass FK: Die Alzheimersche Krankheit: Ein pathologischer Alterungsvorgang des Gehirns? *Acta Gerontol* 1972; 2:359–367.

23 Histocompatibility Locus Antigens and Alzheimer's Disease

Roy L. Walford

Teresa Fortoul

THE GENE PRODUCTS OF THE MULTIPLE LOCI of the HLA histocompatibility complex show significant disequilibrium with a number of human diseases. These include most of the autoimmune diseases, a few malignancies, diseases primarily metabolic or endocrinologic in origin (hemochromatosis, 17-hydroxylase deficiency), and others. The first HLA typing of a series of 34 Alzheimer patients in the age range 64–92 years by Henschke and associates (1) revealed an increased frequency of the antigen HLA-Cw3 ($P < .05$, uncorrected) and a nonsignificant increase in HLA-B7. The second study, by Cohen and associates (2), reported increases in B7, Cw3, and DRw4. On the basis of these results a collaborative HLA typing of 55 cases of nonfamilial Alzheimer's, undertaken as part of the 8th International Histocompatibility Workshop (3), revealed a statistically significant increase in B7 and a nonsignificant increase in Cw3. Of note was the fact that the haplotype B7Cw3 ("haplotype" refers to the two antigens occurring on the same chromosome, i.e., in cisposition) was present in 9.1% of the Alzheimer (AD) patients, versus an expected normal population frequency of 0.36%. The difference is highly significant ($P < 10^{-6}$). Furthermore, in the one four-generation family analysis submitted to the workshop, a common haplotype, including the B7Cw3 combination, appeared to be segregating with the disease.

Recently Cohen and associates (4) compared the patterns of cognitive loss in a series of 17 unrelated AD patients divided into groups with or without the B7 antigen. Cognitive loss was assessed by means of a Cognitive Evaluation Battery of 15 subtests. Two groups of subtests measured performance in terms of attention and memory, respectively, and a third measured focal cognitive skills such as reading, writing, and verbal fluency. Although both B7 (+) and B7 (−) AD patients showed equivalent deficits in memory capacity and retrieval from short- and long-term memory, the selective attention scores of B7 (+) patients were significantly lower than those of B7 (−) patients ($P < .001$).

While the above overall data seem to make a convincing case for an HLA association with AD, other studies have found either different associations or no significant association. In a small (18-case) series, Wilcox and co-workers (5) noted an increase in A2 for patients with onset under 60 years of age, and an increase in A1 and A3 for patients with a later age of onset. None of these values reached statistical significance. Among 124 cases including those with both early and late onset, Renvoize and colleagues (6) observed an increased frequency of Bw15. Unfortunately, the frequencies of other HLA antigens were not given in this report, but Bw15 is often associated with Cw3 (the C-locus may not have been typed-for in this study). Among 32 patients typed by Sulkava and associates (7) and 14 by Whalley and associates (8), no significant HLA disequilibria were detected. In two multigeneration families examined by Goudsmit and co-workers (9), there was clearly no segregation of the disease with the HLA haplotypes, even though B7 and Cw3 were present in both families.

In Table 23–1 we have listed the disease and control data for those HLA antigens which in some studies have shown evidence of disequilibrium, plus the total or combined data. Direct comparisons between disease and control HLA frequencies for the combined data are not valid because the ratios of disease to control populations vary between the studies, and the races are not exactly comparable. For example, the report of Sulkava and co-workers (7) adds a far larger percent of controls to the combined control groups than it adds to Alzheimer cases, so the distribution of HLA in the combined controls is more influenced by their (racial stratification) data than is the HLA distribution in the combined disease cases. This dilemma can be handled by calculating relative risk (RR) values, which permits evaluation with different racial groups in a combined analysis (10). These RR values are also given in Table 23–1, and the statistically significant ones are indicated. These figures, at face value, would suggest for example that B7(+) individuals are 50% more likely to develop nonfamilial AD than persons lacking this phenotype and A3(+) individuals are 40% less likely.

Assuming these data reflect not a statistical accident but a real influence of HLA upon AD, the following remarks seem in order. First, since most of the typing was done retrospectively rather than prospectively, it is not possible to distinguish entirely between resistance and susceptibility factors. For example, an increase in B7 might suggest that B7(+) persons are more susceptible, but if the real influence of B7 is to prolong the course of the disease (therefore representing a form of resistance), B7(−) persons will die off sooner; and if one simply HLA-types all available AD patients, B7 will appear increased. Typing data obtained prospectively, i.e., at time of onset or diagnosis, would clarify this situation.

Second, in HLA studies disease diagnosis is crucial because a moderate degree of disease heterogeneity (e.g., incorrect diagnosis) markedly lessens the chance to obtain meaningful correlations. This is a particular difficulty with AD since diagnostic problems definitely exist (11): perhaps a third or more of patients diagnosed using clinical criteria may not show senile plaques (SPs) and neurofibrillary tangles (NFTs) on cortical brain biopsy (12).

The HLA data for AD reveal several interesting features. The *decrease* in A3 and the borderline *increase* in B7 are paradoxical in that A3B7 is a common haplotype, and so A3 and B7 generally increase or decrease together when either is associated with disease, as for example in multiple sclerosis (13). If A3 were in fact associated with resistance and B7 (or the B7Cw3 haplotype) with susceptibility, a pattern of ↓A3 ↑B7 might obtain. The ↓A3 ↑B7, or even ↓A3 normal B7; the apparent increase in frequency of the otherwise rare B7Cw3 haplotype (3); the association of B7 with a selectively greater cognitive function loss (4); the great increase in one study (6) of Bw15, a phenotype often associated with Cw3; and finally the curious (but probably chance) occurrence of B7 and Cw3 in the three multiproband families so far typed, though not segregating with the disease, suggest that HLA genes or genes linked thereto may influence AD, but in a particularly complicated way. Some speculation may at least clarify the possibilities. The increase of A3 in the metabolic disease hemochromatosis may indicate some relation of A3− linked genes to iron transport or metabolism, and perhaps therefore to transport or absorption of other metals (aluminum?). ↓A3 and normal B7 may obtain in a syndrome characterized by adrenal cortical hyperfunction

TABLE 23–1
Frequencies of Certain HLA Phenotypes in Alzheimer's Disease from Five Studies in Percent. Relative Risk Values

HLA Phenotype	Henschke and Associates (1)		Cohen and Associates (2)		Walford and Hodge (3)		Wilcox and Associates (5)		Sulkava and Associates (7)		Total		
	Alz. $N=34$	Contr. $N=239$	Alz. $N=34$	Contr. $N=50$	Alz. $N=55$	Contr. $N=300$	Alz. $N=18$	Contr. $N=342$	Alz. $N=33$	Contr. $N=900$	Alz. $N=174$[a]	Contr. $N=1,831$[a]	Relative Risk
A 1	35	24	26	32	24	27	56	40	22	20	29	26	1.2
2	47	45	47	40	55	45	56	48	47	54	50	50	1.0
3	21	20	21	32	13	22	33	23	38	44	23	33	0.6[b]
B 7	29	21	44	24	36	17	33	27	16	24	32	24	1.5[c]
15	15	10	21	8	2	11	0	9	19	20	11	15	0.7
Cw 3	38	22	35	16	26	20	0	9	32	27	31	27	1.3
6	—	—	—	—	29	17	—	—	13	7	16	8	1.9[c]
DR 3	—	—	18	21	10	21	—	—	—	—	12	21	0.5
4	—	—	41	22	27	22	—	—	—	—	31	22	1.6[c]

[a] For Cw3, $N = 156$ for Alzheimer's, $N = 1,531$ for controls; for Cw6, $N = 122$ for Alzheimer's, $N = 1,250$ for controls. For DR, $N = 89$ for Alzheimer's, $N = 350$ for controls.
[b] $P < .01$.
[c] $P < .05$.

(13). B7 may be associated, furthermore, with some degree of humoral and cellular hyporeactivity.

Further studies of HLA association with AD should consider the following: (1) Evidence, although conflicting, suggests that familial and sporadic AD may be distinct (9, 14, 15). The HLA patterns are not inconsistent with this view, in that only the sporadic cases appear to show statistically significant relationships. Additional studies should therefore be divided not only by familial status but by age of onset or diagnosis (since younger patients tend to be of the familial form). (2) Prospective studies are preferred, but since inclusion of early cases increases the difficulty of diagnosis, further careful retrospective studies may also be useful. In any event, confirmation by autopsy or brain biopsy would probably greatly solidify the HLA association, if it exists. (3) Some HLA-disease associations are more related to clinical course and/or response to treatment than to simple presence or absence of disease. This has not yet been looked at for AD. (4) Possible relations between discriminatory cognitive function loss and genetic markers should be further evaluated.

REFERENCES

1. Henschke PJ, Bell DA, Cape RDT: Alzheimer's disease and HLA. *Tissue Antigens* 1978; 12:132–135.

2. Cohen D, Zeller E, Eisdorfer C, et al: Alzheimer's disease and the main histocompatibility complex (HLA system). *Gerontologist* 1979; 10(pt 2):57.

3. Walford RL, Hodge SE: HLA distribution in Alzheimer's disease, in Terasaki PI (ed): *Histocompatibility Testing*. Los Angeles, UCLA Tissue Typing Laboratory, 1980, pp 727–729.

4. Cohen D, Eisdorfer C, Walford R: Histocompatibility antigens (HLA) and patterns of cognitive loss in dementia of the Alzheimer type. *Neurobiol Aging* 1982; 2:277–280.

5. Wilcox CB, Caspary EA, Behan PO: Histocompatibility antigens in Alzheimer's disease: a preliminary study. *Eur Neurol* 1980; 19:262–265.

6. Renvoize EB, Hambling MH, Pepper MD, et al: Possible association of Alzheimer's disease with HLA-Bw15 and cytomegalovirus infection. *Lancet* 1979; i:1239.

7. Sulkava R, Koskimies S, Wikstrom J, et al: HLA antigens in Alzheimer's disease. *Tissue Antigens* 1980; 16:191–194.

8. Whalley LJ, Urbaniak SJ, Darg D, et al: Histocompatibility antigens and antibodies to viral and other antigens in Alzheimer pre-senile dementia. *Acta Psychiatr Scand* 1980; 61:1–7.

9. Goudsmit J, White BJ, Weitkamp LR, et al: Familial Alzheimer's disease in two kindreds of the same geographic and ethnic origin. *J Neurol Sci* 1981; 49:79–89.

10. Woolf B: On estimating the relation between blood group and disease. *Ann Hum Genet* 1955; 19:251–255.

11. Masters CL, Gajdusek DC, Gibbs CJ Jr: Problems of case ascertainment and diagnosis in the epidemiology of dementia occurring in geographic isolates and worldwide, in Mortimer JA, Schuman LM (eds): *The Epidemiology of Dementia*. Cambridge, Oxford University Press, 1981, pp 155–170.

12. Zeisel S, Reinstem D, Corkin S, et al: Cholinergic neurons and memory. *Nature* 1981; 293:187–188.

13. Bertrams J: HLA and disease associations. *Behring Inst Mitt* 1978; 62:69–92.

14. Ford EHR: Complex patterns of inheritance in human disease. *Nature* 1978; 272:755–756.

15. Moreau-Dubois M, Brown P, Goudsmit J, et al: Biologic distinction between sporadic and familial Alzheimer's disease by an in *vitro* cell fusion test. *Neurology* 1981; 31:323–325.

CLINICAL DIAGNOSIS AND DIFFERENTIAL DIAGNOSIS OF ALZHEIMER'S DISEASE AND RELATED DISORDERS

24

Clinical Presentation, Diagnosis, and Symptomatology of Age-Associated Cognitive Decline and Alzheimer's Disease

BARRY REISBERG

THE CLINICAL SYNDROME OF ALZHEIMER'S DISEASE (AD), sometimes referred to as primary degenerative dementia (PDD) (1), is characterized and identified by its unique onset, course, and presentation. Until recently, these features of the illness process had not been fully detailed; hence, clinicians diagnosed AD by excluding other conditions rather than by reference to its own unique features (2–4). These features, which have been detailed elsewhere (5–7), are briefly reviewed in this chapter.

GLOBAL CLINICAL SYMPTOMATOLOGY

The clinical symptomatology of persons with cognitive decline consistent with normal aging or AD varies with the magnitude or stage of cognitive impairment. Within each stage, symptomatology is fairly consistent. The global clinical characteristics, and the psychological test concomitants of each stage of cognition in normal aged and in those with mild to severe AD, can be seen in the Global Deterioration Scale (GDS) for age-associated cognitive decline and AD described in Table 24–1 (7, 8). The reader should study this table carefully, since it provides the only detailed description of the clinical symptomatology of progressive cognitive impairment in normal aging and AD in this volume. A less detailed description of the symptomatology in the forgetfulness, confusional, and dementia phases can also be found in Section 1 of this text. The discussion below enlarges upon, without replicating, the descriptions found in Section 1 of this volume and in Table 24–1. In reading this chapter, the reader is urged to refer back to Table 24–1 frequently.

Clinicians must recognize the variability of prognostic concomitants in the evolutionary phases of progressive cognitive decline. These prognostic features will be discussed below. However, if the patient has been correctly diagnosed, then the presence of a particular stage of cognitive impairment does imply that the patient must already have experienced the preceding stages and symptoms. In all cases, the condition's progress is gradual, and all patients who are correctly diagnosed and who are not the victims of secondary disease processes spend periods of several months to years in each global stage.

TABLE 24-1
Global Deterioration Scale (GDS) for Age-Associated Cognitive and Alzheimer's Disease

GDS Stage	Clinical Phase	Clinical Characteristics	Psychometric Concomitants
1 No cognitive decline	Normal	No subjective complaints of memory deficit. No memory deficit evident on clinical interview.	Average or above average performance for age and WAIS vocabulary score on 3 of 5 Guild (23) memory subtests.
2 Very mild cognitive decline	Forgetfulness	Subjective complaints of memory deficit, most frequently in following areas: (a) forgetting where one has placed familiar objects; (b) forgetting names one formerly knew well. No objective evidence of memory deficit on clinical interview. No objective deficits in employment or social situations. Appropriate concern with respect to symptomatology.	Below average performance for age and WAIS vocabulary score on 3 of 5 Guild subtests.
3 Mild cognitive decline	Early confusional	Earliest clear-cut deficits. Manifestations in more than one of the following areas: (a) patient may have gotten lost when traveling to an unfamiliar location; (b) co-workers become aware of patient's relatively poor performance; (c) word and name finding deficit become evident to intimates; (d) patient may read a passage or a book and retain relatively little material; (e) patient may demonstrate decreased facility in remembering names upon introduction to new people; (f) patient may have lost or misplaced an object of value; (g) concentration deficit may be evident on clinical testing. Objective evidence of memory deficit obtained only with an intensive interview conducted by a trained geriatric psychiatrist. Decreased performance in demanding employment and social settings. Denial begins to become manifest in patient. Mild to moderate anxiety accompanies symptoms.	One standard deviation or greater below-average performance for age and WAIS vocabulary score on 3 of 5 Guild memory subtests. Often no errors on the Mental Status Questionnaire (MSQ) (24).
4 Moderate cognitive decline	Late confusional	Clear-cut deficit on careful clinical interview. Deficit manifest in following areas: (a) decreased knowledge of current and recent events; (b) may exhibit some deficit in memory of one's personal history; (c) concentration deficit elicited on serial subtractions; (d) decreased ability to travel, handle finances, etc. Frequently no deficit in following areas: (a) orientation to time and person; (b) recognition of familiar persons and faces; (c) ability to travel to familiar locations. Inability to perform complex tasks. Denial is dominant defense mechanism. Flattening of affect and withdrawal from challenging situations occur.	Frequent mistakes on 3 or more items on MSQ.

174

			Deficits evident on brief MSQ assessment.
5 Moderately severe decline	Early dementia	Patient can no longer survive without some assistance. Patient is unable during interview to recall a major relevant aspect of their current lives: e.g., their address or telephone number of many years, the names of close members of their family (such as grandchildren), the name of the high school or college from which they graduated. Frequently some disorientation to time (date, day of week, season, etc.) or to place. An educated person may have difficulty counting back from 40 by 4s or from 20 by 2s. Persons at this stage retain knowledge of many major facts regarding themselves and others. They invariably know their own names and generally know their spouses and children's names. They require no assistance with toileting or eating, but may have some difficulty choosing the proper clothing to wear and may occasionally clothe themselves inappropriately (e.g., put shoes on the wrong feet, etc.)	
6 Severe cognitive decline	Middle dementia	May occasionally forget the name of the spouse upon whom they are entirely dependent for survival. Will be largely unaware of all recent events and experiences in their lives. Retain some knowledge of their past lives but this is very sketchy. Generally unaware of their surroundings, the year, the season, etc. May have difficulty counting from 10, both backward and sometimes, forward. Will require some assistance with activities of daily living, e.g., may become incontinent, will require travel assistance but occasionally will display ability to travel to familiar locations. Diurnal rhythm frequently disturbed. Almost always recall their own name. Frequently continue to be able to distinguish familiar from unfamiliar persons in their environment. Personality and emotional changes occur. These are quite variable and include: (a) delusional behavior, e.g., patients may accuse their spouse of being an imposter; may talk to imaginary figures in the environment, or to their own reflection in the mirror; (b) obsessive symptoms, e.g., person may continually repeat simple cleaning activities; (c) anxiety symptoms, agitation, and even previously nonexistent violent behavior may occur; (d) cognitive abulia, i.e., loss of willpower because an individual cannot carry a thought long enough to determine a purposeful course of action.	5–10 errors on MSO.
7 Very severe cognitive decline	Late dementia	All verbal abilities are lost. Frequently there is no speech at all—only grunting, incontinent of urine; requires assistance in toileting and feeding. Loses basic psychomotor skills, e.g., ability to walk. The brain appears to no longer be able to tell the body what to do. Generalized and cortical neurologic signs and symptoms are frequently present.	

Source: Developed by Barry Reisberg, Steven H. Ferris, and Thomas Crook.

Previous investigations have revealed strong, significant relationships between progressive decline on these global clinical parameters and independent psychometric (7–9), neuroradiologic (10, 11), neurometabolic (12, 13), neuroimmunologic (14), and electrophysiologic (15) assessments.

MULTI-AXIAL CLINICAL ASSESSMENTS

More recent work has indicated that these global stages can also be clinically subdivided into five clinical axes: (I) concentration, (II) recent memory, (III) past memory, (IV) orientation, and (V) functioning and self-care (16).

When properly defined, decline on each of these clinical parameters tends to proceed at a rate consistent with the global stage of cognitive functioning (16). Definitions of these clinical parameters, or "axes," corresponding to the successive stages of global cognitive deterioration can be seen in the Brief Cognitive Rating Scale (BCRS) described in Table 24–2.

Since scores on each of the clinical axes described in Table 24–2 correlate strongly not only with each other but also with the corresponding Global Deterioration Scale (GDS) scores (Table 24–1), the BCRS axes (Table 24–2) provide a brief clinical sketch of the corresponding clinical stage of cognitive functioning. Hence, a patient with moderate cognitive decline in the late confusional phase (GDS-4) (as described in Table 24–1) is likely to show a corresponding degree of impairment on each of the BCRS axes. Specifically, this patient is likely to demonstrate "definite concentration deficit for persons of their background" (Table 24–2, Axis 1, rating score "4"). This concentration deficit can frequently be manifested by asking the patient to subtract serial 7's from 100. These late confusional phase patients will frequently demonstrate not only marked deficits on subtraction of serial 7's, but also deficits in subtraction of serial 4's from 40. As can be seen in Table 24–2, this same patient is, however, likely to be capable of subtracting serial 2's from 20 without difficulty.

This same patient, in the late confusional phase, will likely not recall some major events from the previous weekend and have a "scanty knowledge of current events" (Axis II, rating score "4"). However, this late confusional phase patient is likely to recall the name of the current head of state of the country of residence, as well as the correct personal current address.

As visualized in Table 24–2, this late confusional phase patient is also likely to show corresponding deficits in past memory (Axis III). A common statement about mildly to moderately impaired PDD patients, frequently articulated by patients as well as family members, is that their recent memory has suffered; however, the patients' past memory "remains excellent." This perception is in part a product of the PDD patient's continual necessity to recall events from the recent past, whereas the patient is rarely queried in detail with respect to childhood or early school experiences. On those unusual occasions when a mildly or moderately impaired PDD patient is required to recall details from the past, it is acceptable to frequently resort to the rationalization, "It was so long ago, how can I be expected to remember that?" Hence, deficits in past memory, although present, are not as readily manifest, and are not as troubling for the patient or the patient's family.

The orientation deficits which are most probably manifest at each GDS stage can be seen in Axis IV of the BCRS. Thus, in the late confusional phase (GDS = 4), the patient is likely to err by ten or more days in response to queries on the current date. At this stage the patient can, most probably, still recall the current year, and remains oriented with respect to location.

Functional deficits are particularly notable concomitants of each global stage of deterioration. These deficits are the ones most clearly observed by family members and caretakers of AD patients. In the late confusional phase, characteristic functional deficits are difficulties with handling finances and marketing. Yet these patients not only remain fully capable of *donning* their clothing properly, but also of *choosing* the proper clothing for the season and special occasions.

OTHER CLINICAL FEATURES

In addition to the clinical features described in Tables 24–1 and 24–2, other clinically observable changes accompany the various stages of progressive cognitive decline. The most notable additional clinical features are those related to speech, psychomotor abilities, and mood and behavior (17).

CHANGES IN SPEECH AND LANGUAGE

As shown in Table 24–1, the forgetfulness phase is frequently accompanied by subjective difficulty in recalling names of persons and objects. In the early confusional phase more overt word-finding difficulties occur, and these deficits become evident to spouses and other intimates. Occasionally in this phase, the patient's verbalizations will be interrupted intermittently as the patient gropes for the proper word. Mild stuttering may also occur. In the late confusional phase, the language deficit is most frequently manifested in a notable decrease in verbalizations. The patient becomes notably quieter. Reasons for the late confusional phase patients' unaccustomed reticence are multiple, and include decreased intellectual abilities in general, as well as specific decreased verbal abilities. Such reticence is also compatible with an affective flattening which occurs at this phase. Conversely, some patients react to this increased word-finding deficit in the confusional phase with a tendency to ramble or talk around the point. Thus, ironically, this form of adaptation to the verbalizing deficit may lead to an overall increase in verbalization, although speech precision is compromised.

In the early dementia phase, the earlier reticence becomes an overt paucity of speech. Sentence production remains intact; however, the patient uncommonly offers more than one-sentence responses to queries. Spontaneous speech is also notably decreased. In the middle dementia phase, the patient is no longer capable of speaking in full sentences. Responses tend to be limited to one or, at most, a few words. Patients at this phase who have acquired new languages over the course of their lifetime frequently revert to using words from languages which had been acquired earlier in life. For instance, one man in the mid-dementia phase had been born in Poland, moved to Germany as a child, met his wife, and subsequently moved permanently with her to the United States. This man began addressing his wife not in their current English, nor in their former mutual language, German, but rather in Polish, which was unintelligible to his wife and others in attendance.

In the late dementia phase all verbal abilities are lost; grunting, neologisms, verbigeration, echolalia, and other major language disturbances predominate. (Verbigeration is often mani-

TABLE 24–2
Brief Cognitive Rating Scale (BCRS)

Axis	Rating (Circle Highest Score)	Ordinal Clinical Characteristics
I: Concentration	1	No objective or subjective evidence of deficit in concentration.
	2	Subjective decrement in concentration ability.
	3	Minor objective signs of poor concentration (e.g., on subtraction of serial 7's from 100).
	4	Definite concentration deficit for persons of their background (e.g., marked deficit on serial 7's; frequent deficit in subtraction of serial 4's from 40).
	5	Marked concentration deficit (e.g., giving months backwards or serial 2's from 20).
	6	Forgets the concentration task. Frequently begins to count forward when asked to count backwards from 10 by ones.
	7	Marked difficulty counting forward to 10.
II: Recent memory	1	No objective or subjective evidence of deficit in recent memory.
	2	Subjective impairment only (e.g., forgetting names more than formerly).
	3	Deficit in recall of specific recent events evident upon detailed questioning. No deficit in the recall of major recent events.
	4	Cannot recall major events of previous weekend or week. Scanty knowledge (not detailed) of current events, favorite TV shows, and so on.
	5	Unsure of weather; may not know current president or current address.
	6	Occasional knowledge of some recent events. Little or no idea of current address, weather, and so on.
	7	No knowledge of any recent events.
III: Past memory	1	No subjective or objective impairment in past memory.
	2	Subjective impairment only. Can recall two or more primary school teachers.
	3	Some gaps in past memory upon detailed questioning. Able to recall at least one childhood teacher and/or one childhood friend.
	4	Clear-cut deficit. The spouse recalls more of the patient's past than the patient. Cannot recall childhood friends and/or teachers but knows the names of most schools attended. Confuses chronology in reciting personal history.
	5	Major past events sometimes not recalled (e.g., names of schools attended).
	6	Some residual memory of past (e.g., may recall country of birth or former occupation).
	7	No memory of the past.

TABLE 24–2 (*Continued*)
Brief Cognitive Rating Scale (BCRS)

Axis	Rating (Circle Highest Score)	Ordinal Clinical Characteristics
IV: Orientation	1	No deficit in memory for time, place, identity of self or others.
	2	Subjective impairment only. Knows time to nearest hour, location.
	3	Any mistake in time > 2 hr; day of week > 1 day; date > 3 days.
	4	Mistakes in month > 10 days or year > 1 month.
	5	Unsure of month and/or year and/or season; unsure of locale.
	6	No idea of date. Identifies spouse but may not recall name. Knows own name.
	7	Cannot identify spouse. May be unsure of personal identity.
V: Functioning and self-care	1	No difficulty, either subjectively or objectively.
	2	Complains of forgetting location of objects. Subjective work difficulties.
	3	Decreased job functioning evident to co-workers. Difficulty in traveling to new locations.
	4	Decreased ability to perform complex tasks (e.g., planning dinner for guests, handling finances, marketing, etc.).
	5	Requires assistance in choosing proper clothing.
	6	Requires assistance in feeding, and/or toileting, and/or bathing, and/or ambulating.
	7	Requires constant assistance in all activities of daily life.

Source: Developed by Barry Reisberg, Gerri E. Schwartz, Thomas Crook, and Steven H. Ferris.

fested by repeating the first syllable of a word.) Some patients simply let out infrequent screams. One patient at this stage had a vocabulary consisting entirely of "okay," which she repeated innumerable times when she recognized a family member and in response to stress or other verbalization-provoking phenomena. At some point in this phase, most patients eventually lose all verbal abilities.

CHANGES IN PSYCHOMOTOR ABILITIES

Decreased performance of complex psychomotor tasks (such as sailing ability or complex constructional tasks) does not occur until the early confusional phase. Since these complex motor abilities are not necessarily a part of modern, everyday life, psychomotor deficits may not be noted either by the patient or their relatives at this phase. In the late confusional phase, general motor abilities overtly decline. Most frequently, those who know the patient will note that the patient's gait has slowed, and the patient seems more cautious with respect to movements. In the early dementia phase the slowing of gait and related movements in patients are observable even to a physician unfamiliar with a patient's previous level of functioning.

Although arthritis, mild parkinsonism (18), or other clinical contributors to impaired movement may sometimes coexist in these aged patients, the Alzheimer's process alone is sufficient to account for such observed patient motor changes in this early dementia phase. In the mid-dementia phase, the patient frequently requires assistance with ambulation. Even when assistance is not required, the patient's steps become small and movements markedly halted. Individuals at this phase also frequently have difficulty signing their name properly, even with assistance. Another concurrent psychomotor manifestation is increased difficulty with manipulating silverware; the ability to manage a knife or fork is compromised.

In the late dementia phase patients lose all ability to walk. They cannot even begin to sign their names and are frequently unable to grasp a pen or pencil placed in their hand. They cannot use utensils, and either eat with their hands or must be fed.

CHANGES IN MOOD AND BEHAVIOR

Cognitive changes are accompanied by mood and behavior shifts which vary with the overall severity of the illness. The mild subjective symptomatology of the forgetfulness phase is accompanied by an increase in concern in the patient; anxiety is voiced by the patient (i.e., it is subjective) but is not otherwise clinically manifest.

In the early confusional phase the stresses and demands of a lifestyle which the patient can no longer successfully fulfill result in more overt anxiety manifestations. The latter may be evident to the clinician as well as the patient's kin. In the late confusional phase denial becomes a dominant defense mechanism, and the patient frequently begins adaptive withdrawal from stresses. The net effects of these denial and withdrawal processes is a blunting of emotional response which psychiatrists term a "flattening of affect." The patient becomes less involved in activities, both intellectually and emotionally.

In the early dementia phase this decreased involvement may be accompanied by a mourning process. The patient may suddenly cry for no apparent reason during the day, and then suddenly stop. Concomitantly, denial prevents a patient from explaining such crying episodes. In most cases, however, the patient is probably mourning the loss of his intellect, consciously or unconsciously. The mid-dementia phase is accompanied by overt agitation, which may result from the constant threat of an environment which the patient can no longer successfully negotiate, and which is therefore genuinely dangerous. The stresses and physiologic changes accompanying the illness may result in severe psychiatric disturbances at this stage as well as generalized agitation. Patients may begin talking to themselves. They may experience visual hallucinations, which may be related to their reveries. Frequently patients become paranoid or formally delusional, paranoia the possible result of adaptive suspicion of a world which is becoming frighteningly unfamiliar. Alternatively, the delusions may provide a personal explanation for the anger or memory deficits which have befallen the patient.

In the late dementia phase, patients become relatively passive as they lose the ability to speak and to walk. Under these circumstances agitation is utilized for communication. Excitement or crying out may indicate that the patient is about to have a bowel movement and requires assistance; it might also indicate that the patient has soiled himself or herself. Finally, increased respiration, verbalization, or a scream may indicate that the patient recognizes someone well-known or loved.

INSIGHT AND DENIAL

A complex pattern of stage-specific increased concern, anxiety, and denial, accompanies the evolution of progressive cognitive deficits. Understanding this process is necessary for assessment and clinical differential diagnosis of early age-related memory loss and AD.

"Denial" has been defined as a "defense mechanism, operating unconsciously, used to resolve emotional conflict and allay anxiety by disavowing thoughts, feelings, wishes, needs, or external reality factors that are consciously intolerable" (19 [p. 28]). Denial is betrayed by an obvious disparity between the patient's condition and how the patient reports it; patients often smilingly insist that all is well or that a symptom does not exist (20). Although denial has been a reported component of a very broad spectrum of physical and emotional maladies, the extent to which this mechanism operates as a concomitant of cognitive decline in normal aging and in PDD has apparently only recently been systematically studied (21).

The loss of one's intellectual and general thinking capacities is a tragedy too painful for conscious contemplation. As with any devastating illness or loss, the psychological defense mechanism termed denial operates to prevent full conscious contemplation of the loss which would be emotionally shattering.

The earliest symptoms of cognitive decline in what we term the forgetfulness phase are fully recognized by the patient and those with whom they are in intimate contact, most often their spouse. In a sense, the observational powers of the spouse are validated by the remarkable concordance of both patients and spouses with respect to onset and severity of these very subtle early cognitive symptoms.

Emotionally, these early symptoms evoke a sense of alarm in patients and their spouses. Both recognize increased emotional difficulties which noticeably affect ongoing family relationships. Both patients and intimates become more irritable as a result of these symptoms. Spouses, in particular, are somewhat ashamed of the patients' forgetfulness; however, neither patient nor spouse feels at all helpless at this early stage. Interestingly, at this early stage, the patient becomes not only acutely aware of their cognitive problem, but also acutely, perhaps hyperacutely, sensitive to slight cognitive problems in the spouse.

In general, the patients' reported awareness of their memory deficits tends to peak in the confusional phase. Spouses' awareness of memory problems in the patient tend not to differ markedly from the patients' assessments at this phase. Patients and spouses continue to experience some emotional problems as a result of the patients' memory difficulties. However, increased irritability and shame are transient phenomena which the patient can still suppress at this phase. A sense of helplessness on the part of both the patient and the spouse also develops for the first time in this phase. Confusional phase patients and their spouses can adjust socially to the patients' memory problems by isolating the cognitive symptomatology in terms of its marital and social manifestations. Denial of specific cognitive problems does occur in the confusional phase, however. Specifically, patients, but not their spouses, are unwilling to accept their increasing incapacity to carry out the basic activities of daily living.

In the dementia phase, patients develop a profound denial of cognitive and emotional deficit. The denial appears to occur in precisely those areas of cognition and emotional functioning which are most severely affected. Despite the profound denial, even in the early and mid-dementia phases, patients do appear to display insight with respect to the functioning of their spouses in cognitive and other areas.

Clinically, the denial of cognitive deficit which appears such a notable concomitant of dementia phase symptomatology manifests itself in various ways. A minority of patients find any evaluation of their memory forcing them to confront their deficit too painful an experience for voluntary participation. Some patients refuse to see all physicians in general, and physicians or other professionals who will be evaluating their cognitive status in particular. Other patients brought in for an evaluation become acutely anxious; they may develop an acute anxiety attack or exhibit conversion or dissociative symptomatology. For example, one woman recently responded to all questions put to her by panting and grunting. Other patients refuse any evaluation of their memories and simply leave the office or testing room.

Many other dementia phase patients, although they display marked denial symptomatology, do not exhibit the extreme symptoms described above. For example, a typical patient, when asked, "Who is the president of the United States?" will simply respond with the rationalization, "I don't follow politics very closely." Other rationalizations are also frequent. A dementia phase patient who does not recall the name of the college where the patient earned a degree might explain, "But that was so many years ago; how can you expect me to remember what school I went to 50 years ago?"

Collectively, these rationalizations and other defense mechanisms buttress the dementia phase patients' capacity for denial. The net gain for the patient is the psychological defense which they develop against what would otherwise be exceedingly traumatic emotional concomitants of their illness process.

PROGNOSIS

The prognosis for outpatients with age-associated cognitive decline or AD, who lack other complicating illnesses which might confound the clinical presentation, can be seen in Tables 24–3 and 24–4 (22).

Forgetfulness phase symptomatology does indeed appear to be benign. After approximately 2 years of follow-up, all 16 patients whom we followed remained alive, well, functional community residents. Furthermore, these patients did not demonstrate significant decline on independent clinical cognitive assessments or functional assessments over the follow-up interval.

All 14 patients in the early confusional phase whom we followed also remained alive, well, and community residing after more than 2 years. However, these patients had declined significantly on clinical cognitive assessment scores.

The late confusional phase patients showed serious decline over the follow-up interval. Two of the 11 patients whom we followed were deceased and 1 was institutionalized at the time of follow-up. The remaining 8 showed significant decline on clinical cognitive and mental status questionnaire (MSQ) assessments.

The early dementia phase was also associated with marked deterioration after a 2-year interval. Of six patients followed, one was deceased and two were institutionalized. Of the remaining three, decline on the functional assessments was evident, although because of the small number of survivors, this decline did not reach statistical significance.

These prognostic data can provide us with a definition of the clinical boundaries between primary degenerative dementia, consistent with AD, and of age-associated cognitive decline, consistent with normal aging. Clearly, the forgetfulness phase is benign and does not fit the definition of a degenerative, slowly progressive condition. Equally clearly, late confusional phase, or more severe symptomatology, is consistent with a progressive degenerative condition. Early confusional phase symptomatology is less prognostically clear-cut, and hence provides

TABLE 24–3
Follow-up Intervals, Residential Status at Follow-up, and Mortality Differentiated by Initial GDS Scores

GDS Score (Initial Assessment)	Follow-up Interval (mo)		Residential Status at Follow-up and Mortality
	Mean ± S.D.	Range	
2	27.18 ± 3.71	23–33	16 Community residing 0 Deceased 0 Institutionalized
3	27.36 ± 5.46	18–34	14 Community residing 0 Deceased 0 Institutionalized
4	27.54 ± 5.18	21–37	8 Community residing 2 Deceased 1 Institutionalized[a]
5	23.17 ± 5.78	16–32	3 Community residing 1 Deceased 2 Institutionalized[a]
Total	26.81 ± 4.94	16–37	41 Community residing 3 Deceased 3 Institutionalized[a]

Source: Reisberg B, Schulman E, Ferris SH, et al. (22).

[a] In nursing homes.

a borderline condition midway between benign senescent forgetfulness and a degenerative illness consistent with AD.

When patients do succumb to AD, they generally develop a secondary infection or illness which results from their diminished capacity to care for themselves. Pneumonia, secondary to aspiration or exposure, is one of the most frequent immediate causes of death. Infected decubital ulcerations are another frequent cause of mortality. Although it has been

TABLE 24–4
Initial and Follow-up Scores on Assessment Parameters (Mean ± S.D.) for Community-Residing Survivors

GDS	N	MSQ Score		Clinical Cognition Assessment Scores		Functional Assessment Inventory Scores	
		Pre	Post	Pre	Post	Pre	Post
2	16	0.25 ± 0.45	0.13 ± 0.34	12.94 ± 1.44	13.19 ± 2.61	6.00 ± 0.00	6.37 ± 0.72
3	14	0.64 ± 1.08	1.36 ± 1.08	14.71 ± 2.64	15.71 ± 2.89[b]	6.21 ± 0.58	7.36 ± 1.65
4	8[d]	3.00 ± 2.20	5.87 ± 1.73[a]	16.50 ± 3.21	22.13 ± 2.47[b]	9.25 ± 2.05	13.83 ± 2.51
5	3[d]	7.33 ± 2.08	8.33 ± 0.58	18.66 ± 3.79	19.33 ± 2.52	12.66 ± 1.53	16.00 ± 1.73
Total	41[d]	1.41 ± 2.31	2.27 ± 2.98[b]	14.63 ± 2.96	16.42 ± 4.21[c]	7.54 ± 2.85	8.90 ± 3.82[c]

Source: Reisberg B, Shulman E, Ferris SH, et al. (22).

Significance of baseline vs. follow-up differences on assessment measures: Wilcoxin matched pair signed rank test (from Colton, *Statistics in Medicine,* 1974). Nonparametric, two-tailed probabilities.

[a] $P \leq .05$.
[b] $P \leq .01$.
[c] $P \leq .001$.
[d] Community-residing survivors only.

TABLE 24–5
Differential Diagnoses of Dementias

	Alzheimer's Disease	Senescent Forgetfulness (forgetfulness phase)	Geriatric Depression	Chronic Schizophrenia	Multi-Infarct Dementia
Onset of cognitive impairment	Gradual process extending generally over a period of years if proper history is obtained.	Gradual process extending over a period of several months to years.	Onset generally sudden and associated with present illness episode; however, a "life-long" history of memory problems is sometimes obtained.	An accurate history of onset is generally not obtained. However, if patient is seen between florid episodes of the illness process, then cognitive impairment is generally long-standing, extending for at least several years.	Sudden, "strokelike" onset.
Course of cognitive impairment	Progression of process is noted. Patient eventually becomes severely demented with incontinence, loss of speech, loss of ambulatory ability, and so on.	No subjective or objective evidence of progression.	If associated with present episode, then cognitive symptomatology will remit; if associated with "chronic depression," remains the same. Patients *do not* become severely demented.	If not associated with acute episode of the illness, then cognitive impairment generally continues to worsen over course of decades. Patients do not become incontinent, do not lose ambulatory ability; speech is sometimes severely compromised.	"Stepwise course" with remissions and exacerbations.

Clinical cognitive symptomatology	As described in Tables 24–1 and 24–2. Deficit proceeds relatively uniformly on concentration, recent memory, past memory, functioning and orientation axes.	Subjective complaints of cognitive deficit only. No clinically objective evidence of cognitive deterioration obtained.	Deficits are particularly notable, when present at all in concentration and in functioning. Despite complaints of "memory problems," there may be no objective evidence of deficit whatever. Sometimes patients, despite excellent recent recall, can remember little with respect to their childhood; this latter deficit is most frequently related to active denial.	Deficits in concentration and functioning are notable; memory for past may be denied. Recent memory is frequently intact. Deficits classically described in: concentration, attention, insight, judgment, orientation, and affect.	"Emotional incontinence is frequently noted." E.g., patient may suddenly cry for no apparent reason. Otherwise, clinical symptomatology is variable.
Associated clinical symptomatology	As discussed in text and Tables 24–1 and 24–2.	Very mild anxiety and/or depression are only associated symptoms; alternatively, patient may have no associated clinical symptomatology whatever.	Associated mood disturbances with dysphoria, depression, and sadness. Anxiety is frequently associated. "Vegetative symptoms" also frequently occur. These include: sleep and appetite disturbances (insomnia or hypersomnia; anorexia or hyperphagia). Anergia is another frequent complaint.	History of florid psychotic symptomatology with delusions and/or hallucinations, and/or "suspiciousness," and/or paranoia.	Risk factors for cerebral vascular disease are generally present. May be history of blackouts. Peripheral vascular and cardiovascular disease is frequently present, notably including hypertension.

185

said that patients do not directly die of AD, this is not entirely consistent with clinical experience. Some patients, as progressive brain decay proceeds, become comatose and eventually die in this state. The coma may be preceded by a mild febrile state, but a specific infectious etiology or locus is not always found, even when a complete medical work-up is performed. It is conceivable that diminished hypothalamic function, as well as decreased cortical capacity, are related to this terminal malignant process.

DIFFERENTIAL DIAGNOSIS

As stated in the chapter introduction, the key to the diagnosis and differential diagnosis of age-associated cognitive decline, consistent with normal aging and with AD, from other similar clinical conditions, is recognition of the characteristic clinical features of the illness process. These characteristic features have been described briefly here and references for more detailed descriptions have been provided. Additional salient features in the clinical differential diagnosis of these disorders, from conditions with which they are commonly confused, can be seen in Table 24–5.

ACKNOWLEDGMENT

This work was supported in part by Grant No. AG03051 from the National Institute on Aging of the National Institutes of Health.

REFERENCES

1. American Psychiatric Association: *Diagnostic and Statistical Manual of Mental Disorders,* ed 3. Washington, DC, American Psychiatric Association, 1980.
2. Roth M: Diagnosis of senile and related forms of dementia. *Aging NY* 1978; 7:71–85.
3. Miller NE, Cohen GD: Clinical aspects of Alzheimer's disease and senile dementia: synopsis and future perspectives in assessment, treatment, and service delivery. *Aging NY* 1981; 15:17–35.
4. Gustafson L, Nilsson L: Differential diagnosis of presenile dementia on clinical grounds. *Acta Psychiatr Scand* 1982; 65:194–209.
5. Reisberg B: *Brain Failure: An Introduction to Current Concepts of Senility.* New York, Free Press, 1982, pp 81–122.
6. Reisberg B, Ferris SH: Diagnosis and assessment of the older patient. *Hosp Community Psychiatry* 1982; 33:104–110.
7. Reisberg B, Ferris SH, Crook T: Signs, symptoms, and course of age-associated cognitive decline. *Aging NY* 1982; 19:475–481.
8. Reisberg B, Ferris SH, de Leon MJ, et al: The Global Deterioration Scale (GDS): an instrument for the assessment of primary degenerative dementia (PDD). *Am J Psychiatry* 1982; 139:1136–1139.
9. Reisberg B, Ferris SH, Schneck MK, et al: The relationship between psychiatric assessments and cognitive test measures in mild to moderately cognitive impaired elderly. *Psychopharmacol Bull* 1981; 17:99–101.
10. de Leon MJ, Ferris SH, Blau I, et al: Correlations between CT changes and behavioral deficits in senile dementia. *Lancet* 1979; ii:859.

11. de Leon MJ, Ferris SH, George AE, et al: Computed tomography evaluations of brain–behavior relationships in senile dementia of the Alzheimer's type. *Neurobiol Aging* 1980; 1:69–79.

12. Ferris SH, de Leon MJ, Wolf AP, et al: Positron emission tomography in the study of aging and senile dementia. *Neurobiol Aging* 1980; 1:127–131.

13. Ferris SH, de Leon MJ, Christman D, et al: Positron emission tomography (PET) studies of regional brain metabolism in elderly patients, in Jansson B, Perris C, Struwe G (eds): *Biological Psychiatry.* Amsterdam, Elsevier North-Holland, 1981, pp 280–283.

14. Nandy K, Reisberg B, Ferris SH, et al: Brain-reactive antibodies and progressive cognitive decline in the aged, abstracted. *J Am Aging Assoc* 1981; 4:145.

15. Reisberg B, Ferris SH, Ahn H, et al: Electrophysiologic asymmetry and brain change in primary degenerative dementia, abstracted. *Soc Neurosci* 1981; 7:241.

16. Reisberg B, Schneck MK, Ferris SH, et al: The Brief Cognitive Rating Scale (BCRS): findings in primary degenerative dementia (PDD). *Psychopharmacol Bull* 1983; 19:47–50.

17. Reisberg B, London E, Ferris SH, et al: The Brief Cognitive Rating Scale (BCRS): motoric, speech, and mood concomitants in primary degenerative dementia (PDD). *Psychopharmacol Bull* 1983; in press.

18. Pomara N, Reisberg B, Albers S, et al: Extrapyramidal symptoms in patients with primary degenerative dementia. *J Clin Psychopharmacol* 1981; 1:398–400.

19. American Psychiatric Association: *A Psychiatric Glossary,* ed 3. Washington, DC, American Psychiatric Association, 1969.

20. Martin MJ: Psychiatry and other specialties, in Freedman AM, Kaplan HI, Sadock BJ (eds): *Comprehensive Textbook of Psychiatry.* Baltimore, Williams & Wilkins, 1975, vol 2, p 1740.

21. Reisberg B, Gordon B, McCarthy M, et al: Insight and denial accompanying progressive cognitive decline in the aged, in Melnick VL, Dubler, N (eds): *Senile Dementia of the Alzheimer's Type and Related Diseases: Ethical and Legal Issues Related to Informed Consent,* in press.

22. Reisberg B, Shulman E, Ferris SH, et al: Clinical assessments of age-associated cognitive decline and primary degenerative dementia: prognostic concomitants. *Psychopharmacol Bull* 1983; in press.

23. Gilbert JG, Levee RF: Patterns of declining memory. *J Gerontol* 1971; 26:70–75.

24. Kahn RL, Goldfarb AI, Pollack KM, et al: Brief objective measures for the determination of mental status in the aged. *Am J Psychiatry* 1960; 117:326–328.

25 Differential Diagnosis of Alzheimer's Dementia: Multi-Infarct Dementia

Vladimir C. Hachinski

The term "multi-infarct dementia" was coined to emphasize that when vascular disease is responsible for mental decline, it is largely via small or large cerebral infarcts (1). This is in contradistinction to the still prevailing view that atherosclerosis of cerebral vessels causes critical narrowing, leading to chronic shortage of blood to the brain and, hence, mental deterioration. This misconception lives on in drug advertisements, in some medical journals, and in the lay press. The *New York Times,* for example, explaining the imminent retirement of Finland's president, alleged that "his ailment, a persistent cerebral insufficiency or disturbance of blood supply to the brain, was causing lapses in memory and absentmindedness" (2).

Although atherosclerosis is the commonest underlying cause of cerebral infarctions, these usually lead to focal deficits rather than global intellectual impairment. Nevertheless, vascular disease accounts for 7.7% of cases in several dementia series (3). The relative rarity of multi-infarct dementia notwithstanding, recognizing it is important because of its association with treatable conditions such as severe hypertension and recurrent emboli from either the heart or carotid artery lesions. Appropriate treatment may arrest progression of the dementia and even permit some recovery.

Brain lesions are not additive, they multiply; i.e., a further insult has a greater global effect than the sum of individual lesions, particularly if they occur over a short period of time. Consequently, it also becomes important to recognize and treat vascular factors in patients with Alzheimer's disease (AD), since their brains are more vulnerable and their vascular disease may determine their rate of deterioration.

Clinical Evaluation

Clinical evaluation remains the single most important means of distinguishing AD from multi-infarct dementia. In order to do this systematically, we (4) devised an *ischemic score* consisting of 13 items scoring either 1 or 2 points each (Table 25–1).

On applying this score, the patients fell into two distinct nonoverlapping populations: those scoring seven or above, whom we classified as multi-infarct dementia patients and

TABLE 25–1
Ischemic Score

Feature	Score
1. Abrupt onset	2
2. Stepwise deterioration	1
3. Fluctuating course	2
4. Nocturnal confusion	1
5. Relative preservation of personality	1
6. Depression	1
7. Somatic complaints	1
8. Emotional incontinence	1
9. History of hypertension	1
10. History of strokes	2
11. Evidence of associated atherosclerosis	1
12. Focal neurological symptoms	2
13. Focal neurological signs	2

those scoring four points or less, who were labeled as having primary degenerative dementia or AD.

1. An *abrupt onset* of dementia is highly suggestive of a vascular etiology; however, one must not mistake sudden recognition with abrupt onset. It is not uncommon for patients with decreased mental capacity to decompensate following an operation, trauma, or infection. Also, the illness or death of a spouse will often bring to light a previously unsuspected intellectual decline, as the patient has to cope with a new situation.

2. *Stepwise deterioration* may be induced by multiple infarcts, too small individually to produce a major clinical stroke. In combination these may impair intellectual function (5).

3. A *fluctuating course* may be produced by improvement seen after one cerebral infarct followed by deterioration caused by a new one.

4. *Nocturnal confusion* is a nonspecific symptom occurring most frequently in patients with multi-infarct dementia.

5. *Relative preservation of personality* characterizes multi-infarct dementia patients. Patients with cerebral infarctions may range in their emotions from indifference to undue emotionality, depending on the site of their lesions. By contrast, patients with AD tend to lapse gradually into docility and shallowness of affect and action.

6. *Depression* can occur in virtually every type of major dementia, but is more common in multi-infarct dementia, partly because of the greater preservation of personality and insight in multi-infarct patients as compared to AD subjects.

7. *Somatic complaints* can relate to either depression or the physical discomforts in mobility and sensation caused by cerebral infarction.

8. *Emotional incontinence* is a common feature of pseudobulbar palsy, also characterized by dysarthria, dysphagia, and a brisk jaw jerk. These findings imply bilateral damage to the cortico-bulbar fibers and hence bilateral and usually widespread cerebral lesions.

9. *A history of hypertension* is most commonly found in patients with multi-infarct dementia, particularly those in the younger age group.

10. *A history of strokes* is more common in patients with multi-infarct dementia but by itself does not prove that the etiology of the dementia is vascular. AD patients can have incidental strokes that may worsen but do not account for their dementia. The role of stroke in dementia has been discussed by Wells (6).

11. *Evidence of associated atherosclerosis* is more valuable in the diagnosis of younger than of older patients with dementia. Although the correlation of retinal and peripheral atherosclerosis to cervico-cerebral atherosclerosis is not strong, the presence of extensive atherosclerosis makes multi-infarct dementia more likely.

12. *Focal neurological symptoms* such as visual impairment, or numbness or weakness of the face, arm, or leg, if transient usually represent forewarnings of stroke, and if treated can often prevent a stroke. If the symptoms are persistent, they may represent cerebral infarction. The patient's self-perception of neurologic problems is frequently more subtle than the neurological examination.

13. *Focal neurological signs,* including specific memory disorders, aphasias, agnosias, and alexias (in addition to the more easily recognizable visual, motor, and sensory impairments and reflex changes) are more likely to be due to multi-infarct dementia than to AD. Focal motor, reflex, and visual field defects, in particular, are helpful in establishing a vascular etiology. Sensation is difficult to evaluate in demented patients but abnormalities are most often found in multi-infarct dementias. Symmetrical primitive reflexes such as the palmomental, grasp, snout, sucking, and labioauricular are more common in AD than in multi-infarct dementia.

VALIDITY AND PRACTICALITY OF THE ISCHEMIC SCORE

Although the ischemic score has been used in a number of studies and publications, few papers have addressed the issues of its validity and practicality. Harrison and colleagues (7) were among the first to do so. They divided 52 patients presenting with dementia into a multi-infarct and a primary degenerative group by the use of the ischemic score. They found that focal electroencephalographic changes, angiographic evidence of ischemic areas, and atheromatous disease of the intracranial vessels was more common in the multi-infarct group. They concluded that the ischemic score can identify those patients whose dementia is associated with vascular disease.

Loeb (8), in a chapter on the clinical diagnosis of multi-infarct dementia, concluded that "the ischemic score of Hachinski et al represents an effective clinical tool, but the definite groupings of cases should be evaluated within a broad clinical context." Part of the difficulty in classification lies with a number of cases that have both AD and multiple cerebral infarcts. The ischemic score may identify such mixed cases as being of the multi-infarct type. However, from a clinical viewpoint this is an advantage, since vascular factors are often treatable.

Rosen and co-workers (9) validated the ischemic score in a clinicopathologic study. They found that abrupt onset, stepwise deterioration, a history of stroke, focal neurological signs, and focal neurological symptoms were of prime importance in making the diagnosis of multi-infarct dementia. Hypertension was of secondary importance, while other items were of questionable importance. Since the study was based on 14 cases, it may be best to use the ischemic score as originally devised, since some of the items thought to be not significant in this small series may prove to be so in a larger one. Furthermore, the use of a uniform scoring system allows for standardization and comparability between studies.

The ischemic score is easy and practical to apply once the really difficult part of obtaining a reliable history and performing the examination have been carried out.

Neuropsychological Evaluation

Perez and associates (10) found that by using a discriminant function analysis based on the Wechsler Adult Intelligence Scale (WAIS) they were able to correctly classify 75% of patients into multi-infarct and AD groups. They also found that the degree and pattern of intellectual deficit in multi-infarct dementia was variable, depending on the site, location, extent, and number of cerebral infarctions. In a further study they showed that a discriminant function analysis based on the Wechsler Memory Scale classified 100% of patients correctly (11). Since the correctness of classification was judged only in relation to the ischemic score, however, these results should be considered promising but preliminary.

Neurophysiological Evaluation

Electroencephalographic findings in dementia and the use of evoked responses in the clinical differentiation of AD, multi-infarct, and other dementias is discussed elsewhere in this book.

Computerized Tomography of the Brain

This procedure and its uses and limitations in the differential diagnosis of dementia are discussed in Chapter 33. The point is that the mere demonstration of multiple cerebral infarcts does not prove the diagnosis of multi-infarct dementia. First in the diagnosis is to establish that there is global mental impairment rather than focal neurological problems. The value of the CT scan lies in providing confirmatory evidence for a vascular etiology. The extent of mental impairment with multiple cerebral infarcts depends on a number of factors, including the location, extent, nature, and chronicity of lesions.

Nevertheless, a high ischemic score correlates well with suggestive findings on CT scanning. Frackowiak and colleagues (12) found that among eight patients with an ischemic score of 8 or above, five had evidence of cerebral infarcts or focal sulcal pools (suggesting previous cerebral infarction); one patient had evidence of periventricular low white matter attenuation, often associated with hypertension (13); two had infarcts, focal sulcal pools, and periventricular low white matter attenuation; and two patients did not manifest these findings. One patient without vascular CT scan findings but with an ischemic score of 10 was proven to have multi-infarct dementia at autopsy, suggesting that the ischemic score is a more sensitive index of multi-infarct dementia than CT scanning.

Cerebral Blood Flow and Metabolic Studies

These are discussed elsewhere in this book. Of particular interest is the evidence from simultaneous cerebral blood flow and oxygen metabolism studies regarding chronic cerebral hypoperfusion as an important mechanism in vascular dementia. But if this were so, one would expect an increased oxygen extraction rate with ischemia. No significant elevation of directly measured oxygen extraction ratio has been found in vascular dementia (12), further supporting the view that vascular disease manifests not as a chronic global cerebral ischemia but truly as a multi-infarct dementia (1).

CONCLUSION

The majority of cases of AD can be distinguished from patients with multi-infarct and mixed dementias through the use of a clinical ischemic score; computerized tomography of the brain is a useful adjunct to the ischemic score in making the differentiation. Neuropsychological, neurophysiological and cerebral blood flow, and metabolic studies are also potentially useful in distinguishing AD from multi-infarct dementia.

REFERENCES

1. Hachinski VC, Lassen NA, Marshall J: Multi-infarct dementia: a cause of mental deterioration in the elderly. *Lancet* 1974; ii:207–209.
2. Wiskari W: Finland expecting a leadership shift. *New York Times,* October 4, 1981, p 4.
3. Wells CE: *Dementia,* ed 2. Philadelphia, Davis, 1977.
4. Hachinski VC, Iliff LE, Zilhka E, et al: Cerebral blood flow in dementia. *Arch Neurol* 1975; 32:632–637.
5. Marshall J: A survey of the management and non-surgical treatment of cerebrovascular disease, in Vinken PJ, Bruyn CW (eds): *Handbook of Clinical Neurology,* vol 12. New York: Elsevier–North Holland, 1972, pp 447–455.
6. Wells CE: Role of stroke in dementia. *Stroke* 1978; 9:1–3.
7. Harrison MJG, Thomas DJ, Du Boulay GH, et al: Multi-infarct dementia. *J Neurol Sci* 1979; 40:97–103.
8. Loeb C: Clinical diagnosis of multi-infarct dementia. *Aging NY* 1980; 13:251–260.
9. Rosen WG, Terry RD, Fuld PA, et al: Pathological verification of ischemic score in differentiation of dementias. *Ann Neurol* 1980; 7:486–488.
10. Perez FI, Rivera VM, Meyer JS, et al: Analysis of intellectual and cognitive performance in patients with multi-infarct dementia, vertebrobasilar insufficiency with dementia, and Alzheimer's disease. *J Neurol, Neurosurg Psychiatry* 1975; 38:533–540.
11. Perez FI, Stump DA, Gay JRA, et al: Intellectual performance in multi-infarct dementia and Alzheimer's disease: a replication study. *Can J Neurol Sci* 1976; 3:181–187.
12. Frackowiak RSJ, Pozzilli C, et al: Regional cerebral oxygen supply and utilization in dementia: a clinical and physiological study with oxygen-15 and positron tomography. *Brain* 1981; 104:753–778.
13. Zeumer H, Schonsky B, Sturm KW: Predominant white matter involvement in subcortical arteriosclerotic encephalopathy (Binswanger's disease). *J CAT* 1980; 4:14–19.

26 Differential Diagnosis of Alzheimer's Dementia: Affective Disorder

CHARLES E. WELLS

DIFFERENTIATING ALZHEIMER'S DEMENTIA (AD) from affective disorders (or recognizing their concurrence) is at times vexing, and because of this, the topic has attracted a good deal of attention in the recent medical literature. It should be recognized, however, that the vast majority of patients with AD do not give the appearance of suffering from a primary affective illness, nor do most patients with primary affective disorders appear demented. Nonetheless, problems and mistakes in diagnosis occur with sufficient regularity that they warrant serious scrutiny. Although questions may occasionally arise in differentiating mania from dementia, most problems concern the differentiation of depressive spectrum disorders from dementia, and these latter will be the focus of this chapter.

Although both AD and depressive disorders have a high incidence in the elderly, we have surprisingly little data on how often mistakes in their diagnosis occur. Most of our information comes from studies of younger subjects, in whom the incidence of AD is much lower. Two excellent studies from university hospital services in Great Britain demonstrated that the original diagnosis of presenile dementia often could not be substantiated when these patients were carefully followed up after an interval of several years (1, 2). Regrettably, the causes for these mistaken diagnoses were not reported in detail, and thus aside from putting us on guard, they do not assist us in our efforts to avoid making such mistakes in our daily practice. Unfortunately, we lack comparable follow-up studies in elderly subjects, in whom Alzheimer's dementia is diagnosed much more frequently.

The obverse is also true: dementia may be mistaken for affective disorders, especially depression and especially early in its course. Liston (3) reported, for example, that a primary diagnosis of a depressive spectrum disorder had frequently been made in patients who were later found to have presenile dementia. Liston did not, however, critically explore the origin of these early mistakes in diagnosis and inform us how often such affective diagnoses might have been justified on the basis of clinical observations and how often they may have been catchall diagnoses, made because the physician was uncertain about the disease process or failed even to consider the possibility of dementia in these younger patients.

Cognitive changes have been well established in depression. Folstein and McHugh (4), for example, demonstrated the frequency of cognitive losses in elderly patients with depression, going so far as to suggest naming this cognitive loss "the dementia syndrome of depression." They too, however, failed to inform us of how often these cognitive losses resulted in serious differential diagnostic questions, and how often they might be regarded only as one aspect, albeit an important one, of an otherwise typical depressive episode.

To complicate matters further, the differential diagnostic problem is not always simply a question of whether the patient has AD *or* depression; sometimes it is a question of whether the patient has dementia *and* depression. In these difficult clinical situations, the physician must try to assess the contribution of an affective disorder to the overall clinical picture in the patient who has demonstrable organic disease, and must then decide how vigorously to treat the affective component in the patient who has established dementia.

As will be readily perceived, from a practical standpoint the serious danger here lies in the clinician's failure to recognize and diagnose affective disorders (or other so-called functional psychiatric disorders) when they are important in the patient's symptomatology, not in the clinician's failure to make an early diagnosis of Alzheimer's dementia. The course of AD will be changed not at all as a consequence of its early recognition and diagnosis, however satisfying that early diagnosis may be to the clinician. In contrast, the course of affective disorders can usually be changed dramatically by early diagnosis and treatment; indeed appropriate treatment may in certain cases be life-saving.

The important question then is: What clinical clues can help the physician to correctly reach the diagnosis of affective disease in the patient who appears in many ways to be primarily demented? Or, to put the question differently: What clinical features allow the physician to recognize pseudodementia, a clinical syndrome that has been described as "a caricature or burlesque, not an imitation, of dementia" (5)? Subsequent studies have indicated, however, especially in the elderly, that depressive pseudodementia may indeed mimic dementia with considerable accuracy (6).

Most of what we know about this difficult area of differential diagnosis is based on scattered reports of individual cases. The clinician who attacks these problems must do so largely with the tools of clinical observation; ancillary diagnostic procedures, though sometimes helpful, cannot establish the correct diagnosis for the clinician, and indeed they depend for their correct interpretation on the clinician (7). In most instances, careful attention to details of the history and clinical observation will lead the physician to the correct diagnosis, although conversely the passage of time must be invoked sometimes to prove or disprove a tentative diagnostic hypothesis.

I have suggested elsewhere (8) that depression (in the young as well as in the elderly) is misdiagnosed as dementia most often because many clinicians still tend to accept cognitive loss in itself as diagnostic of an organic brain syndrome. In the elderly patient, this pattern of thinking leads to a diagnosis of AD rather than one of depressive disorder. In fact, cognitive loss is a feature of many psychiatric syndromes and is by no means confined to the organic brain syndromes alone. As noted, Folstein and McHugh (4) highlighted the frequency of impaired cognition during episodes of depression in the elderly. More recently, Weingartner and associates (9) reported both qualitative and quantitative changes in information processing during depressive episodes even in middle aged subjects. Physicians must then learn that although cognitive impairment is the hallmark of the organic brain syndromes, cognitive impairment alone is insufficient to establish such a diagnosis.

Most of the time, mistakes in diagnosis can be avoided if the physician pays careful attention to the details of history and clinical observation. To be successful in this context, however, the physician must approach the task in a manner that differs from the diagnostic approach emphasized in most teaching today. Contemporary psychiatric diagnosis emphasizes the importance of establishing specific criteria for diagnosis, an emphasis that should in no way be criticized. Depression will continue to be misdiagnosed as dementia, however, if the diagnostic criteria for dementia are applied uncritically. Indeed, the problem arises largely because a certain percentage of patients with primary affective disorders satisfy the stated diagnostic criteria (10) for dementia more exactly than the diagnostic criteria for affective disorders. If errors are to be avoided, clinicians must look just as carefully at key elements in the history or clinical presentation that do *not* fit with the usual presentation and course of dementia as they do at the features that do conform. As I (5) emphasized elsewhere, pseudodementia is suspected first usually because of the incongruity of several of its clinical features; and as Good (11) wrote, diagnostic errors are often the result of "a disregard of discrepant findings, such as evidence of preserved memory function despite errors on formal mental status testing and laboratory studies that [provide] little or no confirmation of considered physical diagnoses."

MEDICAL HISTORY

Study of the relatively scant medical literature dealing with this topic suggests that two historical features are especially useful in the differential diagnosis. First, most recorded cases of depressive pseudodementia in the elderly describe a relatively abrupt onset and a rapid progression of symptoms, with the victim often progressing to an appearance of profound dementia over a period of only two or three months. This is not the course of most diseases that cause dementia, and certainly it is not the course of AD. Whenever a patient appears to have grown profoundly demented over a period of only a few months, serious consideration should be given to the possible diagnosis of depression. If the electroencephalogram (EEG) is also normal, the possibility of a primary depression should be considered even more seriously, because the EEG is usually abnormal in both Creutzfeldt–Jakob disease and in the metabolic diseases that cause dementia, which are probably the most frequent causes of rapidly progressive dementia.

Second, the physician should always consider a diagnosis of depression if there is a previous history of depressive illness episodes. A previous depressive episode certainly does not preclude the development of dementia, but if other features of the clinical picture are at variance with that usually seen with dementia, the possibility of a primary depressive disorder should get serious scrutiny.

CLINICAL OBSERVATIONS

With regard to clinical observations, incongruity of two sorts should suggest a diagnosis of pseudodementia in the patient who appears demented. First, most patients with diffuse cerebral dysfunction, due to AD or other causes, exhibit a decline in function in multiple cognitive spheres on the mental status examination. If function appears profoundly impaired only on certain aspects of the mental status examination and essentially intact on others, the physician should consider the possibility of a nondementing psychiatric disorder.

Second, there should be a certain congruence between the severity of cognitive impairment as demonstrated by the mental status examination and the patient's behavior, especially for those behaviors which depend on cognition. For example, one would not expect a patient who is disoriented for time and place on questioning to be able to learn the locations of the hospital room and the snack bar (and the route between them) with apparent ease. Nor would one expect a demented patient to learn to recognize physicians and nurses soon after hospital admission but to have difficulty recognizing close family members. Variability from time to time in performance is expected in demented patients, but persistent incongruity is not.

Another aspect of clinical observation has been highlighted by Cavenar and associates (12). They pointed out that even in the absence of specific symptoms to suggest depression, the physician's empathic response to the patient may suggest and lead to the recognition of a depressive disorder, even though the patient's presentation points otherwise to an organic diagnosis. The physician must then weigh in subjective responses to interaction with the patient as well as to more clearly observable and definable features.

ANCILLARY DIAGNOSTIC PROCEDURES

Ancillary diagnostic procedures are sometimes helpful but are seldom critical in differentiating between depression and dementia in elderly subjects. Some, such as electroencephalography and CT-scanning, which are especially useful in young and middle-aged subjects, are particularly liable to misinterpretation in the elderly. The CT scan may, for example, reveal considerable cortical atrophy and ventricular enlargement in elderly subjects who have no evidence of dementia; conversely, only moderate atrophic changes may be demonstrated in patients with severe dementia. Ancillary diagnostic procedures must always be interpreted in light of the overall clinical picture, and interpreted by clinicians who are well aware of their pitfalls.

Two procedures deserve mention here in addition to the more commonly used ancillary diagnostic measures. The first of these is the dexamethasone suppression test. Rudorfer and Clayton (13) reported its usefulness in a patient with severe cognitive impairment who also appeared depressed. Failure of this patient's cortisol levels to drop as expected following administration of dexamethasone emboldened them to use ECT for treatment of depression, with prompt recovery to normal function following. These investigators suggested that a medically unexplained abnormal dexamethasone suppression test in a patient with recent cognitive impairment should prompt vigorous treatment for depression. Unfortunately, the results of the dexamethasone suppression test have not yet been reported for patients with proven AD alone, so that we do not know at present how often this test may be falsely positive.

The other procedure deserving of consideration is the diagnostic amytal interview. Snow and Wells (14) reported its helpfulness in a withdrawn and uncooperative patient who appeared both depressed and demented. Under the influence of the barbiturate, this patient was much more vocal in expression of her depressive symptomatology, so that a diagnosis of depression appeared warranted. In this patient, aggressive treatment of the depression then led to considerable improvement, despite the presence of underlying AD.

In summary, there are no simple rules or measures to guarantee that an affective disorder will not be missed in the elderly patient who gives the appearance of being demented. Probably the best precaution is for the physician to maintain a high index of suspicion for depression and to pursue the possibility of depression vigorously whenever historical, observational, or ancillary diagnostic features are at variance with those usually present in AD. Sometimes, even though the diagnosis of a depressive disorder cannot be established with certainty, treatment for depression should be urged because it may be effective. In other cases, only observation over time will allow a definite diagnosis. In few other areas of medicine today are the observational skills of the physician by themselves so important in the establishment of a firm and accurate diagnosis.

REFERENCES

1. Nott PN, Fleminger JJ: Presenile dementia: the difficulties of early diagnosis. *Acta Psychiatr Scand* 1975; 51:210–217.
2. Ron MA, Toone BK, Garralda ME, et al: Diagnostic accuracy in presenile dementia. *Br J Psychiatry* 1979; 134:161–168.
3. Liston EJ Jr: Occult presenile dementia. *J Nerv Ment Dis* 1977; 164:263–267.
4. Folstein MF, McHugh PR: Dementia syndrome of depression. *Aging NY* 1978; 7:87–93.
5. Wells CE: Pseudodementia. *Am J Psychiatry* 1979; 136:895–900.
6. McAllister TW, Price TRP: Severe depressive pseudodementia with and without dementia. *Am J Psychiatry* 139:626–629, 1982.
7. Wells CE: The differential diagnosis of psychiatric disorders in the elderly, in Cole JO, Barrett JE (eds): *Psychopathology in the Aged.* New York, Raven, 1980, pp 19–31.
8. Wells CE: Refinements in the diagnosis of dementia. *Am J Psychiatry* 139:621–622, 1982.
9. Weingartner H, Cohen RM, Murphy DL, et al: Cognitive processes in depression. *Arch Gen Psychiatry* 1981; 38:42–47.
10. American Psychiatric Association: Diagnostic and Statistical Manual of Mental Disorders, ed 3. Washington, DC, American Psychiatric Association, 1980.
11. Good MI: Pseudodementia and physical findings masking significant psychopathology. *Am J Psychiatry* 1981; 138:811–814.
12. Cavenar JO Jr, Maltbie AA, Austin L: Depression simulating organic brain disease. *Am J Psychiatry* 1979; 136:521–523.
13. Rudorfer MV, Clayton PJ: Pseudodementia: use of the DST in diagnosis and treatment monitoring. *Psychosomatics* 23:429–431, 1982.
14. Snow SS, Wells CE: Case studies in neuropsychiatry: Diagnosis and treatment of coexistent dementia and depression. *J Clin Psychiatry* 42:439–441, 1981.

SECTION VII

PSYCHOMETRIC DIAGNOSIS AND DIFFERENTIAL DIAGNOSIS OF ALZHEIMER'S DISEASE AND RELATED DISORDERS

27 Psychometric Differentiation of the Dementias:
An Overview

PAULA ALTMAN FULD

THE PROBLEM OF DIFFERENTIATING among the dementias can be viewed primarily as the problem of distinguishing Alzheimer's disease (AD) from dementia resulting from multiple strokes. AD, which involves the formation of senile plaques (SPs) and neurofibrillary tangles (NFTs) in the cells of the cerebral cortex and the hippocampus, accounts for 50% of all dementia patients who come to autopsy (1, 2).

Although these microscopic changes may be unevenly distributed early in the course, they later affect all parts of the cortex except the primary sensory and motor areas (3). A histo-pathological diagnosis of AD is made in a dementia patient when large numbers of SPs are widespread in the cerebral cortex. Neurochemical studies have shown that AD patients have a deficiency in the cholinergic neurotransmitter system of the brain (4–6).

Because of the nonfocal nature of AD, psychometric testing should show impairment of all higher cortical functions to the extent that they require nonautomatic perceptual and cognitive operations. Simple sensory and motor functions, and simple or automatized mental functions, should be unimpaired. Thus, an accountant with AD may retain the ability to do arithmetic far longer than most patients would, and a patient's ability to merely repeat sentences tends to be preserved longer than the ability to understand them. The greater the novelty or complexity of a task, the more confusion it should cause beyond that experienced by unimpaired individuals of the same age. In contrast to the isolated deficits often seen in patients with focal brain lesions, this excessive difficulty should not be limited to one type of stimulus, sensory modality, or problem. Because the hippocampus is earlier and more densely involved than the cortex (3), impairment of memory should usually have appeared insidiously before other kinds of dysfunction.

The dementia associated with cerebrovascular disease is called multi-infarct dementia (MID), which is thought to result when 50–100 g of brain tissue have been damaged (1). MID accounts for about 22% of dementia cases and, together with AD, accounts for a further 13% (mixed cases) (1, 2).

Many AD patients have some cerebral infarcts. It is unknown to what extent the presence of fewer than 50–100 g of infarcted tissue in the brains of AD patients affects the presentation or course of these cases, and to what extent other combinations of diseases with MID will produce serious dementias.

In MID or mixed cases, the damage to the brain is usually visible to the naked eye at autopsy and appears multifocal, in contrast to the generalized cortical atrophy seen in AD. The most common form of MID, however, is the *lacunar state,* which consists of small lesions usually sparing the cortex and resulting in enlargement of the ventricles (2). This condition, as well as other "subcortical dementias" such as parkinsonism (7, 8), progressive supranuclear palsy (9, 10), or normal pressure hydrocephalus (11, 12), should result in minimal or mild dementia with some slowing of responses, in contrast to AD. Studies comparing dementia patients' scores on the Wechsler Adult Intelligence Scale (WAIS) and its predecessor, the Wechsler Bellevue Test, have found that probable AD patients tend to do less well than patients with MID, although MID patients do less well than nondemented hospital patients. The verbal–performance IQ discrepancy is also said to be greater in AD than in MID (13, 14).

In a study of institutionalized elderly dementia patients who came to autopsy, a system of scoring the clinical features of strokes (15) was shown to identify patients with MID or mixed pathology accurately (16). This scoring system could not distinguish between MID and the patients with mixed pathology, and it is probably most accurate with older patients who are not acute stroke patients.

Although MID patients sometimes present with striking signs of focal brain damage, such cases seem surprisingly infrequent. MID patients appearing for dementia evaluation are generally not acutely ill stroke patients; they often present without a clear stroke-related history and with relatively mild impairments. When dementia evaluation is requested in a patient with a recent stroke, monthly or quarterly evaluations should be done until results appear stable. In patients with seizures, test results may continue to fluctuate unpredictably so long as there is seizure activity occurring from time to time.

Even if some MID patients show signs of focal abnormality on neuropsychological testing, the unpredictable and multifocal nature of this disease should make the configuration of test scores for each patient less similar from patient to patient than one might expect for AD. Although patients with AD may show great variability (17), a specific pattern of relative strengths and weaknesses among patients' scores on various tests appears to exist and may be maintained from the time plaques and tangles become widespread throughout the cortex until the patient becomes too impaired to respond to standardized test procedures.

Such a pattern has been identified in the age-corrected scores obtained by patients on seven WAIS subtests. The content of these subtests is as follows:

- The *Information* and *Vocabulary* tests require verbal recall of general information and the ability to define or give synonyms for words. These tests tend to depend heavily on information acquired in the past.
- The *Similarities* test requires the patient to tell how two things are alike. Giving a category name is a common response. The *Digit Span* test requires the patient to repeat increasing series of digits forwards or backwards.
- The *Digit-Symbol* (coding) test requires the patient to copy symbols rapidly from a digit symbol coding key to empty boxes beneath a random series of digits. The *Block Design* test requires the patient to copy increasingly difficult designs involving red and white blocks.
- The *Object Assembly* test involves jigsaw puzzles made from drawings of familiar things (18).

When these subtests are grouped as indicated above, and when the age-corrected scale scores are averaged as necessary to obtain a single score for each pair, the four resulting scores reveal a profile in some dementia patients which is highly specific for AD as compared with other dementias.

Figure 27–1 shows this profile. It has been identified not only in two groups of consecutive AD patients (center and right panels), but also in a group of normal young adults with temporary cholinergic deficiency (left panel) induced by the administration of scopolamine for an earlier study. This figure is derived from the median subtest scores of those who displayed the profile, only. If all individuals tested were included, the profile would still be apparent but would be less dramatic. As presented, Figure 27–1 illustrates the profile as it actually appears in a particular patient's test results. The profile of scores seen in Figure 27–1 may be expressed as follows:

$$\text{If } A = [\text{Information and Vocabulary}] \div 2,$$
$$B = [\text{Similarities and Digit Span}] \div 2,$$
$$C = [\text{Digit-Symbol and Block Design}] \div 2,$$
$$\text{and } D = \text{Object Assembly},$$
$$\text{then } A = A > B > C \le D, \quad A > D.$$

The magnitude of the differences between the scores is not taken into account in determining whether a particular patient is positive for the profile.

This pattern has been shown to be highly specific for AD, compared with other dementias, in a group of all consecutive testable dementia patients (including those scoring zero on some subtests after standard administration) from a series of 138 dementia evaluations. Figure 27–1 shows the profiles when this series was divided into an initial and a replication group (center and right panels), consisting of 61 and 77 patients respectively. I have found only two false positives among dementia patients. Also, despite its resemblance to what might be expected from normal aging, it has been found in less than 1% of 390 nondemented individuals aged 75–85 whom I have studied using age-corrected scale scores on these WAIS subtests.

Figure 27–1. WAIS age-corrected scaled score profile of scopalamine-treated young adults* and two groups of consecutive Alzheimer dementia patients. *Data from David Drachman collected for Drachman and Leavitt (19).*

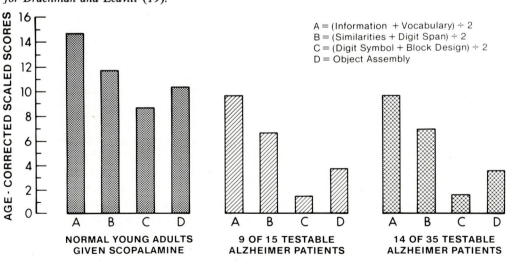

An earlier study of two biopsied AD patients, compared with two patients with Korsakoff's syndrome from cerebral aneurysm excision, showed WAIS test results which distinguished the two types of patients (18). The test scores of the two AD patients can be shown to be consistent with the Fuld profile (20). Several additional older studies have provided WAIS data on dementia patients but did not focus on the problem of differentiating between AD and MID (21–25). Perez and associates found nothing that differentiated their AD and MID patients replicably except their education (26). The lack of consistent criteria for the presumptive diagnosis of AD from study to study makes it difficult to integrate the results. The current availability of research diagnostic criteria as well as better radiological and laboratory techniques to help identify patients with other dementias may improve the comparability of future studies.

Previous experience suggests that the Fuld profile will identify about 50% of all testable AD patients. Because experience in its use is limited, thus far, the presence of the Fuld profile in a patient's test data should lead to a statement such as, "The pattern of strengths and weaknesses exhibited by this patient on seven subtests of the WAIS is typical of a group of patients with AD." It is important to keep in mind that failure to display the profile does not rule out AD, even if the patient was fully tested. It is also essential to remember that a similar profile could occur with focal damage, especially to the right parietal region or nearby. This must be ruled out as thoroughly as possible by administering an adequate battery of sensoricortical and motor tests as well as tests of a variety of cognitive abilities.

The neuropsychological test battery used for dementia evaluation at the Albert Einstein College of Medicine is presented in Table 27–1. This battery is heavily loaded with tests for older adults so cautious statements can be made about relative strengths and weaknesses shown in different test performances. The battery can be altered by the experienced examiner to ensure that a particular referral question can be answered and to test hypotheses about unusual cases. Normally, however, it is given in the same order to all patients in one 3-hour session. The length of the examination is a positive feature in that it provides an opportunity for detailed behavioral observation and amasses a sufficient quantity of data to deal with complex questions and subtleties. Other neuropsychological test batteries and their use have been described by Lezak (27), Russell (28), and Golden (29), as well as in Smith and Phillipus (30), Pirozzolo and Lawson-Kerr (31), and Filskov and Boll (32).

Although studies of the possible contribution of most of the battery in Table 27–1 to the differentiation of the dementias are not yet complete, observations from its clinical use with hundreds of dementia patients may be helpful:

1. AD patients typically do extremely poorly on the WAIS Digit-Symbol substitution subtest and the Raven Colored Progressive Matrices, a novel test of visuo-spatial reasoning. If they can understand the instructions at all, they will usually "lose set" after doing a few items. Reinstruction will rarely prove helpful for long. Patients with other dementias may have difficulty at first but will sometimes catch on after reinstruction and may perform appropriately, if slowly thereafter. Self-corrected errors are probably less likely in AD than in other dementias. If a patient has *some* serious impairments but can do the Raven test at a level consistent with his more preserved abilities, he probably does not have AD, even as a contributor to the picture. Exceptions may be seen early in the course in patients who had careers or longstanding hobbies which involved habitual use of visuospatial abilities (carpentry, jewelry or other handcrafting, sewing, radiology, surgery, drafting).

2. The Block Design subtest (copying designs using red and white blocks) is very difficult

TABLE 27–1
Neuropsychological Test Battery for Dementia Evaluation

Visual acuity (reading distance) with glasses
Wide Range Achievement Test
    Reading (words)
    Arithmetic (level 1)

Mental status: Dementia rating
    Blessed et al. (3)
    Kahn et al. MSQ (52)
    Mattis Dementia Scale (50)

Wechsler Adult Intelligence Scale (WAIS)
    Information   Digit Symbol
    Vocabulary   Block Design
    Similarities   Object Assembly
    Digit Span   Performance IQ[a]
      Verbal IQ[a]

Raven's Matrices (colored or standard)

Telling time (Fuld clocks without numbers)

Gates–MacGinitie reading: Speed and accuracy test
    Level D

Language screening
    Naming
      10 easy objects
      9 colors
      12 body parts
    Sentence Repetition: Spreen and Benton
    Token Test (comprehension): Spreen and Benton
    Word fluency: Drachman and Leavitt
      categories (19)
    Auditory discrimination and phoneme articulation

Visual fields
    Single
    Double simultaneous stimuli

Auditory
    Single (acuity)
    Double simultaneous stimuli

Fine motor coordination
    Purdue pegboard

Sensoricortical
    Stereognosis
    Face–hand (eyes open and eyes closed)
    Two-point discrimination

Learning and Memory

Fuld Object-Memory Evaluation (38)	*Buschke–Fuld verbal list (53)*
Storage	Storage
Recalls	Recalls
Consistency	Consistency
Response to reminders	Recognition
Delayed recall	
Recognition	

[a] IQ's estimated from tests listed.

for most AD patients, even early in the course. Patients often can construct only the simplest item, although a few can also do an additional easy one. Their ability to draw from memory or copy pictures of simple objects (ice cream cone, shoebox, football) and geometric figures (circle, triangle, square) does not usually seem grossly disordered at first; errors in detail may occur and geometric figures may be misnamed by the patient, but drawings will be recognizable. If a patient can do one of the more difficult block designs or earn an age-corrected scale score of 5 or more, she probably does not have AD. Exceptions may be seen as above.

    3. Few advanced AD patients can repeat more than three digits backward, although their ability to repeat digits forward may be excellent. A patient who can repeat five digits backward is probably unlikely to have AD as part of the picture.

    4. Few AD patients can tell time without gross errors on schematic drawings of clocks without numbers, even when "easy" times are involved (3:00, 6:15, 9:30, 11:45) and the minute hand is one-third longer than the hour hand. If a patient can do this without at least one significant error, the patient probably does not have AD.

5. AD patients typically do not have striking language impairments early in the course. They can usually name at least nine of ten common objects presented and can repeat sentences on the Spreen–Benton Sentence Repetition Test at or near the level appropriate for their age and education. Comprehension of spoken commands (Spreen–Benton Token Test), however, is often below the ability to repeat, possibly in part because of the combination of visual search and memory demands involved in this unique method of testing comprehension. The ability to read single words (Wide Range Achievement Test) is usually at or near the level appropriate to education and estimated premorbid intelligence, although reading comprehension will be impaired (Gates–MacGinitie Test).

Prose written by AD patients tends to be somewhat vaguer and less well organized than formerly but does not necessarily display serious mechanical errors early in the course.

6. AD patients can usually follow simple left-right commands until very late in the course.

7. Sensory and motor functions seem unimpaired in the majority of AD patients although confusion may interfere with testing.

8. All statements about the likelihood of AD should be qualified by the words "at present." A patient who does not show evidence of AD when tested may be developing it. Patients who do not show the AD test profile when first tested frequently do so a year or more later: the uneven distribution of plaques and tangles in minimally involved brains may progress to the typical widespread distribution after a time, or newly impaired patients may be more variable in their test performance (more vulnerable to stress?) than they will later appear.

The foregoing observations seem to support the view stated earlier that AD involves impairment of all higher cortical functions to the extent that they are not habitual or automatic, while simple sensory and motor functions tend to remain unimpaired.

One important aspect of dementia that must be discussed is memory. Memory impairment is probably present to some degree in all brain disease, and differential impairments have been shown for patients with Korsakoff's syndrome versus Huntington's chorea (33) and versus herpes encephalitis (34).

Few memory tests provide normative data for older adults, yet norms are essential because recall becomes more difficult with aging. The Guild Memory Scale, similar to the Wechsler Memory Scale, has cutoff scores for adults over 60 (35). The Fuld Object-Memory Evaluation also provides data on elderly community residents vs. nursing home residents. This test employs a unique procedure which guarantees attention to the stimuli, even on the part of patients with sensory or language handicaps. This is done by presenting ten real objects in a bag for naming by touch or at sight with later incidental and intentional recall. Five extended recalls are elicited with reminding, as necessary, after each (36). After the reminders on each trial, the patient is asked to say words rapidly in one of five categories to minimize recall from immediate memory (19). The Fuld test provides normative data on storage, retrieval, consistency of retrieval, and responsiveness to reminders as well as data on delayed recall and recognition (retention) and word fluency (37,38). Data are provided for institutionalized versus community-residing 70–79 versus 80–89 year olds. Two forms are available. Word fluency data are given separately for males and females. Data showing whether differences exist between elderly AD and MID patients on this test will become available when additional autopsies on tested nursing home residents are obtained (12).

The Buschke–Fuld selective reminding test for evaluating verbal memory and learning is frequently used with AD patients participating in drug treatment trials (39–44). These patients are often relatively mildly impaired in that they do learn during the 8–12 trials generally given, but they recall significantly less than normal age-matched controls. Normative data will soon be available (Samuel Brinkman, personal communication; John Largen, personal communication; Harvey Levin, personal communication).

AD patients seem to differ from Korsakoff patients, most schizophrenics, normal elderly, and other hospital patients tested in that they tend to make many inappropriate intrusions during a multitrial attempt to learn such a list of 12 unrelated words. These intrusions are often semantically *un*related to the items on the list and may not even be real words. Phonemic and other distortions in grammatical form are often seen. Such intrusion into memory tests and intrusions into other tests have recently been reported to be a distinguishing feature of AD (45,46) and the number of intrusions has been shown as highly sensitive to cholinergic booster therapy in patients with early AD (47).

The frequency and types of intrusions vary across tests. Although intrusions have been related to cholinergic deficiency and SPs of autopsied AD patients, and occur in over 89% of testable AD patients (46), they are frequently seen with other clinical entities, such as MID and aphasia. Immediate perseverations seem to be about twice as frequent as delayed perseverations (intrusions) in aphasics (48), but immediate perseveration is not common in AD until late in the course (49). The observation of delayed perseverations or intrusions should therefore raise the possibility of AD, but this phenomenon must be further studied before the potential of intrusions in relation to the differential diagnosis of dementia can be realized.

The Mattis Dementia Scale (50) is included in the dementia battery because it allows the examiner to continue to obtain data on patients who become untestable on most other instruments as the disease progresses. It has been reported not to contribute to the differentiation of the dementias (51), but it can be helpful in quantifying an overall level of deterioration against which to view other tests results (12).

Because considerable research on the psychometric characteristics of the dementias is currently in progress, the potential contribution of these tests to the differentiation of the dementias is increasing. As part of an evaluation by a neuropsychologist, the results of these tests can help answer such questions as:

1. Does the patient have *any* acquired impairment of intellectual ability?
2. Does this impairment seem to be typical of Alzheimer-type dementia, or do the test results raise the question of some other contributor to intellectual impairment?
3. Has the patient deteriorated (or improved) since last seen (if baseline scores were obtained on a previous occasion)?

Experienced clinical neuropsychologists combine the results of psychometric tests with the history and clinical impression from detailed behavioral observations to help answer these and other questions regarding behavioral, intellectual and affective changes with dementia and other brain damage. They also help differentiate dementia or other brain damage from psychiatric disorders.

The value of a referral to a psychologist depends in part on the prior experience and interests of the psychologist as well as on the effectiveness of communication between referring physician and psychologist. To arrive at mutually understood and answerable referral questions, extensive dialogue at the time of referral is essential. When appropriate referral questions have been delineated, testing can be optimally planned and a report written so as to maximize the contribution of the psychometric evaluation.

REFERENCES

1. Tomlinson BE, Blessed G, Roth M: Observations on the brains of demented old people. *J Neurol Sci* 1970; 11:205–242.

2. Jellinger K: Neuropathological aspects of dementias resulting from abnormal blood and cerebrospinal fluid dynamics. *Acta Neurol Belg* 1976; 76:83–102.

3. Blessed G, Tomlinson BE, Roth M: The association between quantitative measures of dementia and of senile change in the cerebral grey matter of elderly subjects. *Br J Psychiatry* 1968; 114:797–784.

4. Davies P, Maloney AJF: Selective loss of central cholinergic neurons in Alzheimer's disease. *Lancet* 1976; ii:1403.

5. Bowen DM, Smith CB, White P, et al: Senile dementia and related abiotrophies: biochemical studies on histologically evaluated human postmortem specimens. *Aging NY* 1976; 3:361–378.

6. Perry EK, Tomlinson BE, Blessed G, et al: Correlation of cholinergic abnormalities with senile plaques and mental test scores in senile dementia. *Br Med J* 1978; 2:1457–1459.

7. Boller F. Mizutani T. Roessmann V, et al: Parkinson's disease, dementia and Alzheimer disease: clinicopathological correlations. *Ann Neurol* 1980; 7:329–335.

8. Loranger AW, Goodell H, McDowell FH, et al: *Brain* 1972; 95:405.

9. Albert ML, Feldman RG, Willis AL: The "subcortical dementia" of progressive supranuclear palsy. *J Neurol Neurosurg Psychiatry* 1974; 37:121–130.

10. Kimura D, Barnett HJM, Burkhart G: Psychological test pattern in progressive supranuclear palsy. *Neuropsychologia* 1981; 19:301–306.

11. Katzman R: Normal pressure hydrocephalus. *Aging NY* 1978; 7:115–124.

12. Fuld PA: Psychological testing in the differential diagnosis of the dementias. *Aging NY* 1978; 7:185–193.

13. Rabin A: Psychometric trends in senility and psychoses of the senium. *J Gen Psychol* 1945; 32:149–162.

14. Hopkins BA, Roth M: Psychological test performance in patients over sixty: II. Paraphrenia, arteriosclerotic psychosis and acute confusion. *J Ment Sci* 1953; 99:451–463.

15. Hachinski VC, Iliff LD, Zilhka E, et al: Cerebral blood flow in dementia. *Arch Neurol* 1975; 34:632.

16. Rosen WG, Terry RD, Fuld PA, et al: Pathological verification of ischemic score in differentiation of dementias. *Ann Neuro* 1980; 7:486–488.

17. Miller E: *Abnormal Aging: The Psychology of Senile and Presenile Dementia*. London, Wiley, 1977.

18. Fuld, PA: Test profile of cholinergic dysfunction and of Alzheimer-type dementia. Submitted for publication, 1983.

19. Drachman DA, Leavitt J: Memory impairment in the aged: storage versus retrieval deficit. *J Exp Psychol* 1972; 93:302–308.

20. Sim M, Turner E, Smith WT: Cerebral biopsy in the investigation of presenile dementia. *Br J Psychiatry* 1966; 112:119–125.

21. Ron MA, Toone BK, Garralda ME, et al: Diagnostic accuracy in presenile dementia. *Br J Psychiatry* 1979; 134:161–168.

22. Botwinick J, Birren J: Differential decline in the Wechsler–Bellevue subtests in the senile psychoses. *J Gerontol* 1951; 6:365–368.

23. Roth M, Hopkins BA: Psychological test performance in patients over sixty: I. Senile psychosis and the affective disorders of old age. *J Ment Sci* 1953; 99:439–451.

24. Crookes TG: Indices of early dementia on WAIS. *Psychol Rep* 1974; 34:734.

25. Storrie MC, Doerr, HO: Characterization of Alzheimer type dementia utilizing an abbreviated Halstead-Reitan Battery. *Clin Neuropsychol* 1980; 2:78–82.

26. Perez FI, Stump DA, Gay JRA, et al: Intellectual performance in multi-infarct dementia and Alzheimer's disease: a replication study. *Can J Neurol Sci* 1976; 3:181–187.

27. Lezak M: *Neuropsychological Assessment.* New York, Oxford University Press, 1976.

28. Russell EW, Neuringer C, Goldstein G: *Assessment of Brain Damage: A Neuropsychological Key Approach.* New York, Wiley, 1970.

29. Golden CJ: *Diagnosis and Rehabilitation in Clinical Neuropsychology,* Springfield, Thomas, 1978.

30. Smith WL, Phillipus MJ: *Neuropsychological Testing in Organic Brain Dysfunction.* Springfield, Thomas, 1969.

31. Pirozzolo FJ, Lawson-Kerr K: Neuropsychological assessment of dementia, in Maletta GJ, Pirozzolo FJ (eds): *The Aging Nervous System.* New York, Praeger, 1980.

32. Filskov SB, Boll TJ: *Handbook of Clinical Neuropsychology.* New York, Wiley, 1981.

33. Meudell PA, Butters N, Montgomery K: Role of rehearsal in the short-term memory performance of patients with Korsakoff's and Huntington's disease. *Neuropsychologia* 1978; 16:507–510.

34. Mattis S, Kovner R, Goldmeier E: Different patterns of mnemonic deficits in two organic amnestic syndromes. *Brain* 1978; 6:1179–1191.

35. Crook T, Gilbert JG, Ferris S: Operationalizing memory impairment for elderly persons: the Guild Memory Test. *Psychol Rep* 1980; 47:1315–1318.

36. Fuld P, Buschke H: Stages of retrieval in verbal learning. *J Verbal Learning Verbal Behav* 1976; 15:401–410.

37. Fuld PA: Guaranteed stimulus-processing in the evaluation of memory and learning. *Cortex* 1980; 16:255–271.

38. Fuld PA: *The Fuld Object-Memory Evaluation.* Chicago, Stoelting Instrument Co, 1981.

39. Peters BH, Levin HS: Memory enhancement after physostigmine treatment in the amnesic syndromes. *Arch Neurol* 1977; 34:215–219.

40. Peters BH, Levin HS: Double-blind study of physostigmine in memory impairment. *Neurology* 1978; 397.

41. Peters BH, Levin HS: Effects of physostigmine and lecithin on memory in Alzheimer's disease. *Ann Neurol* 1979; 6:219–221.

42. Sitaram N, Weingartner H, Caine E, et al: Choline: selective enhancement of serial learning and encoding of low imagery words in man. *Life Sci* 1978; 22:1555–1560.

43. Muramoto O, Morihiro S, Hideo S, et al: Effect of physostigmine on constructional and memory tasks in Alzheimer's disease. *Arch Neurol* 1979; 36:501.

44. Davis KL, Mohs RC, Tinklenberg J, et al: Cholinomimetics and memory: the effect of choline chloride. *Arch Neurol* 1980; 37:49.

45. Smith CM, Swash M: Possible biochemical basis of memory disorder in Alzheimer disease. *Age Ageing* 1979; 289–293.

46. Fuld PA, Katzman R, Davies P, et al: Intrusions as a sign of Alzheimer dementia: chemical and pathological verification. *Ann Neurol* 1982; 11:155–159.

47. Thal L, Fuld PA, Masur DM, et al: Oral physostigmine and lecithin improve memory in Alzheimer's disease. *Ann Neurol,* in press.

48. Yamadori A: Verbal perseveration in aphasia. *Neuropsychologia* 1981; 19:591–597.

49. Sim M, Sussman I: Alzheimer's disease: its natural history and differential diagnosis. *J Nerv Ment Dis* 1962; 135:489–499.

50. Mattis S: Mental status examination for organic mental syndrome in the elderly patient, in Bellak L, Karasu TB (eds): *Geriatric Psychiatry*. New York, Grune & Stratton, 1976, pp 77–121.

51. Hersch EL: Development and application of the extended scale for dementia. *J Am Geriatr Soc* 1979; 27:348–354.

52. Kahn RL, Goldfarb AJ, Pollack M, et al: Brief objective measures for the determination of mental status in the aged. *Am J Psychiatry* 1960; 117:326–328.

53. Buschke H, Fuld PA: Evaluating storage, retention, and retrieval in disordered memory and learning. *Neurology* 1974; 24:1019–1025.

28 Psychometric Assessment in Alzheimer's Disease

THOMAS CROOK

PERFORMANCE TESTS AND BEHAVIOR RATING SCALES have two principal applications in both the study and treatment of Alzheimer's disease (AD). First, such measures are of value in establishing the presence and magnitude of the cognitive deficit that is the hallmark of AD. Of course, that is not the same as establishing a diagnosis of AD, since the cognitive deficit may result from other organic or functional factors. Second, psychometric measures provide a basis for assessing change in the severity of AD symptomatology over time or in response to intervention.

In both applications, psychometric instruments may offer greater objectivity and precision than is provided by unstructured clinical assessment or patient report. Patient reports of memory dysfunction, for example, may be more closely related to depression than to actual cognitive impairment (1). On the other hand, there are major limitations to every psychometric instrument now used with AD to assess symptomatology.

A major problem with performance tests is that most instruments bear little relation to the actual behavioral deficits seen in AD. A test may provide a measure of a theoretical construct thought to underly a particular behavioral deficit but, to my knowledge, none of the tests now used has been carefully validated against performance outside the laboratory in relevant tasks of daily life. For example, patients with AD present with specific behavioral deficits ranging from a tendency to misplace objects around the home, to an inability to recall the name of an individual following introduction, to an inability to recognize close family members.

On the basis of such deficits, a clinician or researcher may invoke the psychological construct *memory* and may employ a memory test of some sort to measure the severity and course of the deficit. In most cases, the test employed will have been developed for entirely different applications and will have nothing whatever to do with the actual behavioral deficits that characterize AD. This sort of assessment strategy is particularly problematic when used to evaluate the effects of treatment. For example, reports appear in the literature with unfortunate regularity suggesting that a particular drug may be effective in AD because it has been shown to improve scores on a memory test. Reports of this sort often generate a certain enthusiasm even though the author may not have attempted to demonstrate that the drug has in any way diminished actual clinical problems for which treatment was initiated. Such reports are particularly likely to generate enthusiasm when the tests employed derive from arcane theories of cognition or require complex electronic gadgetry.

In developing tests for use in AD, the logical starting point is provided by the actual behavioral symptoms that incapacitate the individual and bring him or her to the physician for treatment. A satisfactory test may either employ similar stimulus materials and essentially provide a controlled replication of the behavioral deficit, or the test may be abstract and bear no resemblance whatever to the behavioral deficit, provided performance on the measure is shown closely correlated with relevant behavior outside the laboratory. There is, however, an advantage to the former approach, since it is generally recognized that tests must appear to measure the ability being assessed to function properly in practical situations (2). For example, the elderly patient who appears for evaluation after forgetting the names of familiar people or losing his way home from the store may be less than enthusiastic when faced with a memory assessment task requiring retention of seemingly irrelevant information or performance of alien tasks.

Among the tests that do relate directly to the behavioral symptoms of AD is a brief screening instrument labeled the Misplaced Objects Task (3), a facial recognition task (4), a verbal learning task based on recall of material from a grocery shopping list (5), learning and memory tasks based on name–name and name–face associations (6), and a digit-span task requiring recall using a telephone dialing apparatus (7). While these measures require a great deal more development to satisfy recognized standards for psychological tests (8), they illustrate that psychometric measures can, in fact, be modeled quite closely on many actual behavioral deficits which characterize AD.

Ideally, psychometric assessment in AD should be multimodal. A complete assessment of symptomatology requires not only performance tests such as those listed above but also carefully constructed behavior rating scales completed by a psychiatrist or psychologist, and measures of the individual's actual performance in activities of daily living completed by family members for outpatients, or by the nursing staff for institutionalized patients. Patient reports are also of value where impairment is not too severe, provided a carefully constructed scale is used that takes into account the often powerful response biases in AD. State-of-the-art psychometric instruments for each mode of assessment are provided elsewhere (9).

In summary, psychometric instruments may be of value to both the clinician and researcher, provided they reflect the actual behavioral impairments associated with AD rather than an abstract psychological construct. The behavioral deficits in AD are concrete and, unfortunately, often tragic in magnitude.

References

1. Kahn RL, Zarit SH, Hilbert NM, et al: Memory complaint and impairment in the aged. *Arch Gen Psychiatry* 1975; 32:1569–1573.
2. Anastasi A: *Psychological Testing,* ed 2. New York, Macmillan, 1961.
3. Crook T, Ferris SH, McCarthy M: The Misplaced Objects Task: a brief test for memory dysfunction in the aged. *J Am Geriatr Soc* 1979; 27:284–287.
4. Ferris SH, Crook T, Clark E, et al: Facial recognition memory deficits in normal aging and senile dementia. *J Gerontol* 1980; 35:707–714.
5. McCarthy M, Ferris SH, Clark E, et al: Acquisition and retention of categorized material in normal aging and senile dementia. *Exp Aging Res* 1981; 7:127–135.
6. Clark E, Ferris S, McCarthy M, et al: Associational learning and memory tasks associated with brain impairments. *Neurobiol Aging,* in press.

7. Crook T, Ferris SH, McCarthy M, et al: The utility of digit recall tasks for assessing memory in the aged. *J Consult Clin Psychol* 1980; 48:228–233.

8. American Psychological Association: *Standards for Educational and Psychological Tests,* rev ed. Washington, DC, American Psychological Association, 1974.

9. Crook T, Ferris SH, Bartus R: *Assessment in Geriatric Psychopharmacology.* New Canaan, Powley, 1982.

29 Early Detection of Incipient Alzheimer's Disease: Some Methodological Considerations on Computerized Diagnosis

ROLAND J. BRANCONNIER
DONALD R. DEVITT

WELLS (1) HAS DEFINED DEMENTIA as a clinical syndrome associated with chronic, diffuse cerebral hemispheric dysfunction that, when pervasive, is characterized by intellectual deterioration, memory impairment, disordered abstract thinking, defective judgment, poor impulse control, personality changes, and lability of affect. While dementia can result from a large variety of underlying specific diseases, several carefully conducted differential diagnostic studies have shown that in the population over 65 years of age, 50–70% of all cases of dementia are due to Alzheimer's disease (AD) (2–4).

AD is (at present) a chronic, progressive, and irreversible neurological disease. It is characterized histopathologically by the presence of dense concentrations of neuritic plaques and neurofibrillary tangles (NFTs) in the cerebral cortex and by granulovacuolar degeneration of the hippocampus (5). Marked biochemical changes hallmarked by reduced glucose utilization and synthetic activity of choline acetyltransferase have also been observed (6, 7). Clinically, AD carries a prognosis of a 50% reduction in remaining life expectancy and is ranked as the fifth leading cause of death, accounting for 100,000 to 120,000 deaths per year, in the United States (8).

Recent investigations have demonstrated that the extent of pathological changes in brain structure, biochemistry, and metabolism are correlated with the severity of cognitive impairment in AD (6, 7, 9, 10). Such observations have led Roth (11) to conclude that there may be a neuropathological threshold separating cognitively normal from clinically demented subjects. Thus, the early detection of the cognitive dysfunction associated with threshold of incipient AD (IAD) is critical for the initiation of therapeutic intervention to minimize the functional disability of these patients. Unfortunately, the early detection of IAD by psychometric methods has been impeded by absence of a diagnostic screening instrument that is sensitive as well as valid and reliable (12, 13).

DESIGN OF A COMPUTERIZED DIAGNOSTIC SCREENING BATTERY FOR IAD

The initial step in the construction of a new diagnostic battery is to delineate a set of design criteria for the instrument. Thus, in the design of the diagnostic screening battery for IAD, the following framework was used:

1. Target for evaluation those cognitive deficits that occur with high frequency in IAD.
2. To maximize systematic variance, ascertain the precise nature of each deficit and choose tests or combinations of tests that maximize performance discriminability between the normal aged and the IAD patient.
3. To minimize the error variance of the tests, conduct administration and scoring by computer.
4. The test battery should yield a diagnostic measure of high predictive value for IAD.

DETERMINING THE TARGET SYMPTOMS OF IAD

While many investigators and clinicians have described the symptoms of AD, few have provided detailed information about the symptomatic progression of the disease. An exception is the detailed study of Sjögren and co-workers (14).

These investigators have divided AD into three clinically distinct stages. Presented in Table 29–1 are the stages, with the most frequently observed symptoms. Focusing on the cognitive deficits only, Stage I—the point at which the pathological threshold is exceeded—is characterized by incipient dementia, mnestic disturbance (including anomia), and spatial disorientation.

At Stage II, the dementia now becomes more pronounced, with marked mnestic disturbance and spatial disorientation. In addition, disorientation for time, place, and person as well as many focal neurological disturbances such as visual agnosia, aphasia, agraphia, alexia, and apraxia become superimposed on the earlier symptoms.

Stage III is the terminal stage of the disease, where cognitive activity is absent and the clinical picture is dominated by decerebrate vegetative status. These findings agree with contemporary descriptions of the stages of the disease as detailed by Reisberg and associates (15). Thus, the cognitive deficits that should be targeted for testing are incipient dementia, memory impairment, amnestic aphasia, and spatial disorientation.

MAXIMIZING SYSTEMATIC VARIANCE: DEFINITION AND ASSESSMENT OF COGNITIVE DEFICITS IN IAD

INCIPIENT DEMENTIA

While Sjögren and co-workers (14) do not define the term "incipient dementia," clearly it connotes a decline in intellectual capacity. Since this deficit is considered the principal cognitive symptom of AD, a description of the structure of intelligence and its vulnerability to normal aging are presented.

Intelligence is not a unitary process. Horn and Cattell (16) have described two broad categories of intelligence, fluid (Gf) and crystallized (Gc) intelligence. Gf is nonverbal, is independent of education, and is measured by tests of figural and inductive reasoning. In

TABLE 29–1
Stages of Alzheimer's Disease

Symptoms	Frequency of Occurrence (%)
Stage I	
A. Incipient dementia	100
B. Mnestic disturbance (anomia)	100
C. Spatial disorientation	100
D. Reduced spontaneity	83
E. Fixed forward stare	61
Stage II	
A. Progressive dementia	100
B. Mnestic disturbance	100
C. Generalized disorientation	100
D. Aspontaneity	100
E. Amnestic aphasia	100
F. Perseveration	89
G. Sensory aphasia	83
H. Agraphia	83
I. Alexia	77
J. +2 muscle tonus	77
K. Gait disturbance	72
L. Apraxia	72
M. Dysarthria	67
Stage III	
A. Decerebrate vegetative status	100
B. +3 hypokinesis	100
C. Emotional lability	100

Source: Data from Sjögren et al. (14).

contrast, Gc is the ability to use habits of judgment based on experience, is dependent on education, and is measured by tests of general information and knowledge of specific topics.

The effects of normal aging on Gf and Gc are discordant. A large body of evidence suggests that while Gf declines from maturity onward, the Gc dependent functions are concomitantly increasing (17–19). Indeed, Goldstein and Shelly (20) have demonstrated that verbal abilities in normal aged are superior to young normals. These findings suggest that the intellectual deterioration associated with IAD would presumably be characterized by a global decline of both Gf and Gc dependent functions. In contrast, the normal aged would be expected to exhibit a selective decline of Gf with preserved Gc. Moreover, since verbal abilities improve with aging while declining in IAD, tests of general verbal ability should provide optimal discriminability of intellectual deterioration in IAD patients.

Nelson and McKenna (21) have reported that word-reading ability in dementia is retained until the degree of dementia is moderately severe. Since word-reading ability has been demonstrated to be highly correlated with intelligence as measured by the Wechsler Adult Intelligence Scale (WAIS) (22) in normal subjects, reading ability scores in dementia should provide an estimate of premorbid intelligence when contrasted against current levels of performance on the WAIS. The word-reading test developed by Nelson and McKenna (21) to test this hypothesis was the Nelson Adult Reading Test (NART).

In English, there are two types of words: "regular" and "irregular." Regular words such as "nave" can be read by a literate adult by applying the rules of grapheme/phoneme representation and pronunciation, despite a lack of familiarity with these words. In contrast, irregular words such as "subtle" do not follow the above rules and, therefore, correct pronunciation is dependent on familiarity.

The NART is composed of 50 irregular words that are to be read aloud. Scoring consists of the numbers of errors of pronunciation that are made. In the initial standardization, normal subjects were administered both the NART and the WAIS, and NART scores were used to predict verbal, performance, and full-scale IQ. The same procedure was then repeated in a group of patients with dementia. Results of this study showed that while dementia patients had significantly lower IQ scores on the WAIS, the NART scores were not different (21). Since this initial study was reported, the findings have been replicated and norms provided for predicted–obtained IQ discrepancies (23, 24). Thus, the NART–WAIS combination appears to be a sensitive indicator of dementia.

In the version adapted to the screening battery for IAD, intellectual deterioration is assessed by administering the NART and obtaining a predicted verbal IQ based on the regression equations of Nelson (23). The WAIS information, Similarities, and Vocabulary subtests are then administered and prorated to yield an estimate of obtained verbal IQ. These subtests were chosen for prorating because Duke (25) has shown that these three tests combined correlate with full verbal IQ at $r=.96$. In addition, each subtest was shortened according to the method of Satz and Mogel (26), a modification that also results in a high correlation with full verbal IQ (26, 27). Only the verbal IQ is evaluated, as this measure is loaded on Gc and, thus, has greater discriminability than either performance or full-scale IQ for IAD. The discrepancy score between predicted and obtained verbal IQ is the parameter of intellectual deterioration.

Mnestic Disturbance

The impairment of anterograde memory is a cognitive deficit associated with both normal aging and IAD (28, 29). Kral (30) has focused attention on the distinct symptomatology, course, and prognosis of memory dysfunction related to each.

The memory impairment characteristic of normal aging is what Kral (30) calls "benign senescent forgetfulness" (BSF). The nature of the deficit is the inability to recall unimportant or minor details of an episode while the episode itself can be recalled. Moreover, the failure to recall specific details is not permanent and the data might be recalled on a different occasion. The progression of BSF is slow and carries no prognostic significance about mortality.

In contrast to this benign form of memory loss is malignant memory loss. This memory dysfunction is characterized by a global inability to recall not only the details of a recent episode, but also the episode itself. The malignant form of memory loss, typical of dementia, progresses rapidly, and is prognostic of a markedly reduced life span.

To place the observations of Kral (30) within the context of modern learning and memory theory, a brief discussion of the structure and assessment of human memory is necessary to provide a conceptual framework for his findings.

The current concept of the structure of human memory is that it consists of four distinct stores each with characteristic storage capacity, a facility with which items are retrieved, and resistance to forgetting. They are sensory, primary (PM), secondary (SM), and semantic memory (31).

In the laboratory, the assessment of memory is concerned with a quantitative analysis of the temporal retention of verbal or nonverbal information. There are three methods of assessing retention; two are direct—recognition and recall—and the third, relearning, is indirect (32). All three methods can be used with a variable interval between learning and the test of retention. Thus, a memory test that has a retention interval > sensory memory but < secondary memory is a test of "immediate" memory and is approximately equivalent to PM. Tests of short-term memory (STM) and long-term memory (LTM) are, to different degrees, dependent on SM (31). In the literature, recall performance is assessed most frequently, recognition less frequently, and relearning infrequently.

Tulving and Pearlstone (33) have drawn a distinction between what is in memory and what can be retrieved, i.e., availability versus accessibility. It has been demonstrated repeatedly that recall is highly correlated with degree of initial storage, but is an insensitive indicator of what is available in memory (34, 35). In contrast, recognition performance is sensitive and can often detect availability of previously learned material when recall (accessibility) fails to do so (36, 37).

Anderson and Bower (38) have proposed a search-recognition hypothesis to explain why recognition is a more sensitive indicator of retention than recall. Recall is a two-step process requiring both the implicit search for an available target item in memory followed by the recognition that the item is correct. In recognition, only one step is required. The target item is presented and must only be identified as an available item in storage. The apparent superiority of recognition over recall results from retrieval (accessibility) failure due to ineffective search.

Applying the conceptual model to BSF, the principal effect of normal aging on memory is characterized by a selective disruption of retrieval from, while sparing storage into, SM. This interpretation is supported by the preponderance of experimental evidence showing that increasing age is associated with deterioration of recall performance while recognition remains unaffected (39). In contrast to BSF, the malignant memory loss seen in IAD is distinguished by a failure of both the storage and retrieval mechanisms of SM. Since recall and recognition are dependent on the availability of information, performance on both would be expected to be impaired. Indeed, this has been confirmed recently by Miller and Lewis (40). Since recognition is impaired in IAD but unaffected in normal aging, assessment of recognition should provide optimal discriminability of memory dysfunction specific to IAD.

To assess availability of information in SM, a two-step process is necessary. In the first step, new information must be stored. In the second, the recognition test for this material must be applied.

For the IAD battery, storage is accomplished by utilizing the technique of selective reminding (41). The procedure consists of the presentation of a list of ten nouns, all belonging to a single category, at a rate of one item every 2 seconds. Following presentation of the entire ten-item list, the patient is asked to recall as many nouns as possible in any order (free recall). If the patient fails to recall some of the items, the patient is selectively reminded of only those items missed on the previous trial. The patient is then asked to recall the entire list. This procedure is repeated until either all ten items are recalled on two consecutive trials without reminder or ten trials have elapsed.

After the criterion is reached, availability of the material learned during selective reminding is tested by a subject-paced, continuous recognition paradigm. A series of 20 words are presented to the patient. Ten of the words are target items learned previously, while the other ten are distractors not part of the original list. Each word is displayed one at a time, accompanied by a question asking if the item was or was not part of the list of items learned. The patient's task is to decide if the item belonged to the list by making a yes response if it was, or a no response if it was not. Order of target presentation and distractors is randomized and balanced for category frequency (42). Scoring of this continuous recognition task consists of determining the number of correct classifications of targets (hits) and incorrect classifications of distractors as targets (false alarms). Hits and false alarms are then converted to hit and false alarm rates and used to determine the response criterion (β) and criterion-free estimate of sensitivity (d') by application of signal detection theory (43). As the d' statistic is dependent on availability, this is the parameter of malignant memory impairment in IAD.

AMNESTIC APHASIA

Aphasia, the disorder of language secondary to brain pathology, is not a consequence of the normal aging process. Indeed, as described above, some language-related functions may improve with aging (44). For example, category instance fluency (CIF) tests utilizing both free and cued recall production of exemplars of specific categories have shown that the retrieval of lexical material is not affected by normal aging (45, 46). Likewise, Waugh and Barr (47) have demonstrated that normal elderly are slightly faster than young normals in a naming-latency task that assessed the speed of retrieval of words from the internal lexicon. Thus, in normal aging the ability to retrieve lexical material does not deteriorate.

In contrast to normal aging, aphasia is a frequently observed symptom of AD (28). Moreover, the progression and symptomatology of aphasia in AD is characteristic (48).

In Stage I, the principal aphasic symptom of AD is a specific type of anomia or word-finding disturbance (49). The anomia is characteristic in that confrontation naming of objects is well preserved with a marked impairment in the ability to generate category instances. As the disease progresses to Stage II, verbal output becomes "empty" with circumlocutory speech that reflects an increasingly impoverished lexical base. However, while both expressive and receptive lexical aspects of language are deteriorating rapidly, confrontation naming is only minimally impaired, and syntactic processes are not affected (48). At this stage, echolalia, the involuntary repetition of words spoken by others, is also common (50). The total pattern of aphasia at Stage II, reduction in lexical stock with preserved syntax and repetition, has led Schwartz and associates (51) to conclude that the linguistic disturbance of advanced AD is a mixed sensorimotor transcortical aphasia in which the intact speech areas are isolated from the higher cortical functions. At Stage III, all linguistic functions are lost and a global aphasia results.

The observation by Benson (49) that in IAD confrontation naming is preserved while category generation is impaired has psycholinguistic implications. Collins and Loftus (52) have proposed that semantic information is structured into two systems, a lexicon for words and a conceptual network. The lexicon is organized by the way words sound while the conceptual network is structured by conceptual relatedness or semantic distance. Each word in the lexicon is linked to at least one concept in the conceptual network. Thus, a concept can be interfaced with a word that is used to designate the concept. Concerning IAD, this would suggest that there is a breakdown of the conceptual network (category generation) while the lexicon remains intact (confrontation naming). Indeed, Warrington (53) has shown that the breakdown of the conceptual network in dementia is systematic and characterized by, first, a loss of specific followed by general concepts. For example, the concept of "robin" would be lost before "bird," and "bird" before "animal." Since the conceptual network is disrupted in IAD but remains unaffected in normal aging, assessment of CIF should provide optimal discriminability of the word-finding disturbance specific to IAD.

In the CIF tests used for the clinical assessment of word-finding disturbance, generation of as many exemplars from a category defined by a specific concept or letter is required (49). The performance criterion is either the number of instances generated with a specified time limit or the time taken to produce a specified number of instances (39). While these methods are adequate to detect gross word-finding disturbances, it is questionable if they are sufficiently sensitive to discriminate minimal deficits. The sensitivity problem can be corrected, however, by employing a chronometric performance criterion based on latency to respond (54).

The paradigm chosen to assess word-finding disturbance is the CIF paradigm proposed by Freedman and Loftus (55). The paradigm consists of presenting the patient with a category name followed by a single letter, then requiring the patient to provide an exemplar of the category beginning with the specified letter. In the IAD version, the patient is presented with a series of 24 category–letter pairs. Six instances of each of the following four categories— a fruit, a bird, a country, and a metal—were chosen from the category norms of Battig and Montague (42). Each of the six letters of each category was obtained by selecting the first letter of the category items with the highest rank-order frequencies. For example, in the category fruit, the first rank-order response is "apple." Therefore, the letter "A" was chosen.

Each trial begins with the presentation of the category for 2 sec. After a 0.25-second delay, a letter is presented. The onset of the letter stimulus initiates a reaction timer and the overt verbal response triggers a voice-activated relay that terminates the display and stops the reaction timer. Category–letter pairs are randomized and a variable 3-, 5-, or 7-second intertrial interval (ITI) is imposed. Reaction time data for each trial are subjected to logarithmic transformation, summed, and the geometric mean obtained. Incorrect responses and omissions are not included. The use of geometric mean is preferred over the median because the median lacks the sampling stability of the mean (56). Thus, the geometric mean is a chronometric performance criterion of CIF that is the parameter of word-finding disturbance in IAD.

Spatial Disorientation

Factor analytic studies of primary mental abilities have demonstrated that there exists a factor of broad visualization (BV) involving spatial concepts and orientation (19). Moreover, longitudinal investigation of BV has revealed that spatial ability is stable and does not decline with normal aging, when generational differences are taken into account (57). However, Gaylord and Marsh (58), using the spatial task of Shepard and Meltzer (59), showed that normal elderly are significantly slower at mental rotation than young normals. The observed mental rotation rates were 17.7 and 9.6 degrees of rotation/sec, or an elderly/young performance ratio of 1.84:1. Recently, Cerella and associates (60) have reported similar results, showing an age-related decline of 1.70:1. Thus, the significance of these findings is that while subtle chronometric deficits in spatial performance are observed in normal aging, manifest spatial orientation is well preserved.

Geographic (or topographic) disorientation is a form of visual agnosia that results from a disturbance of the comprehension of spatial concepts (61). It is characterized by diminished ability to orient places on maps, estimate distances accurately, and find routes in both familiar and new places (62). Because of the devastating effect geographic disorientation has on functional capacity, it is often the first recognizable symptom of AD (28). Indeed, Sjögren and co-workers (14) reported that 100% of their Stage I AD patients had an obvious impairment in the ability to orient in space, while orientation for time was well preserved. The defect is so striking that Reisberg and colleagues (15) have suggested that a positive finding of geographic disorientation is virtually pathognomic of IAD when observed in an elderly patient as part of a constellation of idiopathic cognitive dysfunctions. Since manipulation of spatial information is markedly impaired in IAD while it is only minimally affected in normal aging, assessment of speed of mental rotation should provide optimal discriminability of spatial disorientation.

As cited earlier, the most sensitive method of assessing spatial ability appears to be the speed of mental rotation paradigm of Shepard and Meltzer (59). The basic test involves the serial presentation of two pictures of a three-dimensional object and requires the subject to determine if both objects are congruent. As the angular orientation of the second object is varied systematically, the researchers demonstrated that there was a linear increase in decision time as a function of degrees of rotation. The slope of the function relating decision time to angular displacement is considered a pure measure of the speed of mental rotation (63).

The version adapted for the IAD battery is similar to the modification of the Shepard–Meltzer paradigm used by Cooper (64). In this modification, a two-dimensional line is rotated. This method was chosen because a two-dimensional rotation concept is more readily comprehensible than a three-dimensional.

The patient is presented with a series of 24 arrow-pairs. At the beginning of each trial, an arrow (S1) that originates in the center of the display and radiates either 0, 90, 180, or 270 *d* is presented for 0.5 second. After an interstimulus interval of 0.1 second, a second arrow (S2) is presented that is rotated either 0, 90, or 180 *d* from S1. The patient's task is to determine if S1 and S2 are congruent and to respond on a keyboard by pressing yes or no. The onset of S2 initiates a reaction timer and the overt motor response simultaneously terminates the display of S2 and stops the reaction timer. Each test has 24 trials, 8 of which are congruent and 8 of which are rotated at 90 and 180 *d*. Permutations of all possible arrow-pairs are randomized and a variable 3, 5, or 7-second ITI imposed. The performance criterion is the slope (degrees of rotation per second) calculated from the linear regression of degrees of rotation versus logarithmically transformed reaction time for the correct responses. Thus, the slope of the function relating decision time to angular displacement is the parameter of spatial disorientation in IAD.

A summary of the test battery selected for the early detection of IAD is outlined in Table 29–2.

ERROR VARIANCE AND THE COMPUTER

Selecting performance criteria that provide optimal discrimination between cognitive changes associated with normal aging and IAD maximizes the between-group systematic variance. However, the efficacy of maximizing systematic variance can be attenuated unless procedures are implemented to minimize error variance.

Errors of measurement are a principal source of error variance (65). Measurement error can be reduced by increasing the reliability of administration and decreasing human subjectivity in test scoring (66). Both of these objectives can be accomplished by using computerized testing procedures. Moreover, the recent advances in economical and powerful microcomputer hardware, coupled with easy to use BASIC language, have made reduction of measurement error through computerized psychometric assessment generally feasible.

TABLE 29–2
Screening Battery for Early Detection of Incipient Alzheimer's Disease

Symptom	Test	Performance Criterion
Intellectual deterioration	Verbal IQ Reading ability	Predicted–observed verbal IQ discrepancy
Mnestic disturbance	Selective reminding recognition	d' statistic
Amnestic aphasia	Category instance fluency	Mean recall latency
Spatial disorientation	Speed of mental rotation	Slope (degrees/sec)

DIAGNOSTIC TESTS AND PREDICTIVE VALUE THEORY

The purpose of a diagnostic screening test is to discriminate between the presence or absence of a disease. The reliability of a test, for this purpose, can be described by the sensitivity and specificity of the instrument when the test is applied to a selected sample of diseased and nonafflicted subjects (67). Sensitivity is the incidence of true-positive results observed when the test is given to patients with an independently confirmed diagnosis of the disease. Likewise, specificity is the incidence of true-negative results observed when the test is given to subjects who are known to be disease-free (68). However, when a diagnostic test is to be used in an unselected population, it is important to know the probability of obtaining a positive test result from a subject who, in fact, has the disease. This probability cannot be estimated directly from experimental sensitivity and specificity alone, since the predictive value of a positive result is a function of the prevalence of the disease in the population (69). This can be demonstrated by using predictive value theory, a mathematical algorithm based on Bayes's theorem (70).

From Bayes's formula, the *a priori* probability of a disease in the population (prevalence) is $P(\theta_1)$. The *a priori* probability of nondisease in the population is $P(\theta_2)$. The probability of a positive test result in a patient with the disease (sensitivity of the test) can be expressed as $P(R/\theta_1)$ while the probability of obtaining a positive test result in a patient without disease is $P(R/\theta_2)$. It then follows that the *a posteriori* probability of disease given a positive test result (predictive value of a positive result) (PV pos) is:

$$P(\theta_1/R) = \frac{P(\theta_1)P(R/\theta_1)}{P(\theta_1)P(R/\theta_1) + P(\theta_2)P(R/\theta_2)}$$

Thus, it can be shown that if a diagnostic test has an experimental sensitivity and specificity of 95%, the PV pos will vary from 16% to 95% when the prevalence of the disease in the population to which the test is applied increases from 1% to 50%.

In practical application, three parameters can be manipulated to increase the PV pos test result. First, PV pos, as mentioned above, is dependent on disease prevalence. While prevalence in the population cannot be controlled, the application of the diagnostic instrument can be limited to those patients who are suspected of having the disease, thereby increasing the prevalence of the disease in the testing situation. Second, PV pos is correlated to the specificity, but not the sensitivity of a test (71). Since most test scores are not binary, but can be expressed in some form of continuous scale, relative sensitivity and specificity can

TABLE 29–3
Predictive Value Analysis of the Short Portable Mental Status Questionnaire (SPMSQ)

	Score >4 (+)	Score <4 (−)
Raw data		
Diagnosed OBS	43	37
Not OBS	4	129
$X^2 = 74$, $P < .001$		
Prevalence-adjusted data		
Diagnosed OBS	2,700	2,300
Not OBS	2,850	92,150

Prevalence of OBS = 5%
Sensitivity = (43/80)(100)   = 54%
Specificity = (129/133)(100) = 97%
Predictive value (+) = (.54)(.05)/[(.54)(.05)] + [(.95)(.03)] = 49%

be manipulated by the selection of a referent or cutoff point that minimizes false-positive and false-negative results while maximizing specificity (72, 73). Third, specificity can be improved by utilizing more than one test and requiring a positive result from all tests to indicate the presence of disease. While this will tend to reduce sensitivity, specificity and thus PV pos will be maximized (71).

The significance of predictive value can be illustrated by an example. The Short Portable Mental Status Questionnaire (SPMSQ) of Pfeiffer (74) is purportedly a useful instrument for the diagnosis of organic brain syndrome (OBS) in the elderly. The top half of Table 29–3 presents Pfeiffer's data (74) to validate the SPMSQ. As can be seen, the chi-square analysis of the data, using a referent value of 4, shows the SPMSQ valid for detecting the presence of OBS. However, the conclusion of discriminative validity of the scale is based on an experimental OBS prevalence rate of 38% (80/213). The lower half of Table 29–3 presents the same data subjected to predictive value analysis. The relative sensitivity and specificity of SPMSQ, calculated from the experimental data, are 54% and 97%, respectively. Using a prevalence rate of 5% for pervasive OBS in the 65+ population (75), the experimental data are adjusted to show the expected number of positive and negative outcomes per 100,000 cases when the SPMSQ is applied to an unselected population over 65 years of age. Applying Bayes's theorem, a PV (+) = 49% is obtained. This means that for every 100 scores positive for OBS (above the referent value of 4), 51 will be obtained from normal elderly. Thus, the SPMSQ is not a reliable diagnostic instrument to detect the presence of OBS when applied to an unselected population.

SUMMARY

The foregoing has presented several methodological considerations in the design and construction of computerized tests for early detection of AD.

Choice of tests should be governed by the principle of maximizing systematic variance.

For IAD tests, this means choosing tests that offer optimal discrimination between changes in cognitive performance associated with normal aging and AD.

Minimizing error variance prevents the attenuation of systematic variance. As measurement error is a principal source of error variance, using computerized administration and scoring of tests reduces such possibilities for error variance.

For tests that will be employed as diagnostic measures of AD, knowing a test's validity and reliability is not sufficient. Of critical importance is to determine the predictive value of the test when it is applied to an unselected, elderly population.

References

1. Wells CE: Diagnosis of dementia. *Psychosomatics* 1979; 20:517–522.

2. Freemon FR: Evaluation of patients with progressive intellectual deterioration. *Arch Neurol* 1976; 33:658–659.

3. Tomlinson BE: The pathology of dementia, in Wells CE (ed): *Dementia,* ed 2. Philadelphia, Davis, 1977, pp 113–153.

4. Seltzer B, Sherwin I: Organic brain syndrome: an empirical study and critical review. *Am J Psychiatry* 1979; 135:13–21.

5. Terry RD: Structural changes in senile dementia of the Alzheimer type. *Aging NY* 1980; 13:23–32.

6. Ferris SH, de Leon MJ, Wolf AP, et al: Positron emission tomography in the study of aging and senile dementia. *Neurobiol Aging* 1980; 1:127–131.

7. Perry EK, Tomlinson BE, Blessed G, et al: Correlation of cholinergic abnormalities with senile plaques and mental test scores in senile dementia. *Br Med J* 1978; 25:1457–1459.

8. Katzman R: The prevalence and malignancy of Alzheimer disease. *Arch Neurol* 1976; 33:217–218.

9. de Leon MJ, George AE, Ferris SH, et al: Grey and white matter–CT correlates of senile dementia of the Alzheimer's type. Read before the 12th International Congress of Gerontology, Hamburg, July 12–17, 1981.

10. Tomlinson BE, Blessed G, Roth M: Observations on the brains of demented old people. *J Neurol Sci* 1970; 11:205–242.

11. Roth M: Senile dementia and its borderlands, in Cole JO, Barrett JE (eds): *Psychopathology in the Aged.* New York, Raven, 1980, pp 205–232.

12. Jacobs JW, Bernhard MR, Delgado A, et al: Screening for mental syndromes in the medically ill. *Ann Intern Med* 1977; 86:40–46.

13. Cohen D, Eisdorfer C: Cognitive theory and the assessment of change in the elderly, in Raskin A, Jarvik LF (eds): *Psychiatric Symptoms and Cognitive Loss in the Aged.* Washington, Hemisphere, 1979, pp 173–282.

14. Sjögren T, Sjögren H, Lindgren AGH: Morbus Alzheimer and Morbus Pick. *Acta Psychiatr Scand Suppl* 1952; 82:68–108.

15. Reisberg B, Ferris SH, Horn R, et al: Patterns of early age associated cognitive decline. Read before the 12th International Congress of Gerontology, Hamburg, July 12–17, 1981.

16. Horn JL, Cattell RB: Age differences in fluid and crystallized intelligence. *Acta Psychol* 1967; 26:107–219.

17. Baer PE: Cognitive changes in aging: competence and incompetence, in Gaitz CM (ed): *Aging and the Brain.* New York, Plenum, 1972, pp 5–13.

18. Cunningham WR, Clayton V, Overton W: Fluid and crystallized intelligence in young adulthood and old age. *J Gerontol* 1975; 30:53–55.

19. Horn JL: Psychometric studies of aging and intelligence. *Aging NY* 1975; 2:19–43.

20. Goldstein G, Shelly CH: Similarities and differences between psychological deficit in aging and brain damage. *J Gerontol,* 1975; 30:448–455.

21 Nelson HE, McKenna P: The use of current reading ability in the assessment of dementia. *Br J Soc Clin Psychol* 1975; 14:259–267.

22. Wechsler D: *Wechsler Adult Intelligence Scale Manual.* New York, Psychological Corp, 1955.

23. Nelson, HE: *Test Manual for the National Adult Reading Test (NART).* Windsor, England, NFER-Nelson Publishing Co, 1982.

24. Nelson HE, O'Connell A: Dementia: the estimation of premorbid intelligence levels using the new adult reading test. *Cortex* 1978; 14:234–244.

25. Duke RB: Intellectual evaluation of brain-damaged patients with a WAIS short form. *Psychol Rep* 1967; 20:858.

26. Satz P, Mogel S: An abbreviation of the WAIS for clinical use. *J Clin Psychol* 1962; 18:77–79.

27. Burns JE, Elias MF, Hitchcock AG, et al: Corroboration of the utility of the Satz–Mogel abbreviated WAIS with hospitalized geriatric patients. *Exp Aging Res* 1980; 6:181–184.

28. Strub RL, Black FW: *The Mental Status Examination in Neurology.* Philadelphia, Davis, 1977.

29. Botwinick J, Storandt M: *Memory, Related Functions, and Age.* Springfield, Thomas, 1974.

30. Kral VA: Senescent forgetfulness: benign and malignant. *Can Med Assoc J* 1962; 86:257–260.

31. Crowder RG: *Principles of Learning and Memory.* Hillsdale, NJ, Erlbaum, 1976.

32. Deese J, Hulse SH: *The Psychology of Learning,* ed 3. New York, McGraw-Hill, 1967.

33. Tulving E, Pearlstone Z: Availability versus accessibility of information in memory for words. *J Verbal Learning Behav* 1966; 5:381–391.

34. Hulicka IM, Weiss RL: Age differences in retention as a function of learning. *J Consult Psychol* 1965; 29:125–129.

35. Slamecka NJ: Recall and recognition in list discrimination tasks as a function of the number of alternatives. *J Exp Psychol (Gen)* 1967; 74:187–192.

36. Schonfield D, Robertson B: Memory storage and aging. *Can J Psychol* 1966; 20:228–236.

37. Harwood E, Naylor GFK: Recall and recognition in elderly and young subjects. *Austral J Psychol* 1969; 21:251–257.

38. Anderson JR, Bower GH: Recognition and retrieval processes in free recall. *Psychol Rev* 1972; 79:97–123.

39. Schonfield D, Stones MJ: Remembering and aging, in Kihlstrom JF, Evans FJ (eds): *Functional Disorders of Memory.* Hillsdale, NJ, Erlbaum, 1979, pp 103–139.

40. Miller E, Lewis P: Recognition memory in elderly patients with depression and dementia: a signal detection analysis. *J Abnorm Psychol* 1977; 86:84–86.

41. Buschke H: Selective reminding for analysis of memory and learning. *J Verbal Learning Verbal Behav* 1973; 12:543–550.

42. Battig WF, Montague WE: Category norms for verbal items in 56 categories: a replication and extension of the Connecticut category norms. *J Exp Psychol* 1969; 80:1–46.

43. Freeman PR: *Tables of d' and B.* Cambridge, Cambridge University Press, 1973.

44. Goldstein G: Psychological dysfunction in the elderly, in Cole JO, Barrett JE (eds): *Psychopathology in the Aged.* New York, Raven, 1980, pp 205–232.

45. Drachman DA, Levitt J: Memory impairment in the aged: storage versus retrieval deficit. *J Exp Psychol (Gen)* 1972; 93:302–308.

46. Eysenck MW: Retrieval from semantic memory as a function of age. *J Gerontol* 1975; 30:174–180.

47. Waugh NC, Barr RA: Memory and mental tempo, in Poon LW, Fozard TL, Cermak LS (eds): *Directions in Memory and Aging.* Hillsdale, NJ, Erlbaum, 1980, pp 251–260.

48. Irigaray L: *Le language des déments.* The Hague, Mouton, 1973.

49. Benson DF: Neurologic correlates of anomia, in Whitaker H, Whitaker HA (eds): *Studies in Neurolinguistics.* New York, Academic, 1979, vol 2, pp 293–327.

50. Stengel E: Psychopathology of dementia. *Proc R Soc Med* 1964; 57:911–914.

51. Schwartz MF, Martin OSM, Saffran EM: Dissociation of language function in dementia. *Brain Lang* 1979; 7:277–306.

52. Collins AM, Loftus EF: A spreading activation theory of semantic processing. *Psychol Rev* 1975; 82:407–428.

53. Warrington EK: The selective impairment of semantic memory. *Q J Exp Psychol* 1975; 27:635–657.

54. Posner MI: *Explorations of Mind.* Hillsdale, NJ, Erlbaum, 1978.

55. Freedman JL, Loftus EF: The retrieval of words from long-term memory. *J Verbal Learning Verbal Behav* 1971; 10:107–115.

56. Guilford JP, Fruchter B: *Fundamental Statistics in Psychology and Education.* New York, McGraw-Hill, 1973.

57. Nesselroade JR, Schaie KW, Baltes PB: Ontogenetic and generational components of structural and quantitative change in adult behavior. *J Gerontol,* 1972; 27:222–228.

58. Gaylord SA, Marsh GR: Age differences in the speed of spatial cognitive process. *J Gerontol* 1975; 30:674–678.

59. Shepard RN, Meltzer J: Mental rotation of three-dimensional objects. *Science* 1971; 171:701–703.

60. Cerella J, Poon LW, Fozard JL: Mental rotation and age reconsidered. *J Gerontol* 1981; 36:620–624.

61. Luria AR: *Higher Cortical Functions in Man.* New York, Basic Books, 1966.

62. Lezak MD: *Neuropsychological Assessment.* New York, Oxford University Press, 1976.

63. Cooper LA, Shepard RN: The time required to prepare for a rotated stimulus. *Memory and Cognition* 1973; 1:246–250.

64. Cooper LA: Demonstration of a mental analog of external rotation. *Percept Psychophysiol* 1976; 19:296–302.

65. Kerlinger FN: *Foundations of Behavioral Research.* New York, Holt, Rinehart & Winston, 1973.

66. Nunnaly JC: *Psychometric Theory.* New York, McGraw-Hill, 1978.

67. Thorner RM, Remein QR: *Principles and Procedures in the Evaluation of Screening for Disease.* Government Printing Office, 1961.

68. Galen RS, Gambino SR: *Beyond Normality: The Predictive Value and Efficiency of Medical Diagnoses.* New York, Wiley, 1975.

69. Sunderman FW, Van Soestbergen AA: Laboratory suggestions: probability computations for clinical interpretation of screening tests. *Am J Clin Pathol* 1971; 55:105–111.

70. Bayes T: An essay toward solving a problem in the doctrine of chance. *Philos Trans R Soc London* 1963; 53:370–418.

71. Vecchio TJ: Predictive value of a single diagnostic test in unselected populations. *N Engl J Med* 1966; 274:1171–1173.

72. McNeil BJ, Keeler E, Adelstein SJ: Primer on certain elements of medical decision making. *N Engl J Med* 1975; 293:211–215.

73. Murphy EA, Abbey H: The normal range: a common misuse. *J Chronic Dis* 1967; 20:79–88.

74. Pfeiffer E: A short portable mental status questionnaire for the assessment of organic brain deficit in elderly patients. *J Am Geriatr Soc* 1975; 23:433–441.

75. Gurland B, Dean L, Cross P, et al: The epidemiology of depression and dementia: the use of multiple indicators of the conditions, in Cole JO, Barrett JE (eds): *Psychopathology in the Aged.* New York, Raven, 1980, pp 37–60.

Section VIII
SPECIAL DIAGNOSTIC PROCEDURES

30 Electroencephalography

EWALD W. BUSSE

TWO NONINVASIVE PROCEDURES ARE BECOMING widely used as a diagnostic evaluative tool for determining the brain status of elderly persons. These are electroencephalography (EEG) and computerized tomography (CT). Both laboratory diagnostic procedures are readily available in most medical facilities. The clinician must learn to appreciate the uses and limitations of these two procedures for individual examinations as well as their interactions, both positive and negative.

Diagnostic tests and procedures are frequently classified as either sensitivity tests or specificity tests (1). A sensitivity test, when normal, permits the physician to confidently exclude the disease. A specificity test, when abnormal or showing a specific type of abnormality, essentially confirms the presence of the disease. The EEG is both a sensitivity and a specificity procedure, but the true diagnostic value of the EEG is frequently largely determined by correlation with the available clinical information. The EEG often helps determine if the presence of brain pathology is unlikely or probable. The EEG is less often helpful in identifying the diagnostic category of a progressive degenerative disorder.

NORMAL EEG AND VARIATIONS

The human EEG undergoes progressive changes with age from birth through senescence. The normal adult EEG recorded while awake displays two distinct components: alpha and beta activity. Alpha activity consists of regular, recurring sinusoidal waves of 8–13 c/s. Normal low-voltage fast activity (beta) is usually 15–35 c/s and is under 20 μV amplitude, usually less amplitude than any alpha activity present. Beta activity can occur in at least three types: frontal, diffuse, and rolandic (2).

ALPHA ACTIVITY

A common characteristic of EEG changes after the age of 65 is the slowing of the dominant alpha frequency and the appearance of slow waves; that is, waves below the usual alpha range. Alpha frequency (the alpha index) declines approximately 0.05 to 0.75 c/s each decade after age 60 (3).

Sex differences, too, occur in elderly subjects. Males have a significantly lower mean alpha frequency than do females of comparable age (4). There is no difference between white Americans and black Americans. The alpha slowing within the range of 8–13 c/s

231

found in elderly community subjects is not paralleled by changes in intellectual performance. Furthermore, there is no relationship between alpha slowing within the normal range and longevity. In addition to the alpha slowing commonly found in late life, scattered slow waves also appear. A slight slowing of the alpha index with scattered 6–8 c/s activity is not pathognomonic for any particular disorder.

BETA ACTIVITY (LOW-VOLTAGE FAST)

It is recognized that there are electroencephalographers who do not believe that beta activity is synonymous with low-voltage fast activity. It is agreed, however, that low-voltage fast activity is most often found in the anterior region of the brain. When it periodically appears in the posterior area of the brain, it is disrupting an alpha activity and is usually associated with an attention response. Fast waves resembling low-voltage fast, but of a higher amplitude, can be produced or enhanced by a wide variety of drugs. At the present time the diagnostic significance of variations in beta activity is of considerable doubt.

Low-voltage fast activity has not been reported to change with age. However, fast waves (that is, waves that are of higher amplitude than low-voltage fast) are more frequent in women than in men and tend to increase in females with the passage of time. Fast activity is present in 23% of females aged 60–79 years but in only 4% of elderly males the same ages.

TEMPORAL FOCI

In addition to the age changes involving alpha activity and the appearance of fast waves, a large percentage of elderly people develop focal activity predominantly involving the left anterior temporal area. Focal abnormalities of EEG, slow waves and sharp waves, appear over the anterior temporal lobe of 30–40% of apparently healthy elderly people. The left anterior temporal area is primarily involved in 70–80%, and in approximately 25% of temporal foci the mid- and posterior temporal leads are active. Bilateral focal patterns are found in 18–20%, and in 4–5% the distribution is more on the right. In the 20 years between 40 and 60 years of age, 20% of subjects show temporal lobe irregularities. After the age of 60, the percentage increases to 30–40%. When this focus is confined to the anterior temporal area, psychological deficiencies have been suspected but have not been unequivocally confirmed. However, when the focal slow activity spreads to involve adjacent areas, mental and behavioral problems are likely and often interfere with good social adjustment.

The localized EEG abnormality is usually episodic and is composed of high-voltage waves in the delta and theta range occasionally accompanied by focal sharp waves. The disturbance is found in the waking record, is maximum in the drowsy state, and disappears in sleep. It is not related to handedness or so-called cerebral dominance, and although it is episodic in nature, it is unrelated to seizures (5).

TEMPORAL LOBE DIFFERENCES AND ERP

Evoked response potentials (ERP) are discussed in detail in Chapter 31. Many studies of elderly individuals have focused on a component of ERP variously labeled "P300" or "late positive component" (LPC). Of particular interest is that the temporal recording sites that are T5 (left posterior temporal) and T6 (right posterior temporal) in the international

10–20 system show the greatest age differential. Young subjects show a hemispheric asymmetry with the right hemisphere (T6) site having the largest LPC and N1 component. Older subjects show no asymmetry other than a slightly longer LPC on the left. It is possible that these temporal lobe differences are in some way related to the temporal lobe differences found in the EEGs (6).

Slowing: Theta and Delta Activity

A slight slowing of the alpha rhythm, that is, with scattered 6–8 c/s waves, is not pathognomonic for any particular disorders (7). However, a moderate amount of slowing within the theta range (4–7 c/s) with rare delta (1–3 c/s) and severe slowing (that is, delta activity approximately 10% of the time) is characteristically found in brain disorders whether the dementia is classified as degenerative or vascular. A good correlation has been demonstrated between EEG slowing and cerebral oxygen consumption and/or cerebral blood flow (8). Diffuse slow activity, more than any other EEG variable, is related to senile intellectual deterioration. This correlation, however, is much better in institutionalized elderly subjects than in community volunteers, as borderline or mild slowing does not necessarily correlate with evidence of intellectual impairment. It is possible that the psychological tests are not sufficiently sensitive to early mental changes, and hence the correlation is not as good (9).

Patients with moderate or severe dementia usually show an alpha frequency below the normal alpha range; that is, frequencies of 7 c/sec or less. Several studies indicate that alpha slowing is accompanied by a decline in cerebral blood flow, metabolism, and mortality (10). Obrist (10) has shown that over a span of 5–7 years the alpha slowing in those who died was double that found in survivors. This observation has been confirmed by other investigators (11, 12).

Increasing Alpha Rhythm

As previously mentioned, normal alpha activity gradually declines in frequency with the passage of time. Throughout the adult lifespan the amount of alpha activity in the EEG over a given amount of time is often influenced by the so-called level of arousal or the levels of anxiety the subject experiences. Relaxation techniques including biofeedback approaches are known to result in an increase in the amount of alpha activity. However, it does not influence its frequency (alpha index). It has been demonstrated that the percentage time of alpha activity can be increased in the older adult, but the biofeedback approach is essentially no different from simple instructions on how to assume a tranquil, image-producing state of mind. Differences among individuals at various ages appear to be related to personality factors (13).

It is sometimes reported that medications "improve," that is, increase, the average alpha frequency. Such observations are often questionable, as alpha frequency analysis is complicated by a number of possible errors such as the unavailability of automatic frequency analysis (14).

Sleep in the Aged

It is claimed that changes in all-night EEG sleep patterns are among the most sensitive age-related physiological variables (10). Although there is considerable individual variation, overall sleep becomes more fragmented and awakenings during the night are longer and more frequent. This is associated with a marked reduction in Stage 4 (high-amplitude slow waves) and a moderate decrease in the amount of time occupied by rapid eye movement (REM) sleep. In addition, there is a significant decline in the number of 12–14 c/s spindle bursts, which are replaced by lower frequency spindlelike rhythms. Feinberg (15) and Prinz and co-workers (16) reported that the amount of decrease of REM sleep and the number of spindles correlated well with performance scores on the Wechsler Adult Intelligence Scale (WAIS) in both normal elderly adults and in groups with evidence of organic brain disease.

Among elderly patients with organic dementia the EEG changes during sleep are similar but more pronounced than those described for normal aging (17).

Reliability of the EEG

The reliability of the EEG as a diagnostic procedure is influenced by numerous factors. The minimal technical requirements for performing clinical EEG have been determined by the American Electroencephalographic Society (18). A minimum of eight channels should be recorded. Sixteen channels of simultaneous EEG recordings is, however, encouraged. The so-called 10/20 system of electrode number and placement is recommended. Both bipolar (scalp-to-scalp) and scalp-to-reference-leads should be used. The clinician is advised to ascertain if the EEG laboratory used is adhering to the standards or routines. Other factors affect the reliability of the EEG; these include prior medication, level of arousal, and cooperation of the subject. In elderly persons the EEG abnormality occasioned by a drug may persist for several months after the medication is discontinued. Finally, EEG slowing may be aggravated by acute metabolic disorders.

Diagnostic Values and Limitations

Electroencephalograms and Autopsy Findings

Müller and Schwartz (19) concluded that diffuse EEG slowing suggested senile Alzheimer's brain disease (AD), while intermittent lateralized slowing strongly suggested "hemodynamic problems due to sclerosis of cerebral arteries." In addition, the authors reported that symmetrical rhythmic delta wave disturbances had special significance. They were suggestive of acute or chronic dysfunction without localization; they were not primarily indicators of epilepsy. The symmetrical rhythmic discharges should be distinguished from the intermittent and persistent lateralized EEG abnormalities.

An interesting observation by Johannesson and associates (20) is that AD cases had EEG abnormalities which progressed slowly. In contrast, the Pick's disease patients had normal EEGs which remained so even late in the course when signs of dementia were marked. These investigators studied not only EEG but regional cerebral blood flow, and correlated the two observations. They concluded that if the EEG is highly abnormal in a case of presenile dementia, this favors the diagnosis of AD. If, on the other hand, a borderline or normal EEG is found, it is highly likely that the patient suffers from degenerative changes, mainly affecting the frontal and temporal lobes of the brain, a process that might represent Pick's disease. This study confirmed the relationship between bifrontal temporal episodes and the occurrence of brain stem changes. No bifrontal delta episodes occurred with a normal brain stem.

EEG AND COGNITIVE IMPAIRMENT IN PRESENILE DEMENTIA

Patients with AD, Pick's disease, and cerebrovascular dementia as well as a variety of other types of presenile organic brain disease were studied by Johannesson and associates (21). Four out of seven of those with Pick's disease had a normal EEG, which distinguished them from those with AD who had a comparable psychometric defect. Those with AD were more likely to have a severe or moderate degree of EEG abnormality than were those with cerebrovascular disease. One consistent observation was made, that the more abnormal the EEG, the more pronounced the intellectual reduction.

THE PRESENILE DEMENTIAS

Although patients with Pick's disease frequently have relatively normal EEGs, patients with Creutzfeldt–Jakob disease are usually abnormal, often with periodic triphasic waves. Early in the disease process of Creutzfeldt–Jakob disease there is disorganization of the EEG with some focal abnormality. As the clinical course of the disease progresses, approximately 90% of patients show periodic records, often with triphasic waves (22). The triphasic waves, although prominent in Creutzfeldt–Jakob disease, are seen in other conditions, notably hepatic and other metabolic encephalopathies.

O'Connor and co-workers (23) maintain that the classifications and clinical description of brain disorders in the senium are unsatisfactory. Hence the differential diagnosis is far from accurate. Furthermore, conventional EEG investigation with visual analysis of the EEG records has not proven sufficiently reliable. This study described a pilot project to test the efficiency of a particular type of computerized EEG analysis in ameliorating this problem.

This approach utilized bipolar EEG recordings and analyzed power and coherence spectra based on 20-second epochs. The power spectrum refers to the amplitude of the EEG waves, while the coherence spectrum compares homologous regions of the hemispheres. Unfortunately, O'Connor and co-workers employed rather standard methods of differentiating their groups of patients into depression, arteriosclerosis, and senile dementia. Of the three groups studied, there were significant differences. The best discriminator between groups was EEG coherence estimates between right parietal and temporal derivation.

SUMMARY

So-called normal aging is accompanied by EEG changes that can be misinterpreted as evidence of brain disorder. Age changes occur both during the waking and sleeping EEG. When such so-called normal age changes become excessive, they are associated with pathology. Diffuse slow waves are usually associated with progressive degenerative dementias. However, the EEG in Pick's disease is likely to remain normal despite evidence of mental impairment, and easily recognized triphasic waves are likely to be found in Creutzfeldt–Jakob disease.

REFERENCES

1. Griner PF, Mayewski RS, Mushlin AL, et al: Selection and interpretation of diagnostic tests and procedures. *Ann Intern Med* 1981; 94:553–600.

2. Dutertre F: Catalogue of main EEG patterns, in Donday M, Gaches J (eds): *Handbook of Electroencephalography and Clinical Neurophysiology.* Amsterdam, Elsevier, 1974, pp 46–79.

3. Busse EW, Wang HS: The electroencephalographic changes in late life: a longitudinal study. *J Clin Exp Gerontol* 1979; 1:145–158.

4. Obrist WD, Busse EW: The electroencephalogram in old age, in Wilson WP (ed): *Applications of Electroencephalography in Psychiatry.* Durham, Duke University Press, 1965, pp 185–205.

5. Busse EW: Brain wave changes in later life. Clinical EEG 1973; 4:152–163.

6. Marsh G: Cognitive and physiological changes with aging, in Busse EW, Maddox GL (eds): *The Final Report, Duke Longitudinal Studies.* New York, Springer, to be published.

7. Busse EW: The aging central nervous system: electroencephalography (EEG), in Busse EW, Maddox GL (eds): *The Final Report, Duke Longitudinal Studies.* New York, Springer, to be published.

8. Obrist WD, Sokoloff L, Lassen NA, et al: Relationship of EEG to cerebral blood flow and metabolism in old age. *Electroencephalogr Clin Neurophysiol* 1963;15:610–619.

9. Wang HS, Busse EW: Correlates of regional blood flow in the elderly community resident, in Harper AM, Jennett WB, Miller JD, et al (eds): *Blood Flow and Metabolism in the Brain.* London, Churchill Livingstone, 1975, pp 8.17–18.

10. Obrist WD: Cerebral blood flow in EEG in normal aging and dementia. in Busse EW, Blazer DL (eds): *Handbook of Geriatric Psychiatry.* New York, Van Nostrand Reinhold, 1979, pp 83–101.

11. Müller HF, Grad B, Englesman F: Biological and psychological predictors of survival in a psychogeriatric population. *J Gerontol* 1975; 30:47–52.

12. Busse EW, Wang HS: Heart disease and brain impairment among aged persons, in Palmore E (ed): *Normal Aging.* Durham, Duke University Press, 1974, vol 2, pp 160–167.

13. Brannon LJ: *The Effect of Increased Alpha Production on the Psychological Functioning of the Elderly,* thesis. Pennsylvania State University, University Park, 1975.

14. Müller HF, Dastoor DP, Klingner A, et al: Amantadine in senile dementia: electroencephalographic and clinical effects. *J Am Geriatr Soc* 1979; 27:9–16,

15. Feinberg I: Functional implications of changes in sleep physiology with age. *Aging NY* 1976; 3:23–41.

16. Prinz PN, Marsh GR, Thompson LW: Normal human aging: relationship of sleep variables to longitudinal changes in intellectual function. *Gerontologist* 1974; 14(5,pt2):41.

17. Feinberg I, Koresko RL, Heller N: EEG sleep patterns as a function of normal and pathological aging in man. *J Psychiatr Res* 1977; 5:107–144.

18. Harner RN (ed): *Guidelines in EEG.* Atlanta, American Electroencephalographic Society, 1980.

19. Müller HF, Schwartz G: Electroencephalograms and autopsy findings in geropsychiatry. *J Gerontol* 1978; 33:504–513.

20. Johannesson G, Brun A, Gustafson I, et al: EEG in presenile dementia related to cerebral blood flow and autopsy findings. *Acta Neurol Scand* 1977; 56:89–101.

21. Johannesson G, Hagberg B, Gustafson L, et al: EEG and cognitive impairment in presenile dementia. *Acta Neurol Scand* 1979; 59:225–240.

22. Lewis J, Burger A, Rowan J, et al: Creutzfeldt–Jakob disease: an electroencephalographic study. *Arch Neurol* 1978; 26:428–433.

23. O'Connor KP, Shaw JC, Ongley CO: The EEG and differential diagnosis in psychogeriatrics. *Br J Psychiatry* 1979; 125:156–162.

31 Average Evoked Potentials in Dementia

Julie V. Patterson
Henry J. Michalewski
Larry W. Thompson

WHILE AN APPRECIABLE PORTION of elderly persons with dementia may be suffering with a reversible disease process (1), the majority of dementing illnesses seen in the elderly are known to result in a progressive and irreversible deterioration of brain tissue. At the present time, virtually all treatments for conditions such as Alzheimer's disease (AD) are palliative in nature. The development of effective therapies has been hindered by an inability to detect the various dementias in their early stages. Early detection would allow potential treatments to be tested at a time when sufficient portions of the central nervous system are still intact and some difference in the clinical picture can be realized. Tests designed for early detection might also be useful for assessing the effect of new treatment therapies attempting to arrest the course of progressive atrophic brain changes.

Electrophysiological techniques such as the average evoked potential (EP) may prove to be helpful in the early detection of dementia, and it is surprising that so few standardized clinical procedures using these methods are currently in use. These techniques have extended our knowledge of brain and behavior relationships, and are gaining widespread clinical attention and support (2). For the full value of EP techniques to be realized, however, technical procedures must become standardized across laboratories, so normative data can be obtained from different age, sex, and diagnostic groups. Efforts to coordinate procedures in various clinical laboratories are currently in progress, and it is likely that normative data will be available in the near future. As these data become available, EP techniques may provide a unique contribution to the clinician's diagnostic armamentarium. Prior research has shown that the EP is exquisitely sensitive to both brain changes and varying levels of behavioral functioning. While specialized laboratory procedures such as computerized axial tomography (CT) and positron emission tomography (PET) provide information regarding structure and metabolism in discrete areas of the brain, EP procedures can provide complementary information regarding the functional integrity of an affected region. Furthermore, as clinical EP techniques become more systematized and routine, information relevant to the detection of early dementia can be obtained in a cost-effective manner.

One major problem in the early diagnosis of dementia in the elderly, where EP techniques may have immediate applicability, is in differentiating dementia from serious depressive illness. Currently administered diagnostic procedures yield a significant number of misclassifications (3–5). In many instances differentiation of functional from organic sources of mental status disorders can occur only upon repeated examination after a time interval, or after a trial of antidepressant medication (6, 7), neither of which is a satisfactory solution to the problem. Even with careful evaluations the misidentification of depressive illness as an organic disorder still occurs (4). The results of studies evaluating EPs in organically impaired persons suggest that even relatively straightforward normative studies may yield sensitive indicators of cerebral dysfunction. The development of such objective, nonintrusive tests, based on electrophysiological measures, could provide an important and economical adjunct to the procedures currently in use.

Scalp-recorded EPs are small-amplitude brain signals elicited by a stimulus or event. Signal averaging techniques have conventionally been used to extract the EP from the EEG. The resulting waveform consists of a series of positive and negative peaks; different but characteristic waveforms are described for auditory, visual, and somatosensory stimulation. Measures of the latency of the various peaks from stimulus onset (milliseconds), and amplitude measures such as peak-to-peak voltages (microvolts) typically are computed to quantify features of the EP waveform. Peaks are generally labeled according to polarity (positive, negative) and approximate latency (e.g., N100 or N1). The peaks or components of the average EP, which range from approximately 1 through 600 msec or more in latency, are thought to reflect neural activity from generators at progressively higher levels of the CNS, ranging from specific areas such as brain stem nuclei to diffuse nonspecific cortical centers.

Sensory stimulation can produce a complex but distinctive waveform. In the auditory EP, for instance, as many as 15 peaks may be recorded if the early, middle, and late components are identified (8). An idealized illustration of an auditory EP is shown in Figure 31–1. The morphology of the EP waveform is affected by the task requirements imposed by the experimental procedure. In passive situations, the stimulus is simply presented to the individual. In this case, stimulus-related or exogenous factors such as intensity and rate have a major influence on the recorded components, particularly in the early portions of the response. In contrast, prominent late components usually appear in the waveform in task situations which require the individual to make a decision about the stimulus. These emitted components are task-related or endogenous in nature, and are more dependent on the cognitive operations performed than on sensory modality or stimulus properties (9, 10). The distinction between stimulus-related and task-relevant EPs is not absolute and portions of the waveform may overlap the two categories. An intermediate class of components is influenced by attentional mechanisms as well as stimulus parameters. The vertex potential, or N1–P2, is in this category (10).

Conceivably, then, by using a combination of EP measures to gather information about the integrity of afferent systems as well as brain processes related to cognition and attention, a mapping of successive stages of mental function may be possible. In the following we will examine the way in which average EP techniques have already been used to assess sensory and mental status and the prospects for future application in the evaluation of dementia.

STIMULUS-EVOKED POTENTIALS

The EP responses described in this section typically have been recorded under passive experimental conditions during presentation of simple auditory, visual, or somatosensory

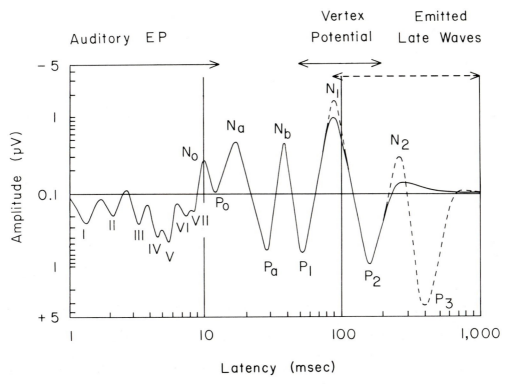

Figure 31–1. Idealized auditory evoked potential (EP) illustrating the various components that may be recorded from the scalp. *Adapted from Hillyard et al. (10) with permission.*

stimuli (e.g., click, flash, or stimulation of the ulnar nerve). While early portions of these waveforms are thought to be related to sensory aspects of the evoking stimulus, later components are considered to reflect more complex processing of incoming information (11). Some components following the early sensory portions of the response, for example, are influenced by factors such as attention and arousal level (12). Generally it has not always been possible to hypothesize which components might be affected in a particular case of degenerative disease or functional process, since the neural generators of portions of the EP are not known precisely (13). This is especially true in the study of phenomena that have diffuse origins such as might occur in dementia, as opposed to those that are localized within a particular cortical structure or neural pathway.

Because the stimulus-evoked potentials have a demonstrated sensitivity to the effects of aging, it is important to take into account these differences when evaluating EPs in organically impaired individuals. Briefly, EP components occurring after approximately 100 msec generally increase in latency and decrease in amplitude with age in both the visual and somatosensory modalities (14–21). Some earlier peaks for the visual EP display prolonged latencies and increased amplitudes with advanced age, whereas early somatosensory components have shown a less consistent trend (16, 17, 19, 21, 22). The auditory EP has not been subject to the same age-related changes extending from adolescence to senescence seen for the visual and somatosensory responses (23), although evidence for increased P1 amplitudes and prolonged P2 latencies with age has been suggested (24, 25). Age-related effects in the EP presumably are linked with possible structural alterations in the brain (26) and changes in perceptual or attentional mechanisms.

In the few studies that have tested organically impaired elderly patients, the comparison of EP findings among groups has been complicated by differences in methodology and recording procedures used by various laboratories. Despite the possible influence of confounding factors that might obscure group differences, several consistent patterns have nevertheless emerged. Individuals with dementing illnesses have consistently had longer latencies and, to a lesser extent, greater amplitudes in the later portions of both the auditory and visual evoked response. In a study of auditory evoked potentials (AEPs), for example, Hendrickson and associates (27) observed prolonged latencies for all but the first of six recorded components (approximately 35–350 msec) in dementia patients compared to controls; latencies of a depressed group were between those for the other two groups. Measures of cognitive function were found to be correlated with peak latency, particularly for the later components of the response. Similarly, in the visual evoked potential (VEP), Visser and co-workers (28) found prolonged latencies and increased amplitudes for several components beyond 100 msec in patients diagnosed as having presenile (Alzheimer-type) or senile dementia. Patient data were compared with a young group of controls, however, and possible differences due to age complicate a direct interpretation of the results. Straumanis and associates (22) noted that patients with organic brain syndrome had prolonged VEP latencies compared with older normals for three components occurring after 100 msec; in contrast, older and young normals differed primarily in the peaks prior to 100 msec. The baseline-to-peak amplitude of a peak appearing at approximately 50 msec was also larger in the patients. Straumanis and colleagues (22) view the early components as related to the transmission of information, whereas the later events are implicated in information processing; significant changes in later events are consistent, then, with the clouded sensorium and diminished cognitive capacity characteristic of dementia patients. Differences in the later components of the EP have also been reported in organic disorders which may present dementing symptoms, such as Down's syndrome (29) and Creutzfeldt–Jakob disease (30), suggesting that changes in EP responses may be similar among different etiologies of organic pathology.

Comparisons of early somatosensory evoked potentials (SEPs) in controls, depressed individuals, and dementia patients have not been conclusive. Levy and co-workers (31), for example, observed a tendency for five peaks measured within the first 100 msec to be longer in dementia than depression, but the differences were significant only for the third peak (39.4 versus 49.9 msec). A ratio measure of the amplitude of the fifth peak to the amplitude of the first peak was smaller in dementia patients. Hendrickson and associates (27), on the other hand, found no significant differences between control, depressed, or dementia cases in SEP responses. While scalp-recorded SEPs may be influenced by slowing at a number of levels between periphery and cortex, no differences in sensory nerve conduction velocity were found between dementia patients and a psychiatric group in a study by Levy (32). There is some dispute over the slowing of motor nerve conduction in dementia patients compared to controls (32, 33), possibly reflecting differences in patient etiology.

Observations of groups of patients with functional disorders have usually yielded a quite different pattern of EP responses than those found in organic syndromes. In psychotic depression, for example, decreased amplitudes for peaks occurring after approximately 100 msec have been reported for both the AEP and the SEP, when responses are compared with those for age-matched controls (34, 35). Similarly, in the visual modality, Perris (36) observed a negative relationship between severity of depression and VER amplitude; Vasconetto and co-workers (21) however, reported larger than normal amplitudes for certain VEP components in endogenous depression. Decreased P1, N1, and P2 latencies have also been found in psychotically depressed individuals (37). Responses for individuals with neurotic depression apparently do not differ from those for normals. While additional studies systematically comparing different diagnostic groups are needed, the findings for AEPs, VEPs, and to a lesser degree SEPs, indicate that even relatively simple EP procedures may be helpful in the differentiation of organic and functional disorders.

Brain Stem Auditory Evoked Response

A group of very early components commonly referred to as far-field potentials can be recorded to simple click stimuli (see Fig. 31–1). The brain stem auditory evoked response (BAER) consists of a group of seven submicrovolt peaks occurring within 10 msec of stimulus onset and conventionally labeled waves I through VII (38–40). Unlike the potentials discussed thus far, each component of the BAER has been associated with possible generators, especially waves I through V. These include the acoustic nerve (wave I); cochlear nuclei (wave II); superior olivary complex and fibers crossing the midline (wave III); lateral lemniscus (wave IV); inferior colliculus (wave V); possibly the medial geniculate (wave VI); and possibly thalamocortical auditory radiations (wave VII) (38, 41–47). In addition to the stability of peak latencies and the reproduceability of the BAER waveform, the presumed correlation of each peak with portions of the auditory pathway has given impetus to the application of the BAER in clinical settings. If, for instance, brain stem tumors or demyelinating diseases such as multiple sclerosis are present, abnormalities in the latencies and amplitudes of certain components may be found depending on the site of pathology (45–49). The overall ability of the BAER to detect brain stem pathology, and pathology within the vicinity of related structures, suggests that BAER procedures might be useful in uncovering changes associated with degenerative diseases.

Recent evidence from anatomical studies raises the possibility that areas of subcortical pathology in AD might be reflected in the BAER. Extensive loss of neurons in the locus ceruleus in individuals with AD has been reported by Bondareff and colleagues (50). Projections between the locus ceruleus and other brain stem regions such as the medial and lateral geniculate, inferior olive, and dorsal cochlear nucleus (51) suggest that abnormal BAERs might be hypothesized in Alzheimer patients. Inhibition of dorsal cochlear nucleus neurons by locus ceruleus stimulation has been reported in animals (52). Neurofibrillary tangles (NFTs) of the Alzheimer type can be found in certain brain stem areas in dementia patients (53, 54). Likewise, certain age-related neuronal and structural changes are also found in the brain stem (55–61). In addition to the function of the locus ceruleus, then, structural changes in other areas of the brain stem may affect the electrical potentials generated within ascending pathways and various nuclei of the auditory system.

At this writing only two studies have reported BAERs in Alzheimer patients. Harkins and Lenhardt (62) equated young normal, elderly normal, and Alzheimer patients on the basis of wave I latency, in an effort to focus on CNS pathology and minimize peripheral hearing losses. They found significantly prolonged wave V latencies and reduced wave V amplitudes in presumed Alzheimer patients compared with both normal groups. While the findings appeared promising, the authors cautioned that the effect of hearing losses on the BAER could not be eliminated. In a later report, increases in central transmission time (wave V latencies minus wave I latencies) and increased wave III latencies were also observed in Alzheimer patients (63). The successful application of the BAER in future studies of degenerative processes requires consideration of its sensitivity to intensity and rate (64, 65); sensorineural, conductive, and retrocochlear hearing disorders (66–68); and age and sex effects (62, 69–74).

Task-Related Potentials

The behavioral impairments accompanying extensive cortical pathology in AD make the late task-related components likely candidates for the differentiation of dementing processes. The P3 or P300 wave, for example, occurring with an approximate latency of 300 msec (300–600 msec), is one of the most prominent of the event-related potentials and has been studied extensively (for reviews see refs. 9, 10). The P3 wave, while difficult to characterize simply, is thought to represent a nonspecific act of decision (75) resulting from CNS functions involving stimulus selection and stimulus processing (9, 12, 76, 77). The latency of P3 seems to be correlated with the time required for stimulus evaluation and categorization. The amplitude of P3 waves is related to stimulus probability, but stimuli must be task relevant (9, 10). The P3 wave is broadly distributed over the scalp, appearing largest over central and parietal locations, and is independent of stimulus modality; precise neural generators of P3 in humans are not known (13), although efforts at localizing the origins of this late component are being attempted in animals (78). The N2 or N200 component, preceding P3, appears to be related to target selection and likelihood of stimulus occurrence, and can be elicited when stimuli are not directly attended by the subject (9).

A typical experimental procedure used to record the late components is the target detection or "oddball" paradigm. The task for the individual is to report an occasional, infrequent target stimulus (e.g., a high-frequency tone) which occurs randomly in a series of frequent, nontarget stimuli (e.g., low-frequency tones). The EPs to target (infrequent) and nontarget (frequent) stimuli are averaged separately. The P3 wave is elicited by the target or oddball stimulus. Since the task demands are not excessive in this paradigm, the possibility of using P3 as an index of mental function, particularly in dementia, has been tested now by several laboratories. As might be expected, some demented patients may have difficulty in performing the task and may respond incorrectly or not at all to the target stimuli. Because P3 has been shown as sensitive to factors of attention, perception, and memory processes, changes in P3 in demented patients may simply be the result of not understanding or forgetting the task. Task comprehension, however, is not viewed as a serious limitation of the test procedures. The large P3 wave seen to targets, compared with nontargets, argues for differential processing of the two types of stimuli (79).

Squires and his colleagues have used the target detection paradigm to evaluate changes in the AEP in patients with neurological and psychiatric disorders (79–81). A total of 151 patients, ranging in age from 19 to 80 years, have been tested and compared with data from normal controls (82). Patient diagnoses were based on clinical evaluation, neuropsychological testing, and scores of 25 or less (out of a possible 30) on the Mini-Mental State exam (MMS) of Folstein and associates (83).

The results for normal aging, analyzed using linear regression, indicated increased P3 latencies with age at a rate of 1.64 msec per year, as well as increased P2 (0.7 msec per year) and N2 (0.8 msec per year) latencies. Changes in the latency of N1 were not significant. Peak-to-peak amplitudes of N1–P2 and N2–P3 were found to decrease with age at a rate of 0.2 μV per year. While similar age-related effects for latency have been reported by other investigators, amplitude results have been less consistent (24, 84–87).

Dementia patients, psychiatric patients, and normals were differentiated most reliably by P3 latency. A summary table of diagnostic classification, number of patients, MMS score, and P3 latency deviation from normal in standard deviation (SD) units for each subgroup of dementia, psychiatric, and nondemented neurological patients is given in Figure 31–2. This figure also shows the P3 latencies for dementia patients, psychiatric patients, and nondemented neurological patients, referred to the regression line for normals. As indicated in Figure 31–2, P3 latencies for dementia patients were significantly longer than those for normals, by an average of 3.61 S.D. units. While P3 amplitude was significantly reduced in dementia patients compared to normals, the differences were less consistent and not as pronounced as for the P3 latency measure. No significant differences between dementia patients and normals were observed for N1 or P2 latencies or amplitudes. Nondemented

Figure 31–2. Diagnostic classification, number of patients (*N*), Mini-Mental State score (MMS), and P3 latency deviation from normal in standard deviation (S.D.) units for each subgroup of dementia, psychiatric, and nondemented neurological patients. Centered around the normal regression line are lines representing one and two standard deviations. *Adapted from Squires et al. (79). Copyright 1980 by the American Psychological Association. Adapted by permission of the publisher and author.*

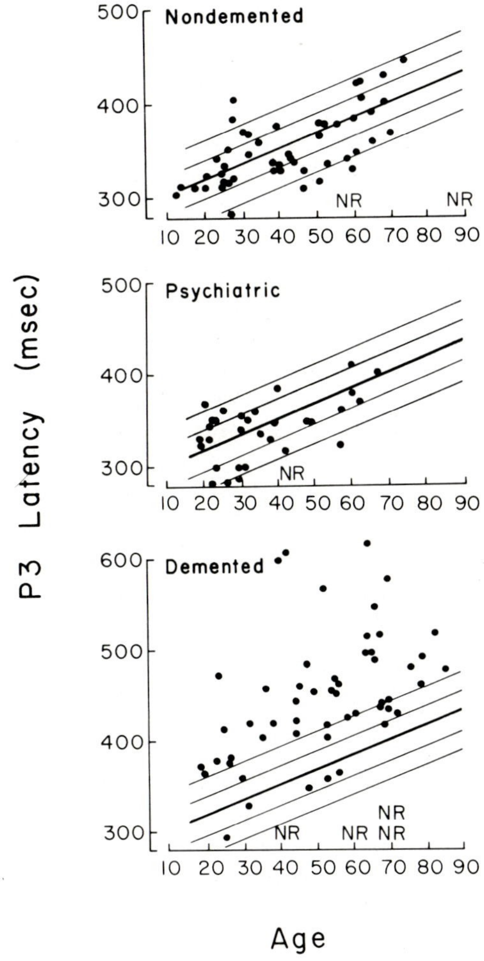

Patient Diagnosis	N	MMS	S.D.
Multiple sclerosis	6	29.5	−.42
Cerebrovascular disease	7	29.3	−.41
Parkinson's disease	5	29.0	.50
Hydrocephalus	5	29.0	.87
Brain tumor	8	29.7	−.52
Trauma	3	28.3	.41
Miscellaneous	17	28.3	.02
Mean	51	28.9	−.03
Depression	12	28.9	−.22
Manic-depression	6	29.0	.16
Acute schizophrenia	4	28.3	.23
Paranoid schizophrenia	11	28.4	−.30
Mean	33	28.7	−.18
Alzheimer-type dementia	13	17.6	2.79
Metabolic encephalopathy	11	16.7	4.09
Hydrocephalus	7	21.2	2.84
Cerebrovascular disease	8	21.3	4.98
Brain tumor	4	19.0	4.20
Multiple sclerosis	2	23.5	8.19
Herpes simplex encephalitis	1	20.0	−.29
Uncertain etiology	12	21.7	3.17
Mean	58	19.6	3.61

patients did not differ from normal individuals on any of the latency or amplitude measures. By using a P3 latency deviation of 2.0 S.D. units above normal as a cutoff for predicting dementia, 80% of the dementia patients were classified correctly; 3% of the psychiatric and 4% of the nondemented neurological patients were misclassified.

Prolonged P3 latencies in dementia patients have been reported in other investigations. Syndulko and colleagues (87) compared 12 dementia patients, ranging in age from 50 to 84 years, to 45 normals. A diagnosis of moderate progressive dementia of unknown etiology (presumed Alzheimer type) was used as the basis of patient selection, as well as MMS scores below 27. The results indicated that ten patients had abnormal P3 latencies (greater than 2.0 standard errors of the estimate [S.E.E.s] above the regression line at the appropriate age) at central and parietal electrode sites; at the frontal site, nine patients showed abnormal latencies. At the parietal derivation, the average deviation from the normal regression line was 3.0 S.E.E. units. The latencies of P2 were prolonged by 2.0 S.E.E.s in five of twelve patients at the parietal site; overall, however, P2 was judged not to add useful diagnostic information since the same patients showed abnormal P3 latencies. No abnormal N1 latencies were observed in the patient group.

Similarly, Brown and associates (85) reported delayed P3 latencies (greater than 2.0 S.D.s above the normal regression line) for seven out of ten diagnosed Alzheimer patients. Data on 15 normals, five multi-infarct dementia patients, three Parkinson's disease patients, and seven depressed individuals were also reported. Three of the multi-infarct cases and one parkinsonian patient had abnormal P3 latencies while none of the depressed patients were outside the normal range. Significant negative correlations were observed between P3 latency and MMS scores, several subtests of the WAIS, and tests of visual organization and retention. No significant correlations were observed between P3 latency and measures of depression.

Prolonged P3 latencies can occur in CNS disorders involving milder degrees of cognitive impairment. Hansch and co-workers (88) found that P3 latencies to target stimuli for 6 out of 20 parkinsonian patients were an average of 2.5 S.E.E.s from the age-matched normal regression line. However, the average deviation from normal for all parkinsonian patients was 1.1 S.E.E.s, yielding an abnormality rate of 30%. While the patients were not diagnosed as clinically demented, moderate degrees of cognitive deficit were indicated by some neuropsychological test scores. Clinical studies of dementia in selected parkinsonian patients have reported similar abnormality rates (89).

In our laboratory, we have examined VEPs in nine depressed patients (61–78 years, mean = 68.1), nine demented patients (57–86 years, mean = 71.6), and nine healthy community volunteers (60–74 years, mean = 68.0) using a visual target detection paradigm (90). Results for the depressed patients and controls have been reported in more detail previously (91). Mini-Mental State scores for the dementia group ranged from 14 to 23, with a mean of 19.3. Visual stimuli included (1) a frequent or background stimulus (the number 6); (2) a task-relevant or target stimulus (the number 9); and (3) novel stimuli consisting of several different randomly drawn patterns (92). Nine blocks of 40 stimuli, consisting of 10% 9's, 10% novel patterns, and 80% 6's, were presented in quasi-random order. The participants were instructed to watch a TV monitor and to press a button as soon as they saw a 9 (target) on the screen. Stimulus duration was 50 msec, with a variable interstimulus interval (minimum of 9 sec) controlled by the experimenter. The VEPs were obtained from midline frontal (Fz), central (Cz), and parietal (Pz) sites, referenced to linked earlobes. Additional electrodes were placed above and below the right eye to monitor ocular movements. Scalp electrical activity was recorded with Grass amplifiers (12-second time constant) and processed with a Nicolet Med-80 computer.

Peak latency from stimulus onset and baseline-to-peak amplitudes for components N2 and P3 to the targets and random stimuli were determined. Separate two-way analyses of variance (ANOVAs) (Group x Electrode) with repeated measures on the second factor were performed on the latencies and amplitudes for each component. Reaction times to targets were analyzed using a one-way between-groups ANOVA. *Post hoc* comparisons of the means were carried out using the Newman–Keuls procedure for multiple comparisons (93).

The group averages of the resulting VEP waveforms to the target stimuli are illustrated in Figure 31–3 for controls, depressed, and dementia patients. The results indicated that the target latencies for P3 were significantly prolonged in the dementia patients (mean = 513.2 msec) compared to controls (mean = 426.4 msec); the P3 latencies of the depressed individuals were between the latencies of the other two groups (mean = 451.2 msec). The same latency effect was observed for N2 (controls = 245.0 msec; depressed = 284.1 msec; and dementia patients = 311.6 msec). Reaction times were prolonged in the demented individ-

Figure 31–3. Group averages for visual evoked potentials (VEP) to targets (the number 9) for controls, depressed, and demented individuals.

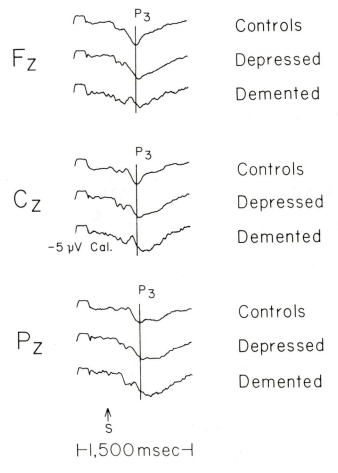

uals (1,427.9 msec) compared to both control (773.6 msec) and depressed (958.7 msec) subjects. The results for the random patterns indicated the N2 latencies were significantly longer in the dementia group (mean = 315.9 msec) than the control group (mean = 263.9 msec); the N2 latencies of the depressed group were between the latencies of the other two groups (mean = 288.2 msec). The P3 latencies for the random patterns were also longer in the dementia patients, but the differences among groups did not reach significance. Amplitude measures for N2 and P3 did not systematically differentiate the groups.

OVERVIEW

The use of EP techniques appears promising in assessing both sensory and cognitive function in dementing type processes. At the present time, the late components of the EP, particularly the P3 wave, seem to provide the most consistent discrimination of patient groups. Many of the studies considered so far have tested patients with presumed AD or dementia of unknown etiology, and the possibility of misdiagnosis cannot be overlooked. The association between EP measures and dementing processes would be strengthened in future studies that also provide histological and other laboratory support of the degenerative pathology involved. Future studies likewise are needed to systematically evaluate the practicality of using EP for differential diagnosis. While the late components appear to be abnormal in organic syndromes regardless of etiology, recent findings suggest that EP methods may be sensitive in differentiating functional from organic syndromes. Additionally, the utility of EP in cases of pseudodementia and mild organic deficit demands further evaluation.

The adoption of the oddball paradigm has contributed significantly to testing a wide range of patient groups with varying intellectual capacities and may serve as a basis of standardization necessary for the collection of normative data. Additional refinements or modifications may, however, be necessary to extend its usefulness. For example, the use of stimuli that can arouse attention or produce orienting responses may add a dimension of meaningfulness to the task that cannot be duplicated with the simple laboratory clicks or tones currently used. The practical value of EP procedures may also be enhanced by the application of specialized neurometric analysis techniques such as those developed and employed by John and colleagues (94, 95). In these procedures, a number of EP measures are combined to optimally discriminate clinical from normal groups. The possibility that dementing illnesses may be reversed or arrested cannot be addressed seriously until techniques are developed for early detection. The role EP methods will play in dementia will be supported by evidence concerning the neural bases of these potentials and further understanding of the dementing process. While potential treatments for dementia await future research, a basic knowledge of the electrophysiological changes accompanying nervous system deterioration may serve to bring us closer to a solution for arresting these destructive effects by providing a relatively simple, noninvasive and objective method of determining functional status in the various stages of dementing illnesses.

REFERENCES

1. Butler RN: The role of NIA. *Aging NY* 1978; 7:5–9.
2. Starr A: Sensory evoked potentials in clinical disorders of the nervous system. *Annu Rev Neurosci* 1978; 1:103–127.

3. Raskin A: Signs and symptoms of psychopathology in the elderly, in Raskin A, Jarvik LF (eds): *Psychiatric Symptoms and Cognitive Loss in the Elderly.* New York, Halstead, 1979, pp 3–18.

4. Roth M: Senile dementia and its borderlands, in Cole JO, Barrett JE (eds): *Psychopathology in the Aged.* New York, Raven, 1980, pp 205–232.

5. Wells CE: Chronic brain disease: an overview. *Am J Psychiatry* 1978; 135:1–12.

6. Crook TH: Psychometric assessment in the elderly, in Raskin A, Jarvik LF (eds): *Psychiatric Symptoms and Cognitive Loss in the Elderly.* New York, Halstead, 1979, pp 207–220.

7. Salzman C, Shader RI: Clinical evaluation of depression in the elderly, in Raskin A, Jarvik LF (eds): *Psychiatric Symptoms and Cognitive Loss in the Elderly.* New York, Halstead, 1979, pp 39–72.

8. Picton TW, Hillyard SA, Krausz HI, et al: Human auditory evoked potentials: I. Evaluation of components. *Electroencephalogr Clin Neurophysiol* 1974; 36:179–190.

9. Donchin E, Ritter W, McCallum WC: Cognitive psychophysiology: the endogenous components of the ERP, in Callaway E, Teuting P, Koslow SH (eds): *Event-Related Brain Potentials in Man.* New York, Academic, 1978, pp 349–441.

10. Hillyard SH, Picton TW, Regan D: Sensation perception, and attention: analysis using ERPs, in Callaway E, Teuting P, Koslow SH (eds): *Event-Related Brain Potentials in Man.* New York, Academic, 1978, pp 223–347.

11. Marsh GR, Thompson LW: Psychophysiology of aging, in Birren JE, Schaie KW (eds): *Handbook of the Psychology of Aging.* New York, Van Nostrand Reinhold, 1977, pp 219–248.

12. Picton TW, Hillyard SA: Human auditory evoked potentials: II. Effects of attention. *Electroencephalogr Clin Neurophysiol* 1974; 36:191–199.

13. Goff WR, Allison T, Vaughan HG Jr: The functional neuroanatomy of event-related potentials, in Callaway E, Teuting P, Koslow SH (eds): *Event-Related Brain Potentials in Man.* New York, Academic, 1978, pp 1–91.

14. Buchsbaum MS, Henkin RI, Christiansen RL: Age and sex differences in averaged evoked responses in a normal population, with observations of patients with gonadal dysgenesis. *Electroencephalogr Clin Neurophysiol* 1974; 37:137–144.

15. Celesia GG, Daly RF: Effects of aging on visual evoked responses. *Arch Neurol* 1977; 34:403–407.

16. Dustman RE, Beck EC: Visually evoked potentials: changes with age. *Science* 1966; 151:1013–1015.

17. Dustman RE, Beck EC: The effects of maturation and aging on the wave form of visually evoked potentials. *Electroencephalogr Clin Neurophysiol* 1969; 26:2–11.

18. Luders H: The effects of aging on the wave form of the somatosensory cortical evoked potential. *Electroencephalogr Clin Neurophysiol* 1970; 29:450–460.

19. Schenkenberg T: *Visual, Auditory, and Somatosensory Evoked Responses of Normal Subjects from Childhood to Senescence,* thesis. Salt Lake City, University of Utah, 1970.

20. Shagass C, Schwartz M: Age, personality, and somatosensory cerebral evoked responses. *Science* 1965; 148:1359–1361.

21. Vasconetto C, Floris V, Morocutti C: Visual evoked responses in normal and psychiatric subjects. *Electroencephalogr Clin Neurophysiol* 1971; 31:77–83.

22. Straumanis JJ, Shagass C, Schwartz M: Visually evoked cerebral response changes associated with chronic brain syndromes and aging. *J Gerontol* 1965; 20:498–506.

23. Beck EC, Dustman RE, Schenkenberg T: Life span changes in the electrical activity of the human brain as reflected in the cerebral evoked response, in Ordy JM, Brizzee KR (eds): *Neurobiology of Aging.* New York, Plenum, 1975, pp 175–192.

24. Brent GA, Smith DB, Michalewski HJ, et al: Differences in the evoked potential in young and old subjects during habituation and dishabituation procedures. *Psychophysiology* 1976; 14:96–97.

25. Pfefferbaum A, Ford JM, Roth WT, et al: Event-related potential changes in healthy aged females. *Electroencephalogr Clin Neurophysiol* 1979; 46:81–86.

26. Scheibel ME, Scheibel AB: Structural changes in the aging brain. *Aging NY* 1975; 11–37.

27. Hendrickson E, Levy R, Post F: Averaged evoked responses in relation to cognitive and affective state of elderly psychiatric patients. *Br J Psychiatry* 1979; 134:494–501.

28. Visser SL, Stam FC, Van Tilburg W, et al: Visual evoked responses in senile and presenile dementia. *Electroencephalogr Clin Neurophysiol* 1976; 40:385–392.

29. Dustman RE, Callner DA: Cortical evoked responses and response decrement in nonretarded and Down's syndrome individuals. *Am J Ment Defic* 1979; 83:391–397.

30. Lee RG, Blair RDG: Evolution of EEG and visual evoked response changes in Jakob-Creutzfeldt disease. *Electroencephalogr Clin Neurophysiol* 1973; 35:133–142.

31. Levy R, Isaacs A, Behrman J: Neurophysiology correlates of senile dementia: II. The somatosensory evoked response. *Psychol Med* 1971; 1:159–165.

32. Levy R, Isaacs A, Hawks G: Neurophysiology correlates of senile dementia: I. Motor and sensory nerve conduction velocity. *Psychol Med* 1970; 1:40–47.

33. Christie JE: Neurophysiology of dementia, in Glen AIM, Whalley LJ (eds): *Alzheimer's Disease: Early Recognition of Potentially Reversible Deficits.* New York, Churchill Livingstone, 1979, pp 90–92.

34. Shagass C, Ornitz EM, Sutton S, et al: Event-related potentials and psychopathology, in Callaway E, Teuting P, Koslow SH (eds): *Event-Related Brain Potentials in Man.* New York, Academic, 1978, pp 443–509.

35. Shagass C, Roemer RA, Straumanis JJ, et al: Evoked potential correlates of psychosis. *Biol Psychiatry* 1978; 13:163–184.

36. Perris C: EEG techniques in the measurement of the severity of depressive syndromes. *Neuropsychobiology* 1975; 1:16–25.

37. Buchsbaum M, Landau S, Murphy D, et al: Average evoked response in bipolar and unipolar affective disorders: relationship to sex, age of onset, and monoamine oxidase. *Biol Psychiatry* 1973; 7:199–212.

38. Jewett DL: Volume-conducted potentials in response to auditory stimuli as detected by averaging in the cat. *Electroencephalogr Clin Neurophysiol* 1970; 28:609–618.

39. Jewett DL, Romano MN, Williston JS: Human auditory evoked potentials: possible brainstem components detected on the scalp. *Science* 1970; 167:1517–1518.

40. Jewett DL, Williston JS: Auditory evoked far-fields averaged from the scalp of humans. *Brain* 1971; 94:681–696.

41. Buchwald JS, Brown KA: The role of acoustic inflow in the development of adaptive behavior. *Ann NY Acad Sci* 1977; 290:280–283.

42. Buchwald JS, Huang CM: Far-field acoustic response: origins in the cat. *Science* 1975; 189:382–384.

43. Huang CM, Buchwald JS: Interpretation of the vertex short-latency acoustic response: a study of single neurons in the brain stem. *Brain Res* 1977; 137:291–303.

44. Schmer H, Feinmesser M: Cochlear action potentials recorded from the external ear in man. *Annal Otol Rhinol Laryngol* 1967; 76:427–435.

45. Starr A, Achor LJ: Auditory brain stem response in neurological disease. *Arch Neurol* 1975; 32:761–768.

46. Starr A, Hamilton AE: Correlation between confirmed sites of neurological lesions and abnormalities of far-field auditory brainstem responses. *Electroencephalogr Clin Neurophysiol* 1976; 41:595–608.

47. Stockard JJ, Rossiter VA: Clinical and pathological correlates of brain stem auditory response abnormalities. *Neurology* 1977; 27:316–325.

48. Robinson K, Rudge P: Abnormalities of the auditory evoked potentials in patients with multiple sclerosis. *Brain* 1977; 100:19–40.

49. Robinson K, Rudge P: The early components of the auditory evoked potentials in multiple sclerosis. *Prog Clin Neurophysiol* 1977; 2:38–67.

50. Bondareff W, Mountjoy CQ, Roth M: Selective loss of neurones of origin of adrenergic projection to cerebral cortex (nucleus locus coeruleus) in senile dementia. *Lancet* 1981; i:783–784.

51. Amaral DG, Sinnamon HM: The locus coeruleus: neurobiology of a central noradrenergic nucleus. *Prog Neurobiol* 1977; 9:147–196.

52. Chikamori Y, Sasa M, Fujimoto S, et al: Locus coeruleus–induced inhibition of dorsal cochlear nucleus neurons in comparison with lateral vestibular nucleus neurons. *Brain Res* 1980; 194:53–63.

53. Ishii T: Distribution of Alzheimer's neurofibrillary changes in the brain stem and hypothalamus of senile dementia. *Acta Neuropathol* 1966; 6:181–187.

54. Ishino H, Otsuki S: Frequency of Alzheimer's neurofibrillary tangles in the basal ganglia and brain-stem in Alzheimer's disease, senile dementia, and the aged. *Folia Psychiatr Neurol Jpn* 1975; 29:279–287.

55. Brody H: An examination of cerebral cortex and brainstem aging. *Aging NY* 1976; 3: 177–181.

56. Hansen CC, Reske-Nielsen E: Pathological studies in presbycusis. *Arch Otolaryngol* 1965; 82:115–132.

57. Kirikae I, Sato T, Shitara T: A study of hearing in advanced age. *Laryngoscope* 1964; 74:205–220.

58. Konigsmark BW, Murphy EA: Volume of the ventral cochlear nucleus in man: its relationship to neuronal population and age. *J Pathol Exp Neurol* 1972; 31:304–316.

59. Machado-Salas J, Scheibel ME, Scheibel AA: Neuronal changes in the aging mouse: spinal cord and lower brain stem. *Exp Neurol* 1977; 54:504–512.

60. Vijayashankar N, Brody H: Aging in the human brainstem: a study of the nucleus of the trochlear nerve. *Acta Anat* 1977; 99:169–172.

61. Vijayashankar N, Brody H. A quantitative study of the pigmented neurons in the nuclei locus coeruleus and subcoeruleus in man as related to aging. *J Neuropathol Exp Neurol* 1979; 38:490–497.

62. Harkins SW, Lenhardt M: Brainstem auditory evoked potentials in the elderly, in Poon LW (ed): *Aging in the 1980s: Psychological Issues.* Washington DC, American Psychological Association, 1980, pp 101–114.

63. Harkins SW: Effects of pre-senile dementia Alzheimer's type on brainstem transmission time. *Int J Neurosci* 1981; 15:165–170.

64. Don M, Allen AR, Starr A: Effect of click rate on the latency of auditory brain stem responses in humans. *Ann Otol Rhinol Laryngol* 1977; 86:186–195.

65. Pratt H, Sohmer H: Intensity and rate functions of cochlear and brainstem evoked responses to click stimuli in man. *Arch Otolaryngol* 1976; 212:85–92.

66. Coats AC, Martin JL: Human auditory nerve action potentials and brain stem evoked responses: effects of audiogram shape and lesion location. *Arch Otolaryngol* 1977; 103:605–622.

67. Galambos R, Hecox K: Clinical applications of the auditory brain stem response. *Otolaryngol Clin North Am* 1978; 11:709–722.

68. Galambos R, Hecox K: Clinical applications of the brain stem auditory evoked potentials. *Prog Clin Neurophysiol* 1977; 2:1–19.

69. Beagley HA, Sheldrake MB: Differences in brainstem response latency with age and sex. *Br J Audiol* 1978; 12:69–77.

70. Michalewski HJ, Thompson LW, Patterson JV, et al: Sex differences in the amplitudes and latencies of the human auditory brainstem potential. *Electroencephalogr Clin Neurophysiol* 1980; 48:351–356.

71. Patterson JV, Michalewski HJ, Thompson LW, et al: Age differences in brainstem auditory evoked response amplitudes and latencies. *Psychophysiology* 1981; 18:161.

72. Patterson JV, Michalewski HJ, Thompson LW, et al: Age and sex differences in the human auditory brainstem response. *J Gerontol* 1981; 36:455–462.

73. Rowe MJ: Normal variability of the brain stem auditory evoked response in young and old subjects. *Electroencephalogr Clin Neurophysiol* 1978; 44:459–470.

74. Stockard JJ, Stockard JE, Sharbrough FW: Nonpathologic factors influencing brainstem auditory evoked potentials. *Am J EEG Technologists* 1978; 18:177–209.

75. Smith DBD, Donchin E, Cohen L, et al: Auditory averaged evoked potentials in man during selective binaural listening. *Electroencephalogr Clin Neurophysiol* 1970; 28:146–152.

76. Hillyard SA, Picton TW: Event-related brain potentials and selective information processing in man. *Prog Clin Neurophysiol* 1979; 6:1–52.

77. Sutton S: P300—thirteen years later, in Begleiter H (ed): *Evoked Brain Potentials and Behavior.* New York, Plenum, 1979, pp 107–126.

78. Wilder M, Farley G, Starr A: Endogenous late positive component of the evoked potential in cats corresponding to P300 in humans. *Science* 1981; 211:605–607.

79. Squires KC, Chippendale TJ, Wrege KS, et al: Electrophysiological assessment of mental function in aging and dementia, in Poon LW (ed): *Aging in the 1980s: Psychological Issues.* Washington DC, American Psychological Association, 1980, pp 125–134.

80. Goodin DS, Squires KC, Henderson BH, et al: Age-related variations in evoked potentials to auditory stimuli in normal human subjects. *Electroencephalogr Clin Neurophysiol* 1978; 44:447–458.

81. Squires K, Goodin D, Starr A: Event related potentials in development, aging and dementia, in Lehmann D, Callaway E (eds): *Human Evoked Potentials.* New York, Plenum, 1979, pp 383–396.

82. Goodin DS, Squires KC, Starr A: Long latency event-related components of the auditory evoked potential in dementia. *Brain* 1978; 101:635–648.

83. Folstein MF, Folstein SE, McHugh PR: "Mini-mental state." *J Psychiatr Res* 1975; 12:189–198.

84. Beck EC, Swanson C, Dustman RE: Long latency components of the visually evoked potential in man: effects of aging. *Exp Aging Res* 1980; 6:523–545.

85. Brown WS, Marsh JT, LaRue A: Event-related potentials in psychiatry: differentiating depression and dementia in the elderly. *Bull Los Angeles Neurol Soc* 1982; 47:91–107.

86. Ford JM, Hink RF, Hopkins WF III, et al: Age effects on event-related potentials in a selective attention task. *J Gerontol* 1979; 34:388–395.

87. Syndulko K, Hansch EC, Cohen SN, et al: Long-latency event-related potentials in normal aging and dementia, in Courjon J, Mauguiere F, Revol M (eds): *Clinical Applications of Evoked Potentials in Neurology.* New York, Raven, 1982, pp 279–285.

88. Hansch EC, Syndulko K, Cohen SN, et al: Cognition in Parkinson disease: an event-related potential perspective. *Ann Neurol* 1982; 11:599–607.

89. Lieberman A, Dziatolowski M, Kupersmith M, et al: Dementia in Parkinson disease. *Ann Neurol* 1979; 6:355–359.

90. Dessonville C, Thompson LW, Michalewski HJ, et al: Visual event–related potentials in dementia and depression. In preparation.

91. Litzelman DK, Thompson LW, Michalewski HJ, et al: Visual event–related potentials and depression in the elderly. *Neurobiol Aging* 1980; 1:111–118.

92. Courchesne E, Hillyard SA, Gallambos R: Stimulus novelty, task relevance and the visual evoked potential in man. *Electroencephalogr Clin Neurophysiol* 1975; 39:131–143.

93. Winer BJ: *Statistical Principles in Experimental Design*. New York, McGraw-Hill, 1971.

94. John ER: Neutrometrics, in *Functional Neuroscience*. Hillsdale, Erlbaum, 1977, vol 2.

95. John ER, Karmel BZ, Corning WC, et al: Neurometrics. *Science* 1977; 196:1393–1410.

32 Neurometric Electroencephalographic Characteristics of Dementia

LESLIE PRICHEP

FRANCISCO GOMEZ MONT

E. ROY JOHN

STEVEN H. FERRIS

IN THE PAST, clinical applications of electrophysiological methods to the evaluation of cognitive impairment have been greatly limited by the necessity to extract features by visually inspecting the data. Thus, results have often been suggestive but inconclusive. With the advent of cost-effective and powerful minicomputers, many investigators have turned their attention to the problem of developing methods to extract, quantify, and analyze features of diagnostic utility from electrophysiological data (1–4).

This chapter will briefly describe the application of quantitative, neurometric evaluation of the electroencephalogram (EEG) to the study of cognitive impairment in elderly patients. Neurometrics (2, 3, 5–9) uses a computer-controlled data acquisition system that gathers reliable artifact-free EEG and evoked-potential data, from the 19 monopolar channels of the International 10/20 Electrode System (10), using a standardized set of conditions (neurometric test battery) which constitute challenges to a wide range of brain functions. Quantitative features of the electrophysiological activity are extracted and compared with norms. Differences between expected and observed values are described statistically in terms of the probability that any observed feature is abnormal.

Methods of cluster analysis (11) can utilize this information to classify individuals objectively independent of *a priori* categorizations. Other multivariate statistical techniques (factor analysis, discriminant analysis, multiple regression analysis) can also be used to identify neurometric profiles characteristic of certain types of patients or to see behavioral correlates of particular patterns of brain function.

The EEG can be fractionated into a frequency spectrum and recombined into four frequency bands: delta (1.5–3.5 c/s), theta (3.5–7.5 c/s), alpha (7.5–12.5 c/s), and beta (12.5–25.0 c/s). The percentage of the total power which is in each frequency band (relative power) is calculated for frontotemporal (F3T3, F4T4), temporal (T3T5, T4T6), central (C3Cz, C4Cz), and parieto-occipital (P3O1, P4O2) regions.

Relative power is used because we have found it to be more reliable than absolute power (9). Careful study of the distribution of relative power in EEG samples recorded from healthy normal subjects across a wide age range revealed systematic changes with age (12) which could be described by simple mathematical rules (5, 13). Using these rules, called "age regression equations," the relative power in each frequency band of every major cortical region can be accurately predicted for a healthy person of any age. Neurometrics uses "Z-transformations" to express statistically the degree of departure from expected normal values for relative power in delta, theta, alpha, and beta frequency bands in each region. Such Z-transformations compare the obtained value for an individual with the predicted normal value for his age and express the degree of departure from normal in terms of probability. A Z-value of 1.00 indicates that the subject is 1 standard deviation (S.D.) above the mean for the corresponding location and wave type. Sixty-eight percent of normal subjects fall within the mean plus or minus 1 S.D., and 95% of normal subjects fall within 2 S.D. of the mean. A Z-value of 0.00 indicates that a particular subject lies precisely at the mean for his age group on that measure. Among other advantages, data represented in this way provide a convenient method to compensate for age differences between two populations.

The neurometric data presented in this chapter are only a portion of the data extracted from two minutes of eyes-closed EEG collected from "normally functioning" adults and cognitively impaired elderly patients (1). Normally functioning healthy adults between the ages of 17 and 90 served as controls. To be eligible for testing there had to be evidence of current self-support/functioning in job/household-related activities, no history of head injury with loss of consciousness, no prior EEG or neurological exam (or known neurological disease), and no subjective complaints about cognitive function. Whenever possible, IQ estimates were obtained. For those patients above the age of 55, all test measures described below for impaired elderly subjects had to be within normal limits.

All subjects selected as impaired patients were at least 55 years old, with a diagnosis of senile dementia, secondary to either Alzheimer's disease (AD), multi-infarct dementia (MID), or mixed AD and MID. The diagnosis was based on clinical history, psychiatric and medical-neurological examinations, and psychological test performance. All impaired subjects had to have a measurable cognitive decline indicated by significantly below-average performance for age and WAIS vocabulary level on the Guild Memory Scale (14).

In addition, all subjects (normal and impaired) had to have discontinued all psychotropic and/or cognitively active medication at least two weeks prior to participation in the study. Finally, a past history of head trauma, brain damage, seizures, mental retardation, or serious neurological disorder; focal signs of significant neuropathology (unless secondary to MID); a significant history of alcoholism; a previous history of schizophrenia, mania, or depression; or severe cardiac, pulmonary, vascular, metabolic, or hematologic conditions were additional bases for exclusion from the present study.

Senile dementia patients can be divided into two main populations according to their neurometric EEG data: those who have generalized slow waves (1.5–7.5 c/sec) and those with normal neurometric EEG profiles.

Table 32–1 presents the means and standard deviations of 32 neurometric EEG frequency variables (4 bands × 8 regions) in both a control and a senile dementia population. Slow waves are increased while alpha and beta waves are decreased in the senile dementia population. The mild cognitively impaired have a pattern similar to the normal pattern, except for a relative deficit of beta. This characteristic increase in slow waves in senile dementia has been widely reported (2, 3, 15); the variance is also increased. If senile dementia were a homogeneous diagnostic category from the point of view of the EEG, we would expect the standard deviations to be smaller in this group than in the control population.

TABLE 32–1

Mean Z-Value and Standard Deviation (in Parentheses) for Each Band in Each Region for "Normal" Control, Mild Cognitive Impairment (GDS = 2), and Senile Dementia Groups (GDS ≥ 3)

	Control		Mild Cognitive Impairment		Senile Dementia	
	Left	*Right*	*Left*	*Right*	*Left*	*Right*
CΔ	0.11(1.0)	0.10(1.0)	0.26(1.3)	0.07(1.2)	0.80(1.3)	0.71(1.2)
TΔ	0.03(1.0)	0.05(1.0)	−0.01(1.2)	−0.11(1.1)	0.81(1.5)	0.66(1.2)
POΔ	0.09(1.1)	0.04(1.1)	0.28(1.3)	0.04(1.2)	0.81(1.2)	0.75(1.3)
FTΔ	0.01(1.1)	0.00(1.0)	0.08(1.2)	−0.20(1.1)	0.74(1.5)	0.42(1.3)
Cθ	0.20(1.0)	0.06(1.0)	0.07(1.4)	0.05(1.4)	1.07(1.3)	1.11(1.3)
Tθ	−0.06(1.0)	−0.05(1.0)	0.27(1.4)	0.06(1.5)	1.27(1.6)	1.10(1.5)
POθ	−0.04(1.0)	−0.11(1.0)	0.03(1.2)	−0.14(1.2)	0.96(1.3)	0.87(1.2)
FTθ	−0.05(1.1)	0.00(1.0)	0.25(1.6)	0.25(1.7)	1.30(1.6)	1.37(1.7)
Cα	0.01(1.1)	0.02(1.0)	0.24(1.4)	0.22(1.4)	0.01(1.2)	0.03(1.2)
Tα	0.02(1.0)	0.03(1.0)	0.22(1.4)	0.08(1.3)	−0.29(1.1)	−0.48(1.1)
POα	0.03(1.1)	−0.03(1.1)	0.20(1.3)	0.06(1.2)	−0.05(1.1)	−0.26(1.2)
FTα	0.02(1.1)	0.09(1.1)	0.36(1.3)	0.27(1.3)	0.13(1.1)	−0.18(1.3)
Cβ	−0.07(1.0)	−0.10(1.0)	−0.61(1.6)	−0.48(1.7)	−1.14(1.2)	−1.21(1.4)
Tβ	−0.02(1.1)	−0.04(1.1)	−0.72(1.7)	−0.42(1.7)	−1.08(1.6)	−0.62(1.5)
POβ	−0.08(1.1)	0.06(1.1)	−0.65(1.5)	−0.28(1.5)	−1.25(1.2)	−0.99(1.1)
FTβ	−0.02(1.1)	−0.09(1.1)	−0.61(1.6)	−0.53(1.8)	−1.11(1.5)	−0.95(1.8)

Key: C = central, T = temporal, PO = parieto-occipital, FT = frontotemporal.

TABLE 32–2

Interhemispheric Coherence in Control and Senile Dementia Patients

	Controls (N = 57)	Seniles (N = 64)
CΔ	−0.042	−0.317
Cθ	−0.204	−0.294
Cα	0.007	−0.105
Cβ	0.163	0.378
TΔ	−0.116	−0.487
Tθ	0.074	−0.024
Tα	−0.344	−0.917
Tβ	−0.177	−0.550
POΔ	−0.315	−0.648
POθ	−0.229	−0.352
POα	−0.361	−1.135
POβ	−0.385	−1.446
FTΔ	0.006	−0.721
FTθ	0.181	−0.263
FTα	−0.130	−0.622
FTβ	0.064	−0.319

Key: C = central, T = temporal, PO = parieto-occipital, FT = frontotemporal.

TABLE 32–3

A. Mean Values of the 32 EEG Variables for Each Cluster

	A $N = 44$	B $N = 34$	C $N = 56$	D $N = 31$
LCΔ	−0.56	0.00	0.88	1.00
RCΔ	−0.42	−0.10	0.83	0.63
LTΔ	−0.70	−0.03	0.77	1.15
RTΔ	−0.65	0.09	0.75	0.82
LPOΔ	−0.70	0.29	0.84	0.97
RPOΔ	−0.78	0.24	0.70	0.92
LFTΔ	−0.43	−0.29	0.71	1.10
RFTΔ	−0.38	−0.36	0.64	0.67
LCθ	−0.61	−0.26	0.73	1.83
RCθ	−0.50	−0.26	0.78	1.72
LTθ	−0.50	−0.37	0.64	2.34
RTθ	−0.56	−0.29	0.67	2.20
LPOθ	−0.78	−0.10	0.59	1.65
RPOθ	−0.78	−0.14	0.45	1.46
LFTθ	−0.24	−0.61	0.61	2.45
RFTθ	−0.21	−0.65	0.88	2.55
LCα	1.20	−0.84	−0.21	0.52
RCα	1.14	−0.66	−0.35	0.72
LTα	1.14	−0.84	−0.24	−0.10
RTα	1.03	−0.90	−0.30	−0.17
LPOα	1.17	−0.86	−0.32	−0.00
RPOα	1.11	−0.82	−0.38	−0.25
LFTα	1.04	−0.73	−0.05	0.52
RFTα	1.01	−0.93	−0.05	0.45
LCβ	−0.53	0.89	−0.62	−2.24
RCβ	−0.64	0.84	−0.50	−2.24
LTβ	−0.91	1.08	−0.26	−2.27
RTβ	−0.90	1.19	−0.13	−1.81
LPOβ	−0.88	1.06	−0.25	−2.10
RPOβ	−0.81	1.14	−0.04	−1.76
LFTβ	−0.63	0.88	−0.42	−2.09
RFTβ	−0.72	1.21	−0.56	−2.20

B. Percentage of Each Group Classified in Each Cluster

	A $N = 44$	B $N = 34$	C $N = 56$	D $N = 31$
% normal	27	22	40	0
% mild cognitively impaired	25	24	24	20
% with senile dementia	16	5	18	48

Key: C = central, T = temporal, PO = parieto-occipital, FT = frontotemporal, L = left, R = right.

TABLE 32–4
Predicted Cluster Membership

Actual Cluster	No. of Cases	Predicted Cluster (%)			
		A	B	C	D
A	44	93	5	2	0
B	34	0	100	0	0
C	55	4	0	93	4
D	31	3	0	7	90

Percent of cases correctly classified: 94%

Table 32–2 presents the mean Z-transformed values for interhemispheric coherence. This variable measures the similarity of brain wave patterns between symmetrically placed electrodes in each of the two cerebral hemispheres. In this table, we see evidence that senile dementia patients show a decrease in interhemispheric coherence.

The larger standard deviations of the senile dementia groups suggest the possibility of identifying senile dementia patient subgroups that share specific neurometric profiles. Table 32–3 presents four such neurometric EEG patterns, identified using empirical classification methods (cluster analysis). There is a high alpha pattern (A), a high beta pattern (B), and a high slow wave pattern (C). All three patterns can be seen in normal controls and in senile dementia patients. However, the fourth pattern (D) is seen only in senile dementia patients. It is characterized by an excess of delta and theta activity, and although both hemispheres are affected, the left hemisphere shows more abnormal values.

The lower section (B) of Table 32–3 presents the probability for each group of being classified into one of the four EEG clusters. As can be seen, 40% of the control subjects fall into cluster C, while 48% of moderate/severe senile dementia patients fall into cluster D. Mild cognitively impaired patients are evenly distributed in the four clusters.

A discriminant function analysis comparing these four clusters was computed. Of the cases, 94% were correctly classified by the analysis, confirming the separation between clusters (see Table 32–4).

The findings reported in this chapter give support for the utility of neurometric, computerized, quantitative EEG analyses and applications of empirical classification methods for the description of subgroups within diagnostic categories. Clusters of individuals with homogeneous neurometric profiles might be expected to be homogeneous in the neurophysiological mechanisms underlying their psychopathology as well as in prognosis and differential response to treatment. Clear subgroups were also identified within the normal control group, one of which resembles a "dementia profile" but with a lower level of severity. This profile may represent a premorbid state of dementia, and longitudinal follow-up of such subjects is urged. An expansion and more detailed description of these data is presented elsewhere (16).

ACKNOWLEDGMENTS

This work was supported in part by National Institute of Aging Grant #1RO1 MH 32577, "Neurometric Assessment of Mental Health in Aging."

REFERENCES

1. Dolce G, Kunkel H (eds): *CEAN: Computerized EEG Analysis.* Stuttgart, Fischer, 1975.
2. John ER: *Functional Neuroscience, vol. 2.* Hillsdale, NJ: Erlbaum, 1977.
3. John ER, Karmel BZ, Corning WC, et al: Neurometrics: numerical taxonomy identifies different profiles of brain functions within groups of behaviorally similar people. *Science* 1977; 196:1393–1410.
4. Kellaway P, Petersen I (eds): *Automation of Clinical Electroencephalography.* New York, Raven, 1973.
5. John ER, Ahn H, Prichep L, et al: Developmental equations for the electroencephalogram. *Science* 1980; 210:1255–1258.
6. Ahn H, Prichep L, John ER, et al: Developmental equations reflect brain dysfunctions. *Science* 1980; 210:1259–1262.
7. John ER, Prichep L, Ahn H, et al: Neurometric evaluation of cognitive dysfunctions and neurological disorders in children. *Prog Neurobiol* 1983; to be published.
8. Prichep L, John ER, Ahn H, et al: Neurometrics: quantitative evaluation of brain dysfunction in children, in Rutter M (ed): *Behavioral Syndromes of Brain Dysfunction in Childhood.* New York, Guilford, 1983, pp 213–238.
9. John ER, Fridman J, Prichep L, et al: Neurometric evaluation of brain electrical activity in children with learning disabilities, in Duffy F (ed): *Dyslexia: Current Status and Future Directions.* Boston, Little, Brown, 1983.
10. Jasper HH: The ten-twenty electrode system of the International Federation. *Electroencephalogr Clin Neurophysiol* 1958; 10:371–375.
11. Dixon WJ, Brown MB: *Biomedical Computer Programs, P Series.* Berkeley, University of California Press, 1979.
12. Matousek M, Petersen I: Frequency analysis of the EEG in normal children and adolescents, In Kellaway P, Petersen I (eds): *Automation of Clinical Electroencephalography.* New York, Raven, pp 75–102.
13. Prichep L, Fridman J, John ER: EEG equations for normal adults. Submitted to *Science,* 1983.
14. Reisberg B, Ferris S, de Leon M, et al: Global deterioration scale for assessment of primary degenerative dementia. *Am J Psychiatry* 1982; 139:1136–1139.
15. Sheridan FP, Yeager GL, Oliver WA, et al: EEG as a diagnostic and prognostic aid in studying the senescent individual: preliminary report. *Gerontol* 1955; 10:53–59.
16. Prichep L, Gomez Mont F, John ER, et al: Neurometric multivariate studies in psychiatric disorders: electroencephalographic characteristics of cognitive impairment and senile dementia. Submitted for publication, 1983.

33 Computed Tomography Studies of Alzheimer's Dementia

MONY J. DE LEON

AJAX E. GEORGE

SUPERIMPOSED UPON THE AGING BRAIN in as many as 10% of the elderly are pathological brain changes which cause dementia (1). While for many years vascular pathologies were considered the principal cause of the gradual dissolution of personality, and cognitive capacity characteristic of the late life dementias, it is now generally recognized (2) that the most common cause is Alzheimer's disease (AD).

PATHOLOGICAL STUDIES OF AD

Histopathological studies have revealed the diagnostic features of AD. Senile plaques (SPs), neurofibrillary tangles (NFTs), and granulovacuolar degenerations (GVDs) are more likely to be found in the brains of AD patients than in the brains of age-matched cognitively normal controls. Correlation between quantitated measures of these pathologic features and measures of cognitive impairment have been reported (3–5). Regionally, these pathologic changes are most likely to be found in the middle and superior temporal gyri and in the hippocampus (6).

Investigations of neurons, although often contradictory, have recently revealed losses in frontal and temporal lobes (2, 2a). Whitehouse and associates (7) reported that the nucleus basalis of Meynert may be involved in AD. This nucleus, located in the basal forebrain, is believed to be a principal extrinsic cholinergic source for the cortex. Its degeneration may account for the AD cholinergic deficit (8) and associated intellectual changes.

Gross pathological evaluations of the AD patient have revealed shrinkage of the cerebral convolutions with widening of the cortical sulci and ventricular dilatation (9, 10). Gross pathological investigations of old normals reveal similar but less extensive changes. According to Tomlinson (6), the most prominent macroscopic changes in AD are found in the frontal and temporal lobes. It is unclear to what extent these regional gross pathologic changes are of diagnostic value.

COMPUTED TOMOGRAPHY OF THE BRAIN

In vivo examinations of morphological brain changes in aging and in AD have to date greatly relied on radiologic measures. The current clinical use of computed tomography

258

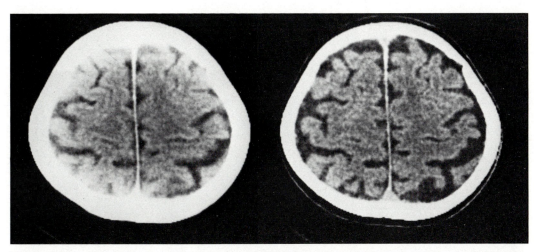

Figure 33–1. Representative CT scan of an AD patient at the high-convexity level of the brain using 1 mm × 1 mm × 10 mm resolution (*left*) and 1 mm × 1 mm × 1.5 mm (*right*). The high resolution scan (*right*) clearly demonstrates the subarachnoid changes.

(CT) in the assessment of patients suspected of having AD is to exclude focal etiologies and to describe the extent of the diffuse brain changes. The structural neuropathologic changes diagnostic of the brain with AD are at a microscopic level beyond the spatial resolving power of CT. (The spatial resolution of most current CT scanners is approximately 1 mm × 1 mm × 10 mm, with some machines capable of increased resolution of 1 mm × 1 mm × 1.5 mm; see Fig. 33–1).

As the pathologic changes found in AD may also be found in the normal aging brain, it has been necessary to search for CT measures that demonstrate these differences. With computed tomography two principal gross pathologic variables have been studied: ventricular dilatation and cortical sulcal prominence. Changes in these brain structures are not unique to AD, and are believed to indirectly reflect changes in brain parenchyma. Both variables have been defined by various CT measurements of ventricular or subarachnoid cerebrospinal fluid (Fig. 33–2). Recent development of the CT scanner and attendant computer software have enabled the more direct investigation of brain parenchyma. As the pathologic data have indicated the regional degeneration of the brain in AD, whether regional parenchymal CT measures can disclose these changes is of interest. For CT, both gray and white matter regions can be visualized (Fig. 33–3), and the attenuation values of these regions can be readily quantitated through computer interactive displays. While this line of investigation is still in its infancy, some preliminary work suggests the potential usefulness of this approach.

CORTICAL ATROPHY AND VENTRICULAR DILATATION

THE NORMAL AGING BRAIN

There appears to be a consistent observation across several different methods of CT scan analysis that both ventricular size and cortical sulcal prominence increase over the lifespan (11–16). It appears that these age-related changes are found for both normal volunteer subjects and neurologic patients diagnosed as normal. For the latter group, this finding is

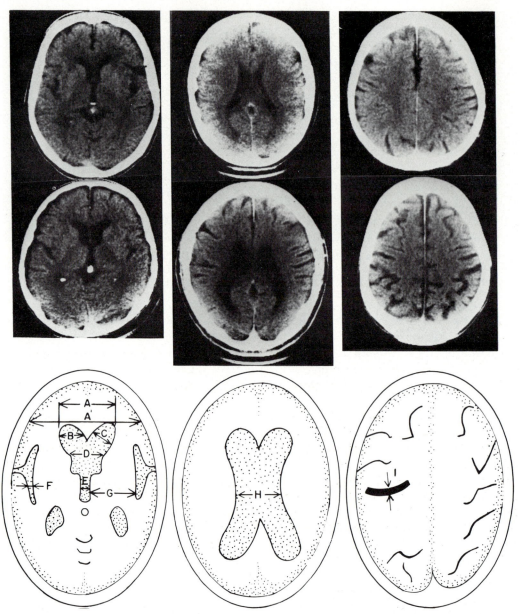

Figure 33–2. Representative CT slices for three levels of brain depicting, from left to right, two ventricular levels and the centrum semiovale level. CT scans on the top row show less atrophic changes than scans on the middle row. The schematics on the bottom row depict commonly used linear measurements.

less interesting, since one would expect an increase in intracranial disease (including the undiagnosed) with increasing age. Furthermore, the use of these neurologically normal patients as controls may inadvertently mask some of the earlier changes associated with AD. With respect to the complex phenomenon of aging, it is important that these age-related

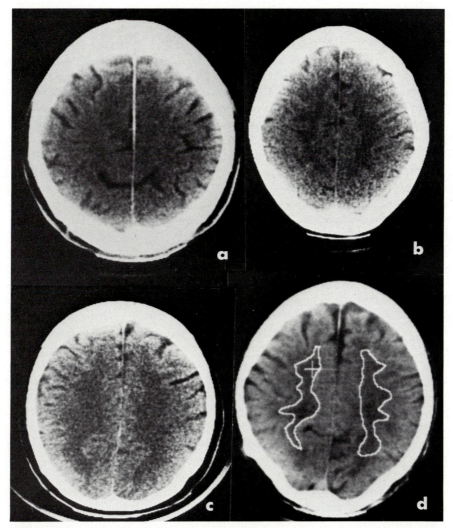

Figure 33–3. Representative CT scans (a–c) depicting gray matter–white matter discriminability at the centrum semiovale level. From left to right there is increasing discriminability (a = poor, b = fair, c = excellent) of the white matter against the background of the medial and lateral gray matter. Scan d depicts white matter regions of interest (ROI) drawn interactively with the computer. These particular ROI's were used to determine the CT attenuation of the white matter.

changes be described by multiple CT measures. However, the relative utility of any single measurement strategy has not been studied. Studies in this area have not attempted to challenge the popular belief that aging always diffusely affects the brain.

There is a trend in these reports to suggest that studies examining limited portions of lifespan (rather than the entire continuum) are less likely to reveal age-related brain changes (17, 18). It does, in fact, remain unclear from these data whether the reported age changes occur gradually throughout the lifespan or are more likely to occur in later years.

THE AD BRAIN

The use of CT in the study of ventricular and sulcal changes in AD has been, in part, disappointing. CT studies of these patients have not been able to establish diagnostic criteria. There have also been several studies which failed to establish how sensitive CT is to brain changes associated with AD. To some extent, this difficulty may be related to criteria used for subject selection. It appears that the studies reporting negative findings have used groups more heterogeneous with respect to age (19, 20) or diagnosis (21, 22) than those studies reporting positive findings.

These positive outcome studies have been able to demonstrate increased atrophy in dementia cases compared with controls and/or relationships between the extent of atrophic change and the extent of cognitive impairment (17, 23–29). For the most part, these studies have identified ventricular changes as more likely than sulcal changes to show relationships with the magnitude of dementia. It does appear, however, that both ventricular and sulcal changes do occur in AD (17, 25, 26).

Methodological constraints related to the CT scan evaluation have possibly prevented the more consistent demonstration of the atrophic changes in AD. In a methodological study, de Leon and associates (26) hypothesized that discouraging results in the search for brain–behavior relationships in AD had been due, at least in part, to coarse clinical rating scales that require judgments about normality in the absence of a normative data base, and the use of objective (linear) measures without known clinical significance or anatomic validation. This present study compared several procedures for evaluating the CT scan, concluding that there are both ventricular and sulcal changes in AD, and that the method used to assess the CT scan is an important determinant of the outcome in the exploration for brain–behavior linkages. De Leon and associates (26) demonstrated that, for the ventricular system, a rank ordering procedure was superior to the traditional clinical rating method and also superior to linear measurements. The rank ordering procedure requires the observer to evaluate each relevant CT slice. Each study is placed in a continuum of increasing pathology, ranging from the most normal, at one extreme, to the most abnormal at the other. Using the ranking method, the observer has the opportunity to compare each study with all other studies. To some extent, this procedure avoids the diagnostic issue of categorizing the normal and the abnormal. Rather, the observer has some flexibility in establishing criteria for estimating the size of complexly shaped structures. The rating procedure requires the observer to categorize the studies, one at a time, into several (usually four) groups. This coarse scaling often disregards fine structural changes, and is heavily dependent on observer experience and bias. New research has shown that the rank ordering procedure is significantly more reliable than the rating procedure when studied across different observers (26).

Cortical evaluations revealed that the subjective rank ordering and rating procedures were statistically equivalent, and that both were superior to the linear measurement technique. Overall, however, the linear measurements seemed to be of little value in this correlation analysis. Ventricular changes seemed more sensitive to the behavioral effects of AD than were cortical changes defined by sulcal prominence (26).

Of possible diagnostic relevance, de Leon and colleagues (26) reported that among linear ventricular measures, the width of the third ventricle was the best correlate of cognitive decline. In later studies of ventricular volume, George and associates (30) offered anatomic evidence validating the use of the third ventricle; the width of the third ventricle, as compared with several commonly reported brain ventricular measures, was the best linear correlate of ventricular volume. "Ventricular volume" is defined as the sum of the areas for all ventricular structures on all CT slices, multiplied by the slice thickness. de Leon and associates have also determined that the ventricular volume is significantly larger in dements as compared with age-matched controls (29) and is correlated with the magnitude of intellectual impairment.

The pathologic significance of dilatation of the third ventricle is not known. Hypothetically, such change may reflect structural changes in adjacent structures. One possibility is that such change reflects the destruction of the nucleus basalis of Meynert. Other indirect evidence comes from an attempt to combine the use of CT and PET. de Leon and associates (31) found significant structure–function relationships primarily when CT or structural measurements were made in the regions surrounding the third ventricle. In other words: the metabolic activity (PET) of frontal and temporal lobes and basal ganglia is consistently correlated with CT structural brain changes from the thalamic and posterior limbs of the internal capsule. Other CT regions more distant from the third ventricle do not show consistent correlation with the PET regions.

CT PARENCHYMAL EVALUATIONS IN AD

Improved scanner capacity to resolve structures spatially, to distinguish between low-contrast tissue, and to facilitate quantitative retrieval of aspects of the visual image have permitted the definition of new brain variables of potential significance.

Naeser and associates (32) reported that the average of CT numbers derived from a sampled region of the centrum semiovale level of the brain was significantly lower in dementia patients than in controls. These investigators studied 14 presenile dementia cases and 6 control patients who had been deemed neurologically normal.

George and associates (28) examined 26 presumed AD outpatients aged 60–84 years, subjectively evaluating the extent to which the gray and white matter could be differentiated. The subjective ratings of the CT scans indicated that the loss of discriminability of the gray and white matter was significantly associated with increasing cognitive impairment. In other words, the visual appearance of the gray and white matter was found to be more homogeneous with increasing cognitive impairment.

De Leon (33) also reported on regional evaluation of subarachnoid cerebrospinal fluid (CSF) distributions. This study examined the basal ganglia level of the brains of 22 AD patients with an average age of 72.1 years. Using the CT computer interactively, estimates were made of the total subarachnoid CSF in frontal, temporal, and parieto-occipital regions, both left and right. For this group of AD patients, it was found that only the measured CSF in the temporal lobes was significantly correlated with the memory tests each patient received. The frontal and posterior regional CSF measures did not show correlation with the magnitude of the memory deficit in AD.

Recently, de Leon and colleagues (34) studied 24 presumed AD outpatients aged 63–81 years. CT attenuation values were derived from gray and white matter regions for four brain levels. The results summarized across all the sampled brain regions indicated that there were consistently significant brain–behavior relationships, especially at the basal ganglia level of the brain. Basal ganglia level was defined as a cut parallel to the canthomeatal line and passing through the pineal. For higher (more dorsal) levels (i.e., centrum semiovale low, centrum semiovale high, and high convexities), the consistency of this effect decreased. The best correlation with a mental status measure was achieved between the attenuation change in both right and left thalamus.

Interestingly, at high convexities the density measures were most consistently correlated with age, which age correlation decreased as one sampled lower (more ventral) brain levels. While these data suggest there may be brain regions more likely to show the effects of age, and other regions more likely to show disease-related changes, care must be taken with these preliminary findings. Foremost, one must assess the effects of the skull on the CT attenuation values derived for the brain. The higher cuts are more influenced by this factor (possibly age-dependent) and the consequence may be to mask disease-related changes also occurring at these brain levels.

CONCLUSION

Traditionally studied measures of ventricular size and cortical sulcal prominence have consistently demonstrated increases in size over the lifespan in normal subjects. In the CT study of dementia and AD in particular, the earlier literature has been somewhat contradictory. More recent evidence suggests that there are ventricular and sulcal changes superimposed on the age-related changes, these disease-related changes being also associated with the magnitude of the cognitive deficit. It appears that the ventricular changes with AD are more salient than are the cortical changes.

Of additional interest are the studies of the third ventricle. There is evidence that this structure is a useful brain correlate of cognitive decline: it may be the best linear ventricular correlate of ventricular volume, and it does not appear to show consistent age-related enlargements (13, 26, 35). It remains unclear why this structure should be such a good indicator of the effects of AD.

Although there are few papers that have reported the use of CT attenuation numbers in the evaluation of brain parenchyma in AD, this line of investigation appears promising. In particular, this type of study will enable the regional analysis of parenchymal changes in AD; such analyses will be of interest given the recent pathologic data suggesting regional changes. In particular, subjective evaluations of parenchyma reveal changes in the relationship between gray and white matter in this disease process. Quantitative regional evaluations of parenchyma at cortical levels are less revealing of pathology than measures taken at ventricular levels, particularly in the region of the third ventricle (thalamus). Interestingly, early reports are that temporal lobe CSF changes show relationships with memory test performances, but that other regions may not. Such evidence argues against the simple diffuse change hypothesis, while regional analyses may offer clues to the progression of AD, and also possibly to recognizing undifferentiated subtypes of presumed AD patients.

REFERENCES

1. Kay DWK: Epidemiological aspects of organic brain disease in the aged, in Gaitz CM (ed): *Aging and the Brain.* New York, Plenum, 1972, pp 15–27.
2. Terry RD: Aging, senile dementia, and Alzheimer's disease. *Aging NY* 1978; 7:11–14.
2a. Terry RD, Peck A, de Teresa R, et al: Some morphometric aspects of the brain in senile dementia of the Alzheimer's type. *Ann Neurol* 1981; 10:184–192.
3. Blessed WF, Tomlinson BE, Roth M: The association between quantitative measures of dementia and of senile change in the cerebral grey matter of elderly subjects. *Br J Psychiatry* 1968; 114:797–811.

4. Farmer PM, Peck A, Terry RD: Correlations among numbers of neuritic plaques, neurofibrillary tangles, and the severity of senile dementia. Read before the 52nd Annual Meeting of the American Association of Neuropathologists, San Francisco, June 11–13, 1976.

5. Tomlinson BE, Kitchner D: Granulovacuolar degeneration of hippocampal pyramidal cells. *J Pathol* 1972; 106:165–185.

6. Tomlinson BE: The structural and quantitative aspects of the dementias, in Roberts PJ (ed): *Biochemistry of Dementia.* New York, Wiley, 1980, pp 15–52.

7. Whitehouse PJ, Price DL, Struble RG, et al: Alzheimer's disease and senile dementia: loss of neurons in the basal forebrain. *Science* 1982; 215:1237–1239.

8. Davies P, Maloney AJR: Selective loss of central cholinergic neurons in Alzheimer's disease. *Lancet* 1976; ii:1403.

9. Tomlinson BE, Blessed G, Roth M: Observations on the brains of demented old people. *J Neurol Sci* 1970; 11:205–242.

10. Corsellis JAN: Aging and the dementias, in Blackwood W, Corsellis JAN (eds): *Greenfield's Neuropathology, ed 3.* Chicago, Year Book, 1976, pp 796–848.

11. Barron SA, Jacobs L, Klinkel W: Changes in size of normal lateral ventricles during aging determined by computerized tomography. *Neurology* 1976; 26:1011–1013.

12. Glydensted C, Kosteljanetz M: Measurements of the normal ventricular system with computer tomography. *Neuroradiology* 1976; 10:205–215.

13. Haug G: Age and sex dependence of the size of normal ventricles on computed tomography. *Neuroradiology* 1977; 14:201–204.

14. Earnest MP, Heaton RK, Wilkinson WE, et al: Cortical atrophy, ventricular enlargement, and intellectual impairment in the aged. *Neurology* 1979; 29:1138–1143.

15. Yamamura H, Ito M, Kubota K, et al: Brain atrophy during aging: a quantitative study with computed tomography. *J Gerontol* 1980; 4:492–498.

16. Zatz LM, Jernigan TL, Ahumada AJ: Changes on computed cranial tomography with aging: intracranial fluid volume. *J Neuroradiol* 1982; 3:1–11.

17. Jacoby RJ, Levy R: Computed tomography in the elderly: II. Senile dementia: diagnosis and functional impairment. *Br J Psychiatry* 1980; 136:256–269.

18. Cala LA, Thickbroom GW, Black J, et al: Brain density and cerebrospinal fluid space size: CT of normal volunteers. *Am J Neuroradiol* 1981; 2:41–47.

19. Kazniak AW, Fox J, Gandell DL, et al: Predictions of mortality in presenile and senile dementia. *Ann Neurol* 1978; 3:246–252.

20. Brinkman SD, Sarwar M, Levin HS, et al: Quantitative indexes of computed tomography in dementia or normal aging. *Neuroradiology* 1981; 138:89–92.

21. Claveria LE, Moseley IF, Stevenson JF: The clinical significance of "cerebral atrophy" as shown by CAT, in DuBoulay GH, Moseley IF (eds): *The First European Seminar on Computerized Axial Tomography in Clinical Practice.* Berlin, Springer, 1977, pp 213–217.

22. Hughes CP, Gado M: Computed tomography and aging of the brain. *Radiology* 1981; 139:391–396.

23. Huckman MS, Fox J, Topel J: The validity of criteria for the evaluation of cerebral atrophy by computed tomography. *Radiology* 1975; 116:85–92.

24. Roberts MA, Caird FI, Grossart KW, et al: Computerized tomography in the diagnosis of cerebral atrophy. *J Neurol Neurosurg Psychiatry* 1976; 39:905–915.

25. de Leon MJ, Ferris SH, Blau I, et al: Correlations between CT changes and behavioral deficits in senile dementia. *Lancet* 1979; ii:859–860.

26. de Leon MJ, Ferris SH, George AE, et al: Computed tomography evaluations of brain–behavior relationships in senile dementia of the Alzheimer's type. *Neurobiol Aging* 1980; 1:69–79.

27. Mersky H, Ball MH, Blume WT, et al: Relationships between psychological measurements and cerebral organic changes in Alzheimer's disease. *Can J Neurol Sci* 1980; 7:45–49.

28. George AE, de Leon MJ, Ferris SH, et al: Parenchymal CT correlates of senile dementia (Alzheimer's disease): loss of grey-white matter discriminability. *Am J Neuroradiol* 1981; 2:205–211.

29. George AJ, de Leon MJ, Rosenbloom S, et al: The relationship of CT ventricular volume to cognitive deficit in senile dementia. *Radiology* 1983, to be published.

30. George AE, de Leon MJ, Rosenbloom S, et al: CT ventricular volume and its relationship to cognitive impairment in dementia. Read before the 11th Annual Meeting of the American Aging Association, New York, Sept 24–26, 1981.

31. de Leon MJ, George AE, Ferris SH, et al: Regional correlation of PET and CT in senile dementia of the Alzheimer type. *Am J Neuroradiol* 1983; 4:553–556.

32. Naeser MA, Gebhardt C, Levine HL: Decreased computerized tomography numbers in patients with presenile dementia. *Arch Neurol* 1980; 37:401–409.

33. de Leon MJ, George AE: Computed tomography in aging and senile dementia, in Mayeux A, Rosen W (eds): *Recent Advances in Neurology.* New York, Raven, 1983, pp 103–122.

34. de Leon MJ, George AE, Ferris SH, et al: Grey matter and white matter CT correlates in senile dementia of the Alzheimer's type. Read before the Tenth Aharon Katzir-Katchalsky Conference on the Aging of the Brain, Mantua, Mar 25–29, 1982.

35. Hahn FJY, Rim K: Frontal ventricular dimensions on normal computed tomography. *Am J Roentgenology* 1976; 126.

34 Cerebral Blood Flow: Use in Differential Diagnosis of Alzheimer's Disease

JOHN STIRLING MEYER

IT HAS BEEN KNOWN for many years that cerebral blood flow (CBF) and oxygen uptake are reduced in both hemispheres in organic dementia (1–15). More recently, it has been shown in dementia that the regional reductions in gray matter flow (F_1) and glucose consumption measured by PET scanning (16, 17) correlate with the disorder of cognition and atrophy of the brain shown by CT scanning.

However, there is evidence of atrophy of the brain in normal aging (18), and measurements of regional CBF (rCBF) and metabolism are more sensitive indicators of organic dementia than CT scanning (13–17). Furthermore, reduction of hemispheric rCBF correlates directly with the degree of impairment of higher cortical function as evaluated by psychological test batteries.

The purpose of the present communication is to review the potential clinical usefulness of rCBF in the differential diagnosis of the common dementias. It was shown (19, 20) some years ago, and has been recently confirmed in five additional cases using the noninvasive ^{133}Xe inhalation method, that following lumbar puncture with removal of 25 ml of CSF, rCBF increases in patients with dementia due to normal-pressure hydrocephalus. To the contrary, removal of CSF causes a further decrease or no change in rCBF in patients with Alzheimer's disease (AD). Apart from its diagnostic usefulness, serial prospective measurements of rCBF in patients with dementia provide an objective measurement of the temporal profile of the dementing process which may be useful in evaluating therapeutic intervention. This is relevant since it is now well known that dementia is becoming a major public health problem in our aging population and objective measurements of the natural history of the disease and any positive effects of therapeutic intervention will be in considerable demand.

The commonest causes of dementia are AD, multi-infarct dementia (MID), and severe depression posing as dementia, or what is termed pseudodementia of depression (21, 22).

In AD there is a metabolic disorder of the neurons of both cerebral hemispheres resulting in decreased neurotransmitter (particularly cholinergic) and protein synthesis, followed later by neuronal atrophy, neurofibrillary degeneration, and neuritic plaques (21).

In MID (19) the dementia results from an accumulation of bilateral cerebral hemispheric infarcts, whereas in the pseudodementia of depression there is no recognizable organic brain pathology. In depressive pseudodementia there is reversible diminution of cognitive function associated with psychomotor retardation, which becomes alleviated as the depressed mood resolves spontaneously or as a result of antidepressant medication. Regional CBF values are tightly coupled with regional brain function and metabolism (23) so that values in organic dementias correlate directly with the degree of dementia and cortical atrophy of the brain (10). Thus, rCBF measurements at rest, during brain work induced by standard behavioral activation, and in response to vasoconstrictor and vasodilator challenges by breathing 5% carbon dioxide in air, or 100% oxygen during rCBF measurements, have been found to be useful for defining which of the disorders, alone or in combination, are responsible for the dementia (13). The vasomotor challenges were made in an effort to define the presence or absence of cerebral arteriosclerosis and infarction, which is likely to be present in MID but not in AD (13, 14).

METHODS

Measurements of rCBF in this laboratory are made by a modification of Obrist's ^{133}Xe inhalation method (24–29). In an earlier paper (13), experience with 60 patients having different types and degrees of dementia was reported. The series included 11 cases of AD, 13 cases of MID, 9 cases with a combination of both AD and MID, with the remainder suffering from other types of encephalopathy including Creutzfeldt–Jakob disease and Wernicke–Korsakoff's dementia. Since reporting these results, many additional patients with AD, MID, and depression were examined. Some of these recent results have been published (26–29) while other studies are in progress. For example, an additional test involved ten patients with AD and six patients with MID, in whom CBF was measured in the steady state as well as during 100% oxygen inhalation to test cerebral vasoconstrictor responsiveness.

The ^{133}Xe inhalation method for measuring rCBF is a modification of the Fick principle. The radioactive xenon is inhaled as the inert indicator, and its washout from the brain permits automatic calculation of fast flow of gray matter (F_1) and slow flow (F_2) of white matter by two-compartmental analysis using a minicomputer. The proportionality of gray matter counts to white matter counts permit estimation of gray matter weight, which correlates with brain atrophy estimated by CT scan (13). A mixture of 3–7 mCi of Xenon ^{133}gas in room air is inhaled by means of a face mask for one minute. Regional clearance curves are monitored for the ensuing 10 minutes by the use of 16 different collimated sodium iodide scintillation detectors placed symmetrically over both cerebral hemispheres and brain stem cerebellar regions. The probes are held in place by means of a helmet which permits them to exert light scalp pressure.

Standard tests of cerebral vasomotor responses (VMR) are carried out by comparing paired measurements of rCBF in the steady state and during inhalation of either 5% carbon dioxide in air for testing vasodilator capacitance, or during 100% oxygen for testing vasoconstrictor capacitance. Testing in this manner provides a safe method for comparative testing of VMR among normal and aged volunteers (13, 14, 17, 25, 28) as well as among patients with cerebral infarction and dementia. End-tidal PCO_2 and PO_2 changes are measured so that these may be correlated for interpreting the results. Regional CBF changes to hypercarbia are customarily expressed as relative percentage: $\Delta F_1/\Delta PECO_2$. This ratio is 3.5 among normal, healthy, young volunteers, but declines to 2 or less by age 80 (28). Regional cerebral vasodilator responses also decrease or disappear after localized cerebral infarction.

Cerebral vasoconstrictive responses to 100% oxygen inhalation are customarily expressed in absolute percentage ΔF_1 since PEO_2 predictably increases from 127 ± 11.9 mm Hg to

634 ± 62.0 mm Hg. In normal volunteers under age 50, $\Delta F_1 = 16.2 \pm 4.8\%$. There is a linear reduction of oxygen-vasoconstrictive responses with advancing age.

Standard behavioral activation testing has been carried out during paired rCBF measurements (19) in patients with moderate to severe dementia. The first measurement (Run 1) was made in quiet darkness, without sleep, as shown by EEG monitoring, routinely carried out during rCBF measurements. The second measurement (Run 2) was made with lights on and eyes open, while counting or attempting to solve simple arithmetical problems and while listening to a musical tape (13).

Another group of 20 patients with early, mild dementia presumed to be due to AD underwent rCBF measurements during testing of Raven's progressive matrices which were carried out during the second run. Results were compared with similar measurements made among 20 normal, healthy control volunteers in the manner previously reported by Maximilian and associates (30).

Results

CBF in Normal Aging

Normal subjects measured while relaxed in the steady state, exhibit declines in values for flow and weight of gray matter (F_1 and W_1) with advancing age (Fig. 34–1). The decrease in F_1 values is about 5ml/100 g of brain/min per decade (14, 24, 25, 31–33). This decrease

Figure 34–1. Effect of normal aging on CBF responsiveness to standard behavior activation tests in normal healthy volunteers without risk factors.

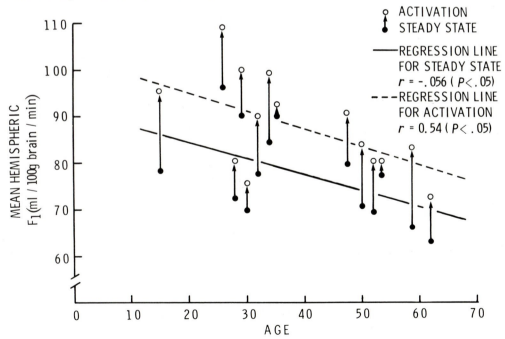

in CBF is due partly to brain atrophy normally occurring with advancing age, and partly to increased cerebrovascular resistance and loss of elasticity of the vessel walls. Atrophy of the brain is evidenced by a decline in W_1 values with advancing age. Loss of elasticity of the cerebral vessels was continued by progressive decreases in VMR with aging during 5% carbon dioxide inhalation (28) and during 100% oxygen inhalation (14). The increase in F_1 values during standard behavioral activation measured among normal volunteers in their sixties did not differ significantly from the results in younger normal subjects (Fig. 34–1).

CBF in Alzheimer's Disease

As shown in Figures 34–2 and 34–3, in the relaxed state patients with moderate to severe AD show diffuse reductions of F_1 values compared with age-matched controls (13). Patients with early AD also show diffuse decreases of F_1 values, but there is some overlap with age-matched controls. Reductions in F_1 values vary directly with the severity of the dementia as judged by psychometric testing (Fig. 34–4), the duration of the dementia (Fig. 34–5), and the degree of brain atrophy measured by CT scanning (Fig. 34–6).

During standard behavioral activation, in moderate to advanced AD there was a significant reduction in CBF increases as compared with CBF increases seen in age-matched normals undergoing the same testing (13).

During the Raven's progressive matrices test the CBF increases were greater, however, in mild AD than in age-matched controls, suggesting that the output or effort of brain work in mildly cortically impaired persons was greater in order to solve these problems (which they were able to do correctly) compared with normals (26).

As shown in Figure 34–7, cerebral vasodilator responsiveness during 5% carbon dioxide inhalation was well preserved in AD (13), but the cerebral vasoconstrictor response during 100% oxygen inhalation was sharply decreased or absent when compared with this response in age-matched normals (14).

Figure 34–2. Percentage difference of regional F_1 values in patients with AD ($N = 11$) compared with young normal volunteers ($N = 55$).

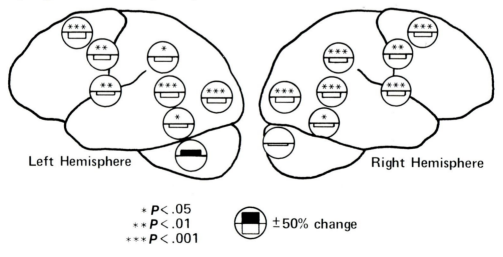

Left Hemisphere   Right Hemisphere

$* P < .05$
$** P < .01$
$*** P < .001$ $\pm 50\%$ change

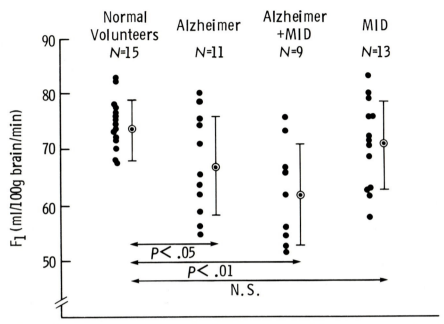

Figure 34–3. Mean hemispheric F_1 values in patients with dementia compared with age-matched normal volunteers.

Figure 34–4. Mean hemispheric F_1 values in relationship to the severity of dementia.

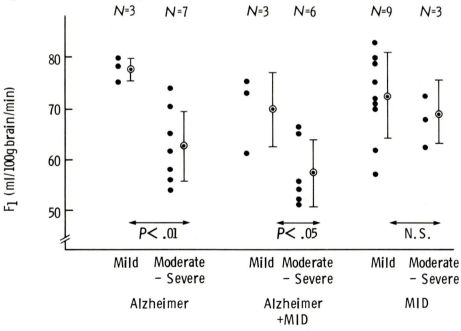

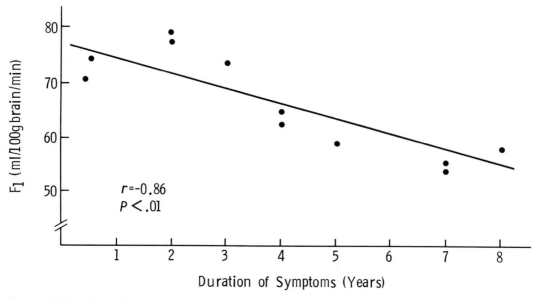

Figure 34–5. Mean hemispheric F_1 values correlated with duration of symptoms in patients with AD.

Figure 34–6. Mean hemispheric F_1 values in AD or AD plus MID, in relationship to computerized tomographic evidence of cerebral atrophy.

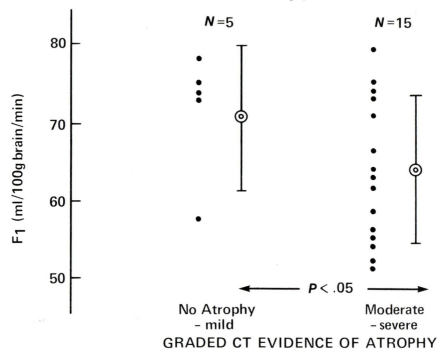

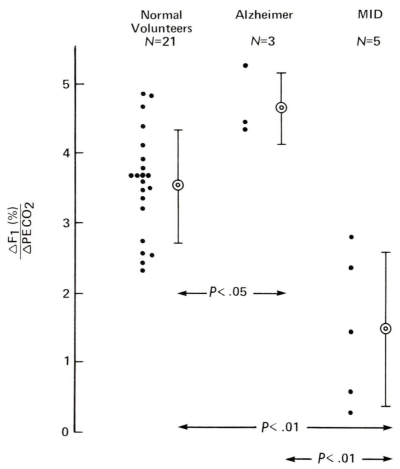

Figure 34–7. CO_2 responsiveness to hypercapnia in patients with AD or MID compared with normal volunteers.

CBF IN MULTI-INFARCT DEMENTIA

As shown in Figure 34–8, in the steady state, patients with multi-infarct dementia showed marked variability in regional flow values, with zones of reduction surrounded by bordering zones of normal or hyperemic (collateral) flow. During standard behavioral activation, there were less marked mean hemispheric increases than seen in age-matched normals and such increases that did occur were patchy (Fig. 34–9).

During tests of vasomotor responsiveness there were reduced responses, with patchy increases during 5% carbon dioxide inhalation and comparably uneven regional vasoconstrictor responses during 100% oxygen inhalation.

CBF IN DEPRESSION

In patients with severe depression, F_1 values are normal or decreased, particularly over the left hemisphere, with invariably normal W_1 values. When there was spontaneous recovery from depression or improvement due to antidepressant medication, any reduced CBF values

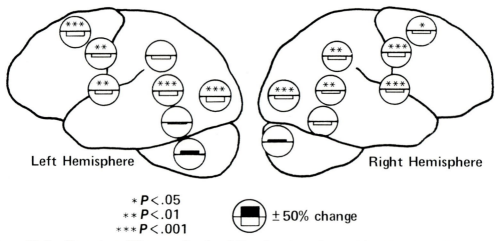

Left Hemisphere   Right Hemisphere

*P < .05
**P < .01
***P < .001

± 50% change

Figure 34–8. Percentage difference of regional F_1 values in patients with MID ($N = 13$) compared with young normal volunteers ($N = 55$).

returned to normal (27). In depressed patients, cerebral vasomotor responsiveness remains normal.

DISCUSSION

Noninvasive, regional cerebral blood flow values have proven to be of practical clinical value in assisting with differential diagnosis of dementia. In normal-pressure hydrocephalus,

Figure 34–9. Regional F_1 changes during multiple psychophysiological activation compared with values at rest in right-handed patients with multi-infarct dementia ($N = 8$); age 64 ± 13 years.

RESTING   : MABP = 98 mm Hg $PECO_2$ = 34.5 mm Hg
ACTIVATION: MABP = 96 mm Hg $PECO_2$ = 34.9 mm Hg

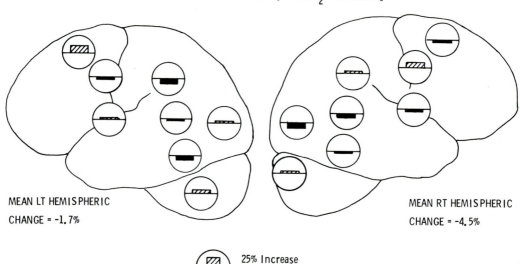

MEAN LT HEMISPHERIC
CHANGE = -1.7%

MEAN RT HEMISPHERIC
CHANGE = -4.5%

25% Increase
25% Decrease

F_1 and W_1 values are diffusely decreased but increase promptly following removal of 15–25 ml of spinal fluid by lumbar puncture. In AD, F_1 and W_1 values are diffusely decreased, correlating with the severity and diffuseness of the disease process; cerebral vasodilator responsiveness to 5% carbon dioxide inhalation is retained, but cerebral vasoconstrictive responsiveness to 100% oxygen inhalation is diffusely reduced or absent. Patients with MID show patchy and asymmetrical reductions of F_1 and W_1 values, with corresponding uneven reductions of cerebral vasodilator responsiveness to 5% carbon dioxide inhalation and of vasoconstrictive responses to 100% oxygen inhalation. These patchy reductions of F_1 values with uneven vasomotor responses confirm that multiple cerebral infarctions are responsible for the dementia.

In psychomotor retardation with pseudodementia due to depression, any decreased F_1 values were primarily over the left hemisphere, cerebral vasomotor responsiveness was preserved, and CBF values increased to normal as the affect improves due either to antidepressive medication or spontaneous recovery.

SUMMARY

There are many causes of dementia but the most common causes of impaired higher cortical function posing as AD are pseudodementia of depression and multi-infarct dementia (MID). Measurement of regional cerebral blood flow (rCBF) by inhalation of ^{133}Xe is a harmless and useful test for establishing differential diagnosis of these dementias. Gray matter flow, and weight of gray matter, are diffusely reduced in moderate to advanced AD compared with age-matched controls in AD. During standard behavioral activation, rCBF shows zero change or smaller increases than seen in age-matched normals; cerebral vasodilator responses to 5% carbon dioxide inhalation are normal, but cerebral vasoconstrictor responses to 100% oxygen are reduced or absent. Patients with pseudodementia of depression show reduced or normal rCBF in the left hemisphere with normal W_1 values and cerebral vasomotor responses. Patients with MID show patchy reductions of F_1 and W_1 of both hemispheres with corresponding regional reductions of vasodilator and vasoconstrictor responses to 5% carbon dioxide or 100% oxygen inhalation. During behavioral activation in MID there are patchy increases of rCBF. Whatever the cause, reductions of rCBF correspond with the severity of the organic dementias.

REFERENCES

1. Freyhan FA, Woodford RB, Kety SS: Cerebral blood flow and metabolism in psychoses of senility. *J Nerv Ment Dis* 1951; 113:449–456.
2. Lassen NA, Feinburg I, Lane MH: Bilateral studies of cerebral oxygen uptake in young and aged normal subjects and patients with organic dementia. *J Clin Invest* 1960; 39:491.
3. Lassen NA, Munck O, Tohery ER: Mental function and cerebral oxygen consumption in organic dementia. *Arch Neurol Psychiatry* 1957; 77:126–133.
4. Ingvar DH, Lassen NA: Activity distribution in the cerebral cortex in organic dementia as revealed by measurements of regional cerebral blood flow, in *Brain Function in Old Age*. Berlin, Springer, 1979, pp 260–268.
5. Gustafson L, Risberg J: Regional cerebral blood flow related to psychiatric symptoms in dementia with onset in the presenile period. *Acta Psychiatr Scand* 1974; 50:516–538.

6. Gustafson L, Risberg J: Regional cerebral blood flow measurements by the [133]Xenon inhalation technique in differential diagnosis of dementia. *Acta Neurol Scand Suppl* 1979; 60(suppl 72):546–547.

7. Gustafson L, Brun A, Ingvar DH: Presenile dementia: clinical symptoms, pathoanatomical findings, and cerebral blood flow, in Meyer JS, Lechner H, Reivich M (eds): *Cerebral Vascular Disease.* Amsterdam, Excerpta Medica, 1976, pp 5–9.

8. Ingvar DH, Gustafson L: Regional cerebral blood flow in organic dementia with early onset. *Acta Neurol Scand Suppl* 1970; 46(suppl 43):42–73.

9. Hachinski VC, Illiff LD, Zilkha E: Cerebral blood flow in dementia. *Arch Neurol* 1975; 32:632–637.

10. Hachinski VC, Larsen NA, Marshall J: Multi-infarct dementia: a cause of mental deterioration in the elderly. *Lancet* 1974; ii:207–209.

11. Simard D, Olesen J, Paulseon OB, Lassen NA, Skinhoj E: Regional cerebral blood flow and its regulation in dementia. *Brain* 1971; 94:273–288.

12. Obrist WD, Chivian E, Cronquist S, et al: Regional cerebral blood flow in senile and presenile dementia. *Brain* 1971; 94:273–288.

13. Yamaguchi F, Meyer JS, Yamamoto M, et al: Non-invasive regional cerebral blood flow measurements in dementia. *Arch Neurol* 1980; 37:410–418.

14. Nakajima S, Meyer JS, Yamamoto M, et al: Effects of normal aging and cerebral infarction on cerebral vasoconstrictor responsiveness to 100% oxygen inhalation, in Meyers JS, Lechner H, Reivich M (eds): *Cerebral Vascular Disease.* Amsterdam, Excerpta Medica, 1981, vol 3, pp 145–151.

15. Perez F, Mathew NT, Stump DA, et al: Regional cerebral blood flow statistical patterns and psychological performance in multi-infarct dementia and Alzheimer's disease. *J Neurol Sci* 1977; 4:53–62.

16. Alavi A, Ferris SH, Wolf A, et al: Determination of regional cerebral metabolism in dementia using F_{18} deoxyglucose and positron emission tomography, in Meyer JS, Lechner H, Reivich M (eds): *Cerebral Vascular Diseases.* Amsterdam, Excerpta Medica, 1981, vol 3, pp 109–112.

17. Meyer JS: Summary of the Tenth World Federation of Neurology International Conference on Cerebrovascular Disease. *Stroke* 1981; 12:147–152.

18. Carlen PL, Wilkinson A, Wortzman G, et al: Cerebral atrophy and functional defects in alcoholics without clinically apparent liver disease. *Neurology* 1981; 31:377–385.

19. Meyer JS, Miyakawa T, Ishihara N, et al: Effect of CSF removal on CBF and metabolism in patients with Alzheimer's disease versus recent stroke. *Stroke* 1977; 8:44–50.

20. Mathew NT, Meyer JS, Hartmann A, et al: Abnormal cerebrospinal fluid–blood flow dynamics: implications in diagnosis, treatment, and prognosis in normal pressure hydrocephalus. *Arch Neurol* 1975; 52:657–664.

21. Katzman R, Terry RD, Bick KL (eds): *Alzheimer's Disease, Senile Dementia and Related Disorders.* New York, Raven, 1978.

22. Hofmeister F, Muller L (eds): *Brain Function in Old Age.* New York, Springer, 1979.

23. Meyer JS, Sakai F, Naritomi H, et al: Normal and abnormal patterns of cerebrovascular reserve tested by ^{133}Xe inhalation. *Arch Neurol* 1978; 35:350–359.

24. Meyer JS, Ishihara N, Deshmukh VD, et al: Improved method for non-invasive measurement of regional cerebral blood flow by ^{133}Xe inhalation: I. description of method and normal values obtained in healthy volunteers. *Stroke* 1978; 9:195–205.

25. Meyer JS: Improved method for non-invasive measurement of regional cerebral blood flow by ^{133}Xe inhalation: II. measurements in health and disease. *Stroke* 1978; 9:205–210.

26. Largen JW Jr, Shaw T, Weinman M, et al: Order effects and responsiveness of regional cerebral blood flow in early putative Alzheimer's disease. *J Cerebral Blood Flow & Metabolism Suppl* 1981; 1(suppl 1):483–484.

27. Mathew RJ, Meyer JS, Francis DJ, et al: Cerebral blood flow in depression. *Am J Psychiatry* 1980; 137:1449–1450.

28. Yamamoto M, Meyer JS, Sakai F, et al: Aging and cerebral vasodilator responses to hypercarbia. *Arch Neurol* 1980; 37:489–496.

29. Obrist W, Thompson HK Jr, Wang HS, et al: Regional cerebral blood flow estimated by ^{133}Xe inhalation. *Stroke* 1976; 6:245–256.

30. Maximilian VA, Prohovnik I, Risberg J: Cerebral hemodynamic response to mental activation in normo- and hypercapnia. *Stroke* 1980; 11:342–346.

31. Shaw TG, Cutaia MM, Mortel KF, et al: Prospective measurements of cerebral blood flow in normal and abnormal aging. *Neurology* 1981; 31:102.

32. Shaw TG, Meyer JS, Sakai F, et al: Effects of normal aging versus risk factors for stroke on regional cerebral blood flow (rCBF). *Acta Neurol Scand Suppl* 1979; 60(suppl 72):462–463.

33. Melamed E, Lavy S, Benton S, et al: Reduction in regional cerebral blood flow during normal aging in man. *Stroke* 1980; 11:31–35.

35 Cerebral Blood Flow and Cerebral Metabolism in Alzheimer's Disease: Technical Considerations

David H. Ingvar

IN THIS CHAPTER it will be demonstrated that the specific degenerative changes found in Alzheimer's disease (AD) are accompanied by a reduction of the cerebral metabolic rate (CMR). Since the oxidative metabolism of the brain regulates the cerebral blood flow (CBF), the CMR reduction leads to secondary CBF reduction: the flow adapts to reduced metabolic demands.

The reduction of the total mean CMR and CBF in organic dementia was initially demonstrated with the Kety–Schmidt nitrous oxide technique (1, 2). In the last two decades *regional* techniques to measure rCBF and rCMR (i.e., regional CBF and regional CMR, respectively) have been developed. These regional techniques have demonstrated that the cerebral metabolic and circulatory consequences of AD are not diffuse. Instead, they show regional, sometimes focal features which correlate with the distribution of the pathoanatomical changes and also with the specific symptomatology of the intellectual deficits (3–6). Thus, with the aid of regional techniques, mainly utilizing rCBF studies, one can consider AD as something other than a diffuse cerebral disorder. In the course of the disease's slow progression, distinct regional features can be recognized. Some of these appear of great value for enhancing our understanding of the pathogenesis and perhaps the etiology of the neuronal changes which underlie AD.

TECHNICAL CONSIDERATIONS

Current methods of measuring global or regional CBF or CMR are based upon tracer techniques. The global CBF method of Kety and Schmidt (1) is based upon the inhalation of nitrous oxide for 10 minutes. By arterial and cerebral venous sampling, two curves are obtained during equilibration of the brain tissue. The area between the curves is used to calculate the flow according to the Fick principle:

$$\text{CBF} = \frac{100 \ V.u.S}{\int_{o}^{u} (A - V)\mathrm{d}t} \ \text{ml/100 g/min}$$

where A and V represent the nitrous oxide content in the arterial and venous blood, respectively, u is time of equilibration (10 minutes), and S is the solubility coefficient for nitrous oxide in the brain tissue.

In two dimensions, rCBF can be measured by ^{133}Xe clearance techniques theoretically related to the nitrous oxide method. The gamma-emitting radioactive gas ^{133}Xe labels the brain either as originally described by intracarotid injection (5), by intravenous injection or inhalation (6). With external recording, usually using a battery of detectors placed at the side of the head, the arrival and subsequent clearance of the isotope is recorded simultaneously from a number of brain regions.

Calculating rCBF may be accomplished from the clearance curves, utilizing the "stochastic" method, with the formula:

$$rCBF = \frac{(H_0 - H_{10})}{A_{10}} \times \lambda \times 100 \text{ ml}/100 \text{ g/min}$$

where H_0 and H_{10} represent the initial and the 10-minute heights, respectively, of the clearance curve, expressed in terms of counts per minute; lambda is the partition coefficient of ^{133}Xe between blood and brain tissue (average for gray and white matter); and A_{10} is the total number of counts under the curve during the 10 minutes of recording. There are other methods of calculating rCBF.

The first part of the clearance curve can be assumed to be monoexponential and then yield an "initial slope index" of flow. Clearance curves may also be analyzed in two monoexponential components, representing the clearance in gray and white matter (for a review see ref. 7).

Alternatively, if ^{133}Xe is administered by inhalation or intravenous injection, other methods of calculation must be used since there is a temporal dispersion of the isotope bolus' arrival to the brain (6). This sets certain limitations for the calculation of fast flows represented early in the clearance curves.

No matter how calculated, all rCBF techniques have important limitations. They are pertinent to describe here because rCBF measurements are used so widely to study patients with organic dementia. First, these techniques are mainly *two-dimensional,* i.e., they look at the brain from one or two sides, each detector looking at a stumped cone of brain tissue. Due to absorption of the gamma quanta in the tissue, the detectors see more of the superficial (cortical) brain layers than deeper parts. With intra-arterial measurements, only brain tissue on one side is counted, that part of the hemisphere perfused by the carotid system. The spatial resolution of the two-dimensional intra-arterial rCBF techniques is about 1 cm; the temporal resolution is about 1–2 minutes with the initial slope method, longer with other methods to calculate the flow.

The inhalation and intravenous ^{133}Xe techniques suffer from additional limitations which must be carefully considered when used in a patient population comprising dementia patients, in which the global flow level may be low. First, the clearance of ^{133}Xe is influenced by pulmonary ventilation which is often faulty in elderly patients, augmenting recirculation of the isotope. Second, large doses of the inhaled isotope in the upper airways may be seen by the detectors, which contaminate early and important parts of the clearance curves to which fast (cortical) flows may provide an important contribution. Third, there is a "look-through" effect, since both hemispheres are labeled. Finally, Compton scatter of the ^{133}Xe radiation in the tissue precludes strict focal measurements, especially if, as with atraumatic ^{133}Xe techniques, the counting rate per detector is relatively low, making it impossible to use narrow collimation and discrimination windows. All these factors have recently been the object of a critical review (8).

A three-dimensional rCBF technique using ^{133}Xe inhalation and single photon emission tomography (SPECT) has recently been developed by Stokeley, and collaborators (9). This instrument has the capacity to measure rCBF in all brain regions, even subcortical structures, in three slices of the head. It also enables repeated measurements, which is of significant value in dynamic studies of brain functions at rest and during various forms of activation.

CMR and rCMR methods can be only very briefly touched upon here. CMR for oxygen and glucose is measured together with nitrous oxide determinations of the CBF. From the arterial and cerebral venous samples, the respective concentration and arteriovenous differences (AVD) for oxygen and glucose are obtained. The cerebral metabolic rate of oxygen ($CMRO_2$) is then calculated according to the formula:

$$CMR_{O_2} = CBF \times AVD_{O_2} \, ml/100 \, g/min$$

Since *regional* AVDs cannot be obtained in humans—and only with great difficulty in animals (10)—other approaches have been developed to measure rCMR. Briefly, they imply "autoradiography" of the human brain *in vivo* by means of dual photon emission tomography (DPECT). With the aid of short-lived positron-emitting radioisotopes, administered in suitable forms to the patient, the distribution of the isotope in the head can then be pictured. Using ^{18}fluoro-deoxyglucose (FDG) the $rCMR_{gluc}$ is measured in accordance with principles worked out by Sokoloff (11–13). With $^{15}O_2$, both rCBF and $rCMRO_2$ can be determined (14). These techniques are of immediate interest for dementia research, especially since they picture metabolism in all regions of the brain. The few results published so far have in many ways confirmed and elaborated what has been found with ^{133}Xe rCBF techniques (15).

GLOBAL CBF AND CMR IN ORGANIC DEMENTIA

With the Kety technique it was shown in 1958 that organic dementia is accomplished by a reduction of $CMRO_2$ and—as already was then assumed—a secondary reduction of CBF. The measurements did not give any evidence that Alzheimer patients, showed signs of cerebral ischemia. Thus, the CMR and CBF reductions in AD were interpreted as a consequence of reduced metabolic and circulatory demands of the type now known to be characteristic of this disorder (2).

It was also found by means of psychometric testing that the CMR and CBF reduction was grossly proportional to the loss of intellectual functions. The lowest CMR and CBF values were found in severely deteriorated cases; here the reduction approached the metabolic and circulatory diminution encountered in stupor and coma (6).

One further observation with the nitrous oxide technique in organic dementia merits emphasis. Lassen and co-workers (16) showed a hemispheric difference. The CMR and CBF reduction was slightly more pronounced on the left side, a finding attributed to a greater involvement of the left (dominant) hemisphere than the right. Later studies with bilateral rCBF measurements as well as with $rCMR_{gluc}$ techniques have not confirmed this interesting hypothesis. However, the role of the two hemispheres in relation to the symptoms of dementia has not been entirely clarified as yet.

It should also be recalled here that the global CMR and CBF reduction in AD patients is also accompanied by a slowing of the EEG, again proportional to the clinical symptomatology (17).

STUDIES OF rCBF AND rCMR IN ALZHEIMER'S DISEASE

The intra-arterial ^{133}Xe clearance technique used with multiple detectors provided the first possibility of studying the distribution of the flow reduction in AD as well as in other forms of dementia, and in mental disorders in general. These studies, started in the early 1960s, have demonstrated three findings.

First, it was confirmed that the total mean rCBF (i.e., the hemispheric mean rCBF calculated from all the detectors used) showed a reduction proportional to the magnitude of the intellectual deficit. Thus, one of the major findings with the nitrous oxide technique was confirmed (3, 18).

Second, when detailed psychometric analyses of the patients were performed, regional correlations appeared (4). Memory reductions—sometimes the only prominent symptom in early cases—correlated with a low flow in temporal regions. Agnosia-apraxia and confusional symptoms correlated with low flows in occipito-parieto-temporal areas. Speech disturbances, often a late sign, also correlated with rCBF. Those with expressive forms of aphasia showed more anterior low flows, and those with receptive aphasia showed more posterior reductions (19).

The third main finding was that the rCBF reductions correlated with distribution of degenerative neuronal changes in the cortex, i.e., with degenerative changes on the lateral part of the cortex, that part of the brain mainly measured by the two-dimensional rCBF techniques (20).

Gustafson (18) has found additional correlations between psychiatric symptomatology in patients with dementia with early onset and the rCBF landscape.

In many patients with AD confirmed at autopsy, it was often found that the rCBF values recorded over the Rolandic region, over the pre- and postcentral sulcus, as well as over the middle part of the Sylvian fissure were relatively high (21). This "Rolandic ridge" in the rCBF landscape indicated that the neuronal degeneration appeared to spare primary sensory regions as well as the precentral motor cortex. Pathoanatomical studies by Brun have confirmed this hypothesis and also that the visual cortex in the occipital lobe is relatively less affected by the neuronal degenerative changes (Chap. 4). These interesting findings appear to explain why basic motor and sensory functions often remain intact even in later stages of the disease. Could it be that the constant sensory input and motor output keep the regions mentioned more active and hence less prone to degeneration? Or do these cortical regions have other forms of transmittor mechanisms which make them less vulnerable?

ACTIVATION STUDIES

The results described thus far in this chapter were obtained in patients *at rest:* measurements were carried out in silence, and patients had a pad placed over their eyes and were neither spoken to nor asked to solve any problems (22).

When psychological testing was performed, it was found that the demented patients could not activate their association areas, frontally and postcentrally, as normals do (23).

This important finding should be related to the well-known reduction in capacity for abstract thinking so characteristic in Alzheimer patients. In further studies with the inhalation technique this has been confirmed and elaborated (6).

Considering the regional features of the rCBF landscape in AD, we investigated the possibility of analogous, regional correlations with the EEG abnormalities found in AD (24). In general, the answer was negative. Although regional EEG changes were not found, it could clearly be shown that the more advanced the signs were of intellectual reduction, the more abnormal was the EEG.

Differential Diagnosis

Although numerically the most frequent cause of dementia, AD is obviously not the only form. It is then possible by using rCBF—or CMR—measurements to differentiate between AD and other clinical etiologies of organic or functional dementia? We shall consider four such disorders relevant for differential diagnosis.

Pseudodementia. In so-called pseudodementia, i.e., severe depression accompanied by a marked reduction of normal intellectual abilities, a normal mean hemispheric rCBF has been found. Thus, a normal rCBF finding may help to exclude the Alzheimer diagnosis (25).

Pick's Disease. This rare disorder is accompanied by degenerative changes, especially in temporal and frontal structures. Its clinical signs are in many ways different from those shown by Alzheimer patients as pointed out by Gustafson (18). In addition, even fairly advanced cases may show a normal EEG (24). rCBF measurements in such patients (with both intra-arterial and inhalation techniques) have indicated that the flow reduction may consequently be more pronounced frontotemporally in Pick patients than in Alzheimer cases (25). However, these differences are often encountered at about the same low flow level, and even if they appear in groups of patients confirmed at autopsy, it is always difficult in an individual case to interpret a given rCBF pattern, especially if obtained with inhalation or intravenous ^{133}Xe injection.

Cerebrovascular Forms of Dementia. These form a very varied group. The so-called multi-infarct dementia often differs clinically from Alzheimer dementia. Patients have an episodic history with stroke-like onset followed by some recovery. Other forms are related to hypertension and give rise to *status lacunaris.* Some of these patients may resemble Alzheimer cases, but bilateral rCBF measurements often reveal asymmetries between the hemispheres, which is rare in Alzheimer cases. Regional or suggestive focal flow diminutions may also be encountered in organic dementia of cerebrovascular origin, and sometimes such regional rCBF diminutions may show a clear-cut relation to the focal neurological symptoms which may present in the patient or may have been previously manifest (25).

Normal-Pressure Hydrocephalus. A condition which may be operable in some cases, it is another diagnosis to be excluded from the Alzheimer group. So far, only a few such patients have been studied with the rCBF technique, and the flow landscape has not shown any specific features. During periods with symptoms of intellectual reduction, the flow is low. Patients who improve following operation show some increase in their rCBF (26, 27).

CONCLUDING REMARKS

The extensive studies carried out during the last decade, especially with rCBF methods, have demonstrated that the degenerative neuronal changes characterizing AD are accompanied by secondary reductions of rCBF, coupled with the basic neuronal degeneration and its consequences for the cerebral metabolism.

One of the main rCBF findings in AD is that the flow reductions are not uniform and diffuse but show regional features. These regional features are coupled with the underlying neuronal loss and indeed also with the clinical symptomatology. In addition, it was found that regions with a low flow and consequently severe neuronal degeneration could not be activated during psychological testing, which may explain poor performance during such tests.

Concerning the use of rCBF measurements in the clinical diagnosis of AD, the question may be summarized thus. A finding of global reduction of CBF or mean rCBF in a given patient with symptoms of dementia provides a quantitative index of cerebral functional reduction. A normal CBF or mean rCBF, on the other hand, together with a normal rCBF distribution, can have some diagnostic importance since signs of intellectual reduction which the patient manifests may be due to the pseudodementia of depression.

Concerning other uses of rCBF techniques in the differential diagnosis of AD, they should be considered limited. This is due partly to the inherent limitations of the rCBF techniques, especially the atraumatic modifications, in the capacity to explore the fast flows of the cerebral cortex, and particularly the limitations imposed by the two-dimensional nature of the rCBF methods.

It appears now that the rCBF studies in organic dementia, including AD, have initiated a new era in dementia research. Briefly, one might say that the rCBF era is to an increasing extent overshadowed by the advent of three-dimensional rCMR and rCBF measurements using single or dual photon emitting isotopes and emission tomography. With these techniques, all parts of the brain including subcortical structures will be measured simultaneously, and this will undoubtedly clarify many not-yet understood aspects of AD and other cerebral disorders producing intellectual reduction.

ACKNOWLEDGMENTS

The author was supported by the Swedish Medical Research Council (project no. B82-04X-00084-18A) and the Wallenberg Foundation, Stockholm.

REFERENCES

1. Kety SS, Schmidt CF: The nitrous oxide method for determination of cerebral blood flow in man: theory, procedure, and normal values. *J Clin Invest* 1948; 27:476–483.

2. Schmidt CF: *The Cerebral Circulation in Health and Disease.* Springfield, Thomas, 1950.

3. Ingvar DH, Gustafson L: Regional cerebral blood flow in organic dementia with early onset. *Acta Neurol Scand Suppl* 1970; 46 (suppl 43):42–73.

4. Hagberg B, Ingvar DH: Cognitive reduction in presenile dementia related to regional abnormalities of the cerebral blood flow. *Br J Psychiatry* 1976; 128:209–222.

5. Lassen NA, Ingvar DH: The blood flow of the cerebral cortex determined by radioactive krypton 85. *Experientia* 1961; 17:42–43.

6. Risberg J: Regional cerebral blood flow measurements by ^{133}Xe-inhalation: methodology and applications in neuropsychology and psychiatry. *Brain Lang* 1980; 9:9–34.

7. Lassen NA, Ingvar DH: Radioisotopic assessment of regional cerebral blood flow. *Prog Nucl Med* 1972; 1:376–409.

8. Ingvar DH, Lassen NA: Atraumatic two-dimensional rCBF measurements using stationary detectors and inhalation or intravenous administration of xenon 133. *J Cereb Blood Flow Metabol* 1982; 2:271–274.

9. Stokeley EM, Sveinsdottir E, Lassen NA, et al: Design considerations for a single photon dynamic computer-assisted tomograph (DCAT) for imaging brain function in multiple cross-sections. *J Comput Assist Tomogr* 1980; 4:230–240.

10. Gleichmann U, Ingvar DH, Lassen NA, et al: Regional cerebral cortical metabolic rate of oxygen and carbon dioxide, related to the EEG in the anesthetized dog. *Acta Physiol Scand* 1962; 55:127–138.

11. Sokoloff L: Localization of functional activity in the central nervous system by measurement of glucose utilization with radioactive deoxyglucose. *J Cereb Blood Flow Metabol* 1981; 1:7–36.

12. Reivich M, Kuhl D, Wolf A, et al: The (18-F)fluoro-deoxyglucose method for the measurement of local cerebral glucose utilization in man. *Circ Res* 1979; 44:127–137.

13. Phelps ME, Huang SC, Hoffman EJ, et al: Tomographic measurement of local cerebral glucose metabolic rate in humans with (F-18)2-fluoro-2-deoxy-d-glucose: validation of method. *Ann Neurol* 1979; 6:371–388.

14. Frackowiak RSJ, Jones T, Lenzi GL, et al: Regional cerebral oxygen utilization and blood flow in normal man using oxygen-15 and positron emission tomography. *Acta Neurol Scand* 1980; 62:336–344.

15. Alavi A, Ferris S, Wolf A, et al: Determination of regional cerebral metabolism in dementia using F-18 deoxyglucose and positron emission tomography. *Exp Brain Res Suppl* 1982; suppl 5:187–195.

16. Lassen NA, Feinberg I, Lane MH: Bilateral studies of cerebral oxygen uptake in young and aged normal subjects and in patients with organic dementia. *J Clin Invest* 1960; 39:491–500.

17. Obrist WD, Sokoloff L, Lassen NA, et al: Relation of EEG to cerebral blood flow and metabolism in old age. *Electroencephalogr Clin Neurophysiol* 1963; 15:610–619.

18. Gustafson L, Risberg J: Regional cerebral blood flow related to psychiatric symptoms in dementia with onset in the presenile period. *Acta Psychiatr Scand* 1974; 50:516–538.

19. Gustafson L, Hagberg B, Ingvar DH: Speech disturbances in presenile dementia related to local cerebral blood flow abnormalities in the dominant hemisphere. *Brain Lang* 1978; 5:103–118.

20. Brun A: Alzheimer's disease and its clinical implications, in Platt, D (ed): *Geriatrics.* Berlin, Springer, 1982, vol 1, pp 343–390.

21. Ingvar, DH, Lassen NA: Activity distribution in the cerebral cortex in organic dementia as revealed by measurements of regional cerebral blood flow, in Hoffmeister F, Müller C (eds): *Brain Function in Old Age.* Berlin, Springer 1979, pp 268–277.

22. Ingvar DH: "Hyperfrontal" distribution of the cerebral grey matter flow in resting wakefulness: on the functional anatomy of the conscious state. *Acta Neurol Scand* 1979; 60:12–25.

23. Ingvar DH, Risberg J, Schwartz MS: Evidence of subnormal function of association cortex in presenile dementia. *Neurology* 1975; 25:964–974.

24. Stigsby B, Johannesson G, Ingvar DH: Regional EEG analysis and regional cerebral blood flow in Alzheimer's and Pick's diseases. *Electroencephalogr Clin Neurophysiol* 1981; 51:537–547.

25. Gustafson L, Risberg J: Regional cerebral blood flow measurements by the ^{133}Xe inhalation technique in differential diagnosis of dementia. *Acta Neurol Scand Suppl* 1979; 60 (suppl 72):546–547.

26. Ingvar DH, Schwartz MS: The cerebral blood flow in low pressure hydrocephalus, in Lundberg N, Pontén U, Brock M (eds): *Intracranial Pressure.* Berlin, Springer, 1975, vol 2, pp 153–159.

27. Gustafson L, Hagberg B: Recovery in hydrocephalic dementia after shunt operation. *J Neurol Neurosurg Psychiatry* 1978; 41:940–947.

36 The PET Scan in the Study of Alzheimer's Disease

STEVEN H. FERRIS
MONY J. DE LEON

POSITRON EMISSION TOMOGRAPHY (PET) is a new imaging technique for studying human brain function *in vivo* (1). The PET scan is somewhat analogous to the CT scan (computed x-ray transmission tomography) since an imaging device and computer construct tomographic images of the brain. However, a major difference is that PET images represent regional brain *function,* not brain structure. Thus, when a positron-emitting analogue of glucose is used as a tracer, quantitative measurements of regional brain metabolism may be obtained (2).

The potential neuroscientific applications of PET are numerous. It may be used to study normal brain function (3–6) and brain dysfunction in psychiatric or neurologic disease (7, 8). Other applications include the study of brain–behavior relationships and, using suitable tracers, the study of neuropharmacology or neurochemistry. Finally, of particular relevance to aging and senile dementia is the potential of the PET technique as a diagnostic tool.

BRAIN METABOLISM IN DEMENTIA

Changes in whole-brain metabolism in aging and senile dementia were first reported many years ago using the Kety–Schmidt technique (9). These early studies indicated lower rates of cerebral blood flow (CBF) and oxygen consumption during advanced age (10) and even lower rates in senile dementia (11). A subsequent study failed to show a decline in CBF and oxygen consumption in normal aging, but dementia patients routinely had significantly lower values (12). Dementia patients also showed a sharp reduction in cerebral glucose metabolism. More recent studies utilizing the ^{133}Xe method for regional CBF have confirmed an overall blood flow reduction in dementia, particularly in the temporal, parietal, and frontal brain regions (13, 14). Prior to development of the PET scan technique, however, *regional* metabolic measurements in humans could not be obtained. Recent PET studies of dementia, in particular studies of Alzheimer's disease (AD), have demonstrated strong reductions in regional glucose utilization correlated with the severity of the cognitive impairment (15–19). In this chapter we describe the application of PET to the study of dementia and review the status of current findings.

PET METHODOLOGY

The PET technique requires the synthesis of a positron-emitting tracer for the physiologic process to be studied. In human studies, ^{18}F-2-deoxy-2-fluoro-D-glucose (FDG) is the current tracer compound for brain metabolism; more specifically, for determining rates of glucose utilization. The PET-FDG procedure permits quantification of the rate of glucose metabolism in any discrete, identifiable part of the brain within the spatial resolution constraints of current-generation tomographic systems (2). The FDG is "trapped" in the cells as a 6-phosphorylated derivative and is not further metabolized. The trapping rate is proportional to the metabolic rate, which is assumed to reflect neuronal activity. By quantifying the concentration of radionuclide in the tomographic scan, determining the arterial time course of FDG and glucose, and using an operational equation derived from the mathematical model for glucose metabolism (20), the rate of glucose utilization may be quantified in mg/100 g of brain tissue per minute. There is evidence of a relationship among neuronal function, rate of local cerebral glucose metabolism (rCGM), and rate of regional cerebral blood flow (rCBF) (21).

In synthesizing the FDG tracer, the radionuclide (^{18}F) is first prepared using a cyclotron. The half-life of this radionuclide is approximately 110 minutes. Tomographic scans are obtained with a positron emission scanner, such as the PETT-III system at Brookhaven National Laboratory. This first-generation scanner has a spatial resolution of approximately 1.7 cm^3 (full width half maximum). During the scan, the patient remains stationary while the gantry rotates about the head and performs a series of linear and angular scans. Before the scan, a short intravenous cannula for blood sampling is inserted at the wrist, and the hand is warmed in order to provide arterialized venous blood samples. The bolus of tracer is administered intravenously. Average doses of the radionuclide range from 5 to 10 mCi/mg FDG. Thirty to 45 minutes after the injection (the time required for plasma equilibration of FDG), serial 10-mm transverse scans are obtained parallel to the canthomeatal (eye–ear) reference line. Usually at least five serial scans are obtained. With the PETT III, each positron emission scan takes 10–14 minutes. Thus, on the average, the studies last 1.5–2 hours.

In the current New York University–Brookhaven PET dementia project, we determine various brain regions of interest by carefully matching the CT scans of all experimental subjects with their positron emission tomographs. Since PET images have relatively poor spatial resolution, and since the functional nature of the images can lead to incorrect or subjective anatomic judgments, PET regions are defined operationally by first identifying regions on corresponding CT scans. The coordinates of the CT regions are then transferred to the PET images, and mean rates of glucose metabolism are computed for each region of interest.

PET STUDIES OF DEMENTIA

The objective of the PET dementia project is to study *in vivo* changes in regional brain metabolism occurring in normal aging and senile dementia, comparing normal elderly subjects to both young normal subjects and to patients with dementia. Patients with either AD or multi-infarct dementia (MID) have been studied, as well as patients with geriatric depression ("pseudodementia"). Current results for AD are based upon data from 24 patients

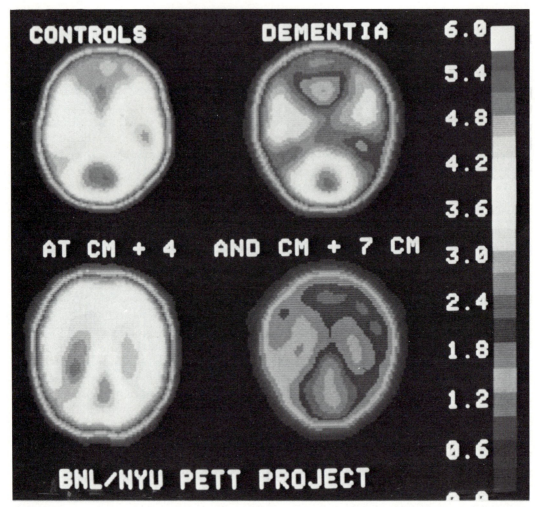

Figure 36–1. Representative PET scans for a normal elderly control subject (*left*) and an AD patient (*right*) at two brain levels: level of the basal ganglia (CM + 4 cm, top) and level of the centrum semiovale (CM + 7 cm, bottom). The tone scale at right represents the rate of glucose utilization (mg/100 g/min).

and 21 elderly control subjects (18). The dementia severity range of the AD patients is mild to very severe, but most have mild, moderate, or moderately severe cognitive impairment.

Some representative PET scans are shown in black and white in Figure 36–1. In these images, ordinarily color-coded, the "hotter" colors (red end of the scale) represent greater metabolic activity than the "cooler" colors (blue end of the scale). Two brain levels are represented, the "level of the centrum semiovale" (bottom), above the ventricular system, 7 cm above the canthomeatal (CM) reference plane (CM + 7); and the somewhat lower "level of the basal ganglia" (top), which cuts through the ventricular system, 4 cm above the CM plane (CM + 4). It is apparent from these images that the rates of glucose utilization are lower in the AD patient than in the elderly control subject.

For the AD and normal subject groups, the mean rates of glucose utilization for four regions of interest at the basal ganglia level (frontal, caudate, thalamus, and temporal) and three regions of interest at the centrum semiovale level (frontal, parietal, and white matter) were determined. For all regions at both levels, the metabolic rates were significantly lower in the AD group than in the controls ($P < .01$). The degree of diminution in the AD group ranged from 18 to 30%. The extent to which the degree of diminution in rate of glucose utilization is related to severity of AD symptomatology was also examined by computing correlation coefficients between objective measures of cognitive function and metabolic rates. Results indicated a consistent, moderate degree of relationship between degree of impairment and reduction in regional brain metabolism ($P < .05$) (18).

Another correlational analysis examined the extent to which changes in regional glucose utilization are related to CT density changes in the same regions (18). Preliminary results did not indicate a consistent pattern of relationship between structural and metabolic changes in each region, but suggested that CT density changes in certain subcortical regions may be correlated with more widespread metabolic changes in cortical areas (22). Another analysis examined whether the metabolic changes in AD may be accounted for by structural changes, as visualized by CT. When the PET values for certain regions were mathematically adjusted to the degree of CT density change for the same region, the correlations between metabolic rates and severity of AD were unchanged (22). This result suggests that the reduction in metabolic rate in AD may represent a true deficit in metabolism, rather than a secondary result of structural loss.

We have also begun to examine the extent to which the diminution in glucose utilization in AD may be of diagnostic value. A series of discriminant classification analyses have been carried out to determine the accuracy with which individual subjects can be classified as AD patients or normals based only upon their regional glucose utilization values. For predictions based on single PET regions of interest, the overall classification accuracy ranges from 70 to 80%.

CURRENT CONCLUSIONS AND FUTURE DIRECTIONS

In summary, current PET results demonstrate significant reductions in regional brain metabolism in AD and show that the degree of diminution is correlated with the severity of the disease. Furthermore, preliminary results suggest that the PET-FDG technique may eventually become a valuable diagnostic tool. Other studies have examined regional brain metabolism in young and old normal subjects (19), and current projects are studying elderly subjects with depression and MID. These studies will further elucidate the diagnostic potential of regional metabolic measurements.

The PET dementia research program recently has taken a major leap forward with the introduction of a greatly improved PET scanner plus the use of a glucose tracer with a shorter half-life. The new PET VI system has improved sensitivity and spatial resolution (less than 1 cm³). With this fast, four-detector ring machine, seven slices are obtained simultaneously in a period of only minutes. When used in conjunction with ^{11}C-deoxyglucose, a positron-emitting tracer with a half-life of only 20 minutes, up to three PET studies can be conducted on one subject on the same day. Thus, studies of the AD-related changes in regional metabolism are possible during various sensory or cognitive tasks (functional mapping) or following administration of potentially effective pharmacologic agents. With these advances, the PET technique will become an important tool for research on the study and treatment of AD.

Acknowledgments

This research was supported by Grant NS 15638 from the National Institute of Neurological and Communicative Disorders and Stroke, National Institutes of Health.

References

1. Wolf, AP: Special characteristics and potential for radiopharmaceuticals for positron emission tomography. *Seminars in Nuclear Medicine* 1981; 11:2–12.

2. Reivich M, Kuhl DE, Wolf AP, et al: The (^{18}F) fluorodexoxyglucose method for the measurement of local cerebral glucose utilization in man. *Circ Res* 1979; 44:127–137.

3. Greenberg JH, Alavi A, Hand P, et al: Metabolic mapping of functional activity in human subjects with the (^{18}F) fluorodeoxyglucose technique. *Science* 1981; 212:678–679.

4. Huang SC, Phelps ME, Hoffman EJ, et al: Noninvasive determination of local cerebral metabolic rate of glucose in man. *Am J Physiol* 1980; 238:69–82.

5. Phelps ME, Kuhl DE, Mazziotta JC: Metabolic mapping of the brain's response to visual stimulation: studies in humans. *Science* 1981; 211:1447–1448.

6. Reivich M, Greenberg JH, Alavi A, et al: The ^{18}F fluorodeoxyglucose method for measuring lcmR$_g$l in man: effects of physiological stimuli, in Passonneau JV, Hawkins RA, Lust WD, et al (eds): *Cerebral Metabolism and Neural Function.* Baltimore, Williams & Wilkins, 1980.

7. Farkas T, Reivich M, Alavi A, et al: The application of ^{18}F-2-deoxy-2-fluoro-D-glucose and positron emission tomography in the study of psychiatric conditions, in Passoneau JV, Hawkins RA, Lust WD, et al (eds): *Cerebral Metabolism and Neural Function.* Baltimore, Williams & Wilkins, 1980, pp 403–408.

8. Kuhl DE, Phelps ME, Kowell AP, et al: Effects of stroke on local cerebral metabolism and perfusion: mapping by emission computed tomography of ^{18}FDG and ^{13}NH$_3$. *Ann Neurol* 1980; 8:47–60.

9. Kety SS, Schmidt CF: The nitrous oxide method for the quantitative determination of cerebral blood flow in man: theory, procedure, and normal values. *J Clin Invest* 1948; 27:476–483.

10. Kety SS: Human cerebral blood flow and oxygen consumption as related to aging. *Res Publ Assoc Res Nerv Ment Dis* 1956; 35:31–45.

11. Frehan FA, Woodford RB, Kety SS: Cerebral blood flow and metabolism in psychoses of senility. *J Nerv Ment Dis* 1951; 113:449–456.

12. Birren JE, Butler RN, Greenhouse SW: *Human Aging: A Biological and Behavioral Study.* Government Printing Office, 1963.

13. Hagberg B, Ingvar DH: Cognitive reduction in presenile dementia related to regional abnormalities of the cerebral blood flow. *Br J Psychiatry* 1976; 128:209–222.

14. Lassen NA, Ingvar DH: Radioisotope assessment of regional cerebral blood flow. *Prog Nucl Med* 1972; 1:376–409.

15. Farkas T, Ferris SH, Wolf AP, et al: ^{18}F-2-deoxy-2-fluoro-D-glucose as a tracer in the positron emission tomographic study of senile dementia. *Am J Psychiatry* 1982; 139:352–353.

16. Ferris SH, de Leon MJ, Wolf AP, et al: Positron emission tomography in the study of aging and senile dementia. *Neurobiol Aging* 1980; 1:127–131.

17. Ferris SH, de Leon MJ, Christman D, et al: Positron emission tomography (PET) studies of regional brain metabolism in elderly patients, in Perris C, Struwe G, Jansson B (eds): *Biological Psychiatry 1981.* Amsterdam, Elsevier North-Holland, 1981, pp 280–283.

18. Ferris SH, de Leon MJ, Wolf AP, et al: Positron emission tomography, in Mayeux R, Rosen WG (eds): *The Dementias*. New York, Raven, 1983, pp 123–129.

19. Ferris SH, de Leon MJ, Wolf AP, et al: Regional metabolism and cognitive deficits in aging and senile dementia, in Samuel D, Algeri S, Gershon S, et al (eds): *Aging of the Brain*. New York, Raven, 1983, pp 133–142.

20. Sokoloff L, Reivich M, Kennedy C, et al: The (C^{14})-deoxyglucose method for the measurement of local cerebral glucose utilization: theory, procedure, and normal values in the conscious and anesthetized albino rat. *J Neurochem* 1977; 28:897–916.

21. Reivich M: Blood flow metabolism couple in brain dysfunction and metabolic disorders. *Res Publ Assoc Res Nerv Ment Dis* 1974; 53:125–140.

22. de Leon MJ, Ferris SH, George AE, et al: The combined use of positron emission tomography and computed tomography evaluations in senile dementia. Read before the Tenth Aharon Katzir-Katchalsky Conference on the Aging of the Brain, Mantua, Mar 25–29, 1982.

SECTION IX

CLINICAL SYNDROMES ASSOCIATED WITH ALZHEIMER'S DISEASE

37 Alzheimer's Disease and Parkinson's Disease:
Clinical and Pathological Associations

François Boller

ALZHEIMER'S DISEASE (AD) AND IDIOPATHIC PARKINSON'S DISEASE (PD) both affect mainly the elderly, and some patients may have both diseases. This paper summarizes recent evidence suggesting that the two conditions are found together in a greater number of cases than would be expected on the basis of the prevalence of the two diseases, and that far from being only fortuitous or related to age, this association may reflect a common, albeit unrecognized, pathological mechanism. As will be seen, the evidence for this hypothesis is based on the clinical and neuropathological study of PD patients who also had AD. Substantially less data are currently available concerning the converse of this problem (i.e., the number of patients with AD who also have PD).

CLINICAL AND NEUROPATHOLOGICAL FEATURES
OF AD IN PATIENTS WITH IDIOPATHIC PD

Idiopathic PD is a relatively well-defined entity: it is generally accepted that the main neuropathological lesion responsible for idiopathic PD is a degeneration of the dopaminergic cells of structures located in the upper midbrain (mainly the substantia nigra) which also show gliosis and characteristic round hyaline cytoplasmic inclusions known as Lewy bodies (1). Because Lewy bodies are characteristic of this condition, the term "Lewy body PD" is sometimes used synonymously with "idiopathic PD." Idiopathic PD is also characterized, from a neuropathological standpoint, by the absence of neurofibrillary tangles (NFTs) in the brain stem. NFTs are, instead, characteristic of postencephalitic parkinsonism. Clinically, PD is characterized by motor symptoms including tremor, akinesia, rigidity, and loss of postural reflexes (2). Mental status changes were originally said to be absent in PD but, as pointed out in a recent review (3), many authors think that dementia is a frequent (30–50%) feature of the disease. Furthermore, although the mental status changes in PD have not always been described in detail, recent studies (3) have indicated that the dementia found in PD patients is similar in its qualitative aspects, as well as its course and progression, to the dementia of AD.

Until recently, the possible pathological basis of this dementia had received little attention. The first suggestion that there might be cortical changes in a sizeable percentage of

PD patients can probably be found in the neuroradiological studies of Svennilson and associates (4), who demonstrated cerebral atrophy by pneumoencephalography in a sizeable percentage of PD candidates for thalamotomy. This was later confirmed by other pneumoencephalographic studies (5, 6) as well as by CT scan studies (7).

Cortical atrophy has also been noticed on autopsy studies. Alvord (8), while reviewing the neuropathology of idiopathic (Lewy body type) PD, pointed out that this cortical atrophy in PD is probably greater than one would expect for an individual of the same age; he also recalled the observation of Woodard (9) showing that many patients with Lewy bodies (many of whom did not have "parkinsonism," i.e., clinical signs of PD) also had histological evidence of AD as shown by increased granulovacuolar degeneration. Alvord concluded "exactly how the correlation will work out with those who have parkinsonism and Lewy bodies remains to be seen, but one can predict that many will have Alzheimer's disease" (8 [p. 133]). It can therefore be stated that Alvord was the first to hypothesize that demented PD patients may also have AD.

In a later study, which included material from both Seattle and Palo Alto, Alvord and collaborators (10) studied "cerebral cortical degeneration"—an index based on the presence of typical AD changes, i.e., NFTs, senile plaques (SPs), and granulovacuolar degeneration (GVD)—in PD patients. They first pointed out that PD patients were more demented, on average, than age-matched controls without PD. They also noted that in Lewy body PD, the degree of parkinsonism is correlated with the degree of neuronal loss in the substantia nigra, while the degree of dementia correlates with the degree of cerebral cortical degeneration.

A review of the literature suggests that, in the years that followed the work of Alvord and his colleagues, several neuropathologists were aware of the association between PD and AD. For example, Victor (11), discussing a paper presented at a symposium on AD (12), mentioned that at least one-third of PD patients who come to autopsy have lesions "characteristic of AD." Others, however, continue to think that the association between PD and AD is only chance. Several groups of researchers, however, have attempted to throw some light on this controversy (13–20).

In a letter to the editor of the Lancet, Hakim and Mathieson (16) pointed out that during the autopsy of a patient with PD and progressive dementia, they found changes in the brain characteristic of both PD and AD. This prompted them to perform a retrospective review of the brains of 21 cases of PD and an equal number of appropriately matched controls. They found that histological features indistinguishable from those of AD were more common in the brains of patients with PD than in the brains of age-matched controls. In particular, SPs were seen in 20 out of 21 cases of PD, and in only 4 out of 21 of the controls, while NFTs were seen in, respectively, 18 PD patients and 6 controls.

In an article that appeared the following year, Hakim and Mathieson (17) further detailed their finding in 34 consecutive cases of patients with idiopathic PD, compared to an equal number of controls matched for sex and age, who showed neither traumatic nor vascular pathology. Clinical data concerning presence or absence of dementia, as well as type and amount of medications taken, and type and severity of symptoms were abstracted from the hospital charts. They found that 19 of the 34 cases of PD (56%) had clinical evidence of mental symptoms ranging from fading memory and mild confusion to clear-cut dementia. It is interesting to note that very few of their patients had received L-Dopa, presumably because most of the cases had died before L-Dopa came into wide clinical use. Four of the 34 (12%) patients had had a pneumoencephalogram; all four were demented, and in all four cases cerebral atrophy had been noted. Only 6% of the controls had clinical evidence of dementia.

On neuropathological examination they found histological features indistinguishable from AD in a very high number of PD cases (33 out of 34 patients with PD). These consisted of SPs in the hippocampus, found in 29 out of the 34 cases of PD (87%) and in 5 out of the 34 controls (15%); of NFTs, found in the hippocampus of 29 PD patients and 7 controls; and of granulovacuolar changes, found in the hippocampal neurons in 88% of PD cases and 21% of the controls. In addition, 15 control cases and 27 PD cases were thought to show some neuronal cell loss in their cortex. As indicated, only one PD case appeared free of all the neuropathological changes usually associated with AD. No attempt was made to correlate the presence and severity of dementia with the presence and severity of Alzheimer-type changes in the neocortex.

In a study performed independently, Boller and associates (14, 15) studied patients who had died with a pathological diagnosis of PD at Case Western Reserve University Hospital (Cleveland, Ohio) and at the hospital of the University of Pennsylvania (Philadelphia, Pennsylvania) between the years 1963 and 1978. Out of a total of 10,585 autopsies performed during that time, 36 cases with adequate samples from the cerebral cortex and midbrain were included in the study. Pathological specimens and clinical records were reviewed independently. The clinical data were ascertained from the clinical charts on the basis of mental status examination by house officers and staff, and by notes of nurses and other health personnel. Particular attention was paid to (1) alertness, attention, appearance, affect, and orientation for place and time; (2) language and language-related functions, including writing; (3) calculating and constructional abilities; (4) immediate memory (digit span), recent memory (ability to learn new material), and long-term memory for past events; (5) "abstracting" abilities (explanation of similarities and differences, ability to interpret proverbs); and (6) insight. On the basis of their performance, patients were subdivided into those with normal mental status, mild dementia, and severe dementia.

The pathological diagnosis was based on the examination of at least four sections obtained at autopsy from the cerebral cortex (including the hippocampus) after they had been appropriately stained. The density of SPs was determined independently by three investigators in ten consecutive randomly chosen fields. The number of NFTs was recorded separately for allocortex and neocortex. The following changes were considered consistent with the histopathological diagnosis of AD: (1) presence of more than one senile plaque in combination with neocortical NFTs; (2) more than ten SPs in the absence of neocortical NFTs; and (3) ten or more neocortical NFTs in the absence of SPs. The diagnosis of AD was made only when one of these changes was associated with dementia.

Out of the 36 patients, only 29 had records sufficiently detailed to establish their mental status. Nine of the patients had severe dementia. Detailed examination of their higher cortical functions showed that the nine patients had a rather consistent mental status profile. Their ability to sustain attention was normal or mildly decreased. Responses tended to be slow. Affect was often labile but there was no elation or severe depression. Orientation for time and place was invariably impaired. Speech was usually abnormal, showing the characteristic hypokinetic dysarthria of PD. Although no true aphasia was noted, some patients had problems naming uncommon objects and comprehending complex sentences. When writing was legible, sentences were found to be orthographically and syntactically correct. Oral and written calculations, as well as drawing or copying of simple forms, were consistently impaired. Ability to recall recent events was severely disrupted; immediate memory (digit span) and the ability to recall past events were moderately affected. Ability to state similarities and differences was moderately impaired but proverb interpretation was often correct. Most patients were appropriately aware of their motor and cognitive disabilities.

There were also seven patients who had mild dementia. All had slow responses, mild disorientation, and impaired memory for recent events. Performance on other tests was adequate. It was felt that the performance of these patients resembled more "benign senescent forgetfulness" (21, 22) than true dementia. Mental status in the remaining 13 patients was normal except, in most cases, for slower responses.

On neuropathological examination, 15 of the 36 patients (41%) had histological changes compatible with the neuropathological diagnosis of AD. All nine patients with severe dementia, and three of the seven patients with mild dementia, had pathological changes consistent with AD. Of the 13 patients with normal mental status, 3 (23%) showed histological changes characteristic of AD. Another noticeable feature was that while the age of onset, age of death, and severity of PD did not differ significantly between patients with and those without AD, survival was significantly shorter for those with severe dementia and AD than for those with normal mental status and no AD.

A survey of autopsies performed in the same period (1963–1978) in the hospitals of Case Western Reserve University and the University of Pennsylvania in individuals of an age comparable to the PD population showed that 161 patients had dementia and histological changes consistent with a diagnosis AD. This corresponds to a prevalence of AD in this age-matched population of 5.1%, which is six times lower and statistically different from that found among the PD patients (33.0%). The prevalence of PD in the same population was 1.19%.

Another recent study has examined the possible role of subcortical structures in the dementia of PD (20). It was found that demented PD patients show a marked neuronal cell loss in the nucleus basalis of Meynert, a structure known to be affected in AD patients. Nondemented idiopathic PD patients showed only a slight cell loss.

As can be seen from the preceding review, there is considerable evidence drawn from neuropathological and clinical studies (ref. 18 and Chap. 38 of this volume) suggesting that a sizeable number of PD patients demonstrate clinical and neuropathological changes indistinguishable from AD.

CLINICAL AND NEUROPATHOLOGICAL FEATURES OF PD IN PATIENTS WITH AD

The above studies present strong evidence in favor of an association between PD and AD. As far as the incidence of PD-like symptoms in patients with AD is concerned, numerous clinicians have made remarks concerning the frequent development of "extrapyramidal" features resembling PD in AD patients. This includes the report by Drachman and Stahl (23); Parkes and associates (24); Pearce (25); Sjögren and associates (26); and Pomara and associates (27). The latter report points out that the majority of AD patients do not display all the extrapyramidal symptoms and signs normally associated with PD, and that even AD patients who show some parkinsonian traits tend only to develop a mild picture. From the point of view of neuropathology, we have already alluded to the findings of Woodard (9), who stated that Lewy bodies could be found in 10% of 96 brains of patients who showed neuropathological features of AD. In a control group of 77 persons of comparable age without dementia or PD symptoms, Lewy bodies had not been identified in any individual.

A few reports of AD patients in whom Lewy bodies were found at autopsy have been published (28, 29); however, in many of those cases the presence of PD symptoms was either not stated or was specifically noted as absent.

It must be pointed out that the association between PD and AD is not universally accepted. Several clinical studies of PD have argued that dementia may be an infrequent occurrence. The recent paper by Matthews and Haaland (30) exemplifies such a position; several older papers have come to the same conclusion (for a review, see ref. 3). From the point of view of neuropathology, Heston (31) has recently reviewed the file of 2,204 autopsies performed in the Minnesota State Hospital system. Among all the autopsied patients, he studied in some detail 304 who had a diagnosis of primary dementia. He studied neuropathology reports and reviewed the actual neuropathological material (tissue in paraffin blocks) "in any questionable cases." Among those patients were 12 cases with PD. In the same autopsy survey, Heston noticed that there were 18 cases of idiopathic PD in which dementia was not prominent. He stated that SPs and NFTs characteristic of AD were found in a neuropathological examination of the probands in about the numbers expected, given the age of the subjects, and therefore denied that pathological changes similar to AD are found in a significant percentage of patients with PD.

It could be argued that the negative findings of clinical studies such as that of Matthews and Haaland (30) are due to a bias in patient selection, since that report was based on an outpatient population. Similarly, one could state that some other negative clinical studies (for a review, see ref. 3) were performed at a time when not much attention was being paid to the presence of dementia. Finally, there is now a longer survival in patients with PD due to improved medical care and the introduction of dopaminergic drugs. The negative neuropathological findings of Heston (31) may be explained by the fact that apparently no special stains were made to seek SPs or NFTs. Certainly one can conclude that at present the issue remains controversial.

IMPLICATIONS OF THE ASSOCIATION BETWEEN AD AND PD

Should future studies confirm the association of the two diseases, very little is known about the reason they should be thus associated. The exceptional occurrence of SPs and NFTs in processes such as Pick's disease or Huntington's disease indicates that AD cannot be considered a nonspecific complication of chronic degenerative diseases. Hakim and Mathieson (17) noted that failure of the dopaminergic system in nigrostriatal pathways in PD is well established, and similarly, it is known that enzymes related to acetylcholine metabolism are diminished in the brains of patients with AD, especially in the cerebral cortex. Those two systems appear linked since some neurons in the caudate and putamen are cholinergic, and acetylcholinesterase is present in the dopaminergic neurons of the substantia nigra, caudate nucleus, and putamen. In addition, animal studies (17a) show that nigrostriatal dopaminergic neurons form direct inhibitory synapses on cholinergic intraneurons of the striatum, so that a defective dopaminergic system, as in PD, may cause overactivity of the cholinergic system.

No matter what the reason is for the association between PD and AD, it appears that there are two distinct forms of PD, the first being characterized clinically by the association of PD symptoms with severe dementia, and pathologically by the presence of subcortical PD changes, and cortical changes consistent with AD; in the second, pathological changes are limited to the basal ganglia, and patients do not exhibit dementia. This conclusion has been reached independently by Lieberman and co-workers (18) on the basis of clinical data, and by Boller and co-workers (15) on the basis of neuropathological studies.

A recent article attempted to provide a unifying hypothesis for the cause of amyotrophic lateral sclerosis, PD and AD (13). The article does not review the overlap between these diseases or the cases in which more than one of the two conditions is associated. It argues, however, that "each of the three conditions is due to lack of a disorder-specific neurotrophic hormone which could be elaborated or stored in the target of the affected neurons." It would be released by the postsynaptic cell and then exert its effects in a retrograde fashion after being taken up by the presynaptic terminal. In the lower motor neuron syndromes of amyotrophic lateral sclerosis, failure of muscle cells to release the appropriate motor neurotrophic hormone would result in impaired function of anterior horn cells. In PD, the neurotrophic failure would be characterized by inability of striatal cells to provide the required dopamine neurotrophic hormone, with resulting impairment of substantia nigra cells. In AD, the abnormality would lie in failure of the hippocampus and cortical cells to supply the relevant cholinergic neurotrophic hormone, with resulting impairment of medial septal and nucleus basalis neurons. As Appel (13) points out, aside from nerve growth factor, no neurotrophic hormones have been identified and purified so far. His theory, however, appears eminently testable and could lead to rational therapy of these diseases.

Finally, Rossor (19) recently pointed out that, from a neuropathological and biochemical standpoint, AD and PD seem to share several features: they both show a loss of ascending projections (respectively, cholinergic cortical projections in AD; dopaminergic striatal projections in PD) and they both show a loss of noradrenergic projections from the locus ceruleus. The cells of the locus ceruleus, of the substantia nigra, as well as of other structures involved in AD and PD (substantia innominata and septal nuclei) show a similar organization of their connections: these connections (dendrites) appear to be uniform, with extensive generalized intermingling of axons and dendrites, which contrasts with the highly specialized dendritic configuration of other cerebral structures. It has been postulated that structures including cells with generalized connections ("isodendritic") may belong to a system (so-called isodendritic core) that extends from the spinal cord to the forebrain (for a review, see ref. 32). Rossor (19) hypothesized that PD and AD may both represent a disorder of the isodendritic core and may therefore be seen as different parts of a continuous spectrum. This hypothesis led Rossor to several interesting implications. One could predict that in both AD and PD, loss of cells could be observed in other portions of the isodendritic core such as the reticular formation of the spinal cord, the raphe nuclei, the hypothalamus, and the intralaminar thalamic nuclei. Furthermore, this hypothesis raises the possibility that replacement treatment with appropriate neurotransmitters could delay secondary cell loss.

CONCLUSION

This chapter has shown that many data suggest that AD and PD are indeed associated, not by chance, but by a common pathogenetic mechanism. One would conclude that a useful direction for future research would be to pay considerable attention to this association in epidemiological or neuropathological study of either condition. At the present time, both disorders are of undetermined etiology and any clue that might explain the occurrence of one of the two conditions might be used in furthering our understanding of the other.

ACKNOWLEDGMENTS

Research supported in part by the Veterans Administration Medical Research Council.

REFERENCES

1. Greenfield JG, Bosanquet FD: The brainstem lesions in parkinsonism. *J Neurol Neurosurg Psychiatry* 1953; 16:213–226.

2. Klawans HL, Kramer J: The movement disorders: diseases of the basal ganglia, in Rosenberg RN (ed): *Neurology,* New York, Grune & Stratton, 1980, pp 266–296.

3. Boller F: Mental status of patients with Parkinson disease. *J Clin Neuropsychol* 1980; 2:157–172.

4. Svennilson E, Torvik A, Lowe R, et al: Treatment of parkinsonism by stereotactic thermo-lesions in the pallidal region. *Acta Psychiatr Neurol Scand* 1960; 35:358–377.

5. Gath I, Jorgensen A, Sjaastad O, et al: Pneumoencephalographic findings in parkinsonism. *Arch Neurol* 1975; 32:769–773.

6. Selby G: Cerebral atrophy in parkinsonism. *J Neurol Sci* 1968; 6:517–559.

7. Schneider E, Fischer PA, Jacobi H, et al: The significance of cerebral atrophy for the symptomatology of Parkinson's disease. *J Neurol Sci* 1979; 42:187–197.

8. Alvord EC: The pathology of parkinsonism: II. An interpretation, with special reference to other changes in the aging brain. *Recent Adv Parkinson's Dis* 1971; 8:131–161.

9. Woodward JS: Concentric hyaline inclusion body formation in mental disease: analysis of 27 cases. *J Neuropathol Exp Neurol* 1962; 21:442–469.

10. Alvord EC, Forno LS, Kusske JA, et al: The pathology of parkinsonism: a comparison of degeneration in cerebral cortex and brainstem. *Adv Neurol* 1974; 5:175–193.

11. Victor M: Discussion of "subcortical dementia." *Aging NY* 1978; 7:194.

12. Katzman R, Terry R, Bick KL (eds): *Aging NY* 1978; 7.

13. Appel SH: A unifying hypothesis for the cause of amyotrophic lateral sclerosis, parkinsonism, and Alzheimer disease. *Ann Neurol* 1981; 10:499–505.

14. Boller F, Mizutani T, Ruessmann R, et al: The dementia of Parkinson's disease (PD): clinical-pathological correlation (abstr). *Neurology* 1979; 29:508.

15. Boller, F, Mizutani T, Ruessmann R, et al: Parkinson disease, dementia, and Alzheimer disease: clinicopathological correlations. *Ann Neurol* 1980; 7:329–335.

16. Hakim AM, Mathieson G: Basis of dementia in Parkinson's disease. *Lancet* 1978; ii:729.

17. Hakim AM, Mathieson G: Dementia in Parkinson disease: neuropathologic study. *Neurology* 1979; 29:1209–1214.

17a. McGeer PL, Hattori T, Singh VK, et al: Cholinergic systems in extrapyramidal function, in Yahr MD (ed): *The Basal Ganglia.* New York, Raven, 1976, pp 213–222.

18. Liberman A, Dziatolowski M, Kupersmith M, et al: Dementia in Parkinson disease. *Ann Neurol* 1979; 6:335–359.

19. Rossor NN: Parkinson's disease and Alzheimer's disease as disorders of the isodendritic core. *Br Med J* 1981; 283:1588–1590.

20. Whitehouse PJ, Hedreen JC, White CL III, et al: Basal forebrain neurons in the dementia of Parkinson disease. *Ann Neurol* 1983; 13:243–248.

21. Kral VA: Benign senescent forgetfulness. *Aging NY* 1978; 7:47–51.

22. Kral VA, Dorken H: Comparative psychological study of hyperkinetic and akinetic extrapyramidal disorders. *Arch Neurol Psychiatry* 1951; 66:431–442.

23. Drachman DA, Stahl S: Extrapyramidal dementia and levodopa. *Lancet* 1975; i:809.

24. Parkes JD, Marsden CD, Rees JE, et al: Parkinson's disease, cerebral arteriosclerosis, and senile dementia. *Q J Med* 1974; 43:49–61.

25. Pearce J: The extrapyramidal disorder of Alzheimer's disease. *Eur Neurol* 1974; 12:94–103.

26. Sjögren T, Sjögren H, Lindgren AGH: Morbus Alzheimer and Morbus Pick: a genetic, clinical, and pathoanatomical study. *Acta Psychiatr Neurol Scand Suppl* 1952; 82:1–152.

27. Pomara N, Reisberg, R, Albers S, et al: Extrapyramidal symptoms in patients with primary degenerative dementia. *J Clin Psychopharmacol* 1981; 1:398–400.

28. Forno LS, Barbour PJ, Norville RL: Presenile dementia with Lewy bodies and neurofibrillary tangles. *Arch Neurol* 1978; 35:818–822.

29. Rosenblum WI, Ghatak NR: Lewy bodies in the presence of Alzheimer's disease. *Arch Neuro* 1979; 35:170–171.

30. Matthews CG, Haaland KY: The effect of symptom duration on cognitive and motor performance in parkinsonism. *Neurology* 1979; 29:251–256.

31. Heston LL: Genetic studies of dementia, in Mortimer J, Schuman F (eds): *The Epidemiology of Dementia*. New York, Oxford University Press, 1981, pp 101–114.

32. Ramon-Moliner E: Specialized and generalized dendritic patterns, in Santini M (ed): *Golgi Centennial Symposium Proceedings*. New York, Raven, 1975, pp 87–100.

38 Parkinsonian Dementia and Alzheimer's Dementia:
Clinical and Epidemiological Associations

ABRAHAM N. LIEBERMAN

PARKINSON'S DISEASE (PD) IS A CHRONIC DISORDER of the central nervous system (CNS) of variable progression and severity. The annual incidence rate of PD is approximately 20 per 100,000 population, and the prevalence rate is approximately 200 per 100,000 (1). Clinically, the disease is characterized by rigidity, a resting tremor, bradykinesia, and gait disorder (2). There may also be speech impairment, dysphagia, sialorrhea, seborrhea, orthostatic hypotension, and urinary incontinence. Not all of these features are necessarily present in a particular individual. Pathologically, the disease is characterized by degeneration of the pigmented neurons in the substantia nigra and, to a lesser degree, degeneration of the neurons in the caudate nucleus, the putamen, and the globus pallidus.

A large body of human and animal experimentation has demonstrated that a decrease of dopamine in the nigra and the striatum is specific for PD and is responsible for the clinical symptomatology (3). Repletion of striatal dopamine, through the administration of its immediate precursor levodopa, has significantly altered the course of the disease (4). While levodopa treatment does not halt disease progression, treated patients live, on average, 3 more years; they no longer die early in the disease of complications of immobility (5).

Originally, dementia was not associated with PD, but recently there has been a growing awareness of their association. It should be noted, however, that many other kinds of mental changes besides dementia may occur among PD patients. Some of these changes consist of minor disturbances in memory or cognition, disturbances that may be no different from those in other elderly individuals (6). Some of the mental changes consist of drug related episodic confusional states (7–10); some relate to the depression that frequently accompanies PD (11, 12) and some are frank dementias. The depression often associated with PD is considered an integral part of the disease, and it has been postulated that losses of central monoamines predispose these patients to depression.

PREVALENCE OF DEMENTIA IN PARKINSON'S DISEASE

The prevalence of dementia among PD patients as reported in the literature ranges between 20% and 80% (13–18). There are several explanations for these disparate rates: one is that the population of surveyed PD patients with dementia is not representative of the general population of PD patients. Thus, higher prevalence rates for dementia would be expected from studies surveying PD patients from chronic disease hospitals, as opposed to those surveying PD patients from outpatient clinics. Another explanation is that in some series, all PD patients exhibit some mental changes and are conveniently regarded as demented. Thus, higher prevalence rates for dementia would be expected in studies failing to distinguish dementia from drug induced organic confusional syndromes or failing to distinguish between dementia and the mild disturbances in mentation that accompany depression. Cognizant of the aforementioned pitfalls, several recent studies have been undertaken to determine the prevalence of dementia in PD.

Marttila and Rinne (15) studied dementia in a PD population consisting of all traceable patients in a defined geographical area. The prevalence of dementia in that study was found to be 129 patients in a population of 444 (29%). Martin and associates (13), in a survey of 100 patients referred for levodopa treatment, found that 23 of the patients exhibited moderate to severe dementia. Lieberman and associates (16) studied dementia in a group of 520 PD patients attending an outpatient clinic at the New York University Medical Center (NYUMC). Dementia was defined, for the purposes of the NYUMC study, as a permanent change in cognition, abstraction, reasoning, judgment, and memory. Assessment of all patients included an evaluation of recent and long-term memory, and of higher intellectual functions including tasks of orientation, general information, spelling, digit span backward, addition, subtraction, interpretation of proverbs, similarities, and word definitions. Patients with a dementia ascribable to alcoholism, drug ingestion, craniocerebral trauma, vascular disease, multiple cerebral infarcts, or illness other than PD were excluded. Patients who showed transient breakdowns under stress, experienced nocturnal confusion, or showed impairment on no more than two tasks of higher intellectual function were considered to have mild dementia. Patients experiencing confusion, disabling impairment of memory, or performance errors on more than three tasks of higher intellectual function were considered to have moderate dementia. Patients unable to recognize familiar places, and to act or speak coherently were considered to have advanced dementia. Along with the 520 test subjects were 470 living spouses who served as age-matched controls, also assessed for dementia.

Among the 520 PD patients, we found that 168 (32%) showed moderate or advanced dementia. Although the demented patients were older than the nondemented patients (70.5 versus 65.5 years), dementia was ten times more prevalent among PD patients than among the controls. Conversely, the prevalence of moderate to advanced dementia among the controls was similar to that reported for other populations of the same age (19). In addition to being older than the nondemented PD subjects, the demented patients developed PD at a later age, and had the PD for a shorter period of time. In 19 patients (11%) the dementia antedated the PD. Atypical parkinsonian features, amyotrophy, cerebellar outflow tremor, and pyramidal tract signs, were equally frequent among demented and nondemented PD patients. There was no difference in the prevalence of dementia between the 459 patients treated with levodopa and the 61 who were not so treated. But, among the levodopa treated PD patients, the demented PD patients improved less. While 56 of the 153 demented patients (37%) treated with levodopa developed reversible mental changes, 17 of the 306 nondemented patients (6%) developed some degree of reversible mental changes. And while 42 of the 168 demented patients (25%) were noticeably depressed (requiring psychiatric consultation, medication, or electroconvulsive therapy), fully 107 of the 306 nondemented patients (33%) were comparably depressed.

In a similar study involving PD outpatients, Sroka and colleagues (18) found that 26 of 93 PD patients (28%) were also demented. In this study, all patients had computed tomography (CT) scans; the scans were compared with age-matched controls without PD or dementia. In this situation, 100% of all PD patients with dementia had abnormal CT scans, while only 37% of the PD patients without dementia, and 44% of the controls, had abnormal scans. Among the PD patients with dementia, 92% of the abnormal scans showed cerebral atrophy consisting of both ventricular and sulcal enlargement (40%), sulcal enlargement only (40%), or ventricular enlargement only (12%). Only 8% of the abnormal scans showed cerebral infarction. These findings suggest that PD patients with dementia are more likely to have cerebral atrophy. The converse is not true, however, and the presence of cerebral atrophy does not necessarily indicate dementia (18, 20). In this study, unlike the NYUMC study, there was a higher prevalence of dementia among patients with atypical parkinsonian features as compared to patients with typical parkinsonian features.

The foregoing seems to establish that dementia is frequently associated with PD. From these studies, however, it is not clear whether all patients who develop PD are at risk for developing dementia or whether the group who develops PD and dementia represents a distinct subset of the PD population. From the cited data and other corroborative literature two separate groups of PD patients can be extrapolated with some degree of confidence: one, a younger group, with an exclusive motor disorder having a longer and more benign course plus a better response to levodopa, and the second, an older group, with a motor-followed by a cognitive disorder, with both a more fulminant course and a poorer response to levodopa. The clinical overlap between these two groups is such that one cannot reliably predict who will become demented.

RELATIONSHIP BETWEEN PARKINSON'S DISEASE WITH DEMENTIA AND ALZHEIMER'S DISEASE

Hakim and Mathieson (21) reviewed the clinical and necropsy data on 34 PD patients, and noted that 19 (56%) had some degree of dementia compared to 2 (6%) in age- and sex-matched controls. These authors also noted that the incidence of histological features indistinguishable from Alzheimer's disease (AD) was considerably higher in PD patients than in controls. Thus, only one of the 34 PD patients (3%) appeared wholly free of the histological changes of AD, compared to 12 of the controls (35%).

Alvord and colleagues (22), on the other hand, defined two groups of PD patients. In one group, there was a correlation between the degree of neuronal loss in the nigra and the severity of the motor symptoms. In the second group, there was more cortical degeneration and less nigral degeneration. The clinical and pathological features of the second group more closely resembled AD, and there was less of a correlation between the degree of neuronal loss in the nigra and severity of motor symptoms. Boller and associates (17) reviewed the clinical and necropsy data on 29 patients with idiopathic PD. These researchers found that 16 patients (55%) had some degree of dementia with AD-related pathological features of senile plaques (SPs) and neurofibrillary tangles (NFTs). Boller and associates also suggested that there may be two forms of PD: one form with neuropathological changes limited to the basal ganglia and no dementia; the second with the basal ganglia changes of PD and cortical changes of AD, characterized by the association of motor symptoms and dementia.

The patients with PD and dementia may be, in fact, part of a spectrum of degenerative disorders (23–25). Thus, Pearce (23) investigated 65 unselected patients referred to a neurological unit of a general hospital with an organic dementia and noted that 40 (62%) showed parkinsonian features. Pearce suggested that, just as mental changes may develop among patients with PD, so parkinsonian features may develop among patients with AD. Pearce suggested that there may be a cortical (supranuclear) pathway of importance in regulating dopamine at a lower level in the basal ganglia, and that this supranuclear type of basal ganglia dysfunction is responsible for the parkinsonian features in patients with AD.

There is controversy as to whether the mental changes seen among PD patients are related to basal ganglia and brain stem (subcortical) or cortical changes. Thus, Albert and co-workers (26) differentiated the subcortical dementias from the cortical dementias by the preservation of language-dependent activities and perceptual skills in the subcortical dementias. Albert and co-workers noted the presence of a subcortical dementia among patients with progressive supranuclear palsy (PSP), a disorder with parkinsonian features, a preponderance of pathological changes in the brain stem and basal ganglia, and relative sparing of the cortex. These investigators hypothesized that the mental changes of PSP were a consequence of the pathological changes in the subcortical region. While the dementia of PD has many clinical features in common with the dementia of PSP, because of the occurrence in PD of pathological changes in both cortical and subcortical regions, the dementia of PD cannot be attributed solely to the subcortical changes.

DIFFERENTIAL DIAGNOSIS

Parkinson's disease with dementia should be distinguished from a number of conditions.

THE LACUNAR STATE

The lacunar state, a clinical syndrome associated with mental changes, pseudobulbar palsy and a gait disorder may be seen in patients with hypertensive or diabetic vascular disease (27). Pathologically, the brains of these patients contain lacunas, multiple irregular small cavities, from 0.5–15.0 mm in size, distributed bilaterally throughout the brain stem, basal ganglia, and internal capsule. Lacunas result from occlusion of small penetrating arteries. In most patients, while individual lesions do not cause recognizable symptoms and signs, cumulatively they may produce a picture which can be mistaken for PD. Indeed, so striking is the resemblance that, in the past, many patients with the lacunar state were thought to be parkinsonian on the basis of their vascular disease, the so called "arterio-sclerotic parkinsonism." Vascular disease is not now felt to be a cause of parkinsonism and the term "arteriosclerotic PD" has been abandoned. The lacunar state may be differentiated from PD by the steplike onset of symptoms in the lacunar state, and by the lack of symptom response to levodopa. When steplike symptom onset is absent, or when PD coexists with the lacunar state (both being not infrequent disorders of aging) then differentiating between the two states is impossible.

BRAIN TUMORS

Brain tumors rarely present with only extrapyramidal symptoms. Sciarra and Sprofkin (28) were able to find only 12 out of 474 patients (2.5%) with brain tumors who presented with only extrapyramidal symptoms. Indeed, most basal ganglia tumors are asymptomatic until they result in ventricular obstructions with signs of increased intracranial pressure.

However, a mass lesion (not necessarily arising in the basal ganglia) should be suspected in any parkinsonian patient with a relatively rapid course (several weeks to months), particularly if the symptoms are associated with other symptoms of a mass lesion: headaches, drowsiness, seizures. Computed tomography (CT) with intravenous infusion of iodinated contrast is mandatory in such patients.

PROGRESSIVE SUPRANUCLEAR PALSY

PSP is a disorder characterized by supranuclear ophthalmoplegia, pseudobulbar palsy, dysarthria, rigidity, dystonia of the neck, and dementia (29). Early in the disease, if the eye findings are not well developed, PSP may be mistaken for PD with dementia.

RIGID FORM OF HUNTINGTON'S DISEASE

On rare occasions, Huntington's disease (HD) may present with rigidity and bradykinesia. Although the rigid form is more commonly seen in children, it does appear in adults. Thus, among 50 adult patients with HD examined by us, only one (2%) had the rigid form (30). A family history of HD is essential for differentiating the rigid form of HD from PD with dementia.

STRIATONIGRAL DEGENERATION

Striatonigral degeneration (SND) is a disorder characterized by rigidity, tremor, bradykinesia, and a gait disturbance which is clinically indistinguishable from PD (31). Pathologically, the disorder is characterized by a preponderance of changes in the striatum, with relatively fewer changes in the substantia nigra, the inverse of the situation in PD. Interest in this disorder has grown because patients with SND do not respond to levodopa.

NORMAL-PRESSURE HYDROCEPHALUS

Normal-pressure hydrocephalus (NPH) was originally described by Adams and colleagues (32), who reported three cases of dementia and a gait disturbance resembling PD associated with enlarged ventricles under normal cerebrospinal fluid pressure. There was improvement in both dementia and gait disturbance after ventricular shunting. The clinical features and the radiological and isotropic criteria necessary to make the diagnosis have been reviewed by several authors, but there is controversy as to the specificity of these criteria. Clinically, dementia is the most prominent symptom in NPH, and it may range from relatively mild mental changes to severe psychomotor retardation resembling akinetic mutism; the dementia usually develops at a relatively rapid pace. The gait disturbance may appear before or after the onset of dementia and varies from a shuffling parkinsonian gait with short steps and difficulty in initiating movements, to an inability to lift either foot and walk normally: "a magnetic gait." Deep tendon reflexes are brisk and pyramidal tract signs may be present. Most patients with NPH are incontinent of urine. Normal-pressure hydrocephalus may be differentiated from PD by the response of NPH patients to shunting, or by the response (of PD patients) to levodopa. It should be noted, however, that while many patients meet all the criteria of NPH, only a few benefit from ventricular shunting.

RELATIONSHIP OF PARKINSON'S DISEASE WITH DEMENTIA TO THE PARKINSONISM-DEMENTIA COMPLEX OF GUAM

The parkinsonism-dementia complex is confined to the Chamorros of the Island of Guam (33, 34). The Guam parkinsonism-dementia complex begins early, the average age of onset being 54 years (the range is 32–77 years), and it involves males more than females in a 2 to 1 ratio; it is characterized by an invariably fatal course beginning with a progressive dementia followed by extrapyramidal dysfunction. Not infrequently, the Guam parkinsonism-dementia complex is associated with a neurological picture indistinguishable from amyotrophic lateral sclerosis (ALS). Guam parkinsonism-dementia, Guam parkinsonism-dementia with ALS, and Guam ALS (without clinical parkinsonism) occurs with high frequency among the Chamorros (up to 15% of the population). Neuropathological studies of 48 ALS and 45 parkinsonism-dementia patients showed that in addition to the lesions of classical ALS, all 48 Guam ALS patients had histological features of PD in varying degrees of severity, although not all clinically manifested parkinsonism, and 17 of the 45 parkinsonism-dementia patients had additional histological features of ALS, although—again—not all clinically manifested ALS. This unique confluence of three degenerative processes: dementia, extrapyramidal dysfunction, and amyotrophy strongly suggests that a single process may underlie them all. Guam parkinsonism-dementia ALS complex to a certain extent resembles some cases of Creutzfeldt–Jakob disease, a disorder known to be caused by a slow virus (see Chap. 39).

MANAGEMENT

There is no specific therapy for the dementia associated with PD. Moreover, PD patients with dementia tolerate all antiparkinsonian drugs poorly—frequently developing, in addition to their dementia, a toxic confusional syndrome: delusions, hallucinations, and aggressive behavior. The toxic confusional syndrome, but not the dementia, is reversible upon discontinuing the drug. Any antiparkinsonian drug should be used cautiously (and at a lower dose) in a demented parkinsonian patient; the physician must make a careful judgment as to whether the improvement in mobility in the patient secondary to the use of the drug is commensurate with the increased risk of the patient's developing a toxic confusional syndrome.

REFERENCES

1. Kurland LT, Kurtzhe JF, Goldberg ID, et al: Parkinsonism, in Kurland LT, Kurtzhe JF, Goldberg ID (eds): *Epidemiology of Neurologic and Sense Organ Disorders*. Cambridge, Harvard University Press, 1973, pp 41–63.

2. Lieberman A: Parkinson's disease: a clinical review. *Am J Med Sci* 1974; 267:66–80.

3. Bernheimer J, Birkmayer W, Hornykiewicz O, et al: Brain dopamine and the syndromes of parkinsonism and Huntington. *J Neurol Sci* 1973; 20:415–455.

4. Cotzias GC, Papavasiliou PS, Gellene R: Modification of parkinsonism: chronic treatment with L-dopa. *N Engl J Med* 1969; 280:337–345.

5. Yahr MD: Evaluation of long-term therapy in Parkinson's disease: mortality and therapeutic efficacy, in Birkmayer W, Hornykiewicz O (eds): *Advances in Parkinsonism.* Basel, Roche, 1976, pp 435–443.

6. Loranger AW, Goodell H, McDowell F: Intellectual impairment in Parkinson's syndrome. *Brain* 1972; 95:402–412.

7. Goodwin FK: Psychiatric side effects of levodopa on man. *JAMA* 1971; 218:1915–1920.

8. Jenkins RB, Groh RH: Mental symptoms in parkinsonian patients treated with L-dopa. *Lancet* 1970; ii:177–180.

9. Sacks OW, Kohl MS, Messeloff CR: Effects of levodopa in parkinsonian patients with dementia. *Neurology* 1972; 22:516–519.

10. Sweet RD, McDowell H, Feigenson JS: Mental symptoms in Parkinson's disease during treatment with levodopa. *Neurology* 1976; 26:305–310.

11. Mindham RHS: Psychiatric symptoms in parkinsonism. *J Neurol Neurosurg Psychiatry* 1966; 33:188–368.

12. Mayeux R, Stern Y, Rosen J, et al: Depression, intellectual impairment, and Parkinson disease. *Neurology* 1981; 31:645–650.

13. Martin WE, Lowenson RB, Resch JA: Parkinson's disease: clinical analysis of 100 patients. *Neurology* 1973; 23:783–790.

14. Pollock M, Hornabrook RW: The prevalence, natural history, and dementia of Parkinson's disease. *Brain* 1966; 89:429–448.

15. Marttila RJ, Rinne UK: Dementia in Parkinson's disease. *Acta Neurol Scand* 1976; 54:431–441.

16. Lieberman A, Dziatolowski M, Kupersmith M: Dementia in Parkinson disease. *Ann Neurol* 1979; 6:355–359.

17. Boller F, Mizutani T, Roessmann, U, et al: Parkinson disease, dementia, and Alzheimer disease: clinico-pathological correlations. *Ann Neurol* 1980; 7:329–335.

18. Sroka H, Elizan TS, Yahr MD, et al: Organic mental syndrome and confusional states in Parkinson's disease: relationship to computerized tomography signs of cerebral atrophy. *Arch Neurol* 1981; 38:339–342.

19. Wang HS: Dementia of old age, in Smith LW, Kinsbourne M (eds): *Aging and Dementia.* New York, Spectrum, 1977, pp 1–4.

20. Selby G: Parkinson's disease, in Vinken PJ, Bruyn GW (eds): *Handbook of Clinical Neurology.* Amsterdam, North-Holland, 1968, vol 6, pp 173–211.

21. Hakim AM, Mathieson G: Dementia in Parkinson disease: a neuropathologic study. *Neurology* 1979; 29:1209–1214.

22. Alvord FC, Forvo LS, Kusske JA: The pathology of parkinsonism: a comparison of degeneration in cerebral cortex and brain stem. *Adv Neurol* 1974; 5:175–193.

23. Pearce J: The extrapyramidal disorder of Alzheimer's disease. *Eur Neurol* 1974; 12:94–103.

24. Parkes JD, Marsden DC, Rees JE: Parkinson's disease, cerebral arteriosclerosis, and senile dementia. *Q J Med* 1974; 1969:49–61.

25. Gottfries CG, Adolfsson R, Aquilonius SM, et al: Parkinsonism and dementia disorders of Alzheimer type: similarities and differences in Parkinson's disease, in Rinne UK, Klinger M, Stemm G (eds): *Current Progress, Problems, and Management.* New York, Elsevier North-Holland, 1980, pp 197–208.

26. Albert ML, Feldman RG, Willis AL: The "subcortical dementia" of progressive supranuclear palsy. *J Neurol Neurosurg Psychiatry* 1974; 37:121–130.

27. Fisher CM: Lacunas: small, deep cerebral invarcts. *Neurology* 1965; 15:774–784.

28. Sciarra D, Sprofkin BE: Symptoms and signs referable to the basal ganglia in brain tumor. *Arch Neurol Psychiatry* 1953; 48:450–461.

29. Steele JC, Richardson JC, Olszewski J: Progressive supranuclear palsy. *Arch Neurol* 1964; 10:333–358.

30. Lieberman A, Neophytides A, Casson I, et al: Huntington's disease. *NY State J Med* 1979; 79:1188–1190.

31. Adams RD, Van Bogaert L: Striatonigral degeneration. *J Neuropathol Exp Neurol* 1964; 23:584–608.

32. Adams RD, Fisher CM, Hakim AM, et al: Symptomatic occult hydrocephalus with "normal" cerebrospinal fluid pressure: a treatable syndrome. *N Engl J Med* 1965; 273:117–126.

33. Elizan TS, Hirano A, Abrams B: Amyotrophic lateral sclerosis and parkinsonism dementia complex of Guam. *Arch Neurol* 1966; 14:356–368.

34. Chen L: Neurofibrillary change on Guam. *Arch Neurol* 1981; 38:16–18.

39 Relation to Creutzfeldt–Jakob Disease and Other Unconventional Virus Diseases

ANDRÉS M. SALAZAR
PAUL BROWN
D. CARLETON GAJDUSEK
CLARENCE J. GIBBS, JR.

SINCE THE DISCOVERY OF THE TRANSMISSIBLE NATURE of kuru and Creutzfeldt–Jakob disease (CJD) (1, 2), there has been much speculation about the possible role of slow viruses in other degenerative conditions of the central nervous system (CNS) and particularly in Alzheimer's disease (AD). In this chapter, we review clinical, epidemiologic, pathologic, and experimental evidence suggesting an association between AD and the slow virus diseases, particularly CJD (see Table 39–1).

The typical clinical and pathologic spectra of kuru and CJD have been described elsewhere, and will not be detailed here (3–6). Briefly, kuru is a subacute degenerative disease of the brain restricted to the remote Fore linguistic group and their neighbors of the eastern highlands of Papua New Guinea. Clinically, it is characterized by severe cerebellar ataxia and characteristic involuntary movements including a characteristic tremor and mass reflex, and progress to death in 6–24 months. The pathological hallmarks are neuronal loss and gliosis, fibrillary amyloid plaques, and spongiform change. The neuropathological similarity of kuru to the gliosis and neuronal loss of scrapie, a progressive neurologic disorder occurring in sheep, gave encouragement to the long-term observation of animals inoculated in transmission attempts. Subsequently, the similarity of the experimentally transmitted kuru with severe spongiosis to CJD led to the transmission of CJD to chimpanzees and monkeys (1, 2) and established the concept of slow virus infections in humans. Creutzfeldt–Jakob disease, originally described as "spastic pseudosclerosis" in 1921, occurs worldwide and is usually a fulminant presenile dementia including pyramidal, extrapyramidal, and/or cerebellar signs, myoclonus, and typical periodic, paroxysmal sharp waves on the EEG. The disease is transmissible to various species of laboratory animals including chimpanzees, monkeys, goats, cats, guinea pigs, and mice, with variable, host-dependent incubation periods averaging 2–3 years in primates. Although much has been learned about the unconventional viruses causing scrapie, kuru, and CJD, the chemical structure of these agents is still unidentified (6–8).

TABLE 39-1
Relation of Alzheimer's Disease to CJD, Kuru, and Scrapie

Clinical Similarities
  Similar ages of onset (10)
  Presence of presenile dementia
  Presence of myoclonus (10, 11, 12, 14)
  Presence of periodic EEG (8, 14, 16, 17, 18)
  Joint occurrence in single families (10)
  Joint occurrence in one individual (13)
  Autosomal-dominant inheritance of familial forms (10, 11, 22, 23)
  Conjugal occurrence (10)

Pathologic Similarities
  Spongiform change in Alzheimer's (13, 31, 32)
  Amyloid plaques
    Occur in 100% of AD, 70% of kuru, 9% of CJD (25)
    Morphologic spectrum overlaps in AD, kuru, CJD, scrapie (25)
    Reproducible in scrapie-infected mice (30)

Transmission Experiments
  Spongy encephalopathy transmitted to primates from only 2 patients with familial AD (34, 35)

Other Experiments
  Animal model of dementia: Genetically controlled scrapie in mice (29)
  Paired helical filament inducing factor in AD (37)
  Induction of cell fusion by CJD and familial AD (38)
  Decreased choline-acetyltransferase in AD and scrapie (42)
  Serum neurofilament autoantibody in 55% of CJD, 25% of AD (40, 41)

CLINICAL SIMILARITIES OF AD AND CJD

In the differential diagnosis of cortical dementia, once vascular, neoplastic, traumatic, toxic-metabolic, and conventional infectious etiologies have been excluded, AD is the most common diagnosis. However, CJD must always be considered among the presenile dementias, particularly if the dementia progresses rapidly, or if myoclonus, extrapyramidal, or cerebellar findings appear. Not infrequently, there is sufficient clinical similarity between CJD and AD so that only pathologic examination establishes the diagnosis.

Both conditions have similar average ages of onset: 67 years with a range of 40–89 years for AD, and 60 years with a range of 35–84 years for CJD (occasional much younger cases have been reported for both). Although the duration of AD is usually much longer (8 years as compared to 8 months), the range of duration overlaps in both conditions (1–120 months for CJD versus 10–300 months for AD). AD may be slightly more common in females (M–F ratio 0.6), whereas CJD incidence is non-gender specific (8–10).

Perhaps the most troublesome symptom is myoclonus, which has long been recognized as one of the clinical hallmarks of CJD but has been described in occasional patients with AD as well, particularly AD of the familial type (10–14). Thus far, there is no way to distinguish the myoclonus of AD from that of CJD. Even the presence of periodic paroxysmal sharp wave complexes on the EEG, typical in CJD, has been reported in at least eight patients with pathologically confirmed AD (14–18).

The repeated occurrence of CJD and AD within different members of one family and also the apparent evolution of some cases of AD into a clinicopathologic picture typical of CJD, confuses the distinction between the two diseases. Gaches and associates (13) recently described two cases with overlapping signs of CJD and AD. One case, a 43-year-old man with a 4-year history of slowly progressive simple dementia underwent a brain biopsy pathologically confirming the clinical diagnosis of AD, but then deteriorated rapidly, developed myoclonus and a periodic EEG; on repeat biopsy, he showed the typical spongiform change of CJD. Subsequent necropsy confirmed the combined pathologic changes of AD and CJD, with senile plaques (SPs) and neurofibrillary tangles (NFT), as well as spongiform change (13). The joint occurrence of the two diseases in these cases suggests more than a fortuitous association.

FAMILIAL OCCURRENCE

The familial occurrence of AD and CJD has been reviewed in detail recently by Masters and co-workers (10) and provides some of the most convincing evidence for the etiologic relationship of the two conditions. In an analysis of 73 families with CJD and 52 other families with AD, these authors found four families in which one member had pathologically confirmed CJD, and at least two other members had AD (10, 11, 19, 20). In 17 other families with a total of 88 AD-affected members, at least 30 members of these families had a relatively rapid course with myoclonus or other movement disorder, suggesting a diagnosis of CJD. Most of these cases showed the typical changes of AD on pathologic examination; none had the spongiform change characteristic of CJD. Conjugal cases of CJD or AD, or cases related through marriage have been rare, although there is one report of pathologically confirmed CJD in a woman whose husband was almost simultaneously ill with confirmed AD (10).

Familial cases constitute about 10–15% of both AD and CJD, and their clinical and pathologic pictures are virtually indistinguishable from their respective sporadic forms. The mean age at death of familial CJD is somewhat younger than in both sporadic CJD and familial AD (51, 58, and 56 years, respectively). The familial forms of both diseases demonstrate a tendency for a decrease in age of onset in members of succeeding generations, and generations are not usually skipped. Concordance among twins has been the rule in AD, although discordant monozygotic twins have also been reported (11, 17, 21).

Notwithstanding the above reports of discordant twins, both diseases occur in a pattern consistent with autosomal dominant inheritance (10, 11, 22). CJD thus becomes the prime example of an "inherited" infectious disease, although we cannot as yet distinguish between a genetically determined viral susceptibility, increased viral exposure, vertical transmission of the virus through the sperm or ovum, or some other as yet unknown mechanism (8, 10, 23).

The pattern of disappearance of kuru in New Guinea (4) strongly suggests that contamination through the ritual of endocannibalism was the only route of transmission of the disease, and that genetic predisposition and vertical transmission are unlikely. Although kuru had been common in children years earlier, the age of onset of new cases has gradually increased over the past 20 years such that only villagers old enough to have participated in the ritual cannibalism (which ceased about 1959) have developed the disease. Likewise, none of the hundreds of infants born to kuru-affected mothers, but mothers likewise too young to have participated in such rituals, has become ill to date. Whether some of these children will develop kuru or another form of presenile dementia as they enter their fourth or fifth decade remains to be seen, but such transmission cannot explain the hundreds of pediatric cases of kuru seen in the early days of kuru investigation.

PATHOLOGIC SIMILARITIES

AD, CJD, kuru, and scrapie all show neuronal loss and gliosis, as well as amyloid plaques, although there is continuing controversy as to the meaning of the various forms of amyloid plaque deposition in each disease (24–26). Amyloid plaques occur to some degree in virtually all cases of AD, in 70% of kuru cases, and in a much smaller proportion of cases of CJD (9%). This latter is notably evident in an unusual familial variant of transmissible CJD with dementia, prominent cerebellar signs, and typical spongiform change (Gerstman–Straussler syndrome) in which the morphology of the amyloid plaque is intermediate between the fibrillary type of kuru and the neuritic senile plaques (SPs) of AD. Masters and associates (25) also found 22 other cases of clinically typical, transmissible, spongiform CJD with the amyloid and neuritic SPs characteristic of AD. Amyloid plaque deposition in these cases was increased out of proportion either to the occasional NFTs seen or the expected number of plaques in nondemented age-matched controls, making it unlikely that these cases represent the fortuitous joint occurrence of AD and CJD. Amyloid plaques occur more frequently in cases of CJD or kuru with a longer duration of illness, and thus the plaques may represent a relatively nonspecific, secondary, immunological host response to disease. Their morphology likewise appears to be determined by duration of illness, with a spectrum stretching from no plaques seen in short duration cases of CJD (6 months); through kuru type or amyloid SPs occurring in longer duration CJD (14 months), kuru, scrapie, and short duration AD; to neuritic type SPs seen mostly in the very long duration cases of AD (25). While the time sequence of this progression remains controversial (27), it still suggests that the amyloid plaque in its various forms shares a common pathogenesis in these diseases. Studies with scrapie in mice have also demonstrated that the type of pathologic changes seen are determined largely by virus and host genetics (28–30). The pathogenesis and possible significance of the amyloid plaque is discussed in more detail elsewhere in this volume and by Masters and associates (25).

Conversely, the principal pathologic change of CJD, spongiform change, has also been described in cases which were otherwise clinically and pathologically typical of AD (13, 31, 32). The spongiform changes in three of these patients were ultrastructurally very similar to those of CJD, although transmission experiments were not performed with tissue from these patients. As has been emphasized elsewhere, the typical spongiform change of transmissible CJD is often difficult to distinguish from other forms of vacuolation not associated with transmissibility, and such findings must be regarded with caution (7, 33).

TRANSMISSION EXPERIMENTS

The most direct potential demonstration of the relation of AD and CJD would be the transmission of a spongiform encephalopathy to primates from the brains of patients with confirmed pathologically familial AD. Two such transmissions have been reported (34), but neither has been confirmed in repeat experiments using the frozen, stored original brain tissue. The results may be real, the result of laboratory error, or even represent the simultaneous occurrence of the CJD agent in a patient with AD. Given the clinical and pathologic overlap described above, these results are not wholly unexpected, as spongiform change may simply be a characteristic of the transmissible form of a broader spectrum of disease. Brain tissue suspensions from 76 other patients with either sporadic or familial AD have been inoculated into nonhuman primates, and of these, at least 52 have been under observation long enough to be considered negative transmission experiments. Goudsmit and associates (35) reviewed this subject in detail and concluded that the transmissibility of AD has not yet been demonstrated with any reasonable degree of certainty. Again, failure to transmit disease under these conditions may relate not to the absence of virus, but to other factors such as virus strain; host genetics, age, and endocrine-metabolic changes; facilitating toxins; or exceptionally prolonged incubation period.

OTHER EXPERIMENTAL DATA

Abnormal fibrillary structures (scrapie-associated fibrils) have been observed by electron microscopy (EM) in subfractions of synaptosomal preparations from brains of scrapie-affected mice and hamsters, although they have not been found on EM examination of the brains themselves (36). They are morphologically dissimilar to normal brain fibrils but do bear a resemblance to amyloid, including the type of amyloid present in plaques from patients with AD.

They appear to be different, however, from the structures interpreted as paired helical filaments (PHFs) observed in human fetal neuron cultures inoculated with AD brain extracts or spinal fluid (37). These latter filaments, induced by a so-called "PHF assembly factor" that passes through a 250-nm filter, sediments between 40S–80S and is sensitive to both heat and ultraviolet radiation, are in turn not morphologically identical to the PHFs in the AD brain. The significance of these experimentally induced filamentous structures to the pathogenesis of amyloid plaques and to PHF in the NFTs of naturally occurring AD remains problematical and subject to continuing research.

Moreau-Dubois and colleagues (38) have reported the induction of cell fusion in a genetic complementation assay using mouse neuroblastoma and mouse fibroblast cell lines by suspensions of brain from over 65% of cases of CJD, about 30% of neurologic disease controls, and only 1 of 25 nonneurologic disease controls. Subsequent studies have also shown a percentage of positives among familial AD of 59%, as opposed to 17% of cases with sporadic AD. The significance of these findings is still unclear, but they do demonstrate a biologic similarity between familial AD and CJD, as well as reinforce the apparent distinction between familial and sporadic AD suggested by genetic studies, and by the transmission experiments reported above (10, 11, 35, 39).

Sotelo and associates (40) and more recently Bahmanyar and associates (41) have demonstrated an autoantibody to neurofilaments in the serum of 55% of patients with CJD, 54% of patients with kuru, but only 8% of healthy controls. Preliminary experiments have indicated that approximately 10–15% of sera from patients with AD or other neurologic diseases are also positive.

Finally, neurotransmitter studies by McDermott and colleagues (42) have demonstrated a deficiency of choline acetyltransferase in the brains of scrapie-infected animals, as has also been repeatedly demonstrated in AD. It is most likely that this change is secondary in both diseases, but it does represent another shared feature, and again suggests a common pathogenesis.

CONCLUSIONS

The transmissibility of AD has not yet been convincingly demonstrated, yet there is a growing body of clinical, pathological, epidemiological, and experimental evidence suggesting a possible etiologic relationship between AD and CJD, particularly in familial AD. There is overlap in both the clinical and pathologic features of both diseases. The association of AD with other genetic, toxic metabolic, traumatic, immunologic, and age-related factors discussed in detail elsewhere in this volume does not exclude virus infection, perhaps by a ubiquitous unconventional virus, as a possible etiology. Much has been learned about the role of virus strain and host genetics in determining the variety of clinical and pathologic manifestations of disease in animals infected with the unconventional viruses (28, 30, 43, 44) but much remains to be explored about the role of toxic, metabolic, endocrine, age, and immunologic factors in shaping the final clinical and pathologic form of these infections in a given host.

REFERENCES

1. Gajdusek DC, Gibbs CJ, Alpers M: Experimental transmission of a kuru-like syndrome to chimpanzees. *Nature* 1966; 209:794–796.
2. Gibbs CJ Jr, Gajdusek DC, Asher DM, et al: Creutzfeldt–Jakob disease (spongiform encephalopathy): transmission to the chimpanzee. *Science* 1968; 161:388–389.
3. Gajdusek DC, Zigas V: Degenerative disease of the central nervous system in New Guinea: the endemic of "kuru" in the native population. *N Engl J Med* 1957; 257:974–978.
4. Gajdusek DC: Unconventional viruses and the origin and disappearance of kuru. *Science* 1977; 197:943–960.
5. Roos R, Gajdusek DC, Gibbs CJ Jr: The clinical characteristics of transmissible Creutzfeldt–Jakob disease. *Brain* 1973; 96:1–20.
6. Traub RD, Gajdusek DC, Gibbs CJ Jr: Transmissible virus dementia: the relation of transmissible spongiform encephalopathy to Creutzfeldt–Jakob disease, in Kinsbourne M, Smith L (eds): *Aging and Dementia*. New York, Spectrum, 1977, pp 91–172.
7. Masters CL, Gajdusek DC: The spectrum of Creutzfeldt–Jakob disease and the virus-induced subacute spongiform encephalopathies. *Recent Adv Neuropathol* 1982; 2:139–163.
8. Brown P: An epidemiologic critique of Creutzfeldt–Jakob disease. *Epidemiol Rev* 1980; 2:113–135.
9. Heston LL, Mastri AR, Anderson VE, et al: Dementia of the Alzheimer type. *Arch Gen Psychiatry* 1981; 38:1085–1090.
10. Masters CL, Gajdusek DC, Gibbs CJ Jr: The familial occurrence of Creutzfeldt–Jakob disease and Alzheimer's disease. *Brain* 1981; 104:535–558.
11. Cook RH, Ward BE, Austin JH: Studies in aging of the brain: IV. Familial Alzheimer disease: relation to transmissible dementia, aneuploidy, and microtubular defects. *Neurology* 1979; 29:1402–1412.
12. Faden AL, Townsend JJ: Myoclonus in Alzheimer disease. *Arch Neurol* 1976; 33:278–280.
13. Gaches J, Supino-Viterbo V, Foncin JF: Association des maladies d'Alzheimer et de Creutzfeldt–Jakob. *Acta Neurol Belg* 1977; 77:202–212.
14. Jacob H: Muscular twitching in Alzheimer's disease, in Wolstenholme GEW, O'Connor M (eds): *Alzheimer's Disease and Related Conditions*. London, Churchill, 1970, pp 75–93.

15. Brown P, Cathala F: Creutzfeldt–Jakob disease in France, in Prusiner S, Hadlow W (eds): *Slow Transmissible Diseases of the Nervous System.* New York, Academic, 1979, vol 1, pp 213–228.

16. Ehle AL, Johnson PC: Rapidly evolving EEG changes in a case of Alzheimer's disease. *Ann Neurol* 1977; 1:593–595.

17. Gloor P: EEG characteristics in Creutzfeldt–Jakob disease. *Ann Neurol* 1980; 8:341.

18. Watson CP: Clinical similarity of Alzheimer and Creutzfeldt–Jakob disease. *Ann Neurol* 1979; 6:368–369.

19. Ball MJ: Features of Creutzfeldt–Jakob disease in brains of patients with familial dementia of the Alzheimer type. *Can J Neurol Sci* 1980; 7:51–57.

20. Rice GPA, Paty DW, Ball MJ, et al: Spongiform encephalopathy of long duration: a family study. *Can J Neurol Sci* 1980; 7:171–176.

21. Davidson EA, Robertson EE: Alzheimer's disease with acne rosacea in one of identical twins. *J Neurol Neurosurg Psychiatry* 1955; 18:72–77.

22. Cathala F, Chatelain J, Brown P, et al: Familial Creutzfeldt–Jakob disease: autosomal dominance in 14 members over 3 generations. *J Neurol Sci* 1980; 47:343–351.

23. Dickinson AG, Frazer H: An assessment of the genetics of scrapie in sheep and mice, in Prusiner S, Hadlow W (eds): *Slow Transmissible Diseases of the Nervous System.* New York, Academic, 1979, vol 1, pp 367–385.

24. Chou SM, Martin JD: Kuru plaques in a case of CJD. *Acta Neuropathol* 1971; 11:150–155.

25. Masters CL, Gajdusek DC, Gibbs CJ Jr: Creutzfeldt–Jakob disease virus isolations from the Gerstmann–Straussler syndrome, with an analysis of the various forms of amyloid plaque deposition in the virus-induced spongiform encephalopathies. *Brain* 1981; 104:559–587.

26. Pro JD, Smith CH, Sumi SM: Presenile Alzheimer disease: amyloid plaques in the cerebellum. *Neurology* 1980; 30:820–825.

27. Wisniewski HM, Terry RD: Re-examination of the pathogenesis of the senile plaque. *Neuropathol* 1973; 2:1–26.

28. Dickinson AG, Fraser H: Scapie—pathogenesis in inbred mice: an assessment of host control and response involving many strains of the agent, in Ter Meulen V, Katz M (eds): *Slow Virus Infections of the Central Nervous System.* New York, Springer-Verlag, 1977, pp 3–14.

29. Dickinson AG, Fraser H, Bruce M: Animal models for the dementias, in Glen, Whaley (eds): *Alzheimer's Disease.* Edinburgh, Churchill Livingston, 1981.

30. Fraser H: Neuropathology of scrapie: the precision of the lesions and their diversity, in Prusiner S, Hadlow W (eds): *Slow Transmissible Diseases of the Nervous System.* New York, Academic, 1979, vol 1, pp 387–405.

31. Flament-Durand J, Couck AM: Spongiform alterations in brain biopsies of presenile dementia. *Acta Neuropathol* 1979; 46:159–162.

32. Mancardi GL, Mandybur TI, Liwncz BH: Ultrastructural study of the spongiform-like abnormalities in Alzheimer's disease. *J Neuropathol Exp Neurol* 1981; 40:360.

33. Masters CL, Richardson EP: Subacute spongiform encephalopathy (Creutzfeldt–Jakob disease): the nature and progression of the spongiform change. *Brain* 1978; 101:333–334.

34. Rewcastle NB, Gibbs CJ Jr, Gajdusek DC: Transmission of familial Alzheimer's disease to primates. *J Neuropathol Exp Neurol* 1978; 37:679.

35. Goudsmit J, Morrow CH, Asher DM, et al: Evidence for and against the transmissibility of Alzheimer's disease. *Neurology* 1979; 30:945–950.

36. Merz PA, Somerville RA, Wisniewski HM, et al: Abnormal fibrils from scrapie infected brain. *Acta Neuropathol* 1981; 54:63–74.

37. Crapper-McLachlan DR, de Boni U: Etiologic factors in senile dementia of the Alzheimer type. *Aging NY* 1980; 13:173–181.

38. Moreau-Dubois MC, Brown P, Goudsmit J, et al: Biologic distinction between sporadic and familial Alzheimer disease by an *in vitro* cell fusion test. *Neurology* 1981; 31:323–325.

39. Goudsmit J, White BJ, Weitkamp LR, et al: Familial Alzheimer's disease in two kindreds of the same geographic and ethnic origin. *J Neurol Sci* 1981; 49:79–89.

40. Sotelo J, Gibbs CJ Jr, Gajdusek DC: Autoantibodies against axonal neurofilaments in patients with kuru and Creutzfeldt–Jakob disease. *Science* 1980; 210:190–193.

41. Bahmanyar S, Gajdusek DC, Sotelo J, et al: Longitudinal spinal cord sections as substratum for anti-neurofilament antibody detection. *J Neurol Sci* 1982; 53:85–90.

42. McDermott FR, Fraser H, Dickinson AG: Reduced choline-acetyltransferase activity in scrapie mouse brain. *Lancet* 1978; ii:318–319.

43. Gibbs CJ Jr, Gajdusek DC, Amyx H: Strain variation in the viruses of Creutzfeldt–Jakob disease and kuru, in Prusiner S, Hadlow W (eds): *Slow Transmissible Diseases of the Nervous System.* New York, Academic, 1979, vol 2, pp 87–110.

44. Wisniewski HM, Moretz RC, Lossinsky MS: Evidence for induction of localized amyloid deposits and neuritic plaques by an infectious agent. *Ann Neurol* 1981; 10:517–522.

40 Age-Associated Changes and Dementia in Down's Syndrome

KRYSTNYA E. WISNIEWSKI

HENRYK M. WISNIEWSKI

DOWN'S SYNDROME (DS), with characteristic phenotypic and genotypic expression, continues to be the major known cause of mental retardation (MR). The recent estimate of the incidence rates for Down's syndrome indicate the disorder's occurrence in 1/1,000 live births, as compared with 1.33/1,000 live births in 1960 (1). The majority of DS cases show severe or profound MR. Only 5.5% of DS patients have an IQ of more than 70, and only 10.6% have an IQ of 60 or greater (2). The recent interest in early stimulation of infants and increased pressure on educators may bring new statistical data.

The phenotypic expression of DS can be categorized into major and minor signs of abnormalities. The major signs include mental retardation; visual, auditory, speech, and fine motor coordination impairment; growth retardation; microcrania, flat occiput, and various dysmorphic features (slanting eyes, flat nasal bridge, narrow palate, short neck and hands, incurved fingers, gap between 1st and 2nd toes, and abnormal dermatoglyphics). Hypotonia, another major sign of DS, may be seen only up to the second decade; nystagmus is more commonly seen after the first decade of life.

The minor signs of abnormalities, numbering more than 60, are less pathognomonic for DS. Those DS patients with fewer than 10 major signs (often associated with *de novo* partial trisomy) we propose to call atypical DS (for an example of atypical DS seen by us see ref. 3).

In reviewing the cytogenetic advances in DS during recent years, Mikkelsen (4), indicated that the distal segment of the long arm of chromosome 21 seems to be responsible for phenotypic variation, and that severity of the syndrome is inversely proportional to the size of the segment loss. The distal segment is considered to encode the gene for cytoplasmic superoxide dismutase (SOD); this reported observation is based on work by Tan and associates (5). These studies utilized mouse/human somatic cell hybrids to assign the locus of an enzyme subsequently shown to be SOD to human chromosome 21. Other studies also demonstrate a 50% increase of SOD in RBC, platelets, polymorphonuclear granulocytes, lymphocytes, and skin fibroblasts in the complete trisomy 21 syndrome (6–13). Based upon analysis of partial chromosome 21 translocations, there appears to be a limited region of the distal arm of chromosome 21 which is required for the phenotypic expression of DS (8, 14). Several patients have been described with DS, partial translocation, trisomy 21, and normal levels of SOD (15–18). Whether the elevated levels of SOD in DS contributes to the phenotype of accelerated aging is unknown at the present time. The intracellular concentrations of peroxide and SOD are potentially capable of pathological interaction with many structural cell elements such as protein, lipids, and polynucleotides, and they have been implicated in pathological aging (19). Another subject of investigation in DS is abnormality in the immunoendocrine system. It is well known that there is a DS patient susceptibility to infection, malignancy, and endocrinopathy (20, 21). A major subject of investigation, therefore, which is of particular relevance for this textbook, is the mechanism of accelerated aging in DS.

Intellectual and developmental quotients decrease with increasing age in DS (22–26). Also, there is evidence for the appearance of behavioral and neurological changes accompanying aging indicating personality aberrations in the form of apathy, sudden affective changes, deterioration of personal hygiene, loss of vocabulary, and increased incidence and severity of abnormal neurological signs (27–29).

Wisniewski and associates (30) studied 50 unselected institutionalized patients with Down's syndrome to determine the clinical course of precocious aging, and mental and neurological deterioration. The researchers found statistically significant differences in neurological and mental deterioration in patients above age 35, indicating progressive changes in the CNS. A higher incidence of recent memory loss, impairment of short-term visual retention, frontal release signs, hypertonia, hyperreflexia, apraxia, long tract signs, and psychiatric problems was noted in patients over 35 (Table 40–1). Also, the presence of external features of precocious aging was noted in many patients over 35; for example, 30% suffered hearing loss, and 4% suffered hypothyroidism. Of the 50 cohorts studied for karyotype, 96% showed trisomia 21, 2% a mosaic pattern, and 2% translocation. This is comparable to other studies on the occurrence of chromosomal abnormalities in Down's patients.

Recently Wisniewski and co-workers (31) studied another group of 30 institutionalized DS patients with profound (11 patients), severe (11 patients), and moderate (8 patients) MR (mean age 24.8 years; age range 11–42 years). In these patients, the CT scan showed basal ganglia calcification (BGC) (Fig. 40–1) in 8 of the 30 patients and brain atrophy of different degrees in 27 of the 30 patients. Also, clinical evidence of regression and a history of seizures was present in 7 patients (Table 40–2). In this group of patients, calcium homeosta-

TABLE 40–1
Abnormal Responses in the Neurological Examination in 50 Down's Syndrome Patients

Item Description	CA < 35[a]		CA > 35[b]	
	N	%	N	%
Snout reflex	2	7.7	17	70.8
Sucking reflex	0	0	8	33.3
Palmomental signs	7	26.9	17	70.8
Hoffman's signs	0	0	5	20.8
Decreased muscle tone	7	26.9	0	0
Increased muscle tone	7	26.9	12	50.0
Hyperreflexia	8	30.8	19	79.2
Babinski	1	3.9	5	20.8
Absence of Mayer's	13	50.0	19	79.2
Facial muscle hyperreflexia	8	30.8	17	70.8

CA = chronologic age
[a] 26 patients < 35 years of age
[b] 26 patients > 35 years of age

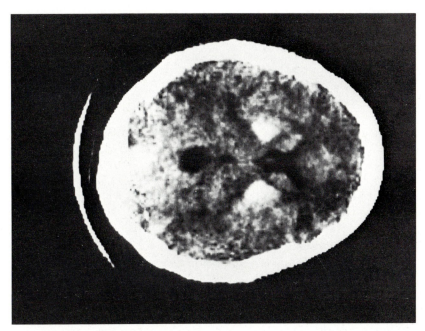

Figure 40–1. A CT scan 7800, 320 matrix at 50–60-mm level from base, showing basal ganglia calcification in a 17-year-old Down's syndrome patient.

tis was investigated in 12 of the 30 DS subjects (total serum and ionized calcium, 25-hydroxy vitamin D and parathormone). None of these studies was abnormal. Absence of evidence of a generalized calcium metabolic disturbance in association with a higher incidence of DS BGC suggests that local brain factors may be causative and may be associated with an acceleration of aging in the DS nervous system.

The same study also looked at the frequency and intensity of histologically detected BGC in 100 DS brains, as a function of age at death. The BGC was demonstrated in all 100 DS brains; this strengthens the hypothesis that BGC may be a characteristic of DS and is a manifestation of premature aging in this disorder. BGC in non-DS persons is usually not apparent until beyond the fifth decade; in the Wisniewski DS postmortem study it was seen at all ages (31). History of regression and dementia are well correlated with the postmortem studies (32) showing accelerated Alzheimer-type brain changes (neuritic plaques and

TABLE 40–2
Clinical Observation and CT Scan Detected Incidence of Basal Ganglia Calcification (BGC) and Hydrocephalus ex vacuo (H.E.) in 30 Down's Syndrome Patients During Life

Age, Yrs	No.	CT BGC (+)	CT BGC (−)	Hydrocephalus ex vacuo (H.E.)[a] o	a	b	c	d	Clinical Regression	Seizures	Extra-pyramidal Signs
10–20	7	3	4	1	3	3			1	1	0
21–30	17	3	14	2	7	6	2		3	3	0
30+	6	2	4			2	3	1	3	3	0

[a] o = normal, a = minimal, b = mild, c = moderate, d = severe.

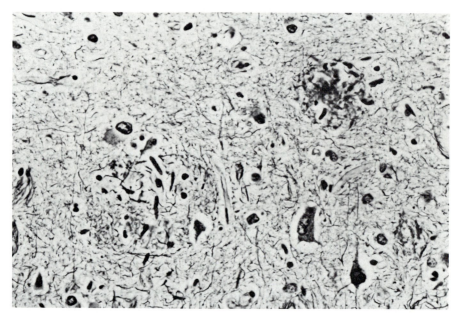

Figure 40–2. Neuritic plaques in the frontal cortex of a 30-year-old Down's syndrome patient; Bodian impregnation × 400.

neurofibrillary changes), and also with postmortem evidence of lipofuscin accumulation (Fig. 40–2). These accelerated Alzheimer's and age-related neuropathologic changes start unusually early in life in DS (33–36). All DS patients over the age of 35 have been found to exhibit Alzheimer dementia–like changes. Malamud (36) found neuritic plaques and neurofibrillary tangles (NFTs) in the brains of a few DS cases in the third decade of life, and Burger and Vogel (37) found neuritic plaques in the second decade of life in some DS patients.

Wisniewski and co-workers (32) recently studied 100 Down's syndrome (DS) brains of patients who died in institutions for chronically ill residents. Only 48% of the individuals were above the age of 30. History of regression (loss of interest in work and surroundings, plus a decrease in cognitive ability, motor function, and personal hygiene) was documented from the medical records in 2 out of 52 (3.84%) below and 14 of 48 (29.1%) above the age of 30. It was found that 9 of 52 (17.3%) below and 41 of 48 (85.4%) above the age of 30, and 48 of 48 (100%) above the age of 35 had plaques and tangles. Neuritic plaques are usually seen earlier than NFTs. The numbers of plaques and tangles correlated well with the history of regression, the duration of regression, and the patient age. Very large numbers of plaques and tangles were found in 19 of 41 (47.5%) brains above the age of 35, out of which 14 of 41 (35%) had a history of regression. There were some DS brains over the age of 35, where the number of plaques and tangles was very small. Morphometric studies are in progress. But recent clinicopathological findings indicate that about 30% of DS patients above 35 years of age show clinical signs and symptoms of dementia, with corresponding pathological changes compatible with Alzheimer's disease (AD). This finding also indicates that not all DS patients develop AD; however, AD develops much earlier in DS and is most likely two to three times more prevalent than in the general population. To prove this hypothesis, a prospective study of a large number of DS patients should be conducted among noninstitutionalized DS clients. In the non-DS population these changes are 14% above the age of 40 years (36) and 100% above the age of 65 (38).

Ultrastructural studies of the neurofibrillary changes and neuritic plaques in DS reveal them to be identical to those observed in AD (35, 39–41). Crapper and co-workers (42) found a disproportionate increase in NFTs occurring in the inferior frontal, middle temporal, and occipital areas of the brain from a Down's syndrome patient, compared to both a nonretarded control, and a 65-year-old demented man dying of AD. Additionally, a severe reduction in the total number of nerve cells in radial columns of the DS brain was noted. The number of Alzheimer's NFTs and the loss of pyramidal neurons from the hippocampus in DS patients exceed those found in normal aging subjects. The relationship between plaques, tangles, and clinical dementia in 24 cases of DS over the age of 30 have been described by Ropper and Williams (43).

Acceleration of age-related changes in the brains of Down's syndrome patients is not uniform in all cases. In DS, the dendritic spines and postsynaptic endings have the essential elements of the neuronal circuit decreased (44). A good clinical review paper discussing this problem is given by Lott (45).

The association between DS and senility is made more intriguing by the epidemiologic demonstration of familial clustering of AD, malignancy, and birth of offspring with DS (46, 47).

Also studied has been brain weight (BW) in 100 DS brains from the collection of Dr. George A. Jervis. Brain weight of DS patients at birth is comparable to that of normal neonates. After mid-infancy, however, DS brain weight is often 2 standard deviations below the mean. The curves for normal brain weights and those in DS can be seen in Figure 40–3 (48).

These findings indicate that (1) in DS there is a retardation of BW at the time of the initial period of brain growth and maturation, and (2) there is a shortening of BW plateau and accelerated age-associated change with decreased BW in DS.

Normally, the time of growth, maturation, and aging reflects the life spans in a given species and is genetically determined. The shorter the period of growth and maturation, the sooner the aging process appears. Down's syndrome, in this sense, is one of the classical models for early growth and maturation delay, along with premature aging.

Brain growth appears to be regulated by a growth hormone-dependent growth factor

Figure 40–3. Brain weights in 100 Down's syndrome patients at death: Relationship to aging.

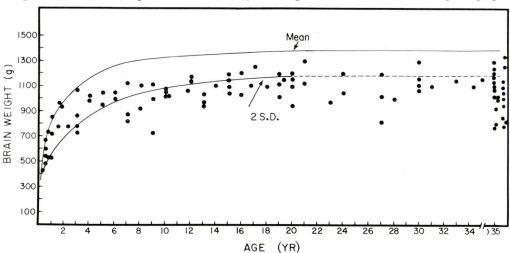

called BGA (brain-growth activity promoting factor). A family of growth hormones dependent on growth promotion of polypeptides has recently been isolated from serum. These hormones, somatomadines, have been found in Down's syndrome fetuses, in lower concentrations than in normals (49), which may be responsible for the retardation of brain growth and the premature start of the aging process. Further studies are needed on DS patients, looking for genetic markers, the results of early treatment with somatomadine, and the effect on the developing brain using the trisomy 16 mouse model of Down, which appears to correspond to human 21 chromosome (50–52).

Recently, research in AD has revealed that the nucleus basalis of Meynert, which consists of large, deeply stained acetylcholinesterase-rich neurons, is selectively damaged. Loss of these cells is associated with a reduction of presynaptic cholinergic cortical markers (53). It will be of great value to study this nucleus and the cholinergic system in DS brains to determine whether further neurochemical and neuropathologic correspondence of these independent, but related, major disease entities pertains.

References

1. Adams NM, Erickson JD, Layde PM, et al: Down's syndrome: recent trends in the United States. *JAMA* 1981; 246:758.

2. Connelly JA: Intelligence levels of Down's syndrome children. *Am J Ment Defic* 1978; 83:193–196.

3. Jenkins EC, Duncan CJ, Wright CE, et al: Atypical Down syndrome and partial trisomy 21. *Clin Genet* 1983; submitted for publication.

4. Mikkelsen M: New aspects of a well-known syndrome (Down syndrome–mongolism). *Eur. J Pediatr* 1981; 136:5–7.

5. Tan YH, Tischfield J, Ruddle FH: The linkage of genes for the human interferon induced antiviral protein and indophenol oxidase-B traits to chromosome G-21. *J Exp Med* 1973; 137:317–330.

6. Sichitiu S, Sinet PM, Lejeune J, et al: Surdosage de la forme dimérique de l'indophénoloxydase dans la trisomie 21, secondaire au surdosage génique. *Hum Genet* 1974; 23:65–72.

7. Sinet PM, Allard D, Lejeune J, et al: Augmentation d'activité de la superoxyde dismutase erythromytairé dans la trisomie pour le chromosome 21. *CR Acad Sci (D)* 1974; 278:3267–3270.

8. Sinet PM, Lavalle F, Michelson AM, et al: Superoxide dismutase activities of blood platelets in trisomy 21. *Biochem Biophys Res Commun* 1975; 67:904.

9. Gilles L, Ferradino C, Foos J, et al: The estimation of red cell superoxide dismutase activity by pulse radiolysis in normal and trisomic 21 subjects. *FEBS Lett* 1976; 69:55–58.

10. Crosti N, Serra A, Rigo A, et al: Dosage effect of SOD-A gene in 21 trisomic cells. *Hum Genet* 1976; 31:197.

11. Feaster WW, Kwok LW, Epstein CS: Dosage effects for superoxide dismutase-1 in nucleated cells aneuploid for chromosome 21. *Am J Hum Genet* 1977; 29:563–570.

12. Brown WT, Dutkowski R, Darlington GJ: Localization and quantitation of human superoxide dismutase using computerized 2-D gel electrophoresis. *Biochem Biophys Res Commun* 1981; 102:675–681.

13. Brown WT, Wisniewski HM: Genetics of human aging. *Rev Biol Res Aging* 1983; 1:81–99.

14. Summit RL: Chromosome 21. Specific segments that cause the phenotype of Down syndrome, in De la Cruz FF, Gerald PS (eds): *Trisomy 21 (Down Syndrome): Research Prospectives.* Baltimore, University Press, 1981, pp 225–251.

15. Kedziora J, Bartosz G, Leyko W, et al: Dismutase activity in translocation trisomy. *Lancet* 1979; i:105.

16. Mattei JF, Baeteman MA, Mattei MG, et al: Superoxide–dismutase-A and chromosome 21, abstract no. p3.19. Abstracts of the Sixth International Congress on Human Genetics, Jerusalem, 1981.

17. Leschot NJ, Slater RM, Joenje H, et al: SOD-A and chromosome 21. *Hum Genet* 1981; 57:220–223.

18. Habedank M, Rodewald A: Moderate Down's syndrome in three siblings having partial trisomy 21q22.2 to qter and therefore no SOD-1 excess. *Hum Genet* 1982; 60:74–77.

19. Sinex FM: The molecular genetics of aging, in Finch CE, Hayflick L (eds): *Handbook of the Biology of Aging.* New York, Van Nostrand Reinhold, 1977, pp 37–62.

20. Walford RL, Barnett EV, Fahey L, et al: Immunological and biochemical studies of Down's syndrome as a model of accelerated aging, in Segre D, Smith L (eds): *Immunological Aspects of Aging.* New York, Dekker, 1981; pp 479–532.

21. Wisniewski K, Jervis GA, Moretz RC: Alzheimer's neurofibrillary tangles in diseases other than senile and presenile dementia. *Ann Neurol* 1979; 5:288.

22. Carr J: *Young Children with Down's Syndrome.* London, Butterworth, 1975.

23. Dameron LE: Development of intelligence of infants with mongolism. *Child Dev* 1963; 34:733–738.

24. Griffiths MI: Development of children with Down's syndrome. *Physiotherapy* 1976; 62:11–15.

25. Koch G: *Down Syndrome; Mongolism.* US, Erlangen in Kommission bei Palm & Enke, 1973.

26. Share J, Webb A, Koch R: A preliminary investigation of the early development status of mongoloid infants. *Am J Ment Defic* 1961; 66:238–241.

27. Dalton AJ, Crapper DR, Schlotterer GR: Alzheimer's disease in Down's syndrome: visual retention deficits. *Cortex* 1974; 10:366–377.

28. Loesch-Modzewski ID: Some aspects of the neurology of Down's syndrome. *J Ment Defic Res* 1968; 12:237.

29. Owens D, Dawson JC, Lowsin S: Alzheimer's disease in Down's syndrome. *Am J Ment Defic* 1971; 75:606.

30. Wisniewski K, Howe J, Williams CG: Precocious aging and dementia in patients with Down's syndrome. *Biol Psychiatry* 1978; 13:619.

31. Wisniewski KE, French JH, Rosen J, et al: Premature basal ganglia calcification (BGC) in Down syndrome. *Ann NY Acad Sci* 1982; 496:179–189.

32. Wisniewski K, Wisniewski H, Wen GY: Plaques, tangles and dementia in Down syndrome. *J Neuropath Exp Neurol* 1983; 42:340.

33. Struwe F: Histopathologische Untersuchungen über Entstehung und Nesen der senilen Plaques. *Z Gesamte Neurol Psychiatr* 1929; 122:291–307.

34. Jervis G: Early senile dementia in mongoloid idiocy. *Am J Psychiatry* 1948; 105:102.

35. Olson MI, Shaw C: Presenile dementia and Alzheimer's disease in mongolism. *Brain* 1969; 92:146.

36. Malamud N: Neuropathology of organic brain syndromes associated with aging, in Gaitz CM (ed): *Aging and the Brain.* New York, Plenum, 1972, pp 63–87.

37. Burger PC, Vogel FS: The development of the pathologic changes of Alzheimer's disease and senile dementia in patients with Down's syndrome. *Am J Pathol* 1973; 73:457–476.

38. Tomlinson BE, Blessed G, Roth M: Observations on the brains of demented old people. *J Neurol Sci* 1970; 11:205–242.

39. Ellis WG, McCulloch JR, Corley CL: Presenile dementia in Down's syndrome: ultrastructural identity with Alzheimer's disease. *Neurology* 1974; 24:101.

40. Schochet SS, Lampert PW, McCormick WF: Neurofibrillary tangles in patients with Down's syndrome. *Acta Neuropath* 1973; 23:342.

41. Wisniewski K, Cobill JM, Wilcox CB, et al: T lymphocytes in patients with Down's syndrome. *Biol Psychiatry* 1979; 14:463.

42. Crapper DR, Dalton AJ, Skopitz M: Alzheimer's degeneration in Down syndrome. *Arch Neurol* 1975; 33:618–623.

43. Ropper AH, Williams RS: Relationship between plaques, tangles and dementia in Down syndrome. *Neurology* 1980; 30:639–644.

44. Suetsugu M, Mehraein P: Spine distribution along the apical dendrites of the pyramidal neurons in Down's syndrome. *Acta Neuropathol* 1980; 50:207–210.

45. Lott IT: Down's syndrome, aging, and Alzheimer's disease: a clinical review. *Ann NY Acad Sci* 1982; 396:15–17.

46. Heston LL: Alzheimer's disease, trisomy 21, and myeloproliferative disorders: associations suggesting a genetic diathesis. *Science* 1977; 196:322–323.

47. Heston LL: Alzheimer's dementia and Down's syndrome: genetic evidence suggesting an association. *Ann NY Acad Sci* 1982; 396:29–37.

48. Blinkov SM, Glezer II: *The Human Brain in Figures and Tables.* New York, Basic Books, 1968, pp 334–337.

49. Sara VR, Hall K, Rodeck CH, et al: Human embryonic somatomadine. *Proc Natl Acad Sci USA* 1981; 78:1–9.

50. Polani PE, Adinolfi M: Chromosome 21 of man, 22 of the great apes and 16 of the mouse. *Dev Med Child Neurol* 1980; 22:223–233.

51. Putz B, Krause G, Garde T, et al: A comparison between trisomy 12 and vitamin A and associated malformation in mouse embryo. *Virchows Arch Pathal Anat* 1980; 368:65–80.

52. Miyabara S, Gropp A, Winking H: Trisomy 16 in the mouse fetus associated with generalized edema and cardiovascular and urinary tract anomalies. *Teratology* 1982; 25:369–380.

53. Whitehouse PJ, Price DL, Struble RG, et al: Alzheimer's disease and senile dementia: loss of neurons in the basal forebrain. *Science* 1982; 215:1237–1239.

SECTION X

PHARMACOLOGIC INVESTIGATIONS INTO THE TREATMENT OF ALZHEIMER'S DISEASE

41 Pharmacologic Treatment of Alzheimer's Disease: An Overview

GORDON S. ROSENBERG

BLAINE GREENWALD

KENNETH L. DAVIS

CHARACTERISTIC HISTOPATHOLOGIC CHANGES IN THE BRAINS OF Alzheimer's disease (AD) patients have been, by this time, well detailed elsewhere in this volume. It is only in recent years, however, that postmortem neurochemical evaluation of AD brain tissue has shed new light on the fundamental pathophysiology of this debilitating illness. The major neurotransmitter systems (cholinergic, noradrenergic, dopaminergic, serotonergic, and GABAergic) have been studied in various brain regions of AD patients (1). Though changes have been reported in all these systems, the most dramatic and consistent finding is a deficit in the acetylcholine (ACh) synthesizing enzyme, choline acetyltransferase (CAT), primarily in the hippocampus and frontal cortex—brain areas associated with memory and cognition (2–21). This deficiency in CAT activity has been positively correlated with impaired performance on mental tasks (8). Evidence corroborating a central cholinergic dysfunction in AD brains includes a deficiency in acetylcholinesterase (AChE), an ACh degradatory enzyme (4, 5, 8, 14, 17, 21–26), as well as decreases in ACh synthesis (10) and content (27). This compelling literature supporting a cholinergic deficit in AD suggests the possibility that pharmacologic agents which augment cholinergic neurotransmission might improve memory and cognition in these patients. This strategy has, in fact, generated great enthusiasm among neurobiologists.

CHOLINERGIC NEUROTRANSMITTER PRECURSORS AND AGENTS

PHARMACOLOGICAL BASES FOR CHOLINERGIC INVESTIGATIONS

Another piece of data consistent with a cholinergic involvement in AD derives from pharmacological investigations of cholinergic agents in human memory. Administration of the anticholinergic scopolamine to young, normal subjects produces a memory deficit quite similar to that observed in drug-free elderly people suffering from an age-related memory loss (28). Such effects are presumed to be specifically related to scopolamine's antimuscarinic

329

properties, and are not secondary to the drug's sedative action, since memory and cognitive effects cannot be reversed by the subsequent administration of amphetamine (29), an attention-enhancing, catecholaminergic agent.

Further implication of ACh's role in human memory is provided by investigations of both physostigmine, an acetylcholinesterase inhibitor, and arecoline, a muscarinic cholinergic direct agonist. Under double-blind conditions these agents enhanced human memory in normal young subjects (30, 31). Physostigmine, in addition, may have an analogous effect in normal elderly people (32).

The pharmacologic mimicry of a syndrome with an antagonist (scopolamine), and its partial reversal with an agonist (physostigmine), strengthens the ACh deficit hypothesis of AD. Of those neurotransmitter systems studied in AD to date, only cholinergic manipulation produces or improves the characteristic AD amnestic syndrome/cognitive impairment. There are several reports of norepinephrine and dopamine-related abnormalities in Alzheimer brains (2, 14, 33–38). These findings are not as consistent or abundant as the CAT data, and upon close scrutiny, many of these studies are flawed by limited diagnostic assessments, lack of control group, and no statistical analysis. Nevertheless, trials of L-dopa and bromocriptine, a dopamine agonist, have been conducted in AD patients and have failed to demonstrate beneficial effects on either memory or cognition (39–42). Additionally, conventional neuroleptics, potent dopamine blockers, do not precipitate a dementia-like picture. Taken together these data, though not refuting possible involvement of and interactions between neurotransmitter systems, support the importance of cholinergic mechanisms in the pathogenesis of the AD memory disorder.

The effect of cholinergic agents on human memory is specific. These drugs influence the subject's ability to store new information in long-term memory. However, cholinergic drugs have minimal effect on the retrieval of information from long-term memory, and no effect on short-term memory processes. Thus, the ability to encode new information into long-term memory (i.e., learning) is the aspect of memory sensitive to cholinergic manipulation (28–31, 43). This learning deficit is a frequent sign in AD (44).

In summary, the postmortem neurochemical AD changes, coupled with the effects of cholinomimetic drugs in enhancing learning, and anticholinergic drugs in precipitating a transient Alzheimer-like dementia, provide a sound rationale for the investigation of cholinomimetic compounds as potential therapies for patients with AD.

One additional note: the cholinergic deficit hypothesis applies to AD only; any study therefore examining drug effects on "dementia" or "cognitive impairment" must be considered carefully for inclusion and exclusion criteria. Particular care must be taken to insure a homogeneous pool of AD patients. It is only this kind of stringent scientific inquiry, utilizing pathophysiologic and histochemical knowledge as well as pharmacologic models, that will reap meaningful breakthroughs in locating the ultimate therapy of this malignant illness.

TREATMENT WITH CHOLINERGIC PRECURSORS

With the aforementioned in mind, it was reasonable to assume that the administration of precursors of ACh, namely choline and lecithin (phosphatidylcholine), might be effective treatments for AD patients. Several lines of evidence support a central effect of these drugs; first, cholinergic precursors increase brain concentrations of ACh (45, 46); second, they have been shown to increase striatal cholinergic transmission (47); and third, precursor administration effectively reduces the abnormal involuntary movements of patients with tardive dyskinesia (48)—a condition that may be characterized by a relative excess of dopamine and hypofunction of ACh in the basal ganglia.

However, results of cholinergic precursor administration to patients with AD and age-related memory loss thus far have not been encouraging (46–61), although several subgroups of patients have demonstrated mild benefit (50, 52, 58, 61). Furthermore, in normal subjects, those individuals whose memory had been enhanced by the administration of intravenous physostigmine, showed no benefit from precursor administration (62). This discrepancy between the effects of physostigmine and choline in memory is in contrast to the qualitatively similar effects of these two drugs to reduce the frequency of abnormal involuntary movements of patients with tardive dyskinesia (48). Thus, one might conclude that the cholinergic neurons of the septo-hippocampal pathway and basalis-cortical projection which have been associated with memory may respond differently to precursor manipulation than the cholinergic interneurons of the striatum that presumably mediate tardive movements.

TREATMENT WITH PHYSOSTIGMINE

An alternative strategy utilizing the acetylcholinesterase inhibitor physostigmine has been employed to ascertain the extent to which the cholinergic deficit in AD could be reversed. Preliminary studies indicate that for nearly every patient, even as little as one dose of intravenous physostigmine enhances memory performance compared to placebo. This enhancement can be as great as a 20% improvement on test scores, potentially a clinically relevant increase, replicable in most subjects (63). Additional studies have reported similar findings (64–67).

The use of physostigmine, as with all precursor strategies, requires an intact presynaptic neuron for ACh synsthesis. However, unlike with the precursor approach, physostigmine does not require the presynaptic neuron to augment ACh synthesis. An important drawback to the clinical utility of physostigmine is its short half-life, and until recently it was not available for oral administration. Clinical trials of oral physostigmine for use in AD have, accordingly, only just begun.

COMBINATION TREATMENT

The search for a cholinergic treatment for the memory loss associated with AD has led some recent investigators to examine broader approaches to the problem of increasing central cholinergic transmission.

The combination of precursor-loading with an anticholinesterase has also been studied. Two of three AD patients on a combination of physostigmine and lecithin improved, compared to baseline, on memory testing, and three of three improved while receiving the combination of physostigmine and lecithin, as compared to lecithin alone (68). Five of nine AD patients demonstrated improved memory on a combination of oral lecithin and tetrahydroaminoacridine (THA), another anticholinesterase, whereas individual treatment with either lecithin or THA failed to improve performance (69, 70). One brief report utilizing pilocarpine and lecithin showed no change on memory testing (71). It should be noted, however, that these studies involved small numbers of patients, and careful dose-response relationships were not established prior to demonstrating a synergistic effect. For example, THA in higher dosages might produce the same effect as lower doses of THA combined with a precursor.

Choline administration has also been combined with treatment with piracetam. Piracetam

(Nootropil) is an agent that may increase the release of ACh in the hippocampus (72) (*see below*). In a single study of this drug combination, a small, nonsignificant improvement in the cognitive abilities of patients with AD was observed (73).

Neuropeptides

A variety of neuropeptides have been shown to have cognitive effects in humans. However, the specificity of these compounds to affect those cognitive processes associated with AD has not been elucidated. The possibility that brain peptides might modulate neurotransmission has led many investigators to explore their potential therapeutic efficacy. While studies of ACTH analogues in elderly impaired individuals have failed to demonstrate clinical benefit (74–78), preliminary findings with vasopressin have been more encouraging. Studies of a vasopressin analogue, 1-desamino 8-D-arginine vasopressin (DDAVP), in elderly subjects have produced measurable improvement in cognitive testing (79). A preliminary study of a few patients with AD has shown reliable enhancement of learning and recall after DDAVP (80). These are exciting results well worth pursuing.

Nootropics

This recently named class of compounds is represented by the prototypical agent called Nootropil or piracetam (2-oxo-pyrrolidine acetamide). Piracetam is a cyclic derivative of gamma-amino butyric acid (GABA). In addition to its CNS effect of increasing ATP synthesis, piracetam may also enhance ACh release in the hippocampus (72). While cognitive functioning has been enhanced in young normals (81), elderly normals (82), and moderately impaired elderly (83), no positive effects have yet been seen in severely demented patients (83–85). As a result of piracetam's potential for increasing the release of ACh from presynaptic neurons, investigations are under way to test its efficacy in combination with cholinergic precursors.

Vasodilators

Dihydrogenated ergot alkaloids (Hydergine), papaverine (Pavabid), and a variety of other vasodilators have been used extensively in the treatment and management of elderly senile patients. Numerous behavioral variables have been reported to improve, including alertness, depression, anxiety, confusion, and general severity of dementia, though the magnitude of these effects have been small (for a complete review of the literature see ref. 86). As of this writing, no objective evidence for improvement in cognitive functioning has been reported. Clearly, when examining the efficacy of vasodilator treatments in dementia, great care must be taken to distinguish between AD and multi-infarct dementias. A rationale for the use of vasodilator treatment is based upon the assumption that the primary cause of the dementia syndrome is arteriosclerotic narrowing resulting in cerebral ischemia, a condition not specifically ascribed to AD. In fact, these drugs, by dilating normal arteries, may "steal" blood away from ischemic areas. Systematic investigations of vasodilator treatment in a homogeneous population of AD patients has not yet been undertaken.

PSYCHOSTIMULANTS

This class of compounds, hypothesized to have "mood elevating" and "attention enhancing" properties, have not been shown to possess any real therapeutic benefit to elderly demented patients. While some reports have suggested that methylphenidate (Ritalin) may improve mood in geriatric populations (87–90), others have not found similar results (91, 92). Other controlled investigations of methylphenidate in normal elderly and memory-impaired elderly have also found no effects on cognition (93, 94).

Pentylenetetrazol (Metrazol), another psychostimulant, has been used in chronic brain syndromes without impressive effect (for a complete review of the literature see ref. 95). No systematic study of this class of compounds has been reported in patients with AD. It is possible that specific subgroups may benefit from one of these compounds, but they remain to be identified.

FUTURE DIRECTIONS

At present there exist no effective pharmacologic therapies for the treatment of patients suffering with AD or age-related memory loss. Several lines of evidence suggest that a variety of pharmacologic compounds may prove to be beneficial and warrant further investigation.

Because of the relative and consistent success of enhancing memory performance with intravenous physostigmine, and the overwhelming neurochemical evidence that AD is a manifestation, at least in part, of a central cholinergic deficit, longer-acting forms of acetylcholinesterase inhibitors may prove to be effective treatments for AD. In addition to oral physostigmine, two other acetylcholinesterase inhibitors, tetrahydroaminoacridine (THA) and di-isofluorphosphate (DFP), are of interest. DFP is a noncompetitive acetylcholinesterase inhibitor with a longer duration of action, but potentially toxic side effects; THA has a half-life intermediate between physostigmine and DFP. It exists in oral form and is almost devoid of side effects (96). In fact, a pilot study indicates that THA enhances cognitive performance in cases of AD (97). Further trials are needed to validate this drug's effects.

Preliminary work utilizing a direct muscarinic cholinergic agonist such as arecoline has been conducted in young normals (31). Arecoline produced improved cognition. If administration of an agonist produces an effect physiologically similar to the effect of ACh released by a functionally intact neuron, then trials utilizing muscarinic receptor agonists in AD should be undertaken. An initial study has shown arecoline to improve memory functioning in AD (66).

Though expectations regarding the therapeutic efficacy of cholinergic precursor–loading in AD have not been realized, combination strategies with precursors and anticholinesterases or nootropics may be viable. It can be hypothesized that one problem in AD may be choline availability for ACh synthesis and neuronal membrane integrity. Lithium carbonate has achieved widespread use in the past decade as both an acute treatment for mania (98), and a maintenance treatment prophylaxis against mania and depression in bipolar affective patients (99). Lithium additionally elevates red blood cell choline (100), possibly by inhibiting choline efflux from the cell. Analogously, increasing brain choline concentrations via precursor loading, coupled with concomitant lithium treatment increasing neuronal choline concentrations, may prove a novel approach toward enhancing cholinergic activity. Unfortunately, although theoretically reasonable, the use of lithium in organic brain syndromes is fraught with dangers of toxicity. Nevertheless, careful surveillance may yet permit trials of lithium/lecithin.

The possibility that increasing the availability of acetyl coenzyme A may augment cholinergic activity has received relatively little attention. However, an approach based on increasing either the concentrations of this compound, or its transport from mitochondria to the cholinergic terminals, might also be worth pursuing.

Somatostatin is a tetradecapeptide first identified as the hypothalamic factor inhibiting the release of growth hormone from the pituitary (101); it is widely distributed in the CNS and may have neurotransmitter-like capability. A decrease in somatostatin immunoreactivity in the cerebral cortex and hippocampus of AD patients has been reported (12, 13), with a parallel loss in CAT activity. Although there is no evidence that somatostatin exists in cholinergic neurons, the parallel loss in CAT and somatostatin, plus animal data demonstrating somatostatin-ACh interactions (101–110), suggest theoretical possibilities regarding a regulatory role of this peptide in central cholinergic activity. Along similar lines, the activity of thyrotropin-releasing hormone, another peptide neuromodulator, has been shown to interact with cortical cholinergic neurotransmission (96). The possibility that neuropeptides may modulate longer-lasting effects on neurotransmission suggests that combined treatment with a cholinomimetic may be a legitimate strategy.

In the future, it is highly likely that other neurotransmitter and neuroregulator deficits will be found in AD. Abnormalities in cholinergic neurons and somatostatin-containing neurons may prove but the tip of the iceberg. For example, a decreased number of neurons in the locus ceruleus, the seat of noradrenergic innervation to the cortex, has recently been reported in several laboratories (111–115), two of which suggest this is a more dramatic finding in presenile and younger senile AD patients (111, 114). The implication that a centrally active adrenergic agonist might partially reverse this noradrenergic deficit raises new therapeutic hopes. The ongoing search for antemortem neurotransmitter markers (e.g., plasma and red cell choline; urinary MHPG; CSF neurotransmitter metabolite concentrations) that might identify subgroups of patients with specific transmitter deficits is an exciting new area of work with great therapeutic ramifications.

Still, any ultimate treatment of AD will have to overcome, either directly or indirectly, the cholinergic deficit. Hence, the development of a safe, orally active, long-lasting cholinomimetic drug for administration to patients with AD would be an important step toward the rational pharmacotherapy of this disorder. Unfortunately, few such compounds are available or have been approved for human investigation.

References

1. Terry RD, Davies P: Dementia of the Alzheimer type. *Annu Rev Neurosci* 1980; 3:77–95.

2. Carlsson A, Adolfsson R, Aquilonius SM: Biogenic amines in brain in normal aging, senile dementia, and chronic alcoholism. *Adv Biochem Psychopharmacol* 1980; 23:295–304.

3. Bowen DJ, Spillane JA, Curzon G, et al: Accelerated aging or selective neuronal loss as an important cause of dementia. *Lancet* 1979; i:11–14.

4. Davies P: Neurotransmitter-related enzymes in SDAT. *Brain Res* 1979; 171:319–327.

5. Davies P, Maloney AJR: Selective loss of central cholinergic neurons in Alzheimer's disease. *Lancet* 1976; ii:1403.

6. Perry EK, Gibson PH, Blessed G, et al: Neurotransmitter enzyme abnormalities in senile dementia. *J Neurol Sci* 1977; 34:247–265.

7. Perry EK, Perry RH, Blessed G, et al: Necropsy evidence of central cholinergic deficits in senile dementia. *Lancet* 1977; i:189.

8. Perry EK, Tomlinson BE, Blessed G, et al: Correlation of cholinergic abnormalities with senile plaques and mental test scores in senile dementia. *Br Med J* 1978; 2:1457–1459.

9. Reisine TD, Yamamura MI, Bird ED, et al: Pre and post synaptic neurochemical alterations in Alzheimer's disease. *Brain Res* 1978; 159:477–481.

10. Sims CR, Bowen DM, Smith CCT, et al: Glucose metabolism and acetylcholine synthesis in relation to neuronal activity in Alzheimer's disease. *Lancet* 1980; i:333.

11. White P, Goodhardt MJ, Kent JP, et al: Neocortical cholinergic neurons in elderly people. *Lancet* 1977; i:668.

12. Davies P, Katzman R, Terry RD: Reduced somatostatin-like immunoreactivity in cerebral cortex from cases of Alzheimer's disease and Alzheimer senile dementia. *Nature* 1980; 288:279–280.

13. Rossor MN, Emson PC, Mountjoy CQ, et al: Reduced amounts of immunoreactive somatostatin in the temporal cortex in SDAT. *Neurosci Lett* 1980; 20:373–377.

14. Yates CM, Allison Y, Simpson J, et al: Dopamine in Alzheimer's disease and senile dementia. *Lancet* 1979; ii:851–852.

15. Bowen DM, Smith CCT, White P, et al: Neurotransmitter-related enzymes and indices of hypoxia in senile dementia and other abiotrophies. *Brain* 1976; 199:459–495.

16. Spillane JA, White P, Goodhardt MJ, et al: Selective vulnerability of neurons in organic dementia. *Nature* 1977; 226:558–559.

17. Yates CM, Simpson J, Maloney AJ, et al: Alzheimer-like cholinergic deficiency in Down syndrome. *Lancet* 1980; ii:979.

18. Rossor MN, Fahrenkrug J, Emson PC, et al: Reduced cortical CAT activity in SDAT is not accompanied by changes in vasoactive intestinal polpeptide. *Brain Res* 1980; 201:249–253.

19. Rossor MN, Iverson LL, Mountjoy CQ, et al: Arginine vasopressin and choline acetyltransferase in brains of patients with Alzheimer type senile dementia. *Lancet* 1980; ii:1367–1368.

20. Perry EK, Perry RH, Gibson PH, et al: A cholinergic connection between normal aging and senile dementia in human hippocampus. *Neurosci Lett* 1977; 6:85–89.

21. Davies P: Studies on the neurochemistry of central cholinergic systems in Alzheimer's disease. *Aging NY* 1978; 7:453–459.

22. Pope A, Hess HH, Lewin E: Microchemical pathology of cerebral cortex in presenile dementias. *Trans Am Neurol Assoc* 1965; 89:15–16.

23. Op den Velde W, Stam FC: Some cerebral proteins and enzyme systems in Alzheimer's presenile and senile dementia. *J Am Geriatr Soc* 1976; 24:12–16.

24. Bowen DM, Smith CCT, White P, et al: Senile dementia and related abiotropies: biochemical studies in histologically evaluated human post-mortem specimens. *Aging NY* 1976; 3:361–378.

25. Perry EK, Perry RH, Blessed G, et al: Changes in brain cholinesterases in SDAT. *Neuropathol Appl Neurobiol* 1978; 4:273–277.

26. Perry R, Blessed G, Perry E, et al: Histochemical observations on cholinesterase activity in the brains of elderly normals and demented (Alzheimer-type) patients. *Age Ageing* 1980; 9:9–16.

27. Richter P, Perry E, Tomlinson B: ACh and choline levels in post-mortem human brain tissue: preliminary observations in Alzheimer's disease. *Life Sci* 1980; 26:1683–1689.

28. Drachman DA, Leavitt J: Human memory and the cholinergic system. *Arch Neurol* 1974; 30:113–121.

29. Drachman DA: Memory and cognitive function in man: does the cholinergic system have a specific role? *Neurology* 1977; 27:783–790.

30. Davis KL, Mohs RC, Tinklenberg JR, et al: Physostigmine: improvement of long-term memory processes in normal humans. *Science* 1978; 201:272–274.

31. Sitaram N, Weingartner H, Gillin JC: Human serial learning: enhancement with arecoline and impairment with scopolamine correlated with performance on placebo. *Science* 1978; 201:274–276.

32. Drachman DA, Sahakian BJ: Memory and cognitive function in the elderly: a preliminary trial of physostigmine. *Arch Neurol* 1980; 37:674–675.

33. Gottfries CG, Rosengren A, Rosengren E: The occurrence of homovanillic acid in the human brain. *Acta Pharmacol Toxicol* 1965; 23:36–40.

34. Gottfries CG, Gottfries I, Roos BE: The investigation of HVA in the human brain and its correlation to senile dementia. *Br J Psychiat* 1969; 115:563–574.

35. Adolfsson R, Gottfries CG, Roos BE, et al: Changes in the brain catecholamines in patients with dementia of the Alzheimer type. *Br J Psychiatry* 1979; 135:216–223.

36. Mann DMA, Lincoln J, Yates PO, et al: Changes in the monoamine containing neurons of the human CSF in senile dementia. *Br J Psychiatry* 1980; 136:533–541.

37. Cross AJ, Crow TJ, Perry EK, et al: Reduced DBH activity in Alzheimer's disease. *Br Med J* 1981; 282:93–94.

38. Yates CM, Ritchie IM, Simpson J, et al: Noradrenaline in Alzheimer-type dementia and Down syndrome. *Lancet* 1981; ii:39–40.

39. Van Woert H, Yahr M, Heninger G, et al: L-dopa in senile dementia. *Lancet* 1970; i:573.

40. Drachman DA, Stahl S: Extrapyramidal dementia and levodopa. *Lancet* 1975; i:809.

41. Kristensen V, Olsen M, Thielgaard A: Levo-dopa treatment of presenile dementia. *Acta Psychiatr Scand* 1977; 55:41–51.

42. Phuapradit P, Philips M, Lees AJ, et al: Bromocriptine in presenile dementia. *Br Med J* 1978; 1:1052–1053.

43. Peterson RC: Scopolamine induced learning failures in man. *Psychopharmacology* 1977; 52:283–289.

44. Torack RM: *The Pathological Physiology of Dementia.* Berlin, Springer, 1978, pp 17–25.

45. Haubrich DR, Wang PFL, Wedeking P: Role of choline in biosynthesis of acetylcholine. *Fed Proc* 1974; 33:477.

46. Cohen EL, Wurtman RJ: Brain acetylcholine: increase after systemic choline administration. *Life Sci* 1975; 16:1095–1099.

47. Ulus IH, Wurtman RJ: Choline administration: activation of tyrosine hydroxylase in dopaminergic neurons of rat brain. *Science* 1976; 194:1060–1061.

48. Davis KL, Hollister LE, Barchas JD, et al: Choline in tardive dyskinesia and Huntington's disease. *Life Sci* 1976; 19:1507–1515.

49. Boyd WD, Graham-White J, Blackwood G, et al: Clinical effects of choline in Alzheimer's senile dementia. *Lancet* 1977; ii:711.

50. Etienne P, Gautier S, Johnson G, et al: Clinical effects of choline in Alzheimer's disease. *Lancet* 1978; i:508–509.

51. Signoret J, Whitely AL, Lhermitte F: Influence of choline on amnesia in early Alzheimer's disease. *Lancet* 1978; ii:837.

52. Etienne P, Gauthier S, Dastoor D, et al: Lecithin in Alzheimer's disease. *Lancet* 1978; ii:1206.

53. Ferris ST, Sathananthan B, Reisberg B, et al: Long-term choline treatment of memory-impaired elderly patients. *Science* 1979; 205:1039–1049.

54. Christie JE, Blackburn IM, Glen A, et al: Effects of choline and lecithin on CSF choline levels and on cognitive function in patients with presenile dementia of the Alzheimer type, in *Nutrition and the Brain.* Barbeau A, Growdon JH, Wurtman RJ (eds): New York, Raven, 1979; pp 377–387.

55. Smith C, Swash M, Exton-Smith A, et al: Choline therapy in Alzheimer's disease. *Lancet* 1978; ii:318.

56. Renvoize EB, Jerram T: Choline in Alzheimer's disease. *N Engl J Med* 1979; 301:330.

57. Peters BM, Levin HS: Effect of physostigmine and lecithin on memory in Alzheimer's disease. *Ann Neurol* 1979; 6:219–221.

58. Vroulis GA, Smith RC, Brinkman S, et al: The effects of lecithin on memory in patients with senile dementia of the Alzheimer's type. *Psychopharmacol Bull* 1981; 17:127–128.

59. Fovall P, Dysken MW, Lazarus LW, et al: Choline bitartrate treatment of Alzheimer-type dementia. *Commun Psychopharmacol* 1980; 4:141–145.

60. Mohs RC, Davis KL, Tinklenberg JR, et al: Choline chloride treatment of memory deficits in the elderly. *Am J Psychiatry* 1979; 135:1275–1277.

61. Mohs RC, Davis KL, Tinklenberg JR, et al: Cognitive effects of physostigmine and choline chloride in normal subjects, in Davis KL, Berger PA (eds): *Brain Acetylcholine and Neuropsychiatric Disease.* New York, Plenum, 1979, pp 237–252.

62. Mohs RC, Davis KL: Choline chloride effects on memory: correlation with the effects of physostigmine. *Psychiatry Res* 1980; 2:149–156.

63. Davis KL, Mohs RC, Davis BM, et al: Enhancement of memory by intravenous physostigmine. *Aging NY* 1982; 19.

64. Muramoto O, Sugishita M, Sugita H, et al: Effect of physostigmine on constructional and memory tasks in Alzheimer's disease. *Arch Neurol* 1979; 36:501–503.

65. Smith CM, Swash M: Physostigmine in Alzheimer's disease. *Lancet* 1979; i:42.

66. Christie JE, Shering A, Ferguson J, et al: Physostigmine and arecoline: effects of intravenous infusions in Alzheimer presenile dementia. *Br J Psychiatry* 1981; 138:46–50.

67. Sullivan EV, Shedlack KJ, Corkin S, et al: Physostigmine and lecithin in Alzheimer's disease. *Aging NY* 1982; 19.

68. Peters BM, Levin HS: Effects of physostigmine and lecithin on memory in Alzheimer's disease. *Ann Neurol* 1979; 6:219–221.

69. Kaye WH, Sitaram N, Weingartner H, et al: Modest facilitation of memory in dementia with combined lecithin and anticholinesterase treatment. *Biol Psychiatry* 1982; 17:275–280.

70. Kaye WH, Weingartner H, Gold P, et al: Cognitive effects of cholinergic and vasopressin-like agents in patients with primary degenerative dementia. *Aging NY* 1982; 19:433–442.

71. Caine ED: Cholinomimetic treatment fails to improve memory disorders. *N Engl J Med* 1980; 303:585–586.

72. Wurtman RJ, Masil SG, Reinstein DK: Piracetam diminishes hippocampal acetylcholine levels in rats. *Life Sci* 1981; 28:1091–1093.

73. Friedman E, Sherman KA, Ferris SH, et al: Clinical response to choline plus piracetam in senile dementia: relation to red cell choline levels. *N Engl J Med* 1981; 304:1490–1491.

74. Ferris SH, Sathananthan G, Gershon S, et al: Cognitive effects of ACTH 4-10 in the elderly. *Pharmacol Biochem Behav* 1976; 5(suppl 1):73–78.

75. Branconnier RJ, Cole JO, Gardos G: ACTH 4-10 in the amelioration of neuropsychological symptomatology associated with senile organic brain syndrome. *Psychopharmacology* 1979; 61:161–165.

76. Willner AE, Rabiner CJ, Feldmar GG: Effect of ACTH 4-10 upon semantic and phonetic retrieval in elderly subjects with memory problems. Read before the Second International Neuropsychological Society European Conference, Noordwijkerhout, Holland, June 1979.

77. Branconnier RJ, and Cole JO: A preliminary data analysis of the effects of Org 2766 on mild senile organic brain syndrome. Report on file with Organon Pharmaceuticals, West Orange, NJ, 1977.

78. Ferris S, Reisberg B, Gershon S: Neuropeptide modulation of cognition and memory in humans. Poon LW (ed): *Aging in the 1980's.* Washington DC, American Psychological Association, 1980, pp 212–220.

79. Legros JJ, Gilot P, Seron Y, et al: Influence of vasopressin on learning and memory. *Lancet* 1978; i:41–42.

80. Weingartner M, Gold P, Ballenger JC, et al: Effects of vasopressin on human memory functions. *Science* 1981; 211:601–603.

81. Dimond SJ, Browers EYM: Increase in the power of human memory in normal man through the use of drugs. *Psychopharmacology* 1976; 49:307–309.

82. Mindus P, Cronholm B, Levander SE, et al: Piracetam-induced improvement of mental performance: a controlled study of normally aging individuals. *Acta Psychiatr Scand* 1976; 54:150–160.

83. Stegink AJ: The clinical use of piracetam, a new nootropic drug: the treatment of symptoms of senile involution. *Arzneim Forsch* 1972; 22:975–977.

84. Abuzzahab FS, Merwin GE, Zimmerman RC, et al: A double-blind investigation of piracetam (nootropil) versus placebo in the memory of geriatric inpatients. *Psychopharmacol Bull* 1978; 14:23–25.

85. Trabant R, Poljakovic Z, Trabant D: Zur Wirkung von Piracetam auf das hirnorganische Psychosyndrom bei zerebrovaskularer Insuffizienze. Ergebnis einer Doppelblindstudie bei 40 Fallen. *Ther Ggw* 1977; 116:1504–1521.

86. Hughes JR, Williams JG, Currier RD, An ergot alkaloid preparation (hydergine) in the treatment of dementia: critical review of the clinical literature. *J Am Geriatr Soc* 1976; 24:490–497.

87. Zahn L: Erfahrungen mit einem zehtralen Stimulans (Ritalin) bei cerebalen Altersveranderungen *Berl Gesundheitsblatt* 1955; 6:419–420.

88. Bachrach S: A new stimulant supplement for the geriatric patient. *J Am Geriatr Soc* 1959; 7:408–409.

89. Bare WW: A stimulant for the aged: observations on a methylphenidate–vitamin–hormone combination (Ritonic). *J Am Geriatr Soc* 8:292–297.

90. Bare WW, Lin DY: A stimulant for the aged: II. Long-term observations with a methylphenidate–vitamin–hormone combination (Ritonic). *J Am Geriatr Soc* 1962; 10:539–544.

91. Darrill FT: Double-blind evaluation of methylphenidate (Ritalin) hydrochloride. *JAMA* 1954; 169:1739–1741.

92. Lehmann HE, Ban TA: Comparative pharmacotherapy of the aging psychotic patient. *Laval Med* 1967; 38:588–595.

93. Crook T, Ferris S, Sathanathan G, et al: The effect of methylphenidate on test performance in the cognitive impaired aged. *Psychopharmacology* 1977; 52:251–255.

94. Gilbert JG, Donnelly KJ, Zimmer LE, et al: Effect of magnesium pemoline and methylphenidate on memory improvement and mood in normal aging subjects. *Int J Aging Hum Dev* 1973; 4:35–51.

95. Prien RF: Chemotherapy in chronic organic brain syndrome: a review of the literature. *Psychopharmacol Bull* 1973; 9:5–20.

96. Hunter B, Zornetzer SF, Jarvik ME, et al: Modulation of learning and memory: effects of drugs influencing neurotransmitters, in Iversen LL, Iversen SD, Snyder SH (eds): *Handbook of Pharmacology.* New York, Plenum, 1977, vol 8, pp 531–578.

97. Summers WK, Viesselman JO, Marsh GM, et al: Use of THA in treatment of Alzheimer-like dementia: pilot study in twelve patients. *Biol Psychiatry* 1981; 16:145–153.

98. Goodwin FG, Zis AP: Lithium in the treatment of mania. *Arch Gen Psychiatry* 1979; 36:840–844.

99. Prien RJ: Lithium in the prophylactic treatment of affective disorders. *Arch Gen Psychiatry* 1979; 36:847–848.

100. Jope RS, Jenden DJ, Ehrlich BE, et al: Erythrocyte choline concentrations are elevated in manic patients. *Proc Natl Acad Sci USA* 1980; 77:6144–6146.

101. Brazeau P, Vale W, Burgos R, et al: Hypothalamic polypeptide that inhibits the secretion of immunoreactive pituitary growth hormone. *Science* 1973; 179:77–79.

102. Guillemin R: Somatostatin inhibits the release of acetylcholine induced electrically in the myenteric plexus. *Endocrinology* 1976; 99:1653–1654.

103. Cohen ML, Rosing E, Wiley KS, et al: Somatostatin inhibits adrenergic and cholinergic neurotransmission in smooth muscle. *Life Sci* 1978; 23:1659–1664.

104. Mendelson WB, Sitaram N, Wyatt RJ, et al: Methscopolamine inhibition of sleep-related growth hormone secretion: evidence for a cholinergic secretory mechanism. *J Clin Invest* 1978; 61:1683–1690.

105. Richardson SB, Hollander CS, Elelto R, et al: Acetylcholine inhibits the release of somatostatin from rat hypothalamus *in vitro*. *Endocrinology* 1980; 107:122–129.

106. Bicknell RJ, Young PW, Schofield JC: Inhibition of the acetylcholine-induced secretion of bovine growth hormone by somatostatin. *Mol Cell Endocrinol* 1979; 13:167–180.

107. Petrusz P, Sar M, Grossman GH, et al: Synaptic terminals with somatostatin-like immunoreactivity in the rat brain. *Brain Res* 1977; 137:181–187.

108. Wood PL, Cheney DL, Costa E: Modulation of the turnover rate of hippocampal acetylcholine by neuropeptides: possible site of action of alpha-melanocyte-stimulating hormone, adrenocorticotrophic hormone, and somatostatin. *J Pharmacol Exp Ther* 1979; 209:97–103.

109. Cohn ML, Cohn M: Barrel rotation induced by somatostatin in the non-lesioned rat. *Brain Res* 1975; 96:138–141.

110. Sorensson DM, Wood PL, Cheney DL, et al: Modulation of the turnover rate of acetylcholine in rat brain by intraventricular injections of thyrotropin releasing hormone, somatostatin, neurotensin, and angiotensin II. *J Neurochem* 1978; 31:685–691.

111. Forno L: The locus coeruleus and Alzheimer's disease. *J Neuropathol Exp Neurol* 1978; 37:614.

112. Mann DMA, Lincoln J, Yates PO, et al: Changes in the monoamine containing neurons of the human CNS in senile dementia. *Br J Psychiatry* 1980; 136:533–541.

113. Forno L, Norville RL: Synaptic morphology in human locus coeruleus. *Acta Neuropathol* 1981; 53:7–14.

114. Bondareff W, Mountjoy CQ, Roth M: Selective loss of neurons of origin of adrenergic projections to cerebral cortex (nucleus locus coeruleus) in senile dementia. *Lancet* 1981; i:783–784.

115. Tomlinson BE, Irving D, Blessed G: Cell loss in the locus coeruleus in senile dementia of the Alzheimer type. *J Neurol Sci* 1981; 49:419–428.

42 The Pharmacological Basis for Cholinergic Investigations of Alzheimer's Disease: Evidence and Implications

DAVID A. DRACHMAN

SINCE THE MID-1970S THERE HAS BEEN a burgeoning of research involving the neuropharmacological and neurochemical aspects of cognitive decline in Alzheimer's disease (AD) and aging. Although several lines of investigation are currently being pursued, studies of the role of central cholinergic impairment have been most productive. A substantial body of information now supports the "cholinergic hypothesis" which suggest that (1) *function of the cholinergic system is necessary (if not sufficient) condition for normal memory and cognitive functions;* and (2) *the behavioral changes observed in Alzheimer's disease and normal aging are specifically related to the decline in cholinergic function.*

EVIDENCE FOR THE CHOLINERGIC HYPOTHESIS

Evidence for this hypothesis comes from several sources. Drachman and Leavitt (1) first demonstrated that central blockade of cholinergic function by the administration of scopolamine to healthy subjects produced a pattern of cognitive impairment which shared many features with the cognitive deficits occurring in aging and dementia. This "scopolamine-induced dementia" has been replicated in humans (2), and has been reproduced in experimental animals as well (3). Further studies showed that the administration of physostigmine, an anticholinesterase, largely reversed the cognitive deficits induced by scopolamine (2,4,5). D-amphetamine, a catecholaminergic CNS stimulant, failed to restore cognitive functions impaired by cholinergic blockade, further demonstrating a degree of pharmacologic specificity for the role of the cholinergic system in memory and cognitive functions.

Within a few years, Davies and Maloney (6) and others (7), demonstrated biochemical abnormalities of the cholinergic system in patients with AD. They found a consistent reduction in cortical choline acetyltransferase (CAT) levels in the brains of patients with AD, both at postmortem and at biopsy, when compared with age-matched controls. These deficiencies in an enzyme necessary for the synthesis of acetylcholine (ACh) have been closely correlated with the extent of neuropathological changes in AD (e.g., the density of the senile plaques [SPs] in the brain), as well as with the degree of impairment on tests of memory and cognitive

340

(M/C) functions (8). Muscarinic ACh receptor-binding is not further diminished in patients with AD compared with age-matched controls, however, which points to a presynaptic cholinergic disorder in this condition (7, 9). By contrast, cortical CAT remains relatively undiminished until advanced old age in the *normal aged* population, although there is a reduction in ACh muscarinic receptor-binding sites (10).

More recently Whitehouse and co-workers (11,12) have demonstrated cell loss and cytopathological abnormalities in the nucleus basalis of Meynert in the brains of AD patients. The consistency and specificity of this finding remain to be established in additional studies. Damage to this structure, which sends diffuse cholinergic projections to the neocortex, might provide a basis for the widespread nature of the CNS disorder in AD, while at the same time demonstrating an anatomically discrete source for cholinergic dysfunction. It is unclear how such a localized lesion could account for the characteristic cortical pathology of AD, making it unlikely that this lesion is more than one component of a diffuse and/or multifocal disorder.

While evidence for impairment of the cholinergic system in AD, and its specific relationship to the behavioral disorder of dementia, is convincing, the etiology and mechanism by which cholinergic impairment occurs in this disease remain obscure. Recent attempts to reverse the cholinergic deficiency in AD by pharmacologic manipulations, as well as other investigative approaches, have begun to provide some insight into the underlying mechanisms of the cholinergic dysfunction.

MECHANISMS FOR THE DECLINE OF CHOLINERGIC FUNCTION IN AD

At least four mechanisms may be considered in the interpretation of diminished cerebral cholinergic function in patients with AD (13).

1. The simplest (and most optimistic) interpretation of the decline of CAT and diminution of M/C function is that there is a *functional decrease in the presynaptic enzymatic machinery needed to synthesize acetylcholine.* Neurons may be intact and functioning normally in other respects, but in this model neurotransmission fails due to impaired synthesis, packaging, or release of acetylcholine.

2. *Anatomic loss or destruction of cholinergic neurons* may be the cause of decreased cortical CAT and impaired cholinergic neuronal function. It is well known that 30–50% of frontal and temporal cortical neurons are lost by age 80 in normal subjects (14), while an even greater proportion of *large* neurons are lost in patients with AD (15). Whether the loss of these neurons, or of neurons in the nucleus basalis as mentioned above, accounts for the decline in cholinergic function is unknown. Alternatively, there may be a major loss of dendritic and axonal arborizations or synaptic connections in neurons whose perikarya remain intact (16). In support of this, Golgi studies in AD have consistently shown a decline in neuronal connections and dendritic spines, and electron microscopic studies have suggested a loss of synapses (17).

3. Cholinergic neurons and their processes may remain relatively intact, but *neuronal functions necessary for signaling*—energy metabolism, axoplasmic flow, maintenance of resting potentials, conduction of impulses, and so on—may be impaired. There is considerable evidence of diminished cerebral blood flow, cerebral oxygen consumption, and cerebral glucose utilization in patients with AD (18). In this context, Blass and Gibson (19) have noted that cholinergic function is *selectively* severely impaired when glucose and pyruvate metabolism are decreased.

4. Evidence can thus be found to support the view that memory and cognitive decline in patients with AD may be due to loss of structure, loss of function, or both structural and functional changes in cholinergic neurons. With either form of impairment, additional secondary effects must also be considered. If information is stored in the brain as patterns of facilitated synaptic connections, maintenance of these neural patterns ("engrams") may depend on the continuing trophic influence of normal synaptic function (13). Interruption of this neuron–neuron interaction may result in decreased connectivity, resulting in *irretrievable "atrophic" loss of information.*

Strategies to Improve Cholinergic Function

If any or several of these mechanisms of cholinergic decline are responsible for the M/C impairment in AD patients, what results might be expected from pharmacologic attempts to enhance cholinergic function? Four strategies are available to attempt to improve function in the cholinergic system. These are (1) the use of large doses of precursors of acetylcholine; (2) administration of anticholinesterase medications; (3) use of muscarinic cholinergic receptor agonists; and (4) administration of drugs that increase other neural activities in cholinergic neurons.

1. Precursors of Acetylcholine. Both choline and lecithin (phosphatidylcholine) have been shown to be effective precursors of ACh in experimental animals. Administration of both substances raises the amount of ACh in the brain of experimental animals (20, 21), and can be shown to increase plasma choline levels in humans (22). The administration of small and large doses of these two precursors both to normal aged and to demented patients has failed to demonstrate any consistent benefit, however (2). In part, this may indicate a failure of choline or lecithin to increase ACh in the cortical neuronal "releasable pool," although there is some evidence that these drugs exert central effects in both tardive dyskinesia and scopolamine-induced dementia (23). In addition, Bartus and co-workers (24) showed that large doses of choline given throughout life may postpone cognitive decline in experimental mice. The *preventative* aspects of this treatment have not been studied in man.

2. Anticholinesterases. The only readily available centrally active anticholinesterase at present is physostigmine. This agent, which prevents the enzymatic hydrolysis of synaptically released ACh, has been administered to normal young subjects (1, 25), elderly subjects (26, 27), and AD patients (2). There is evidence that, in carefully adjusted doses, it may improve cognitive functioning in all three experimental groups. The degree of improvement is modest and variable. This pharmacologic strategy clearly produces significant central cholinergic effects, however, since it sharply improves scopolamine dementia (4). In appropriate doses, it is likely to increase cholinergic activity only at already active synapses, thus providing *specific* amplification of cholinergic activity.

3. Cholinergic Receptor Agonists. Arecoline is believed to act by enhancing muscarinic cholinergic receptor function. Thus, the effect of synaptically released ACh should be specifically augmented in those areas involved in M/C function. So far arecoline has been used experimentally only in normal young subjects, where Sitaram and associates (28) have demonstrated a significant increase in memory function.

4. General Metabolic Enhancers. Piracetam (Nootropil), a gamma aminobutyric acid (GABA) derivative said to increase adenosine triphosphate (ATP) synthesis, has been studied both in animals and in AD patients. In experimental rats, piracetam produced only a small improvement in the retention of a passive avoidance behavior; but the drug, in

combination with choline, produced a sharp improvement of retention (29). A human study of this combination of drugs is currently under way (Ferris, personal communication, 1982).

This review of pharmacologic approaches to the improvement of cholinergic function suggests the possibility that *specific* enhancement of synaptically released acetylcholine may be of benefit in patients with AD. Whether other strategies to augment central cholinergic function will prove useful remains to be determined.

INTERPRETATION OF CHOLINERGIC AGONIST EFFECTS

The information derived from these experimental and therapeutic trials may help to determine which of the four postulated mechanisms are responsible for the cholinergic impairment in AD patients.

First, if cholinergic neural elements are lost, no currently available treatment could restore these elements or, indeed, produce a noticeable improvement in function. Because there is redundancy and plasticity in the brain, however, some benefit could result—probably temporarily—from cholinergic enhancement. As long as sufficient "neural reserve" remained, facilitation of function in intact cholinergic neurons might, by increasing the "gain," moderately improve M/C function (30).

Second, if *synaptic transmission is impaired while neural elements remain intact, facilitation of cholinergic function would be most likely to improve M/C function.* The apparent benefit of physostigmine, although modest, is of interest, supporting this possible mechanism. The failure of both choline and lecithin to improve AD is somewhat contradictory. As mentioned above, however, it may indicate only that precursor supplementation fails to increase ACh in the brain's releasable pool. Alternatively, the failure of a precursor strategy may indicate that memory and cognitive function depend on highly selective patterns of facilitated and inhibited synaptic connectivity; and since precursor supplementation "floods" the cholinergic system in an unselective way, it may obscure meaningful neural signals.

If cholinergic neurons are functionally impaired because of general diminution in metabolic function, therapy directed towards increasing oxidative metabolism, synthesis of cyclic AMP, and assurance of normal electrolytic environments might improve function in cholinergic neurons. The effectiveness of piracetam and choline in aged experimental animals supports this possibility; but its lack of dramatic benefit in AD patients has so far been disappointing (31).

Finally, if the "atrophic" loss of information is important in the M/C decline in AD, a preventative strategy would be necessary. Long-term facilitation of cholinergic function prior to the onset of dementia would be necessary to avoid irretrievable loss of memory and cognitive functions. Although the findings of choline supplementation in aged mice (24) is of interest, there is no evidence that a similar strategy is helpful in human AD.

It must be recognized that any, all, or none of these mechanisms may be involved in the M/C impairment occurring in AD; and that the available pharmacologic strategies may have to be combined, individualized, and fine-tuned to achieve measurable improvement in patients with this condition (31).

There is much evidence in support of the cholinergic hypothesis relating memory and cognitive function to the cholinergic system, and its decline in aging and dementia due to cholinergic disturbances. It is highly unlikely, however, that impairment of cholinergic function is the sole significant disorder occurring in the aged and demented brain. There is evidence that somatostatin is also diminished in AD (32), as is catecholamine function (31), although neither is as severe or as consistent as the cholinergic impairment. Ultimately, attempts to restore function in the cholinergic or other pharmacologic systems by administration of drugs represent patching strategies at best. The ideal therapeutic goal must aim at the prevention or treatment of the underlying biologic disorder—genetic, viral, or biochemical—that results in impairment of neural functioning in AD.

ACKNOWLEDGMENTS

This work was supported in part by the BRSG Grant #6-32472 and the Sterling Morton Research Fund. The author is grateful to Dr. Guila Glosser for assistance in preparation and review of the manuscript.

REFERENCES

1. Drachman DA, Leavitt J: Human memory and the cholinergic system: a relationship to aging? *Arch Neurol* 1974; 30:113–121.

2. Davis KL, Mohs RC, Davis BM, et al: Cholinomimetic agents and human memory: clinical studies in Alzheimer's disease and scopolamine dementia, in Crook T, Gershon S (eds): *Strategies for the Development of an Effective Treatment for Senile Dementia.* New Canaan, Powley, 1981, pp 53–70.

3. Bartus RT, Johnson HR: Short-term memory in the rhesus monkey: disruption from the anticholinergic scopolamine. *Pharmacol Biochem Behav* 1976; 5:39–40.

4. Drachman DA: Memory and cognitive function in man: does the cholinergic system have a specific role? *Neurology* 1977; 27:783–790.

5. Bartus RT: Evidence for a direct cholinergic involvement in the scopolamine-induced amnesia in monkeys: effects of concurrent administration of physostigmine and methylphenidate with scopolamine. *Pharmacol Biochem Behav* 1978; 9:833–836.

6. Davies P, Maloney JF: Selective loss of central cholinergic neurons in Alzheimer's disease. *Lancet* 1976; ii:1403.

7. Perry EK, Perry RH, Blessed G, et al: Necropsy evidence of central cholinergic deficits in senile dementia. *Lancet* 1977; i:189.

8. Perry EK, Tomlinson BE, Blessed G, et al: Correlation of cholinergic abnormalities with senile plaques and mental test scores in senile dementia. *Br Med J* 1978; 2:1457–1459.

9. Davies P, Verth AH: Regional distribution of muscarinic acetylcholine receptors in normal and Alzheimer's-type dementia brains. *Brain Res* 1978; 138:385–392.

10. White P, Hiley C, Goodhardt M, et al: Neocortical cholinergic neurons in elderly people. *Lancet* 1977; i:668–670.

11. Whitehouse PJ, Price DL, Clark AW, et al: Alzheimer disease: evidence for selective loss of cholinergic neurons in the nucleus basalis. *Ann Neurol* 1981; 10:122–126.

12. Whitehouse PJ, Price DL, Struble RG, et al: Alzheimer's disease and senile dementia: loss of neurons in the basal forebrain. *Science* 1982; 215:1237–1239.

13. Drachman DA, Glosser G: Pharmacologic strategies in aging and dementia: the cholinergic hypothesis, in Crook T, Gershon S (eds): *Strategies for the Development of an Effective Treatment for Senile Dementia.* New Canaan, Powley, 1981, pp 35–51.

14. Brody H: An examination of cerebral cortex and brainstem aging. *Aging NY* 1976; 3:177–182.

15. Terry RD, Peck A, DeTeresa R, et al: Some morphometric aspects of the brain in senile dementia of the Alzheimer type. *Ann Neurol* 1981; 10:184–192.

16. Scheibel ME, Scheibel AB: Structural changes in the aging brain. *Aging NY* 1975; 1:11–37.

17. Bondareff W, Geinisman Y: *Loss of Synapses and Decreased Axonal Transport of Glycoproteins in the Septo-dentate Pathway of the Senescent Rat Brain.* Chicago, Northwestern University Press, 1975.

18. Ingvar DH, Brun A, Hagberg B, et al: Regional blood flow in the dominant hemisphere in confirmed cases of Alzheimer's disease, Pick's disease, and multi-infarct dementia. *Aging NY* 1978; 7:203–211.

19. Blass JP, Gibson GE: Carbohydrates and acetylcholine synthesis: implications for cognitive disorders, in Davis KL, Berger PA (eds): *Brain Acetylcholine and Neuropsychiatric Disease.* New York, Plenum, 1979, pp 215–236.

20. Cohen EL, Wurtman RJ: Brain acetylcholine: control by dietary choline. *Science* 1976; 191:561–562.

21. Wurtman RJ, Growdon JH: Dietary control of central cholinergic activity, in Davis KL, Berger PA (eds): *Brain Acetylcholine and Neuropsychiatric Disease.* New York, Plenum, 1979, pp 461–482.

22. Wurtman RJ, Hirsch MJ, Growdon JH: Lecithin consumption raises serum-free-choline levels. *Lancet* 1977; i:68–69.

23. Growdon JH, Hirsch MJ, Wurtman RJ, et al: Oral choline administration to patients with tardive dyskinesia. *N Engl J Med* 1977; 297:524–527.

24. Bartus RT, Dean RL, Goas JA, et al: Age-related changes in passive avoidance retention: modulation with dietary choline. *Science* 1980; 209:301–303.

25. Davis KL, Mohs RC, Tinklenberg JR, et al: Physostigmine: improvement of long-term memory process in normal humans. *Science* 1978; 201:272–274.

26. Drachman DA, Sahakian BJ: Memory and cognitive function in the elderly. *Arch Neurol* 1980; 37:674–675.

27. Drachman DA, Glosser G, Fleming P, et al: Memory decline in the aged: treatment with lecithin and physostigmine. *Neurology* 1982.

28. Sitaram N, Weingartner H, Gillin J: Human serial learning: enhancement with arecoline and choline and impairment with scopolamine. *Science* 1978; 201:274–276.

29. Bartus RT: Age-related memory loss and cholinergic dysfunction: possible directions based on animal models, in Crook T, Gershon S (eds): *Strategies for the Development of an Effective Treatment for Senile Dementia.* New Canaan, Powley, 1981; pp 71–90.

30. Drachman DA: Memory and the cholinergic system, in Fields WS (ed): *Neurotransmitter Function.* Miami, Symposia Specialists, 1977, pp 353–372.

31. Carlsson A: Aging and brain neurotransmitters, in Crook T, Gershon S (eds): *Strategies for the Development of an Effective Treatment for Senile Dementia.* New Canaan, Powley, 1981, pp 93–104.

32. Davies P, Katzman R, Terry RD: Reduced somatostatin-like immunoreactivity in cerebral cortex from cases of Alzheimer disease and senile dementia of the Alzheimer type. *Nature* 1980; 288:279–280.

43 Treatment of Alzheimer's Disease with Choline Salts

Penelope Fovall

Maurice W. Dysken

John M. Davis

A PRINCIPAL AIM OF CLINICAL CHOLINE STUDIES of individuals with Alzheimer's disease (AD) has been the replenishment of brain acetylcholine in these patients. A precursor-loading strategy with choline salts provides the method for these investigations. Brain choline acetyltransferase (CAT) levels have been found to be 70–90% lower than the levels found in normal age-matched controls (1–6). Acetylcholinesterase has also been found to be reduced in the cerebral cortex of Alzheimer patients as compared with age-matched controls (1, 3, 7, 8).

The reduction in CAT, reported by four independent laboratories, is of special significance for a precursor-loading strategy since CAT is considered specific to cholinergic neurons. Related to this evidence are studies that have found normal concentrations of muscarinic acetylcholine receptors in the cerebral cortex of Alzheimer patients (5, 6, 9). Given that the available evidence indicates normal functioning of the postsynaptic cholinergic system, it seemed reasonable to employ loading strategy in order to increase brain acetylcholine levels in these patients. This approach is not without its uncertainties, however. Primary among them is the inference that a major CAT deficit implies a loss of cholinergic neurons. Despite this caveat, the only consistent evidence for a sizable deficit in neurotransmitter markers has been from CAT data (for a review see ref. 10). The hypothesis of a selective loss of cholinergic neurons in the cerebral cortex of patients with AD has thus served as a rationale for the clinical choline studies considered below.

This chapter will critically review these clinical studies of choline treatment of AD patients. Discussion will be directed at this research area as a whole, with reference made to specific studies. Two major issues will be addressed. The first concerns internal validity: does treatment with choline salts significantly affect the behavior of Alzheimer patients? The second concerns external validity: to what extent are these findings generalizable beyond the samples studied? (11, 12)

INTERNAL VALIDITY

The efficacy of choline administration in improving the cognitive and behavioral functioning of Alzheimer patients was tested by a series of studies (Table 43–1). Modest effects of

TABLE 43–1
Design Characteristics

Reference No.	Choline/ Placebo/ Blind	No. S/No. C[a]	Subjects (Ss) Comparison	Dosing No. of Days at No. of g/day
18	Phosphorylcholine as sodium salt/no/?	3/0	Within Ss: all had same tx. sequence	20 at 5 g/day
19	Chloride/no/no	7/0	Within Ss: all had same tx. sequence	21 at 5 g/day 21 at 10 g/day
20	Chloride/no/no	11/0	Within Ss: all had same tx. sequence	1 at 2 g/day 2 at increased 5 at 5 g/day
16	Bitartrate/yes/no	3/0	Within Ss: all had same tx. sequence	14 at placebo 2 at 1 g/day up by 1 g/q2 days, to 8 g/day 10 at dose lowered 14 at placebo
13	Bitartrate/yes/ double	5/0	Within Ss: Ss randomly assigned to 2 tx. sequences	14 at dose-free 14 at placebo[b] 14 at 8 g/day 14 at 12 g/day 14 at 16 g/day 7 at placebo
14	Chloride/yes/ double	9?/9?	Between Ss: choline grp: placebo grp:	56 at 15 g/day 56 at placebo
17	Citrate/no/no	8/8	Between Ss: choline grp: normal grp:	21 at 9 g/day no tx.
15	Bitartrate/yes/ double	10/0	Within Ss: all had same tx. sequence	21 at 9 g/day 7 at washout 21 at placebo

[a] Number of subjects/number of controls.
[b] This placebo period placed after 16 g/day for other tx. sequence.

choline treatment were noted in some AD patients, as revealed by changes in their cognitive and behavioral functioning (Table 43–2, columns 1 and 2). These changes may represent a choline effect, but alternate explanations need to be examined before concluding that the administration of choline is solely responsible. Consequently, emphasis will be given to differences in design characteristics among the studies.

Most informative are studies testing for the effects of choline treatment under controlled conditions. Such studies typically employ a placebo control, and ensure that both patients and staff are blind to the treatment protocol (13–15; Table 43–1, column 1). Two comparison conditions are used in some of these studies (Table 43–1, columns 2 and 3): one type (13, 15) compares patients' placebo performance with their choline performance (within subjects), and the other type randomly assigns patients to two groups: choline and placebo (between

TABLE 43–2
Treatment Outcome Measures

Reference No.	Cognitive Measures	Behavioral Measures	Choline Levels	Side Effects
18	No improvement	Improvement in alertness, physical activity, verbally aggressive	None taken	Nausea, abdominal pain, diarrhea
19	No improvement	Less irritable, more aware of surroundings	None taken	10 g/day: nausea, diarrhea
20	No cognitive measures used	Mild irritability	With 125 g: serum: up 123% after 1 hr, up 129% after 3 hr CSF: 84% higher after 1 hr	Not reported
16	Reproduced design no. 1 of block designs test	No improvement	Plasma: up 341%	Incontinence ($N = 1$)
13	Improvement: word recog. ($N = 5$; $P < .05$)[a]	No improvement	Plasma: up 184% at 12 g	8 g/day: ($N = 1$) anxious, foul fishy odor, nausea, gas
14	No improvement	No improvement	None taken	Not reported
17	Relearning and recall of 30 pictures after delay ($N = 3$)	Improvement in everyday memory ($N = 3$), rated by relatives	None taken	Not reported
15	No improvement	No measurable improvement, but three patients seemed less confused	None taken	Exacerbation of urinary incontinence ($N = 3$), depression ($N = 1$)

[a] Patients were tested five times prior to treatment protocol.

subjects) (14). With no exact knowledge of when or if the choline is administered, treatment expectations of patients and staff are unlikely to effect experimental outcomes.

Cognitive measures show modest improvements substantiated by a test of statistical reliability in one controlled study (13; Table 43–2, column 1). Favorable behavioral outcomes predominate in the non-control studies (no placebo and/or no blind), with no study showing a statistically reliable improvement (Table 43–2, column 2). It is, however, possible that subtle, subclinical cognitive improvement was achieved by administering choline to these patients. At the very least, choline levels were increased over those taken at baseline, and side effects observed (Table 43–2, columns 3 and 4). The question that arises is why the choline effects were not more robust.

The necessity for repeated measurements, especially repeated cognitive testing, can affect test performance in ways that influence treatment results. Requiring patients to repeat a set of cognitive tasks may increase the reliability of behavioral data. Initially, frequent testing may actually interfere with a patient's ability to perform. Most cognitive tests are confrontational and reactive; some patients become upset and anxious, especially during the first few testing sessions; this distress can adversely affect memory task performance. A patient may become disheartened and unwilling to persevere at cognitive tests he/she perceives as simple, but which pose ostensible difficulty. Other patients with mild deficits may show learning effects during the first few testing sessions. Pretesting can minimize test anxiety by allowing patients to become accustomed to testing requirements, and can minimize learning effects in other patients. In either case, such effects are not likely to be confounded with treatment outcomes. The value of pretesting these patients for internal test validity must be weighed against the implications for generalizability of results; this point is further elaborated in the section on external validity.

Of the studies that reported an improvement in cognitive functioning with choline administration (13, 16, 17), only one controlled study (13) reported pretesting patients prior to testing them during treatment. Because pretesting with patients did not show any learning effects, it is unlikely that improvement in cognitive test performance is confounded by learning effects during the study period. Whereas repeated cognitive testing may be affected by patients' reactivity to the measures, repeated behavioral observation can be affected by changes in the way observers rate patient behavior.

Interpretation of choline treatment effects demands awareness of instrumentation changes associated with using an observer-rated behavioral scale. A standardized method for documenting behavioral changes in these patients during treatment is essential, yet has drawbacks that must be made explicit. Under noncontrol conditions, an observer's awareness that a patient is under treatment can obviously bias judgments of patient behavior. Depending on whether he believes the drug will be effective, a rater may inadvertently assign scores that underestimate or overestimate the effect of treatment. Under controlled conditions, there are still systematic errors that may occur with repeated observation. As an observer becomes increasingly familiar with the patients he/she is rating, changes in perception can occur. Among the noncontrol studies, improvement in patients' behavior with choline administration is challenged by the strong possibility that the observers' knowledge of patients' treatment had an effect on their ratings. No scorable improvement in patient behavior was obtained in any of the controlled studies (Table 43–2, column 2). At the same time, some patients did appear to be less confused on choline than on placebo (15). This change, while not substantial enough to be documented according to criteria specified in a rating scale, may still represent a shift in patient behavior. The source of this behavioral shift may not, however, be the choline administration.

An additional factor to consider in interpreting choline treatment outcomes is a change in patient behavior due to maturational changes brought about by the course of the illness. Changes in behavior or cognitive functioning may reflect the fluctuating course observed in many Alzheimer patients, especially in studies lasting more than 3 or 4 weeks. Improvement in cognitive performance and resolution of some patients' confusional status on choline, as compared to placebo, may coincide with a temporary improvement in the dementia state. These studies were not designed to control for this possibility. In fact, the likelihood that a fluctuating disease course is responsible for these effects cannot be ruled out.

In summary, the internal validity question of whether there is a choline treatment effect in Alzheimer patients was addressed by a critical review of strengths and weaknesses among the various studies. A major distinction was made between studies conducted on a double-blind basis with a placebo control, and those that are not. Among the controlled studies, effects are small and confined to individual studies. In considering the non-drug treatment factors that could explain observed cognitive and behavioral effects, it is the fluctuating course of the disease that poses the greatest challenge to the conclusion that choline administration does improve cognitive and behavioral functioning in some patients. If some patients demonstrate a "true" choline effect, there remains the question of how general this effect might be. This issue is addressed in the following section.

EXTERNAL VALIDITY

Limits on the extent to which a choline effect can be generalized are determined by three factors: the degree to which biases in patient selection interact with treatment, the interaction of multiple testing with treatment, and the use of a multiple dosing sequence.

If patient selection procedures differ among studies, more than one type of patient population may be represented. This differential recruitment can result in various patient types who show variation in response to choline treatment. Of the various ways in which some Alzheimer patients differ from others, some characteristics can potentially influence cognitive or behavioral outcomes. Patients who differ in (1) residential status (community dwelling versus institution); (2) severity and duration of disease, especially aphasic disorders; (3) sex and/or (4) age may show dissimilar responses to choline treatment. Regardless of the type of patient who is recruited, it is instructive to know how many complete the treatment protocol. Knowledge of selection and attrition rates provides a global index of the degree to which selection bias may be introduced into any study. A low selection rate (less than 60%) and/or a high attrition rate (greater than 40%) suggest that results may be biased due to an unrepresentative sample patient group.

One way to gauge suspected bias in patient selection is to compare patient characteristics of completers with noncompleters. Differences between these two groups can be useful for suggesting ways to interpret treatment outcomes. Similar reasoning can be used to make comparisons among the three controlled studies. As indicated in Table 43–3, the younger group, which includes few female patients, showed a slight improvement in cognitive test performance. It is possible that characteristics other than age and sex may distinguish this group from the two that did not respond. However, additional information on patient characteristics is incomplete. Another factor that seems unique to the responder group is the extent of pretreatment experience with cognitive test materials, relative to the nonresponders.

Pretesting these patients may minimize learning effects, yet there is the possibility of sensitizing patients to the choline treatment. Patients who have taken a test battery many

TABLE 43–3
Patient Characteristics

Reference No.	Degree of Impairment	Disease Duration	Sex, No. of Males/ No. of Females	Age, Mean; Range
18	Severe	Not reported	?/?[a]	60;48–66
19	Severe	Not reported	?/?	??;70–80+
20	Mild to severe	Not reported	4/7	60;53–67
16	Moderate	Not reported	1/2	82;76–88
13	Mild to moderate	Not reported	3/2	70;55–77
14	Not reported	2+ yr	0/18	73;57–84
17	Mild	2.5–5 yr	?/?	??;59–78
15	Not reported	Not reported	3/7	77;??–??

[a] Unknown.

times may display a subclinical effect tapped by the memory test battery, but which shows no immediate clinical effect in terms of short-term (2 months) day-to-day functioning of Alzheimer patients. This may, in fact, be the case for the one controlled study that reported cognitive improvement (Table 43–2, footnote). Patients in this study were tested five times (three pretestings, two drug-free baseline testings) prior to administration of the treatment protocol. Consequently, this cognitive improvement may represent a facilitated treatment effect operating solely through the sensitizing function of the pretestings. This suggests that the generalizability of a choline effect is limited to slight improvements in patients who are well practiced on the cognitive tasks used to assess such improvement. Such an effect is presumably associated with a particular dose of choline.

It is emphasized that this generalization is warranted only if one dose of choline is tested. Patients treated with more than one dose of choline may, therefore, show a "dose response" that is artifactual. Studies that test more than one dose of choline do so in order to probe for a therapeutic window. An unintended consequence is a cumulative treatment effect. This effect may be associated with the sequence of choline doses, rather than with the particular dose at which an effect was observed. While both nonresponder groups were treated with one dose (14, 15), the responder group was treated with three doses of choline (13). The finding that improved cognitive task performance occurred during the 12 g/day dosing period may have been due to a carryover effect of the 8 g/day dosing period which preceded the 12 g/day. In sum, just as possible interactions between selection and testing factors and treatment may occur, multiple-treatment interactions may operate to restrict the generalizability of treatment outcomes.

In conclusion, the choline treatment studies of Alzheimer dementia patients raise questions of whether choline does favorably affect these patients, and the extent to which such an effect is generalizable. Relatively short-term (under 2 months) choline treatment of some individuals with AD may be accompanied by mild improvement in cognition and behavior. However, this slight improvement is also consistent with the fluctuation in functional level often seen in Alzheimer patients who, nonetheless, deteriorate as the dementia progresses. If choline-related, these slight improvements were not observed in all studies under review.

It would seem that reservations as to the extent to which these effects can be replicated may certainly be anticipated.

References

1. Davies P: Studies on the neurochemistry of central cholinergic systems in Alzheimer's disease. *Aging NY* 1978; 7:453–459.

2. Davies P: Neurotransmitter-related enzymes in senile dementia of the Alzheimer type. *Brain Res* 1979; 711:319–327.

3. Davies P, Maloney AJF: Selective loss of central cholinergic neurons in Alzheimer's disease. *Lancet* 1976; ii:1403.

4. Bowen DM, Spillane JA, Curzon G, et al: Accelerated aging or selective neuronal loss as an important cause of dementia. *Lancet* 1979; i:11.

5. Perry EK, Perry RH, Blessed G, et al: Necropsy evidence of central cholinergic deficits in senile dementia. *Lancet* 1977; i:189.

6. White P, Goodhardt MJ, Keet JP, et al: Neocortical cholinergic neurons in elderly people. *Lancet* 1977; i:668–671.

7. Perry EK, Tomlinson BE, Blessed G, et al: Correlation of cholinergic abnormalities with senile plaques and mental test scores in senile dementia. *Br Med J* 1978; 2:1457–1459.

8. Pope A, Hess HH, Lewin E: Microchemical pathology of the cerebral cortex in presenile dementias. *Trans Am Neurol Assoc* 1965; 89:15–16.

9. Davies P, Verth AH: Regional distribution of muscarinic acetylcholine receptor in normal and Alzheimer's type dementia brains. *Brain Res* 1977; 138:385–392.

10. Terry D, Davies P: Dementia of the Alzheimer type. *Annu Rev Neurosci* 1980; 3:77–95.

11. Campbell DT, Stanley JC: *Experimental and Quasi-experimental Designs for Research.* Chicago, Rand McNally, 1966.

12. Runkel PJ, McGrath JE: *Research on Human Behavior: A Systematic Guide to Method.* New York, Holt, Rinehart & Winston, 1972.

13. Fovall P, Dysken M, Lazarus LW, et al: Choline bitartrate treatment of Alzheimer-type dementias. *Communica Psychopharmacol* 1980; 4:141–145.

14. Renvoize EB, Jerram T: Choline in Alzheimer's disease. *N Engl J Med* 1979; 301:330.

15. Smith CM, Swash M, Exton-Smith AN, et al: Choline therapy in Alzheimer's disease. *Lancet* 1978; ii:318.

16. Etienne P, Gauthier S, Johnson G, et al: Clinical effects of choline in Alzheimer's disease, *Lancet* 1978; i:508–509.

17. Signoret JL, Whiteley A, Lhermitte F: Influence of choline on amnesia in early Alzheimer's disease. *Lancet* 1978; ii:837.

18. Antuono P, Taiuti R, Amaducci L, et al: Preliminary trials of phosphorylcholine in Huntington's chorea and senile dementia, in Barbeau A, Growdon JH, Wurtman RJ (eds): *Nutrition and the Brain.* New York, Raven, 1979, vol 5, pp 331–333.

19. Boyd WD, Graham-White J, Blackwood G, et al: Clinical effects of choline in Alzheimer senile dementia. *Lancet* 1977; ii:711.

20. Christie JE, Blackburn IM, Glen AIM, et al: Effects of choline and lecithin on CSF choline levels and on cognitive function in patients with presenile dementia of the Alzheimer type, in Barbeau A, Growdon JW, Wurtman RJ (eds): *Nutrition and the Brain.* New York, Raven, 1979, vol 5, pp 377–387.

44 Treatment of Alzheimer's Disease with Lecithin

Pierre Etienne

The selective loss of cholinergic neurons in Alzheimer's disease (AD) is well known and this loss may well be related to the severe intellectual deterioration associated with that condition. Accordingly, two main therapeutic strategies have been suggested: (a) inhibition of the degradation enzyme acetylcholinesterase and (b) stimulation of the synthesizing enzyme choline acetyltransferase, by raising substrate (i.e., choline) levels. Suitable central anticholinesterase inhibitors are not yet available for clinical use. For instance, the use of physostigmine is complicated by side effects and a very short duration of action (1). Therefore, several groups of clinicians decided to try the "increased substrate availability" strategy.

Initially, choline itself was used to raise plasma (and brain) choline levels in Alzheimer patients. But shortly afterward, the advantages of lecithin (phosphatidylcholine), a naturally occurring source of dietary choline, were reported (2). (a) Lecithin raises blood choline levels in human subjects, to a greater extent and for a longer period, than an equimolar dose of choline chloride; (b) lecithin does not produce the foul odor concomitant of choline administration in some patients. Unfortunately, lecithin, too, presents some disadvantages. Commercially available lecithin preparations contain a variety of substances in addition to lecithin (phosphatidylcholine) itself. The content of these other substances varies depending upon method of preparation and source of lecithin used: apart from various chemical analogues of phosphatidylcholine, the preparation may also contain impurities such as heavy metals or pesticides originating from the natural source of the lecithin, as well as various trace amounts of chemicals utilized in the process of extraction, purification, and concentration of the substance (3). None of the lecithin preparations currently on the market is composed entirely of pure phosphatidylcholine. In other words, lecithin is not a very clean pharmacological agent.

Overlooking the mysteries around the composition of lecithin preparations, various clinicians decided that a lecithin pilot study in Alzheimer patients was worth a try. The results obtained showed lecithin administration had no remarkable effect on the function of Alzheimer patients despite a twofold to fourfold rise in their plasma choline levels (4, 5). An improvement was suggested in some psychological tests, however, and double-blind trials were undertaken.

Several of these double-blind trials have now been completed and data obtained by various clinical investigators with an aggregate of approximately 100 patients, were recently presented (6–13). The exclusion criteria used to diagnose AD were rigorous; one can safely assume that 75% of these patients had AD. The severity of dementia, length of treatment, lecithin purity, and dosage level per day varied considerably from one study to another, but all treatments were sufficient to raise plasma choline levels at least twofold. The consensus among investigators was that no beneficial or reproducible response had been demonstrated. Despite reservations, however, some observations suggest that lecithin treatment may slow mental deterioration (6). This finding is consistent with the result of studies of aging rodents which show that long-term dietary choline administration could suppress the age-related loss of cortical dendritic spines (Chap. 51) and also preserve retention of passive-avoidance learning (Chap. 53).

REFERENCES

1. Goodman LS, Gilman A (eds): *The Pharmacological Basis of Therapeutics,* ed 5. New York, Macmillan, 1975.

2. Wurtman RJ, Hirsch MJ, Growdon JH: Lecithin consumption raises serum-free choline levels. *Lancet* 1977; ii:68–69.

3. Hanin I: Commercially available "lecithin": proposed guidelines for nomenclature and methodology, in Barbeau A, Growdon JH, Wurtman RJ (eds): *Nutrition and the Brain.* New York, Raven, 1979, vol 5, pp 443–446.

4. Christie JE, Blackburn IM, Glen AIM, et al: Effects of choline and lecithin on CSF choline levels and on cognitive function in patients with presenile dementia of the Alzheimer type, in Barbeau A, Growdon JH, Wurtman RJ (eds): *Nutrition and the Brain.* New York, Raven, 1979, vol 5, pp 377–387.

5. Etienne P, Gauthier S, Dastoor D, et al: Alzheimer's disease: clinical effect of lecithin treatment, in Barbeau A, Growdon JH, Wurtman RJ (eds): *Nutrition and the Brain.* New York, Raven, 1979, vol 5, pp 389–396.

6. Sullivan EV, Shedlack KJ, Corkin S, et al: Physostigmine and lecithin in Alzheimer's disease. *Aging NY* 1982; 19:361–367.

7. Etienne P, Dastoor D, Gauthier S, et al: Lecithin in the treatment of Alzheimer's disease. *Aging NY* 1982; 19:369–372.

8. Heyman A, Logue P, Wilkinson W, et al: Lecithin therapy of Alzheimer's disease: a preliminary report. *Aging NY* 1982; 19:373–378.

9. Pomara N, Goodnick PJ, Brinkman SD, et al: A dose-response study of lecithin in the treatment of Alzheimer's disease. *Aging NY* 1982; 19:379–383.

10. Dysken MW, Fovall P, Harris CM, et al: Lecithin administration in patients with primary degenerative dementia and in normal volunteers. *Aging NY* 1982; 19:385–392.

11. Domino EF, Minor L, Duff IF, et al: Effects of oral lecithin on both blood choline levels and memory tests in geriatric volunteers. *Aging NY* 1982; 19:393–397.

12. Peters BH, Levin HS: Chronic oral physostigmine and lecithin administration in memory disorders of aging. *Aging NY* 1982; 19:421–426.

13. Garcia CA, Tweedy JR, Blass JP, et al: Lecithin and parkinsonian dementia. *Aging NY* 1982; 19:443–449.

45 Combination Treatment of Alzheimer's Dementia

NATRAJ SITARAM

HERBERT WEINGARTNER

WALTER H. KAYE

MICHAEL H. EBERT

RACHEAL EPSTEIN

UNDERSTANDING THE PSYCHOBIOLOGY OF PRIMARY DEGENERATIVE DEMENTIA (PDD) (commonly referred to as Alzheimer's disease) would ideally require an appreciation and detailed knowledge of both the specific type of memory failure(s) as well as the neurochemical correlates of the above cognitive defects. The current state of the art, with respect to psychometric data as well as to results of psychopharmacologic manipulations of memory in dementia, unfortunately lacks such specific understanding or treatment approaches. It is now clear that the specificity claimed originally for loss of cortical choline acetyltransferase in the brains of dementia patients (1, 2) may not hold since a recent autopsy study (3) suggests that a distinct subgroup of PDD patients (characterized by high dementia scores and relatively young age at death) may suffer from a loss of about 80% of locus ceruleus neurons. By and large, treatments based on administration of cholinergic agents have been discouraging.

This chapter will present and discuss some preliminary data pertaining to two issues: (1) a comparison of patients with PDD and normals with respect to their performance on a number of cognitive tasks, in an effort to delineate any specific memory defects that may characterize the disorder, and (2) a trial of a combination treatment of a cholinergic precursor (lecithin) and an orally administered anticholinesterase agent in a small number of PDD patients. The above studies have previously been published in full (4, 5).

NATURE OF MEMORY FAILURES IN PDD

Fourteen patient volunteers (nine males and five females) were selected for study from a much larger sample at the National Institutes of Health (NIH) after extensive systematic and standardized clinical-neurological diagnostic evaluation. All patients had previously functioned well, most of them having ceased to function in an occupational setting at some time during the year preceding the study. All had functioned in a manner that indicated a premorbid intelligence well above normal. The patients studied included five individuals with postgraduate degrees, including a physician, a physicist, a Ph.D. in music, and a lawyer, as well as several business executives. None of the patients studied was an inpatient of an institution. On the basis of detailed historical, clinical, and laboratory data, a diagnosis of PDD (Alzheimer's disease) was arrived at. Diagnoses were established in several stages. All patients had had several detailed neurological examinations prior to a neurological and psychiatric screening evaluation. Patients not included for further study were those whose histories and present cognitive dysfunction and clinical findings could be attributable to other neurological or psychiatric disorders. Generally, subjects selected were in good health. They were not being treated for other medical disorders, nor were they being administered any conflicting form of medication. In addition, those included were assumed in the earliest stage of a progressive dementia. They were all emotionally and behaviorally appropriate, and with some minimal supervision could perform independently many activities including self-care. An equal number of age, education, and socioeconomic status matched control volunteers (where possible, patient spouses) were also recruited and studied. Neither patients nor controls had any history of significant psychiatric disorder. Their average age was 61.2 years (S.D. = 7.9), and their education, 14.1 years (S.D. = 3.2).

A standard battery of psychometric tests, as well as a few specific cognitive tasks, was administered to the subjects. This chapter will briefly highlight the findings of two selected tests, namely, Serial Learning and Prompted Recall Procedure.

SERIAL LEARNING

Subjects were presented with 12 unrelated, commonly occurring words for serial ordered recall. Words used as stimuli were all chosen from the 3,000 most frequently occurring words in the English language. More than half were either "A" or "AA" words using frequency norms of English words. Stimuli were presented at one every 3 seconds. The subject's task was to recall both the presented words and their correct list ordering. After attempting serial reproduction of the list, the subject was presented with the same list in the same order and again attempted serial order recall. This procedure was repeated 10 times, or until the subject had perfectly reproduced all words in their correct list order.

PROMPTED RECALL PROCEDURE

Subjects were presented 14 semantically unrelated common words at a one word/3 sec rate for free recall. After an initial presentation trial and attempted free recall, subjects were presented only those words not recalled on the previous trial. Again, subjects attempted recall of previously remembered words as well as those prior, unrecalled stimuli. After attempted recall of all 14 words, subjects were again selectively reminded of those words missed on the last recall trial. Selective, prompted presentation of words and tests of recall were discontinued after 10 trials or when subjects could recall all 14 words in any order.

The results are shown in Figure 45–1. Patients with PDD appeared to suffer from a profound difficulty in organizing and recalling serially presented material as well as a failure to successfully retain and carry over previously presented words across the span of the 10 trials during the prompted recall procedure.

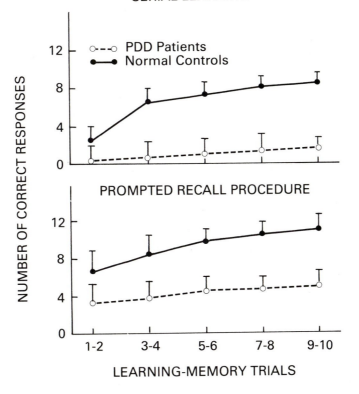

SERIAL LEARNING

PROMPTED RECALL PROCEDURE

o---o PDD Patients
•——• Normal Controls

NUMBER OF CORRECT RESPONSES

LEARNING-MEMORY TRIALS

*Means and standard errors for the serial learning
task (words remembered in correct list order) and
for the prompted recall procedure (number of
words correctly recalled)

Figure 45–1. Word list learning in patients with primary degenerative dementia (PDD) and in normal controls (mean values
and standard errors of the mean).

PHARMACOLOGICAL TRIAL

A recent report by Peters and Levin (6) showing facilitation of memory storage and
retrieval in demented patients by a combination of lecithin and physostigmine appeared to
suggest that additive effects may be achieved by combining a cholinergic precursor and an
anticholinesterase agent. The mechanism of action of such a combination was not and remains
not entirely clear. Nevertheless, the investigators attempted to replicate the above study
using lecithin and tetrahydroaminoacridine (THA) on a group of ten inpatients aged 51 to
71 (mean age, 61.5 years) with PDD. The general characteristics of these patients were
similar to those described in the previous study comparing cognitive differences between
normal controls and PDD patients. Our choice of THA was prompted by a review of the
literature of the 1960s, when it was used extensively by anesthesiologists as an adjunct to
general anesthesia to potentiate the action of succinylcholine, a muscle relaxant (7). THA
also seemed to reverse the symptoms of anticholinergic agents (8). Albert and Glendhill

(9) claimed that THA had predominantly central cholinergic action with few peripheral side effects.

Benveniste and Dyrberg (7), for example, reported an unusually low incidence of vomiting (less than 1%, with a virtual absence of sweating, both cardinal signs of peripheral cholinergic activity) in patients tested even though no peripheral anticholinergic pretreatment had been used. This is in sharp contrast to the often unpleasant side effects noted with physostigmine.

Subjects were treated with lecithin (LE) and THA, administered orally, both separately and in combination under the following four conditions in random order: LE + placebo (for THA), THA + placebo (for LE), LE + THA, placebo (for THA) + placebo (for LE). A minimum of 56 hours elapsed between trials to control for carryover effects. LE was supplied by the American Lecithin Company as Phospholipon 100 (containing 92% pure phosphotidylcholine), mixed in a milkshake to disguise its taste and consistency. The placebo for LE was a mixture of corn oil and graham crackers, and mixed in a milkshake in a manner identical to the active LE. THA and its placebo analogue were administered as capsules. The dosage of THA used was 30 mg and of LE, 60 g, both (or their respective placebos) given in three divided doses at 10:00 P.M. (the night prior to testing), at 8:00 A.M., and at noon, followed by psychological testing at 2:00 P.M. The active study was conducted in double-blind fashion. Prior to the study, patients had a standardized memory test, the Wechsler Memory Scale (WMS), and two baseline trials of a battery of the following memory tests

Serial Learning. Administered as described above in the previous study, except that 10 words were used this time instead of 12.

Prompted Recall Procedure. Again, identical to the one previously described except that only 10 words were used.

Free Recall of Related Words. Subjects were read a list of 32 words, two groups of 16 words each. Each group represented a semantically cohesive group of words indicating a category such as vegetables, sports, parts of the body, and so on. Subjects were instructed to recall as many words as possible immediately after one full list presentation (4).

RESULTS

Wechsler Memory Quotient (WMQ) mean score for the ten patients was 75.9 ± 4.4 (range 57–99). Since the Wechsler Memory Scale was administered prior to the start of the drug trials, it provided a convenient independent measure to correlate with drug test results.

As indicated in Table 45–1, there was no statistically significant difference in the group means of the three tests administered across the four treatment conditions. This was consistent with clinical observations and nursing staff notes, as well as subjective impressions reported by several patient spouses attesting to the lack of improvement. There was, however, a small but nonsignificant trend indicating increased scores on the serial learning task alone, under the LE + THA condition.

The above trend prompted analysis of the serial learning test results alone with respect to whether there was a subgroup of patients who may have demonstrated a measurable improvement. The WMQ score, as stated earlier, provided an independent measure by which

TABLE 45–1
Serial Learning Test Scores in PDD Patients[a]

Test	Placebo	LE Only	THA Only	LE + THA	ANOVA
All patients, $N = 10$	10.1[b] ± 2.0	9.9 ± 2.9	8.5 ± 2.6	14.1 ± 4	$P = $ NS
Patients with "high" WMQ (>79), $N = 5$	12.8 ± 2.6	13.2 ± 5.0	12.3 ± 3.8	22.4 ± 5.6	$P < .05$
Patients with "low" WMQ (<74), $N = 5$	6 ± 2.7	5.6 ± 2.5	4.8 ± 2.8	6 ± 0.8	$P = $ NS

[a] Serial learning scores were computed as the *sum* of the total word pairs across all 10 trials for the subject. Thus, a perfect single-trial score for the 10-word presentation would be 9 pairs, and a perfect 10-trial score would be 90. ANOVA with repeated measures was performed with post hoc Scheffé test. Data for prompted recall procedure and free recall of related words did not show any changes. (See ref. 5 for data.)
[b] Mean ± S.E.M.

patients could be divided in an unbiased fashion. The WMQ correlated significantly and positively with serial learning scores across all four conditions. In addition, a median split based on high (> 79) and low (< 74) WMQ scores revealed that only the high WMQ patients ($N = 5$) had a significant increase in serial learning performance (ANOVA with repeated measures F (3, 24) = 3.05, $P < .05$). Post hoc testing using the Scheffé procedure revealed a selective improvement produced by the combination treatment (LE + THA), during which patients remembered approximately twice as many word pairs, as compared with the other three treatment conditions ($P < .05$). Patients with low initial WMQ, on the other hand, showed no improvement over placebo under any treatment condition.

Further validation of the interaction of the degree of cognitive impairment (as indicated by baseline WMQ scores) with subsequent change (improvement) using the combination (LE + THA) treatment was provided by a significant positive correlation ($r = .71$, $P < .02$) found between WMQ and the increased serial learning score produced by LE + THA combination over placebo (Fig. 45–2).

DISCUSSION

What, if any, is the significance of this small, clinically unobservable but statistically significant improvement of serial learning in a subgroup of PDD patients? Assuming that the finding is replicable, it could indicate the following: The data provides some clinical support for observations by Wecker and Dettbarn (10) that administration of choline alone had no significant effect on rat brain acetylcholine synthesis but that the combination of choline and an anticholinesterase (paraoxon) increased acetylcholine synthesis. This increase was significantly greater than that produced by choline or paraoxon alone. Thus, limited preclinical data supports the possibility that a combination of a cholinergic precursor and cholinesterase inhibitor might have additive effects. Our study confirms this. The above additive effects occur only in mildly impaired patients. This suggests that with increasing severity of dementia in PDD patients, additional factors over and above a simple decrease of choline acetyltransferase may come into being, such as, for instance, a loss of postsynaptic

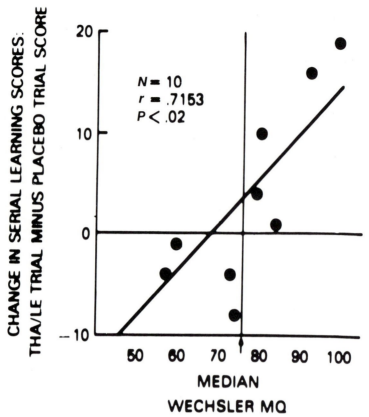

Figure 45–2. Change in memory following lecithin and THA treatment in progressive dementia patients.

muscarinic receptors and/or catecholaminergic depletion. Under these conditions, cholinergic agents may lose whatever efficacy they may have in mildly impaired cases.

REFERENCES

1. Bowen DM, Smith EB, White P, et al: Neurotransmitter-related enzymes and indices of hypoxia in senile dementia and other abiotrophies. *Brain* 1976; 99:459–496.

2. Davies P, Maloney AJF: Selective loss of central cholinergic neurons in Alzheimer's disease. *Lancet* 1976; ii:1403.

3. Bondareff W, Mountjoy CQ, Roth M: Loss of neurons of origin of the adrenergic projection to cerebral cortex (nucleus locus ceruleus) in senile dementia. *Neurology* 1982; 32:164–168.

4. Weingartner H, Kaye W, Smallberg S, et al: Memory failures in progressive idiopathic dementia. *J Abnorm Psychol* 1981: 187–196.

5. Kaye WH, Sitaram N, Weingartner H, et al: Modest facilitation of memory in dementia with combined lecithin and anticholinesterase treatment. *Biol Psychiatry* 1982; 17:275–280.

6. Peters BH, Levin HS: Effects of physostigmine and lecithin on memory in Alzheimer's disease. *Ann Neurol* 1979; 6:219–221.

7. Benveniste D, Dyrberg V: Tetrahydroaminoacridine: clinical use of cholinesterase inhibition in conjunction with succinylcholine. *Acta Anaesthesiol Scand* 1962; 6:1–6.

8. Mendelson C: Central anticholinergic syndrome reversed by tetrahydroaminoacridine (THA) *Med J Aust* 1975; 2:906–909.

9. Albert A, Gledhill W: Improved synthesis of aminoacridines: IV. substituted 5-aminoacridine. *J Soc Chemical Industry* 1945; 64:169.

10. Wecker L, Dettbarn WD: Relationship between choline availability and acetylcholine synthesis in discrete regions of rat brain. *J Neurochem* 1979; 32:961–967.

46 Nootropics

Michael K. Schneck

Nootropics are a new class of psychotropic agents developed in the search for a gamma amino butyric acid (GABA) analogue. The initial compound developed was 2-oxo-pyrrolidine acetamide (piracetam). When tested, this compound failed to demonstrate any GABA-like activity, but did demonstrate central nervous system effects by exerting a therapeutic effect centrally on nystagmus in rats (1).

While many nootropic compounds are now being developed, this review will focus on piracetam as representative of this class of pharmacologic agents, because the vast majority of basic science and clinical studies of nootropics have utilized piracetam. In addition, this review will focus on the utility of nootropics such as piracetam for the treatment of Alzheimer's disease (AD).

Pharmacologic studies of piracetam have demonstrated a number of interesting properties. Early animal studies showed its propensity to increase learning in many situations; it facilitated learning of a Y maze and a water maze by normal, alcoholic, and aged rats (2); and it enhanced brain resistance to severe anoxia in rabbits (3). Rats were protected by piracetam from learning impairment induced by electroconvulsive shock administration (4) and by hypoxia (5). It has been shown to increase the amplitude of certain cortical and transcallosal evoked potentials (6).

Piracetam's actions were not explained by any autonomic, sedative, or stimulant effects in the EEG or on the behavior of these animals. It did, however, increase the ATP/ADP ratio in the brain, thus increasing energy reserves (7). It also increased the turnover of phospholipids in rat brains (8).

Another study demonstrating an enhancement of protein synthesis (9) in cortical nerve cells was reported. Finally, early pharmacologic studies failed to demonstrate any side effects or any toxic effects of this new substance in normal therapeutic doses (1). The lack of toxicity, in addition to its memory enhancing properties, made this new drug a promising avenue of exploration in the treatment of memory disorders of the elderly.

In early double-blind controlled studies with humans, piracetam improved the level of postoperative consciousness in patients undergoing neurosurgery (10), reduced the occurrence and severity of postconcussional symptoms (11), and exerted a protective effect against an assumed hypoxia in patients with artificial pacemakers when the heart rate was reduced (12).

Early European studies all showed improvement in various measures of geriatric patients with the diagnosis of "cerebral arteriosclerosis" (13–16). However, these studies were not well controlled, and the tests gauging improvements were subjectively determined. An early

362

double-blind study by Stegink (17) reported significant improvement in subjectively rated measures such as asthenia, memory, alertness, psychomotor agitation, and perception.

In the area of cognition, Dimond and Brouwers (18) reported a double-blind study of the effect of 400 mg of piracetam daily in 16 healthy, cognitively normal college students. While after 7 days no effect was noted, after 14 days those students on piracetam demonstrated significantly increased performance in certain memory tasks. Mindus and associates (19) studied the effect of piracetam 1.0 g TID in a double-blind placebo controlled study of 19 men and women ranging in age from 47 to 73 years. All subjects had subjective complaints of memory loss, but all were still working and functioning normally in their daily lives. Those patients on piracetam were assessed as "improved" on a global scale as compared to the placebo group. An analysis of their results, however, showed improvement on performance tests, although no specific memory tests were included or observed.

Another double-blind study reported by Abuzzahab and co-workers (20) demonstrated a positive piracetam effect on a clinical global change scale in geriatric hospitalized patients with "deterioration of mental function." Two other double-blind studies reported no improvement (21, 22).

Chouinard and co-workers (23) reported in a double-blind study of 20 elderly psychiatric patients a beneficial effect of piracetam on alertness, socialization, and performance on memory and intelligence tests. While this study was well controlled, and appropriate memory measures were included, it may be criticized because of the 20 patients studied only one was diagnosed as having had a primary organic brain syndrome. Eighteen out of 20 patients were diagnosed as having a schizophrenic or affective disorder in remission, while the remaining patient had a mild organic mental syndrome secondary to alcoholism.

In 1979, Lloyd-Evans and associates (24) reported the results of a major study of piracetam in the treatment of 102 aged patients with mild to moderate brain failure living in geriatric residential homes. Their report highlights several of the technical difficulties in conducting such studies. The study design was a double-blind, placebo-controlled crossover of 800 mg of piracetam TID. Despite close supervision and highly motivated staff in the homes, only 78 of the original 102 patients completed the study. Of these, only 29 remained after disqualification of those who did not show the test marker in the urine. Consequently, only 30% of the patients originally enrolled in the study could be said to have undergone an adequate research trial. Out of the total of 19 tests used in their trial, only one (Designation of Name and Address Test) showed any statistically significant improvement with piracetam when compared with placebo. In addition, this positive finding was only demonstrated for the first 6 weeks of active treatment compared to placebo, and did not extend through the full 12 weeks of the trial. Lloyd-Evans and associates concluded that the improvement seen was so transitory as to be of no positive value.

Branconnier and Cole (25) recently completed a double-blind controlled trial of 40 patients. Twenty subjects received 1.6 g TID of piracetam; the remainder received identical placebo tablets. Here, Branconnier and Cole found a highly significant difference on a test of delayed visual recognition in favor of piracetam. Also, the piracetam group exhibited no loss of retention of visual material acquired before treatment, while the placebo group showed the expected logarithmic forgetting curve. In support of these small positive findings, they reported that an analysis of pre- and post-treatment EEGs demonstrated a reduction in the percentage of delta activity, indicating an overall shift toward faster frequencies after piracetam.

Ferris and associates (26) recently completed a study of 40 geriatric outpatients diagnosed as having mild to moderate Alzheimer-type cognitive impairment. The study design was a double-blind, placebo-controlled crossover trial of 2.4 g TID of piracetam. A preliminary analysis of 20 of the patients has been completed. Of the 37 cognitive test measures evaluated, only two tests showed small significant improvements in favor of piracetam. Thus, most studies utilizing piracetam have demonstrated only subtle positive effects of little clinical significance.

In any case, a rationale in the utility of combining piracetam with a cholinergic precursor in the treatment of AD has been developed in a recent year. It is well known that a large body of scientific evaluations have implicated the cholinergic neurotransmitter system in memory processes (27). Recent neuropathological studies in AD have consistently revealed a sharp reduction in acetylcholine, choline acetyltransferase (CAT), and other enzymes involved in cholinergic neurotransmission (28), as well as a selective reduction in cholinergic neurons. The magnitude of the reduction in CAT has been strongly correlated with the degree of cognitive impairment in AD. Conditions which interfere with cerebral metabolism and impair cerebral carbohydrate oxidation have been shown to cause a decrease in acetylcholine synthesis proportional to the reduction in oxidation (29). Hence, the observed deficits in the synthesis and release of acetylcholine in AD may be secondary to a preexisting metabolic deficiency accompanying the disorder. Accordingly, combining a treatment such as piracetam (enhanced ATP/ADP ratio, improved electrophysiologic functioning, and so on), which remediates the metabolic deficiency, with one that enhances cerebral cholinergic functioning may prove effective in reversing the disease process.

This rationale has recently been considerably strengthened by new findings indicating that piracetam may play a direct role in increasing postsynaptic cholinergic functioning. New animal studies have indicated that piracetam increases the incorporation of ^{32}P into phosphotidylcholine (lecithin) in neurons and glial cells isolated from rabbit cerebral cortex (30). This result implies that piracetam increases the rate of turnover of membrane-bound choline. The investigator in this study also concluded that "the data obtained suggest that piracetam may stimulate excitatory neurons and be involved in the process of synaptic transmission." As stated, a deficiency in the synthesis of acetylcholine in the brain has been strongly related to the development of AD in humans. New data also indicate that the synthesis of brain acetylcholine is reduced in aged mice of two strains (C 57B1 and Balb/c), and that deficits in the cholinergic system may contribute to brain dysfunction which complicate senescence in these animals (Gibson, Peterson, and Jenden, unpublished).

Further support for the hypothesis that piracetam may enhance postsynaptic release of choline derives from the recent work of Wurtman and colleagues (31), who found that piracetam administration in rats caused a significant reduction in hippocampal acetylcholine without significantly modifying choline levels. A reduction in regional brain acetylcholine levels could reflect either slowed synthesis or accelerated release of the transmitter. That piracetam acted by accelerating acetylcholine's release is suggested by its failure to change hippocampal choline levels (32). "If piracetam actually facilitates hippocampal cholinergic neurotransmission, and if this neurochemical effect is related to its reported action on memory," the report concluded, "then it might be possible to amplify its utility by administering it along with choline or lecithin, which enhances acetylcholine's synthesis in and release from rapidly firing cholinergic neurons" (33).

Direct behavioral verification of hypothesized benefits of combined cholinergic precursor therapy and metabolic enhancement has been provided by a recent animal study by Bartus and colleagues (34). Old Fisher 344 rats showed deficits in retention of one-trial, passive avoidance learning. Groups of these rats, 20–28 months of age, received one of four treatments for 1 week: choline, piracetam, choline and piracetam, and saline control. Following the week of treatment, the animals were exposed to a one-trial passive avoidance procedure

TABLE 46-1
Mean Scores on Selective Reminding Task of Four Patients Showing Clinical Response to 1-Wk Treatment with Choline and Piracetam

Measure	Baseline	After 1 Wk	% Change
Storage			
Trial 1	2.25 (1.71)[a]	4.50 (1.73)	100.0
2	4.50 (3.32)	6.25 (3.30)	38.9
3	5.50 (4.20)	8.00 (2.71)	45.5
4	7.25 (2.98)	8.25 (2.22)	13.8
5	7.25 (2.99)	8.25 (2.22)	13.8
Retrieval			
Trial 1	2.25 (1.71)	4.50 (1.73)	100.0
2	3.75 (3.00)	4.25 (0.96)	13.3
3	3.50 (2.39)	5.75 (1.50)	64.3
4	4.25 (1.26)	7.25 (1.71)	70.6
5	4.25 (1.50)	4.50 (3.00)	5.9
Delayed	2.75 (2.75)	4.75 (1.26)	72.7

[a] S.D.s are in parentheses.

and were then tested for retention 24 hours later. Retention for the group receiving choline alone was slightly better than for treatment with saline ($P < .10$). Piracetam alone produced significantly better retention than saline ($P < .02$). However, choline and piracetam was several times better than treatment with piracetam alone ($P < .0001$). Thus, the behavioral effect of increasing cholinergic precursor availability was greatly enhanced by piracetam.

In a pilot study conducted by Reisberg and co-workers (35), seven Alzheimer patients, aged 60 and over, were treated with the combination of piracetam (1.8 g TID) and choline chloride (3 g TID) in a 1-week open trial. Results showed improved mean performance on the memory storage measure of the Buschke verbal learning task for all five Buschke recall trials and for the delayed recall condition. In the same pilot study analogous results were obtained for the memory retrieval measure on four of the five Buschke initial recall trials, and in delayed recall (Table 46-1).

Other test results indicative of recent memory retention, specifically in performance on a task assessing memory for names, were consistent with the findings of Reisberg et al on the Buschke task. Performance on motor and perceptual motor tasks was less consistent, indicating that the memory effects do not appear to have been the product of a simple stimulant effect of the drug combination.

In addition, the study psychiatrist rated four of these seven patients as clinically improved. An analysis of red cell choline and plasma choline data of these patients lends credence to the positive findings. While blood was available for only three of these four patients, their results were found to be significantly different from those of the other three patients. Their initial red cell choline levels were significantly higher than those who did not appear clinically improved (see Table 46-2). Also, the increase in their red cell choline levels following treatment was significantly higher than the increase in the nonresponder group.

These results from an open, uncontrolled study of 1 week's duration need to be researched further in longer controlled studies. Currently, such an undertaking is under way.

In summary, nootropics are a new class of psychoactive drugs. While piracetam has been the only nootropic to undergo clinical testing at present, other more potent nootropics are under development. While further study of these drugs' effects in the brain is needed,

TABLE 46–2
Mean Plasma and RBC Choline Concentrations in Dementia Patients Receiving Placebo or Choline Plus Piracetam for 1 Wk

Treatment	N	Plasma Choline (nmole/ml)	RBC Choline (nmole/ml)
All patients			
Baseline	10	7.1 ± 0.34[a]	12.0 ± 3.33
Choline + piracetam	10	27.5 ± 2.12	34.4 ± 6.35
Responders			
Baseline	3	6.7 ± 1.10	23.8 ± 7.99
Choline + piracetam	3	25.8 ± 4.92	56.4 ± 7.85
Nonresponders			
Baseline	7	7.1 ± 0.34	7.0 ± 0.84
Choline + piracetam	7	28.2 ± 2.44	23.4 ± 3.42

[a] S.E.M.

it appears that nootropics are of little clinical value in the more traditional psychiatric illnesses: schizophrenia, depression, and so on. However, it does appear that nootropics may exert small positive effects on AD, and in combination with cholinergic precursors they may ultimately prove to be of value in the treatment of AD.

References

1. *Nootropil: Basic Scientific and Clinical Data.* Brussels, UCB, 1977.

2. Wolthius L: Experiments with UCB 6215, a drug which enhances acquisition in rats: its effects compared with those of metamphetamine. *Eur J Pharmacol* 1971; 16:283–297.

3. Giurgea LE, Mouravieff-Lesuisse F, Leeman SR: Corrélations électropharmacologiques au cours de l'anoxie oxyprivé chez le lapin en respiration libre ou artificielle. *Rev Neurol* 1970; 122:484–486.

4. Giurgea LE, Mouravieff-Lesuisse F: Pharmacological studies on an elementary model of learning: the fixation on an experience at spinal level: pharmacological reactivity of the spinal cord fixation time. *Arch Int Pharmacodyn* 1971; 191:279–291.

5. Sara SJ, Lefevre D: Hypoxia induced amnesia in one trial learning and pharmacological protection by piracetam. *Psychopharmacologia* 1977; 25:32–40.

6. Buresova O, Bures J: Mechanisms of interhemispheric transfer of visual information in rats. *Acta Neurobiol Exp* 1973; 33:673–679.

7. Pede JP, Shimpfessel L, Crokaert R: The action of piracetam on oxidative phosphorylation. *Arch Int Physiol Biochim* 1971; 79:1036.

8. Gobert JG: Genèse d'un médicament—le piracetam: métabolisation et recherche biochemique. *J Pharm Belg* 1972; 26:281–304.

9. Burnotte RE, Gobert JG, Temmerman JJ: Piracetam (2-pyrrolidinone acetamide) induced modification of the brain polyribosome pattern in aging rats. *Biochem Pharmacol* 1973; 22:811–814.

10. Richardson AE, Bereen FJ: Effect of piracetam on level of consciousness after neurosurgery. *Lancet* 1976; 1110–1111.

11. Hakkarainen H, Hakamies L: Piracetam in the treatment of postconcussional syndrome. *Eur Neurol* 1978; 17:50–55.

12. Lagergren K, Levande S: A double-blind study on the effects of piracetam upon perceptual and psychomotor performance at varied heart rates in patients treated with artificial pacemakers. *Psychopharmacology* 1974; 39:97–104.

13. Boecker M: Clinical trial with UCB 6215 in aged subjects suffering from arteriosclerosis, Pharmaceutical Division report no. CE71A271. Brussels, UCB, 1971.

14. Geraud J: Clinical experts' report on UCB 6215 (piracetam), Pharmaceutical Division report no. CE72B031. Brussels, UCB, 1972.

15. Graux P, Gallet L: Piracetam en sénilité. *Lille Med* 1973; 18:487–488.

16. Weber H: Clinical trial of UCB 6215 in aged people suffering from atherosclerosis, Pharmaceutical Division report no. CE71B031. Brussels, UCB, 1971.

17. Stegink AJ: The clinical use of piracetam, a new nootropic drug: the treatment of symptoms of senile involution. *Arzneim Forsch* 1972; 22:975–977.

18. Dimond SJ, Brouwers EYM: Increase in the power of human memory in normal man through the use of drugs. *Psychopharmacology* 1976; 49:307–309.

19. Mindus P, Cronholm B, Levander SE, et al: Piracetam-induced improvement of mental performance. *Acta Psychiatr Scand* 1976; 54:150–160.

20. Abuzzahab FS, Merwin GE, Zimmermann RL, et al: A double-blind investigation of piracetam (Nootropil) vs. placebo in geriatric memory. *Pharmako psychiatr Neuropsychopharmakol* 1977; 10:49–56.

21. Dencker SJ, Lindberg D: A controlled double-blind study of piracetam in the treatment of senile dementia. *Nord Psykiatr Tidsskr* 1977; 31:48–52.

22. Gustafson L, Risberg J, Johanson M, et al: Effects of piracetam on regional cerebral blood flow and mental functions in patients with organic dementia. *Psychopharmacology* 1978; 56:115–118.

23. Chouinard G, Annable L, Ross-Chouinard A, et al: Ethopropazine and benztropine in neuroleptic-induced parkinsonism. *J Clin Psychol* 1979; 40:147–152.

24. Lloyd-Evans S, Brocklehurst JC, Palmer MC: Piracetam in chronic brain failure. *Curr Med Res Opin* 1979; 5:351–357.

25. Branconnier RJ, Cole JO: Final report of a clinical trial of the efficacy and safety of piracetam in the amelioration of the neuropsychological symptoms associated with mild primary degenerative dementia, April 22, 1980.

26. Ferris SW, Reisberg B, Crook T, et al: Pharmacologic treatment of senile dementia: choline, L-dopa, piracetam and choline/piracetam. *Aging NY* 1982; 19:475–481.

27. Bartus RT, Dean RL III, Beer B, et al: The cholinergic hypothesis of geriatric memory dysfunction: a critical review. *Science* 217; 1982:408–417.

28. Davies P, Maloney AJF: Selective loss of central cholinergic neurons in Alzheimer's disease. *Lancet* 1976; ii:1403.

29. Gibson GE, Blass JP, Jenden DJ: Measurement of acetylcholine turnover with glucose used as a precursor: evidence for compartmentation of glucose metabolism in brain. *J Neurochem* 1978; 30:71.

30. Woelk H: Effects of piracetam on the incorporation of ^{32}P into the phospholipids of neurons and glial cells isolated from rabbit cerebral cortex. *Pharmako psychiatr Neuropsychopharmakol* 1979; 12:251–256.

31. Wurtman RJ, Magil SG, Reinstein DK: Piracetam diminishes hippocampal acetylcholine levels in rats. *Life Sci,* in press.

32. Cohen EL, Wurtman RJ: Brain acetylcholine: increase after systemic choline administration. *Life Sci* 1975; 16:1095–1102.

33. Bierkamper GG, Goldberg AM: Effects of choline on the release of acetylcholine from the neuromuscular junction, in Barbeau A, Growdon J, Wurtman R (eds): *Nutrition and the Brain.* New York, Raven, 1979, vol 5, pp. 243–251.

34. Bartus RT: Pharmacologic manipulations of age-related neurobehavioral dysfunctions, in Enna SJ, Samorajski T, Beer B (eds): *Brain Neurotransmitters and Receptors in Aging and Age-Related Disorders.* New York, Raven, 1981.

35. Reisberg B, Ferris SH, Schneck MK, et al: Piracetam in the treatment of cognitive impairment in the elderly. *Drug Devel Res* 1982; 2:475–480.

47 Neuropeptides in the Treatment of Alzheimer's Disease

STEVEN H. FERRIS

ONE CLASS OF COMPOUNDS CURRENTLY BEING INVESTIGATED for their potential therapeutic value in treating Alzheimer's disease (AD) are the neuropeptides. Many pituitary peptide hormones, or short-chain peptide fragments of these hormones, are present in the brain and have direct CNS effects (1). These neuropeptides are either synthesized in the brain or are transported there from the hypothalamus (2). They are believed to function either as neurotransmitters or as modulators of neurotransmitters (1, 2). Of particular relevance to the processes of attention, memory, and the cognitive deficits of aging are neuropeptides related to ACTH and vasopressin. The current status of ACTH treatment and vasopressin treatment of cognitive deficits has been reviewed in detail elsewhere (3–6). This chapter provides a brief review of the aforementioned clinical research and summarizes the results of two recent studies with AD patients.

ACTH ANALOGUES

ACTH 4–10/MSH (administered by subcutaneous injection) and the more recent oral analogue, ACTH 4–9, are fragments of ACTH with the behavioral effects of ACTH but without peripheral hormonal effects. The animal literature for these neuropeptides has been extensively reviewed (7–10): these compounds facilitate animal learning and retention, block experimentally induced amnesia, and are believed to produce these short-term effects by increasing attention or motivation. The human studies conducted with ACTH analogues have recently been reviewed (3, 11). The literature suggests a general pattern of weak positive effects related to attention, visual memory, or reduction in fatigue.

Ferris and co-workers examined the efficacy of the potentially more potent oral analogue, ACTH 4–9 (Organon 2766). Fifty mildly to moderately impaired senile dementia outpatients, aged 60–85, completed the study. The degree of impairment was documented by means of objective cognitive tests and psychiatric ratings. Patients with significant depression (Hamilton Depression Scale scores greater than 18) or with likely etiologies other than AD were excluded. The study was designed as double-blind multiple crossover so as to evaluate the effects of both single-dose and chronic treatment for four different dosages and a placebo. To evaluate single-dose effects, patients received Treatment A on Day 1 and Treatment B on Day 2. To evaluate the effects of 2 weeks of treatment, Treatment B was continued for Days 3–

15, followed by a return to Treatment A for Days 16–29. Treatment A and B were, respectively, either a particular dosage and a placebo, or two different active dosages. Only 20 of the 50 subjects received a placebo as one of their two treatment conditions. The four dosages used were 20 mg or 10 mg given as single doses, or 10 mg or 5 mg given both morning and night.

Comprehensive behavioral and cognitive assessments were administered on the acute-treatment days and following each 2-week treatment period. The behavioral evaluations included a self-rated mood scale and several geriatric rating scales completed by a psychiatrist. The cognitive battery included a wide variety of memory tasks and perceptual-motor performance tasks. Results indicated that single doses produced a small improvement in visual recall, but slowed simple reaction time and increased fatigue ($P < .05$). However, 2-week treatment produced some small changes in verbal memory, and showed a consistent mood improvement. Specifically, a self-rated mood scale indicated reduced depression and anxiety and showed increased ratings of competence ($P < .05$). Similarly, psychiatric ratings showed reduced depression, increased energy, and increased attention–concentration. Recently, similar antidepressant or mild stimulant effects have been reported in two other studies (for a review see ref. 5). Thus, although the cognitive effects of ACTH 4–9 are minimal, a possible role for this side effect–free compound as a geriatric antidepressant should be examined further.

VASOPRESSIN

Vasopressin is synthesized and secreted by the anterior hypothalamus via the posterior pituitary (10). It has peripheral effects on blood pressure (when given in large doses) and water balance (via its normal action on the kidney) and is therefore also known as an antidiuretic hormone. Animal studies, including work with vasopressin analogues having minimal peripheral activity, have shown that this neuropeptide facilitates learning and increases resistance to extinction for both avoidance and appetitive behavior (9, 10). Vasopressin also antagonizes experimentally induced retrograde amnesias, and animals that lack vasopressin (with hereditary diabetes insipidus) show impairment of learning and memory, both reversed by administration of vasopressin, which has a direct CNS effects in animals. It is believed to exert long-term effects on the consolidation of memory, as opposed to the short-term behavioral effects of ACTH analogues.

In clinical studies with vasopressin, three vasopressin analogues have been examined, LVP (lysine vasopressin), DDAVP (1-desamino-8-D-arginine vasopressin), and DGAVP (des-glycinamide arginine vasopressin). Although the results in nonelderly subjects have not been consistently positive and sample sizes have been generally small, there is clear evidence of CNS activity (4). The vasopressin research with elderly subjects is summarized in Table 47–1. Two studies are suggestive of a positive clinical response: a study with cognitively normal subjects showed consistent improvement across a broad cognitive battery (12), and a recent study of multi-infarct dementia (MID) showed improved memory retrieval and positive behavioral effects (13). On the other hand, results of three studies with AD patients have been much less encouraging (14–16). At the same time, these essentially negative studies were conducted with institutionalized subjects who were generally severely impaired.

In the laboratory, Ferris and co-workers recently completed a study of the effects of LVP in 20 mildly to moderately impaired AD outpatients. In a double-blind crossover procedure, subjects received LVP (10 IU, intranasally) twice daily for 7 days, and a placebo

TABLE 47–1
Vasopressin: Clinical Studies in Aging and Dementia

Reference	Population	Compound	Design (*N*)	Results
Legros et al. (9)	"Normal" elderly	LVP	Parallel (23) 4 wk	Improved cognitive tests
Weingartner et al. (16)	Alzheimer's	DDAVP	Crossover (6)	Some Ss improved memory
Tamminga et al. (14)	Alzheimer's	LVP	Parallel (17)	No memory improvement; reaction time improvement
Bucht et al. (13)	Multi-infarct dementia	LVP	Parallel (20) 3 wk	Improved retrieval, behavior
Tinklenberg et al. (15)	Alzheimer's	DDAVP	Crossover (3) 3–8 days	No changes
		DGAVP	Crossover (1) 5 days	No changes

for 7 days. The order of treatment was randomized. A battery of cognitive tests and behavioral rating scales was administered at baseline, and following each treatment period. Results indicated small but statistically significant improvements on certain memory measures ($P < .05$) interpreted as drug-related improvement in memory retrieval. The psychomotor and attention measures showed no statistically significant improvements. With respect to behavioral measures, of the eight mood factors on a patient-rated mood scale, the factor labeled Carefree ("happy, full of pep, active, cheerful, lively, and carefree") was significantly improved following vasopressin treatment ($P < .05$). Since the study patients were not depressed (and the Depression factor was not significantly changed), the improvement in Carefree may be interpreted as a slight increase in stimulation or arousal.

Since previous negative studies with vasopressin generally employed more severely impaired inpatients, the positive results obtained with the mildly to moderately impaired outpatients suggest that less severely impaired patients may be more responsive to vasopressin treatment. It should be emphasized, however, that the memory improvements and pseudostimulant mood effects observed were not large changes with a clinically significant impact. In other words, results are primarily of theoretical value, since they indicate that vasopressin can produce CNS changes in patients with AD. However, the Ferris findings raise the possibility that more potent, longer-acting vasopressin analogues might have more substantial clinical effects. With respect to the mechanism of action, it remains unclear whether vasopressin acts via a direct CNS effect, or as a weak releaser of ACTH. These two possibilities may also relate to the question of whether vasopressin has a specific memory effect or a more general stimulant effect. This study leaves these issues unresolved, since both memory and stimulant effects seem to have occurred. Whether these two effects are independent or related remains to be determined.

CONCLUSIONS

The ACTH and vasopressin analogues are the only neuropeptides studied thus far as possible treatments for AD. Although current results have not demonstrated clinically significant benefits, both neuropeptides have shown CNS effects. It is hoped that further research, perhaps with more potent analogues, will further define a clinical role for these interesting compounds.

It is also of interest that numerous other neuropeptides have not yet been evaluated for their effects on AD symptoms. These include somatostatin, substance P, the enkephalins, TRH, and cholecystokinin. For each of these substances, a speculative theoretical rationale can be developed which suggests some potential for clinical evaluation; It remains to be seen whether future research with these compounds will lead to successful treatments for AD.

References

1. Guillemin R: Peptides in the brain: the new endocrinology of the neuron. *Science* 1978; 202:390–402.

2. Krieger DT, Liotta AS: Pituitary hormones in brain: where, how and why? *Science* 1979; 205:366–372.

3. Ferris S, Reisberg B, Gershon S: Neuropeptide modulation of cognition and memory in humans, in Poon LW (ed): *Aging in the 1980s: Selected Issues in the Psychology of Aging.* Washington, DC, American Psychological Association, 1980, pp 212–20.

4. Ferris SH, Reisberg B, Schneck MK, et al: Effects of vasopressin on primary degenerative dementia, in Ordy JM, Sladek JR, Reisberg B (eds): *Neuropeptide and Hormone Modulation of Brain Function and Homeostasis.* New York, Raven, in press.

5. Pigache RM: Effects of ACTH-like peptides on cognition and affect in the elderly, in Ordy JM, Sladek JR, Reisberg B (eds): *Neuropeptide and Hormone Modulation of Brain Function and Homeostasis.* New York, Raven, in press.

6. Pomara N, Reisberg B, Ferris SH, et al: Drug treatment of cognitive decline, in Maletta GJ, Pirozzolo FJ (eds): *Advances in Neurogerontology,* vol 2, *Behavioral Assessment and Psychopharmacology.* New York, Praeger, 1981, pp 107–143.

7. Beckwith BE, Sandman CA: Behavioral influences of the neuropeptides ACTH and MSH: a methodological review. *Neurosci Behav Rev* 1978; 2:311–338.

8. de Wied D: Pituitary-adrenal system hormones and behavior, in Schmitt FO, Warden FG (eds): *The Neurosciences.* Cambridge, MIT Press, 1973, vol 3, pp 653–664.

9. de Wied D: Peptides and behavior. *Life Sci* 1977; 20:195–204.

10. van Wimersma Greidanus TB, de Wied D: The physiology of the neurohypophyseal system and its relation to memory processes, in Davison AN (ed): *Biochemical Correlates of Brain Structure and Function.* New York, Academic, 1977, pp 215–248.

11. Pigache RM, Rigter H: Effects of peptides related to ACTH on mood and vigilance in man, in van Wimersma Greidanus T, Rees LH (eds): *Frontiers of Hormone Research, vol 8.* Basel, S Karger, 1981, pp 193–207.

12. Legros JJ, Gilot P, Seron X, et al: Influence of vasopressin on learning and memory. *Lancet* 1978; i:41–42.

13. Bucht G, Adolfsson R, Lancranjan I, et al: Vasopressin in multi-infarct dementia and other neuropsychiatric disorders, in Ordy JM, Sladek JR, Reisberg B (eds): *Neuropeptide and Hormone Modulation of Brain Function and Homeostasis.* New York, Raven, in press.

14. Taminga CA, Durso R, Fedio P, et al: Vasopressin studies in Alzheimer's disease. Read before the Annual Meeting of New Clinical Drug Evaluation Unit Program, Key Biscayne, May 27, 1981.

15. Tinklenberg JR, Peabody CA, Berger PA; Vasopressin effects on cognition and affect in the elderly, in Ordy JM, Sladek JR, Reisberg B (eds): *Neuropeptide and Hormone Modulation of Brain Function and Homeostasis.* New York, Raven, in press.

16. Weingartner H, Gold P, Ballenger JC, et al: Vasopressin enhances memory consolidation in man. *Science* 1981; 211:601–603.

48 Use of Vasoactive Medications in the Treatment of Senile Dementia

Jerome A. Yesavage

SEVERAL RATIONALES FOR THE USE OF vasoactive medications in the elderly have been developed. These rationales have changed rapidly with advancing knowledge of the etiology of dementia. Thus, before a discussion of the various medications, a brief review of general information about the dementias and cerebral blood flow (CBF) would be useful.

It is worthwhile to contrast in detail some important pathological and physiological differences between degenerative and atherosclerotic types of dementias (1, 2). An important point is that some of the degenerative dementias, at least in their early stages, have relatively well-preserved cerebral blood flow (CBF) with minimal loss of nerve cells (3–5). This finding has led to considerable research to attempt to define potential biochemical alterations of aged neurons which might account for a functional impairment leading to deterioration of cognitive abilities. In addition to the work on neurotransmitter metabolism, considerable work with the elderly has attempted to define changes in glucose metabolism which might be responsible for functional impairment of neurons (6). This work is based upon an understanding of the interrelations of cerebral glucose metabolism, oxygen consumption, carbon dioxide production, and regulation of CBF. At mean blood pressures greater than 50 mm Hg, CBF is proportional to brain metabolic activity: increased metabolic activity (e.g., a seizure) burns more glucose, requires more oxygen, and produces more carbon dioxide. The latter is a potent vasodilator, leading to vasodilatation and increased CBF. Investigators have also found a relationship between decline of CBF in aging and slowing of the electroencephalogram (EEG), as well as impaired cognitive test performance (7, 8). Thus, one major theory is that at least some dementias may be related to a primary disorder of neuronal glucose metabolism which then leads to a reduction of CBF and diffuse cerebral impairment.

Despite the arguments for a metabolic basis for dementia, other investigators stress the atherosclerotic component of the disease (9). Studies following this rationale have emphasized data from robust, healthy elderly with no evidence of atherosclerosis. Such elderly have been found to have the same rates of CBF and oxygen consumption as young normals. Furthermore, elderly with mild atherosclerosis without overt symptoms of dementia exhibited reduction of CBF with increased arterial/venous oxygen tension difference. The arterial/ venous oxygen tension difference is a measure of how much oxygen is drawn from the blood by the metabolic activities of an organ such as the brain. An increased difference may mean either increased metabolic demands, unlikely in the elderly, or decreased blood flow due to, say, an atherosclerotic plaque. Thus, before any symptoms had appeared, these patients had evidence of circulatory insufficiency. It is hypothesized that during periods of stress or reduced cardiac output, this insufficiency becomes critical, the patient becomes hypoxic, and neurons are lost. Eventually, due to the death of cells, metabolic demands decline, and there is less arterial/venous oxygen tension difference. Hence, in this theory decline of metabolic rate is secondary to circulatory deficiencies.

Data are not yet available to reject either of the two major theories. It is possible that both processes are active in certain elderly. In any case, these two theories are useful as a rational basis for isolating the two major classes of vasoactive medications used in the dementias.

MEDICATION TYPES

There are myriad compounds which have been purported to ameliorate the wellbeing and mentation of the elderly. Recent reviews discuss nonvasoactive compounds such as neurotransmitter precursors, neuropeptides, and stimulants, all of which have strong rationales behind their use (10). It should also be mentioned that careful differential diagnosis of the reversible medical causes of cognitive decline as well as the knowledgeable use of neuroleptics and antidepressants are essential to the care of the elderly with cognitive deficits (11). This chapter will present the evidence for employing the vasoactive compounds as proposed treatments for dementias (see Table 48–1).

Relating to the two major theories of dementias, one can separate vasoactive drugs for dementia into two classes: drugs which appear to act primarily on cerebral metabolism, then secondarily induce an increase in CBF; and drugs which appear to act primarily on the vasculature. This latter type of drug may be termed a primary or pure vasodilator, while the other type can be referred to as a secondary (or mixed) vasodilator and metabolic agent. Although some medications fall between these two, the distinction appears to have clinical relevance. In a review of 102 studies of both types of agents, the drugs with mixed effects (secondary vasodilators), as a class, had significantly more positive double-blind clinical trials in dementias than did drugs with purely vascular effects (primary vasodilators) (12).

SPECIFIC MEDICATIONS

PRIMARY VASODILATORS

Primary vasodilators have been studied from at least the turn of the century, when nicotinic acid (niacin) was tried as a vasodilator for the elderly. At present, there are a number of primary vasodilators available abroad and in the United States. The individual agents are described below.

Cyclandelate. This is probably the most widely used and studied primary vasodilator, available in both Europe and the United States. The review mentioned above (12) evaluated seven double-blind studies of cyclandelate (13–19). Although six of these studies reported some positive effects (13–18), there was considerable question about its practical use (19).

TABLE 48–1
Cerebrally Vasoactive Drugs by Class

Primary vasodilators (primary action on vasculature)
  Cyclandelate
  Papaverine
  Nylidrin
  Isoxsuprine
  Cinnarizine
  Bencyclane
  Betahistine hydrochloride

Secondary vasodilators (primary action on metabolism)
  Dihydroergotoxine mesylate
  Naftidrofuryl
  Piracetam
  Pyritinol
  Vinca alkaloids

One author has suggested that the drug may have a prophylactic effect, but this remains to be documented (14). Previous studies have found no relationship between positive drug effect and degree of atherosclerosis observed on clinical examination. Future studies attempting to better define a patient population may use computerized axial tomography (CT) to identify cerebral pathology in study groups.

Papaverine. The United States Food and Drug Administration's Peripheral and Central Nervous System Drugs Advisory Committee recently reported that "There is no body of evidence that will support the effectiveness of papaverine and ethaverine for any of their claimed indications" (20). There were questions of bioavailability and few positive double-blind reports. There have been five direct comparisons of papaverine with dihydroergotoxine mesylate, and the latter was superior in all five studies (21–25).

Nylidrin and Isoxsuprine. These structurally similar sympathomimetic amines have been used primarily in peripheral vascular disease. In cerebrovascular disease, studies with isoxsuprine have been less encouraging than those with nylidrin. A recent double-blind placebo controlled trial of nylidrin in senile dementias found statistically significant improvement over placebo in all 11 centers of a multicentered trial involving over 500 subjects (26). This study appears to be the best documentation now available for clinical efficacy of any primary vasodilator. The medication's structure leads to speculation as to its CNS stimulant effects; that is, its amphetamine-like effect, in addition to its peripheral beta receptor activity.

Cinnarizine. This piperazine derivative and its analogue, flunarizine, are potent primary vasodilators (12). The medication's use in dementia is difficult to evaluate since many of the relevant studies have been in patients with transient ischemic attacks or Meniere's disease. It is currently under investigation in the United States for its use in multi-infarct dementias.

Other Primary Vasodilators. Bencyclane has had four clinical trials with mixed results, and betahistine hydrochloride has had one positive trial, in patients with vertebrobasilar artery insufficiency. A recent review (27) has listed a host of other compounds which are potential cerebral vasodilators, including xanthinol niacinate, vasolantin, proxazole, and vitamin E. The same review also discusses the role of anticoagulants in increasing CBF.

SECONDARY VASODILATORS

Several types of medications available worldwide are claimed to be stimulants of cerebral metabolism and secondary cerebral vasodilators. Such medications have been under investigation since the first serious studies of ergotoxine in 1906 (28).

Dihydroergotoxine Mesylate. Dihydroergotoxine mesylate (DEM) is the most widely prescribed medication for the indication of dementia worldwide. Nevertheless, clinicians remain skeptical of its clinical effects. However, at least 22 double-blind placebo controlled studies have shown it to be superior to placebo in this indication (12). Skeptics argue that the medication may improve some psychological tests inconsistently across studies but that the perceived improvements remain quite small. Optimists argue that any change seen in such populations is welcome. Ongoing research is examining the use of higher doses of the medication, as well as the combination of medication with psychotherapy (29, 30).

Naftidrofuryl. This synthetic molecule does not have the long history of the ergot alkaloids; it has recently been under investigation in the United States, where one positive double-blind study has been added to the eight positive well-controlled studies performed in Europe (12). The use of naftidrofuryl is open to the same clinical criticisms of effect as those noted for DEM. Also, as in the case of DEM, the optimal dosage remains unclear. Its usual dose in Europe is 300 mg/day, but studies in the United States have occasionally used higher dosages. At these higher dosages, biochemical effects (reduction of the lactate to pyruvate ratio) consistent with a stimulant effect on cerebral metabolism have been noted in human spinal fluid samples (31).

Vinca Alkaloids. These compounds are used widely in Europe for the same indications as the ergot alkaloids. Although their clinical and biochemical effects seem well documented, they have been studied less than the ergot alkaloids (32). At present, the medication is not slated for testing in the United States.

Piracetam. This synthetic European compound has been shown to have biochemical effects consistent with stimulation of cerebral glucose metabolism. A recent review of the literature of piracetam has documented its very limited clinical utility, which is similar to that of DEM or naftidrofuryl (33); however, in a particularly elegant primate model of aged impairment of memory function, piracetam was shown to be superior to other stimulants of cerebral metabolism, the ergot and vinca alkaloids (34). The same investigator has combined this medication with cholinergic precursors, and in preliminary work has reported effects better than either cholinergic or metabolic agent used alone. The medication is now under investigation (see Chap. 46).

Pyritinol. This medication, available only in Europe, is claimed to have similar metabolic effects as DEM or naftidrofuryl; pyritinol, however, has less well documented results than the other compounds in this class. Its usual formulation is in combination with pyridyl-carbinol, a precursor of nicotinic acid (12).

CONCLUSION AND CLINICAL RELEVANCE

The above statements have summarized the major theories of the etiology of senile dementia and supplied the rationales for the clinical use of primary and secondary vasodilators. Also reviewed were the specific agents in both classes of medication presently available in Europe and the United States. It should be noted that, despite some promising recent work with primary vasodilators, especially nylidrin, the studies reviewed are on the whole more positive for secondary vasodilators than for primary vasodilators. This may be because the metabolic sources of dementia are more common than reversible vascular causes. Further-more, it is still difficult to conceive how a purely vasoactive compound might increase CBF in atherosclerotic vessels or where there is already ischemia and substantial autoregulated vasodilatation (i.e., dilation of cerebral vessels due to large amounts of carbon dioxide). In addition, one could potentially decrease CBF with such agents by increasing peripheral pooling. That is, the CBF could actually drop because the blood has fallen to the lower extremities due to the relaxed vessels there, although this has not been demonstrated to be the case with the commonly used primary vasodilators. There may be some elderly who suffer reversible vasospasm of cerebral arteries as a basis for their intellectual decline; however, there have been no studies to identify this population. Thus, overall, the rationale for the use of primary vasodilators is weak.

In the clinical realm, therefore, one has evidence that secondary vasodilators generally have a better clinical record than primary vasodilators. Accordingly, which secondary vasodi-lator should one choose for a particular patient? In the United States the choice is simple since there is only one such agent available—DEM. In Europe the problem is much more complex since a number of agents are available and there have been no direct comparisons between these drugs in humans. In any case, some general conclusions with respect to the clinical pharmacology of such agents may be more important than the reasons for the specific one chosen.

A primary clinical conclusion is that differential diagnosis of cognitive impairment is essential prior to treatment. One important clinical differential is the identification of depres-sions. This has been discussed at length (35).

A second clinical conclusion is the necessity of carefully monitoring results. Most of the medications take at least 12 weeks to show some effect, and those seen are usually modest. Sometimes the effects may be a slowing of decline rather than an absolute increase in function. A useful general measure for clinical monitoring is the Sandoz Clinical Assessment Geriatric (SCAG) rating (36).

A third clinical conclusion is that the medications seem to work optimally in mildly impaired populations. Although the target population has not been precisely defined, it appears that those who score means of 3 to 5 (mild to moderate) on the SCAG ratings do best. It is unlikely that any subjects with severe forms of dysfunction will respond if one assumes they will still suffer severe loss of neurons and receptors.

A final clinically relevant conclusion is that optimum dosages have yet to be determined for these medications. Although serum level guides have been developed for some neuroleptics, antidepressants, and lithium carbonate, none are yet available for secondary vasodilators. Research in this area should attempt in the future to define the therapeutic window for these medications.

ACKNOWLEDGMENTS

This research was supported by the Medical Research Service of the Veteran's Administration.

REFERENCES

1. Wells C: *Dementia.* Philadelphia, Davis, 1971.
2. Wells CE: Geriatric organic psychoses. *Psychiatr Ann* 1979; 8:57–73.
3. Simard D, Oleson J, Paulson OB, et al: Regional cerebral blood flow and its regulation in dementia. *Brain* 1971; 94:273–288.
4. Treff WM: Das Involutionsmuster des Nucleus Dentatus Cerebelli. *Altern Entwickl* 1974; 18:37–54.
5. Maker HS, Lehrer GM, Weiss C: DNA content of mouse cerebellar layers. *Brain Res* 1973; 50:226–229.
6. Meier-Ruge W, Enz A, Gygax P, et al: Experimental pathology in basic research of the aging brain. *Aging NY* 1975; 2:55–126.
7. Kety SS: Human cerebral blood flow and oxygen consumption as related to aging. *Res Publ Assoc Res Nerv Ment Dis* 1956; 35:31–45.
8. Obrist WD, Chiviane E, Crouquist S, et al: Regional cerebral blood flow in senile and presenile dementia. *Neurology* 1970; 20:315–322.
9. Sokoloff L: Cerebral circulation and metabolism in the aged. *Aging NY* 1975; 2:45–54.
10. Yesavage J: Pharmacotherapy of the aged central nervous system. *Clin Neuropharmacol* 1979; 4:199–220.
11. Hollister LE: Drugs for mental disorders of old age. *JAMA* 1975; 234:195–198.
12. Yesavage J, Tinklenberg J, Berger P, et al: Vasodilators in senile dementias: a review of the literature. *Arch Gen Psychiatry* 1979; 36:220–223.
13. Fine EW: The use of cyclandelate in chronic brain syndrome with arteriosclerosis. *Curr Ther Res* 1971; 13:568–574.
14. Hall P: Cyclandelate in the treatment of cerebral arteriosclerosis. *J Am Geriatr Soc* 1976; 24:41–45.
15. Eichorn O: The effect of cyclandelate on cerebral circulation: a double-blind trial with clinical and radiographic investigations. *Vasc Dis* 1965; 2:305–315.
16. Alderman M, Giardina WJ, Loreniowski S: Effect of cyclandelate on perception, memory, and cognition in a group of geriatric subjects. *J Am Geriatr Soc* 1972; 20:268–277.
17. Ball JAC, Taylor AR: Effect of cyclandelate on mental function and cerebral blood flow in elderly patients. *Br Med J* 1967; 3:525–528.
18. Young J, Hall P, Blakemore CB: Treatment of the cerebral manifestations of arteriosclerosis with cyclandelate. *Br J Psychiatry* 1974; 124:177–180.
19. Westreich G, Alter M, Lundger S: Effects of cyclandelate on dementia. *Stroke* 1975; 6:535–538.
20. Food and Drug Administration: *Drug Bulletin,* November 1979.
21. Baso AJ: An ergot preparation (Hydergine) versus papaverine in treating common complaints of the aged: double-blind study. *J Am Geriatr Soc* 1973; 21:63–71.

22. Einspruch BC: The elderly patient and the nursing home: therapeutic compatibility, scientific exhibit at the annual meeting of the American Geriatric Society, Toronto, Apr 17–18, 1974.

23. Nelson JJ: Relieving select symptoms of the elderly. *Geriatrics* 1975; 30:133–142.

24. Rosen HJ: Mental decline in the elderly: pharmacotherapy (ergot alkaloids versus papaverine). *J Am Geriatr Soc* 1975; 23:169–174.

25. Winslow IE: The hospitalized geriatric patient: guidelines for effective therapy, scientific exhibit at the Annual Meeting of the American Medical Association, Portland, Nov 30, 1974.

26. Gaitz CM, Garetz FK, Goldstein SE, et al: Ergot alkaloids in senile dementia, scientific exhibit at the Annual Meeting of the American Geriatric Society, Washington DC, Nov 1979.

27. Sathananthan GL, Gershon S: Cerebral vasodilators: a review. *Aging NY* 1975; 2.

28. Dale HH: On some physiologic actions of ergot. *J Physiol* 1906; 34:163–208.

29. Yoshikawa M: A dose-response study with dihydroergotoxine mesylate. *J Am Ger Soc* 1983; 31:1–7.

30. Yesavage J, Westphal J, Rush L: Combined pharmacological and psychological treatment for dementias. *J Am Geriatr Soc* 1981; 29:164–171.

31. Yesavage J, Tinklenberg J, Hollister L, et al: Effect of nafronyl on lactate and pyruvate. *J Am Ger Soc* 1982; 30:105–108.

32. Theil P: *La périvincamine dans le monde de la médicine practicienne.* Technical Report 571, Rousell Pharmaceuticals, Paris, January 1975.

33. Reisberg B, Ferris S, Gershon S: Psychopharmacologic aspects of cognitive research in the elderly: some current perspectives. *Interdisc Top Gerontal* 1979; 15:132–152.

34. Bartus R: Four stimulants of the central nervous system: effects on short-term memory in young aged monkeys. *J Am Geriatr Soc* 1979; 27:289–297.

35. Wells CE: Pseudodementia. *Am J Psychiatry* 1979; 136:895–900.

36. Shader RI, Harmatz J, Salzman C: A new scale for clinical assessment in geriatric populations: Sandoz Clinical Assessment Geriatric (SCAG). *J Am Geriatr Soc* 1974; 22:107–113.

49 Psychostimulants in the Treatment of Senile Dementia

Robert F. Prien

CNS STIMULANTS ARE COMPOUNDS that produce central nervous system stimulation as their prominant action. Clinically, they increase motor activity, reduce fatigue, and increase levels of concentration and alertness. Stimulants with psychomotor activating effects are often referred to as psychostimulants.

Stimulants that have been evaluated clinically in senile dementia include methylphenidate, pentylenetetrazol, pipradol, magnesium pemoline, and procaine hydrochloride. All are psychomotor stimulants that increase locomotor activity and stereotypic behavior in rats, and enhance performance on memory or learning tasks in animal studies. Most are adrenergic activators with weak MAO inhibitory activity. The chemical structures of some of the psychostimulants are shown in Figure 49–1.

AREAS OF TREATMENT

Studies of the efficacy of stimulants in senile dementia have focused on three areas of treatment: (1) apathetic and withdrawn behavior; (2) mild depression; and (3) cognitive impairment (particularly of short-term memory). The rationale for evaluating stimulants in these areas has never been systematically formulated. Most likely, investigators assumed that withdrawn, apathetic, and depressed patients with cognitive impairment would benefit from the energizing effects of the drugs. That the drugs increased central adrenergic activity and improved memory retention or learning in animal studies provided additional reason for therapeutic trials.

APATHY AND WITHDRAWAL

Studies indicate that psychostimulants such as methylphenidate and pentylenetetrazol may produce improvement in withdrawn, apathetic senile behavior. These improvements may be reflected as increased interest and involvement in surroundings, decreased lethargy and fatigue, and improvement in self-care. There is no evidence that improvement extends beyond the duration of treatment.

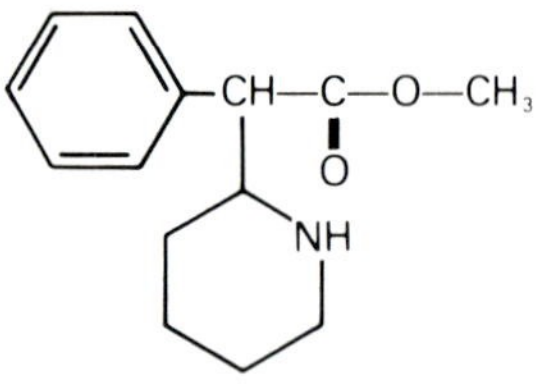

METHYLPHENIDATE

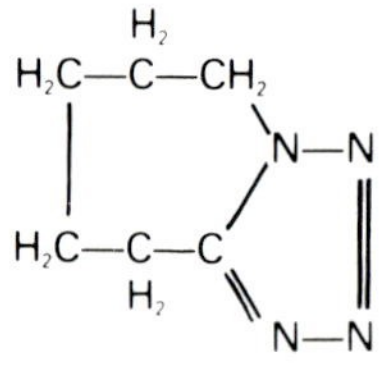

PENTYLENETETRAZOL

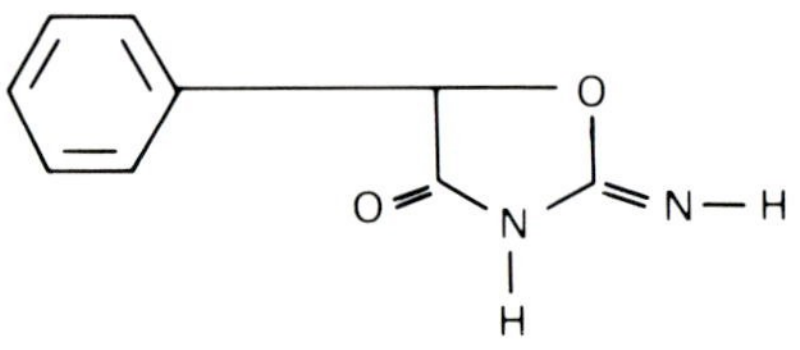

PEMOLINE

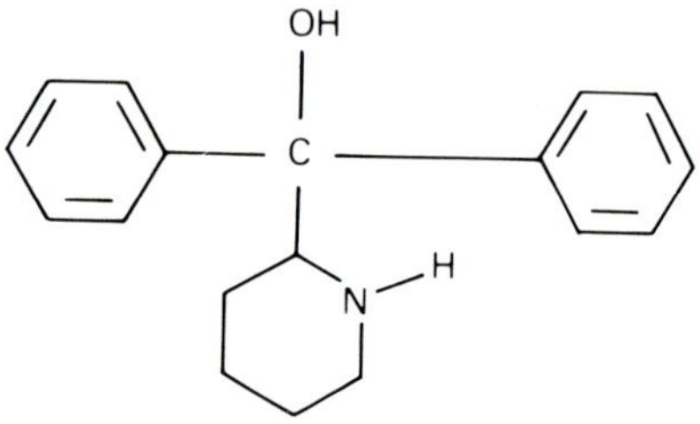

PIPRADOL

Figure 49–1. Chemical structure of four psychostimulants.

Depression

The psychostimulants are thought to act as mood elevators and are considered by some clinicians useful alternatives to the tricyclic antidepressants, which may expose susceptible patients to an unacceptably high risk of adverse cardiovascular and anticholinergic effects. There are, however, few studies comparing stimulants against standard antidepressants in the elderly. To date, methylphenidate is the most carefully studied stimulant for the treatment of depression. Based on the record, in general, there appears to be no advantage to using methylphenidate or other stimulants as a treatment of first choice for depressed geriatric patients; it may be useful with mildly depressed patients who cannot tolerate or are unresponsive to standard antidepressants. However, the introduction of reportedly less toxic antidepressants such as maprotiline and trazodone may ultimately make this use of stimulants unnecessary.

Cognitive Impairment

At various times during the past 25 years, methylphenidate, pentylenetetrazol, procaine hydrochloride, and magnesium pemoline were touted as promising treatments for cognitive dysfunction in the aged (1). These claims were based mainly on findings from animal studies and small-sample open trials with humans. In subsequent controlled trials, however, these agents have failed to demonstrate consistent positive effects and are not currently regarded as useful treatments for cognitive problems with senility.

SPECIFIC DRUGS

METHYLPHENIDATE

Methylphenidate is a sympathomimetic amine with amphetaminelike effects. Numerous uncontrolled trials suggest that methylphenidate may be beneficial for the treatment of apathetic and withdrawn senile behavior (2–7). Nevertheless, further study is required to establish its superiority over placebo. Of four placebo-controlled studies, only one demonstrated a clear advantage of the drug over placebo (8). Results for depression are less positive but suggest that methylphenidate may be a useful treatment for those patients who are not suitable candidates for tricyclic drug therapy (6, 9–13). Attempts to improve memory and cognitive function with methylphenidate have been thus far unsuccessful (14–16).

Methylphenidate is well tolerated at effective dose levels (20–30 mg/day), although insomnia, anorexia, nausea, vomiting, and headache may occur occasionally. Higher dose levels may cause confusion, agitation, paranoid ideation, and a precipitous increase in blood pressure and heart rate.

PENTYLENETETRAZOL

Pentylenetetrazol is a cerebral cortical stimulant with a long history of medical use as a circulatory and respiratory stimulant, convulsive agent, barbiturate antagonist, and treatment for lethargy following recovery from illness and surgery. Therapeutic action has been variously attributed to stimulation of brain stem vasomotor and respiratory centers and cortical psychomotor centers, facilitation of CNS synaptic transmission, and reduction of circulatory lactic acid (17). There are over 50 studies of pentylenetetrazol in senile dementia, including 16 trials comparing pentylenetetrazol against placebo or a comparison drug (1, 17, 18). Although results are mixed, pentylenetetrazol appears to have a beneficial effect on behaviors such as diminished drive, apathy, withdrawal, and attention to self-care. As in the case of psychostimulants, there are as yet no well-defined studies of pentylenetetrazol in depression. Results with cognitive impairment are either negative or equivocal.

At the recommended dosage of 200 to 800 mg/day, pentylenetetrazol appears to be well tolerated, even on prolonged administration. Agitation, nausea, vomiting, and headache are common side effects but seldom interfere with treatment. Again, increased confusion, agitation, paranoid ideation, and blood pressure changes may occur at high dosage.

PIPRADOL

Pipradol is a cyclized amphetamine derivative that shares many of the effects of pentylenetetrazol (17). Alertonic, an elixir containing pipradol, was prescribed from 1957 to 1973 to increase appetite, interest, and mood state, and decrease lethargy and fatigue. Several (uncontrolled) trials in the late 1950s demonstrated beneficial effects on ward behavior of geriatric patients (19–22). In one controlled study on the use of pipradol in senile dementia, high doses of pipradol (5 mg/day) decreased negativistic ward behavior while low doses (2 mg/day) and placebo produced no significant change (23). Likewise, pipradol appears to have no significant effect on mood or memory (24). During the past decade, interest in the drug has declined significantly, and pipradol compounds have been withdrawn from the market in the United States. The drug is still prescribed, however, in some European countries.

PROCAINE

Procaine hydrochloride is a mild stimulant with weak MAO inhibition and local anesthetic action. It is the primary active ingredient in Gerovital-H3, a much publicized solution developed by a Rumanian physician, Aslan, to treat a variety of disorders in the aged, including cognitive impairment and depression (25, 26). There is little evidence to support the use of Gerovital-H3 as a treatment for cognitive dysfunction in senile dementia. Several trials suggest that Gerovital-H3 may be of value in geriatric depression (27–30), but the evidence is far from conclusive. The drug is marketed in Nevada despite objections by the Food and Drug Administration.

MAGNESIUM PEMOLINE

Magnesium pemoline is a cyclized amphetamine with minimal sympathomimetic properties. Early clinical trials (published after a delay of several years) suggested that pemoline therapy could improve memory recall and other cognitive functions in elderly patients (31–33). These findings raised expectations that, at long last, there existed a treatment capable of reversing or halting the intellectual decline associated with senile dementia. The drug's cognitive effects were attributed to its capacity to stimulate production of ribonucleic acid (RNA) within brain cells. This was based on reports that RNA facilitated learning and memory in animals and humans (34, 35). As subsequent trials with pemoline provided consistent negative results (36–38; unpublished data of Freiberg, Cohen, Shulkin at Hahnemann Medical College and Hospital) interest in the drug waned. Most of the drug's modest benefits are now thought to be due to its mild stimulating action (3). A few investigators argue that pemoline should be reevaluated using higher dose levels (39). They point to a study by Bartus (40) in which magnesium pemoline was the most effective of four stimulants in improving short-term memory in aged monkeys. Currently, magnesium pemoline is used almost exclusively with hyperkinetic children.

SUMMARY

CNS stimulants do not appear to alleviate cognitive decline in senile dementia, and seem to exhibit only weak antidepressant properties. Certain stimulants may be useful in the symptomatic treatment of apathetic, withdrawn patients, and may even reduce cognitive impairment exacerbated by lethargy and physical slowing. The drugs do nothing, however, to affect the core symptoms of dementia. It is possible that well-designed studies may ultimately identify subgroups of patients or subtypes of the disorder to respond to one or more of the stimulant agents. Until such data are available, the usefulness of the CNS stimulants in senile dementia would appear to be limited to underaroused (lethargic, motorically depressed) patients who might be expected to benefit from the general stimulating effects of the drugs.

Toxic reactions with the CNS stimulants include cardiovascular and anorectic effects, agitation, activation of psychotic symptomatology, and sleep disturbance. There is the danger that in treating the apathetic, withdrawn patient, inactivity may be replaced by motor agitation and anxiety. The potential for abuse and pharmacological tolerance is also a problem. On balance, however, the toxic risks with the psychostimulants are no greater than the risks associated with other psychopharmacologic agents used to treat senile dementia. What needs to be determined is whether the benefit-to-risk ratio of the psychostimulants warrants their use in preference to other available treatments; this can be determined only with well-controlled clinical studies.

REFERENCES

1. Prien RF: Chronic Organic Brain Syndrome. Washington, DC, Veterans Administration, Department of Medicine and Surgery, 1972.
2. Bachrach S: A new stimulant supplement for the geriatric patient. *J Am Geriat Soc* 1959; 7:408–409.
3. Ban TA: Vasodilators, stimulants and anabolic agents in the treatment of geropsychiatric patients, in Lipton MA, DiMascio A, Killim KF (eds): *Psychopharmacology: A Generation of Progress.* New York, Raven, 1978, pp 1525–1534.
4. Kerenyi AB, Koranyi EK, Sarwer-Foner GJ: Depressive states and drugs: III. Use of methylphenidate in open psychiatric settings and in office practice. *Can Med Assoc J* 1960; 83:1249–1254.
5. Landman ME, Preiseg R, Perlman M: A practical mood stimulant. *J Med Soc NJ* 1958; 55:55–58.
6. Moore DP: Methylphenidate in depression and states of apathy. *South Med J* 1981; 74:347–348.
7. Natenshon AL: Ritonic—a new geriatric supplement for the geriatric patient. *J Am Geriatr Soc* 1960; 8:292–297.
8. Kaplitz SE: Withdrawn, apathetic geriatric patients responsive to methylphenidate. *J Am Geriatr Soc* 1975; 23:271–276.
9. Katon W, Raskind M: Treatment of depression in the medically ill elderly with methylphenidate. *Am J Psychiatry* 1980; 137:963–965.
10. Leitch A, Seager CP: A trial of four antidepressant drugs. *Psychopharmacologia* 1963; 4:72–77.
11. Rickels K, Gingrich RL, McLaughlin FW, et al: Methylphenidate in mildly depressed outpatients. *Clin Pharm Ther* 1972; 13:595–601.
12. Rickels K, Gordon PE, Gansman DH: Pemoline and methylphenidate in mildly depressed outpatients. *Clin Pharm Ther* 1970; 11:698–710.
13. Robin AA, Wyseberg S: A controlled trial of methylphenidate (Ritalin) in the treatment of depressive states. *J Neurol Neurosurg Psychiatry* 1958; 21:55–57.
14. Crook T: Central nervous system stimulants: Appraisal of use in geropsychiatric patients. *J Am Geriatr Soc* 1979; 27:476–477.
15. Crook T, Ferris S, Sathananthan G, et al: The effect of methylphenidate on test performance in the cognitively impaired aged. *Psychopharmacology (Berlin)* 1977; 52:251–255.
16. Gilbert JG, Donnelly KJ, Zimmer LE, et al: Effect of magnesium pemoline and methylphenidate on memory improvement and mood in normal aging subjects. *Int J Aging Hum Dev* 1973; 41:35–51.
17. Lehmann HE, Ban TA: Central nervous system stimulants and anabolic substances in geropsychiatric therapy. *Aging NY* 1975; 2:179–202.
18. Salzman C: Stimulants in the elderly, in Raskin A, Robinson DS, Levine J (eds): *Age and the Pharmacology of Psychoactive Drugs.* New York, Elsevier, 1981, pp 171–180.
19. Begg WA, Reid AA: Meretran, new stimulant drug, *Br Med J* 1956; 1:946–949.
20. Martin KE, Overly GH, Krone RE: Pipradol: combined therapy for geriatric and agitated patients. *Int Rec Med* 1957; 170:33–36.
21. Payne RB, Moore EW: The effects of some analeptic and depressant drugs upon tracking behavior. *J Pharmacol Exp Ther* 1955; 115:480–484.

22. Pomeranze J, Ladek RJ: Clinical studies in geriatrics: III. The "Tonic." *J Am Geriatr Soc* 1957; 5:997–1002.

23. Turek I, Kurland AA, Ota KY, et al: Effects of pipradol hydrochloride on geriatric patients. *J Am Geriatr Soc* 1969; 17:408–413.

24. Shader RI, Harmatz JS, Kochansky GE, et al: Psychopharmacologic investigations in healthy elderly volunteers: effects of pipradol–vitamin (Alertonic) elixir and placebo in relation to research design. *J Am Geriatr Soc* 1975; 23:277–278.

25. Aslan A: Procaine therapy in old age and other disorders (Novocain Factor H_3). *Gerontol Clin* 1960; 2:148–176.

26. Aslan A: Theoretical and practical aspects of chemotherapeutic techniques in the retardation of the aging process, in Rockstein M (ed): *Theoretical Aspects of Aging.* New York, Academic, 1974, pp 1900–1920.

27. Jarvik LF, Milne JF: Gerovital-H_3: a review of the literature. *Aging NY* 1975; 2:203–227.

28. Kurland M, Hayman M: Gerovital-H_3 in the treatment of depression in a private practice population: a double-blind study. Read before the Annual Meeting of the Academy of Psychosomatic Medicine, Scottsdale, Nov. 1974.

29. Ostfeld A, Smith CM, Slotsky BA: The systemic use of procaine in the treatment of the elderly. *J Am Geriatr Soc* 1977; 25:1–19.

30. Zung WWK, Gianturco D, Pfeiffer E, et al: Pharmacology of depression in the aged: evaluation of Gerovital-H_3 as an antidepressant drug. *Psychopharmacol Bull* 1976; 12:50–51.

31. Frehyn FA, Catalano F, Mayo JA: Summary report of clinical investigation of the effects of magnesium pemoline on memory impairment of geriatric patients, cited in Kalinowsky LE, Hippius H: *Pharmacological, Convulsive and Other Somatic Treatments in Psychiatry.* New York, Grune & Stratton, 1971.

32. Plotnikoff N: Learning and memory enhancement by pemoline and magnesium hydroxide. *Recent Adv Biol Psych* 1968; 10:102–120.

33. Plotnikoff N: Pemoline: review of performance. *Tex Rep Biol Med* 1971; 29:467–479.

34. Cameron DE, Solyon L: Effects of ribonucleic acid on memory. *Geriatrics* 1961; 16:74–81.

35. Cameron DE, Svd S, Solyom L, et al: Effects of ribonucleic acid on memory defects in the aged. *Am J Psychiatry* 1963; 120:320–325.

36. Droller H, Bevans HS, Jayaram VK: Problems of a drug trial (pemoline) on geriatric patients. *Gerontol Clin* 1971; 13:269–276.

37. Eisdorfer C, Conner JF, Wilkie FL: Effect of magnesium pemoline on cognition and behavior. *J Gerontol* 1968; 23:283–288.

38. Greenblatt DJ, DiMascio A, Messier M, et al: Magnesium pemoline and job performance in mentally handicapped workers. *Clin Pharmacol Ther* 1969; 10:530–533.

39. Ferris SH: Empirical studies in senile dementia with central nervous system stimulants and metabolic enhancers, in Crook TC, Gershon S (eds): *Strategies for the Development of an Effective Treatment for Senile Dementia.* New Canaan, Powley Associates, 1981, pp 189–208.

40. Bartus RT: Four stimulants of the central nervous system: Effects on short-term memory in young versus aged monkeys. *J Am Geriatr Soc* 1979; 27:289–297.

50 Pharmacologic Treatment of Alzheimer's Disease: Future Directions

NUNZIO POMARA

SAMUEL BRINKMAN

SAMUEL GERSHON

NEVER IN HISTORY has the proportion of elderly to nonelderly been as large as it is today, and never has the suffering and financial drain on families and society from dementia-related problems been as great. In 1980, in the United States alone, the expenditure for nursing home care was 12 billion U.S. dollars (1). This expenditure is expected to rise to 76 billion dollars by 1990 if present U.S. demographic trends continue (2). Since individuals with senile dementia constitute a majority of the nursing home population, any intervention that could produce even a modest improvement in their mental condition and restore some functioning could result in enormous financial savings to society, and preserve the dignity of the afflicted individual. Unfortunately, there is as yet no clinically useful pharmacological agent for the treatment of senile dementia. It is therefore incumbent upon those of us involved in research to reconsider the current pharmacological approaches.

Before the classic studies of Tomlinson and associates (3, 4), memory impairments associated with dementia were generally thought to be due to cerebrovascular insufficiency of atherosclerotic origin. It is not surprising, therefore, that the first attempts at treating these memory impairments used vasodilators and hyperbaric oxygen to increase blood flow, and the supply of oxygen to the brain. Consequently, it was not surprising when these approaches were unsuccessful (5).

As the prevalence of Alzheimer's disease (AD) became more widely recognized (70% of all dementias), experimental treatment strategies emphasized the parenchymal changes, such as impaired neuronal metabolism and alterations in the synthesis and release of neurotransmitters. Pharmacological intervention was therefore directed at correcting or limiting the deleterious effects of these changes in brain function. Of utmost importance in shaping the current pharmacological approaches to the treatment of AD was the demonstration that administration of a dopamine precursor produced dramatic improvements in motor functions of patients with Parkinson's disease (6). This finding represented the first successful attempt at manipulating a neurotransmitter system relatively specifically disrupted in a disorder of the CNS.

Another development that had a significant impact in the field of dementia research was the finding, now replicated in several laboratories, that the brains of AD patients have a marked reduction in choline acetyltransferase (CAT) levels relative to age-matched controls and individuals with a dementia secondary to vascular disease, or multi-infarct dementia (MID) (7–10). That central cholinergic systems play a central role in memory in humans has been well established (11, 12). The memory impairment in AD patients, therefore, was thought to be due to the marked reduction in CAT levels in both the frontal and temporal cortexes. Added support for this view was derived from the report that the CAT deficiencies approximated the distribution of senile (neuritic) plaques and correlated with the severity of dementia before death (13).

Based largely on these findings, numerous clinical trials were conducted to assess the role of cholinergic agents in the treatment of dementia. The primary aim of these clinical trials was directed at increasing the levels of brain acetylcholine by promoting its synthesis with precursor loading agents (choline, lecithin) and/or preventing its enzymatic degradation (physostigmine). Unfortunately, approaches employing cholinergic agents have not been shown to be clinically useful. Therefore, the pertinent question is whether further manipulation of the cholinergic system is likely to result in a useful treatment. The present clinical data clearly do not permit an answer in the affirmative; however, the consistency of the reduction in CAT in AD makes it imperative that the therapeutic manipulation of the cholinergic system be continued. We agree with Davies (14) that additional aspects of central cholinergic functioning need to be explored to fully elucidate the possible utility of cholinergic agents in the treatment of memory disorders.

Although reduced CAT levels are the most impressive and consistent neurotransmitter abnormality in patients diagnosed as having AD, there is increasing evidence that this observation might not be as selective as was initially thought. A reduction in the level of somatostatin, a neuropeptide, has also been described (15). Further, there are numerous reports that the levels of other neurotransmitters (dopamine, serotonin, norepinephrine), may also be reduced in AD (16).

In view of these findings, future therapeutic strategies might involve the pharmacological manipulation of multiple neurotransmitter systems. However, to increase the likelihood that these therapies will be effective, they should not be applied on the basis of a clinical diagnosis of AD alone but should be instead derived on the basis of specific neurotransmitter abnormalities perhaps associated with that particular individual at a particular stage of the disease process.

It is likely that the next decade will witness extensive research in the following areas:

1. Ways of differentiating Alzheimer's individuals from normal controls on the basis of specific *in vivo* neurochemical abnormalities.
2. Attempts at classifying AD into subtypes on the basis of specific neurotransmitter abnormalities.
3. More effective ways of enhancing the activity of central neurotransmitter systems (cholinergic, catecholaminergic).
4. Concurrent pharmacological manipulation of multiple neurotransmitter systems.
5. The elucidation of the possible role of neuropeptides in cognitive processes.

Last but not least, since the neurotransmitter abnormalities could all be secondary to a primary effect of the disease on intraneuronal processes (such as decreased protein synthesis or impaired energy production), increased efforts will also be directed at the understanding of these changes, and at ways of preventing or limiting their deleterious impact on brain function.

Advances in the application of nuclear magnetic resonance (NMR) may soon provide us with a noninvasive and inexpensive means of monitoring minute alterations in cerebral blood flow (17) and metabolism (18).

CHOLINERGIC SYSTEMS

In retrospect, the initial excitement over cholinergic precursor therapy appears to have stemmed from a simplistic view of central cholinergic function, as well as from a prematurely reductionistic view of the selective involvement of the cholinergic system in the pathogenesis of dementia in AD. In all fairness to those who pursued cholinergic precursor therapies with such vigor, the successful alleviation of symptoms in Parkinson's disease by means of dopamine precursors, as well as the safety of choline or lecithin relative to such drugs as physostigmine or arecoline, dictated a thorough evaluation of the efficacy of precursor therapy. Today, it is clear that short-term choline treatment alone is of little clinical value in treating AD (19).

There are many reasons that could explain the poor clinical outcome with cholinergic precursors alone.

1. The enzyme required in the synthesis of acetylcholine, CAT, is the very enzyme depleted in AD. Therefore, simply increasing substrates may not necessarily result in an increase in ACh synthesis.
2. The level of the other necessary substrate in ACh synthesis, acetylCoA, might also be depleted in AD.
3. The uptake of choline by cholinergic neurons might not be affected by increases in the brain levels of this precursor. In this regard, there is some evidence based on animal experiments that the uptake of choline into cholinergic neurons in structures such as the hippocampus and cortex (believed to play a major role in memory processes) is dependent on the activity of a high affinity transport system whose carrier is believed to be saturated at usual plasma choline levels (20). Thus, it has been reasoned that increasing the plasma level of choline may not be of any functional significance. On the other hand, there is evidence that the same high affinity system can be influenced by increases in the rate of neuronal firing (21). Therefore it follows that the utility of precursor therapy (choline, lecithin) is dependent on an ability to simultaneously (concurrently) increase cholinergic neuronal firing.

    Among the most powerful stimulants of the presynaptic cholinergic firing are the postsynaptic muscarinic blockers such as scopolamine and atropine. However, as these agents exert their action by blocking the muscarinic receptors, they can hardly be recommended as a treatment for memory dysfunction. In fact, the administration of these agents has been shown to induce a memory dysfunction analogous to that of AD (12). Therefore, the best approach may be one in which a cholinergic precursor such as choline would be combined with an agent increasing presynaptic cholinergic firing by mechanisms other than blocking muscarinic postsynaptic receptors.

A possible therapeutic approach was suggested by a recent description of presynaptic cholinergic autoreceptors believed to be functionally different from postsynaptic muscarinic receptors in the rat (22). The activation of these autoreceptors by acetylcholine is believed to prevent release of acetylcholine by depolarization of the presynaptic neuron. If this is the case in the human brain, increased ACh synthesis and release may produce little functional gain because of feedback inhibition through presynaptic muscarinic receptors. It may be necessary to block these inhibitory presynaptic receptors selectively in order to produce clinically meaningful improvements in memory.

In the absence of evidence of these presynaptic muscarinic receptors in humans, direct stimulation of the postsynaptic muscarinic receptors (which appear to be preserved in AD) with agents such as arecoline may be meaningful. Arecoline produces improvements in memory in normal young adults (23). Its side effects are similar to those of physostigmine, and therefore may limit its clinical application.

Another factor which may limit the efficacy of muscarinic receptor agonists and other cholinergic agents is the presence of a dysfunction in receptor-mediated responses.

It is well known that the action of acetylcholine at the receptors initiates a series of intraneuronal reactions involving changes in cyclic GMP (cGMP) and in cGMP-dependent kinases. While it is not known whether these processes are affected by normal aging or AD, Lippa and colleagues reported that hippocampal cholinoceptive cells in the aged rat have a dampened firing response to iontophoretically applied acetylcholine (24). This dysfunction appears to be selective for the cholinergic system, since the firing response to glutamate is normal.

Obviously, this electrophysiological impairment of the cholinoceptive receptors needs to be confirmed in man.

One possible way of overcoming the hyporesponsivity of the muscarinic receptor to an agonist was suggested by Davies, who recommended that agents such as thyrotropin-releasing hormone (TRH), believed to enhance muscarinic receptor sensitivity, be investigated in combination with a cholinergic precursor as a possible treatment for cognitive dysfunction (14).

Another possibility of enhancing the efficacy of cholinergic agents was provided by Friedman and colleagues (25). They reported that the combination of choline and piracetam, an agent thought to improve intraneuronal metabolism, led to clinical improvement in a subset of patients. This finding is exciting, as neither agent alone had been found effective in the treatment of dementia. Although this preliminary study did not involve a placebo control or blind arrangements, as it was exploratory in nature, if these results are confirmed in double-blind studies, there may be strong implications for an alternative approach to treatment.

Conclusions

Continued emphasis on cholinergic agents is indicated at this time, and a better understanding of cholinergic neurotransmission may allow for more effective treatment approaches.

At the same time, further work is needed to explore the issue of whether cholinergic precursors might play a role in the prevention of some of the degenerative changes occurring in neurons as a result of normal aging and AD.

There are data indicating that chronic administration of choline might suppress the age-related loss of dendritic spines in animals. Cholinergic precursors which are thought to act by increasing the production of acetylcholine may also increase the amount of phosphatidylcholine, an important component of all neuronal membranes. It has been suggested by

Mervis that increases in phosphatidylcholine may enhance the integrity and stability of neuronal membranes and may account for the suppression of age-related dendritic spine loss, as has been observed following choline administration (26).

There is also one clinical trial in which the administration of a mixture of phospholipids derived from animal tissue to individuals with various types of dementia, including AD, resulted in improvement in some neuropsychological parameters (27).

Clearly, clinical trials involving the long-term administration of cholinergic precursors need to be performed to assess the possible role of these agents in the prevention or attenuation of cognitive dysfunction in the elderly and in AD. Similarly, more rigorous studies are needed to elucidate the role of phospholipids and other compounds such as S-adenosylmethionine (SAM) believed to alter the structure and fluidity of neuronal membranes in the treatment of memory disorders (Stramentinoli and colleagues, personal communication, 1981).

NONCHOLINERGIC NEUROTRANSMITTER SYSTEMS

Although a strong case can be made for the importance of cholinergic dysfunction in the development of cognitive impairment in AD, reductions in the brain levels of dopamine, norepinephrine, and serotonin have also been reported (16). There is also a recent report involving two individuals with a clinical diagnosis of AD who demonstrated a sharp reduction in the levels of homovanillic acid, the main dopamine metabolite, in the CSF, and normal levels of CAT on brain biopsy (28). These findings clearly need to be substantiated, but they do raise doubts about the current practice of selecting individuals for participation in a drug trial solely on the basis of a clinical diagnosis of AD. Ways by which Alzheimer's patients can be further differentiated from each other on the basis of specific neurochemical abnormalities need to be found. As previously stated, there might be cases of AD associated with a selective dysfunction of the dopaminergic neurotransmitter system. If such cases do exist, it might be more appropriate to treat those patients with a dopamine precursor.

Similarly, we know that there are individuals with AD exhibiting extrapyramidal symptoms (EPS) (29). It would be interesting to assess whether these individuals could be differentiated from AD patients with the same cognitive impairment but with no EPS, on the basis of levels of homovanillic acid in the CSF.

Furthermore, given the progressive nature of AD, it is likely that diverse neurotransmitter systems might be affected in each stage of the illness. Pharmacological intervention, if it is to be effective, must be adjusted accordingly.

It is also possible that some of the symptoms of dementia could arise from neurotransmitter imbalances, much in the manner in which DA-ACh imbalances are related to the symptomatology of Parkinson's disease. The role of the GABA-ergic system should also be explored. It is known that agents such as the benzodiazepines, believed to potentiate GABA-ergic activity, produce a memory dysfunction analogous to that produced by the anticholinergic agent, scopolamine. While the effects of scopolamine can be reversed by physostigmine, those deficits produced by diazepam cannot be reversed by this cholinomimetic agent (30).

GABA-secreting neurons are generally inhibitory and are reported to be unaffected in AD (7, 31). In the context of reduced cholinergic, dopaminergic, and possibly serotonergic efficiency, the normal degree of inhibition by GABA-ergic neurons may actually be excessive. Inhibition of this GABA-ergic activity, therefore, may have the net effect of facilitating firing of other neurotransmitter systems to more normal levels.

NEUROPEPTIDES

Although there is no clear theoretical rationale for the administration of neuropeptides to patients with AD, these substances are of considerable interest because of their potential role in memory processes. In his excellent review of the animal literature, deWied (32) pointed out that the administration of vasopressin to amnesic rats produces a prolonged increase in memory ability. The duration of this memory effect far exceeded the presence of the substance in the body. Additionally, vasopressin administration was associated with improvements in both acquisition of new information and retrieval of information acquired before onset of the amnesia in the animals. This finding is important because Miller (33–36) indicated that AD is characterized by deficits in both memory acquisition and retrieval.

Unfortunately, clinical trials to assess the role of these neuropeptides in the treatment of dementia have not been too rewarding (5) and are in great contrast to the impressive animal data.

This discrepancy between the animal and clinical data could be explained if the primary effect of these agents is on general arousal rather than on the cellular processes that underlie learning and memory, as has recently been suggested by Bloom (37). It is well known that agents such as the amphetamines, which also increase arousal, have not been useful in the treatment of AD (see Chap. 49 of this volume) or in reversing the memory disorders induced by scopolamine, a muscarinic blocker (30). Bloom has also pointed out that in rats the effect that vasopressin had on arousal could be eliminated by controlling for blood pressure. This finding points to the need to develop neuropeptides free from peripheral side effects that confound interpretation and yet preserve the clinically desired pharmacological action of these agents. It is also essential to develop animal models more closely related to the clinical entity of AD so that one could more easily extrapolate from animal and behavioral data.

In this regard, it would be useful to assess the role of neuropeptides in reversing the memory dysfunction induced by anticholinergic agents such as atropine or scopolamine. Despite the poor clinical outcome with these agents, alterations in neuropeptide release and function could still play a central role in the symptomatology of AD.

This possibility was raised by reductions in the levels of somatostatin in AD (15). While the clinical significance of this reduction remains unknown, it should be emphasized that the function of neurons utilizing neuropeptides as neurotransmitters may be particularly affected in AD.

The synthesis and release of a neuropeptide is quite different from that of other neurotransmitters such as GABA, dopamine, and serotonin, which are synthesized very rapidly by a slight modification of amino acids by cytoplasmic enzymes. Neuropeptide synthesis and release involves DNA transcription and RNA translation. Additionally, the newly synthesized peptide must then be progressively cleaved to produce the active form of the neurotransmitter, which is then transported for quite a distance from the ribosomes, located in the cell body, to the axon terminals.

It is apparent from these considerations that a disease affecting DNA transcription or RNA translation, or interfering with the transport or release of a neuropeptide could seriously compromise the function of peptidergic neurons.

Crapper and colleagues (38) have reported that Alzheimer's patients undergo a sharp reduction in the fraction of DNA capable of RNA synthesis. Crapper and associates have found that the euchromatin and light chromatic fractions are reduced to 55% of the total DNA, as compared to a 75% reduction in the normal elderly.

These findings are also supported by Mann and colleagues (39). They reported reductions in cytoplasmic RNA presumably secondary to alterations in RNA within the nucleus in AD.

On the assumption that reductions in RNA synthesis might play a role in some of the neurochemical changes associated with AD, such as the reduction in CAT and somatostatin, the behavioral effects of agents known to stimulate brain-RNA and protein synthesis, such as the enkephalins (40) and corticosteroids (41) should be pursued.

The behavioral activity of a newly synthesized potent analogue of somatostatin should also be tested (42).

Conclusions

Pharmacological treatments of AD over the next few years may continue to follow the treatment model of Parkinson's disease, with specific emphasis not only on the cholinergic system but on other neurotransmitter systems that might also be affected in subtypes of the disease. In such cases, the simultaneous manipulations of other neurotransmitter systems may also be indicated. The study of neuropeptides is in an earlier stage of development and is limited by our poor understanding of how these substances act in the brain to organize behavior.

It should be kept in mind that these approaches are symptomatic. They are oriented not to the etiology of the disease but to some aspects of the neurochemistry of the disease. This is also true of Parkinson's disease. However, Parkinson's disease differs from AD in two critical ways: (1) it involves a slower progression; (2) it involves a more circumscribed area of brain pathology and, therefore, a more circumscribed area of behavior. With AD, on the other hand, there is more widespread neuropathology and a more rapid progression (in most cases). In either case, precursor therapy or other neurotransmitter manipulations may alleviate some symptoms while the disease progresses.

Etiologically based treatments, when developed, will be oriented toward arresting or even preventing the disease process. As such, optimum therapy will probably involve a combination of etiologically based medication and symptom-based medication. It should be pointed out that AD may represent an accentuation of age-related neuronal and neurochemical changes. In this case, it might be possible to postpone the onset of the disease by preventing some of these degenerative alterations. As previously stated, there is some preliminary evidence that the long-term administration of cholinergic precursors may be a means of accomplishing this (26).

References

1. News from the National Institute of Health: *Neurobiol Aging* 1981; 2:153–154.
2. Schneider EL, Butler RN: Geriatrics. *JAMA* 1981; 245:2190–2191.
3. Tomlinson BE, Blessed G, Roth M: Observations on the brains of nondemented old people. *J Neurol Sci* 1968; 7:331–356.

4. Tomlinson BE, Blessed G, Roth M: Observations on the brains of demented old people. *J Neurol Sci* 1970; 11:205–242.

5. Pomara N, Reisberg B, Ferris SH, et al: Drug treatment of cognitive decline, in Pirozzolo PJ, Maletta GJ (eds): *Advances in Neurogerontology—Behavioral Assessment and Psychopharmacology.* Praeger Press 1981.

6. Birkmayer W, Hornykiewicz O: Der L-3, 4-dioxyphenyalanin (DOPA): Effekt bei der Parkinson Akinese. *Wien Klin Wochenschr* 1961; 73:787.

7. Davies P, Maloney AJR: Selective loss of central cholinergic neurons in Alzheimer's disease. *Lancet* 1976; ii:1403.

8. Davies P, Katzman R, Terry RD: Regional distribution of muscarinic acetylcholine receptor in normal and Alzheimer's-type dementia brains. *Brain Res* 1978; 138:385–392.

9. Perry EK, Perry RH, Blessed G, et al: Necropsy evidence of central cholinergic defects in senile dementia. *Lancet* 1977; i:189.

10. White P, Hiley CR, Goodhardt MJ, et al: Neocortical cholinergic neurons in elderly people. *Lancet* 1977; i:668–670.

11. Drachman DA, Leavitt J: Human memory and the cholinergic system: a relationship to aging? *Arch Neurol* 1974; 30:113–121.

12. Drachman DA: Memory and cognitive function in man: does the cholinergic system have a specific role? *Neurology* 1977; 27:783–790.

13. Perry EK, Tomlinson BE, Blessed G, et al: Correlation of cholinergic abnormalities with senile plaques and mental test scores in senile dementia. *Br Med J* 1978; 2:1457–1459.

14. Davies P: Theoretical treatment possibilities for dementia of the Alzheimer type, in Crook T, Gershon S (eds): *Strategies for the Development of an Effective Treatment for Senile Dementia.* New Canaan, Powley, 1981, pp 19–34.

15. Davies P, Katzman R, Terry RD: Reduced somatostatin-like immunoreactivity in cerebral cortex from cases of Alzheimer's disease and Alzheimer's senile dementia. *Nature* 1980; 288:279–280.

16. Carlsson A: Aging and brain neurotransmitters, in Crook T, Gershon S (eds): *Strategies for the Development of an Effective Treatment for Senile Dementia.* New Canaan, Powley, 1981, pp 93–106.

17. Battocletti JH, Halbach RE, Salles-Cunha SX, et al: The NMR blood flowmeter—theory and history. *Med Phys* 1981; 8:435–445.

18. Scott AI, Baxter RL: Applications of 13C NMR to metabolic studies. *Annu Rev Biophys Bioeng* 1981; 10:151–174.

19. Brinkman S, Pomara N, Goodnick P, et al: Dose-ranging study of lecithin in the treatment of primary degenerative dementia (Alzheimer's disease). *J Clin Psychopharmacol* 1982; 2:281–285.

20. Jenden D: in Davis KL, Berger PA (eds): *Brain Acetylcholine and Neuropsychiatric Disease.* New York, Raven, 1979, pp 483–514.

21. Sherman KA, Kuster JE, Dean RL, et al: Presynaptic cholinergic mechanisms in brain of aged rats with memory impairments. *Neurobiol Aging* 1981; 2:99–104.

22. Marchi M, Paudice P, Ratteri M: Autoregulation of acetylcholine release in isolated hippocampal nerve endings. *Eur J Pharmacol* 1981; 73:75–79.

23. Sitaram N, Weingartner H, Gillin JC: Human serial learning: Enhancement with arecoline and choline and impairment with scopolamine. *Science* 1978; 201:274–276.

24. Lippa AS, Pelham RW, Beer B, et al: Brain cholinergic dysfunctions and memory in aged rats. *Neurobiol Aging* 1980; 1:13–19.

25. Friedman E, Sherman KA, Ferris SH, et al: Clinical response to choline plus Piracetam in senile dementia: relation to red-cell choline levels. *N Eng J Med* 1981; 34:490–491.

26. Mervis RF, Bartus RT: Modulation of pyramidal cells dendritic spine population in aging mouse neocortex: role of dietary choline. *J Neurop Exp Neurol* 1981; 40:313.

27. Feldman H: Phospholipids in the treatment of dementia. Presented at the International Study Group on the Pharmacology of Memory Disorders Associated with Aging, Zurich, Switzerland April 3–5, 1981 (Abstract)

28. Bowen DM, Sims, NR, Benton JS, et al: Treatment of Alzheimer's disease: a cautionary note. *N Engl J Med* 1981; 305:1016.

29. Pomara N, Reisberg B, Albers S, et al: Extrapyramidal symptoms in patients with degenerative dementia. *J Clin Psychopharmacol* 1981; 1:398–400.

30. Ghoneim MM, Mewaldt SP: Studies on human memory: the interaction of Diazepam, Scopolamine, and Physostigmine. *Psychopharmacol* 1977; 52:1–6.

31. Spillane JA, White P, Goodhardt MJ, et al: Selective vulnerability of neurons in organic dementia. *Nature* 1977; 266:558–559.

32. De Wied D, van Wimermsa Greidanus TB, Bohus B, et al: Vasopressin and memory consolidation. *Prog Brain Res* 1976; 45:181–194.

33. Miller E: On the nature of the memory disorder in presenile dementia. *Neuropsychologia* 1971; 9:75–81.

34. Miller E: Efficacy of coding and the short-term memory defect in presenile dementia. *Neuropsychologia* 1973; 10:133–136.

35. Miller E: Retrieval from long-term memory in presenile dementia: two tests of an hypothesis. *Br Soc Clin Psychol* 1978; 17:143–148.

36. Miller E: Short and long-term memory in patients with presenile dementia (Alzheimer's disease). *Psychol Med* 1973; 3:221–224.

37. Bloom FE: Neuropeptides. *Sci Amer* 1981; 245:148–168.

38. Crapper DR, Quittkat S, de Boni U: Altered chromatin conformation in Alzheimer's disease. *Brain* 1979; 102:483–495.

39. Mann DMA, Neary D, Yates PO, et al: Alterations in protein synthetic capability of nerve cells in Alzheimer's disease. *J Neurol Neurosurg Psychiatry* 1981; 44:97–102.

40. Loh HH, Lee NM, Li CH: Beta-endorphin: stimulation of DNA dependent RNA formation, in Usdin E, Bunney WE, Kline NS (eds): *Endorphins in Mental Health Research,* Oxford University Press, New York 1979, pp 254–259.

41. Etgen AM, Martin M, Gilbert R, et al: Characterization of corticosterone-induced protein synthesis in hippocampal slices. *Neurochem* 1980; 35:598–602.

42. Veber DF, Freidinger RM, Perlow DS, et al: A potent cyclic hexapeptide analogue of somatostatin. *Nature* 1981; 292:55–58.

SECTION XI

NONHUMAN MODELS OF ALZHEIMER'S DISEASE AND SENESCENT FORGETFULNESS

51 Mammalian Pathologic Models

Ronald Mervis

The ideal animal model for Alzheimer's disease (AD) or human senescent forgetfulness should be based upon the triad of evidence—behavioral, morphological, and biochemical—which parallels similar findings in humans. In the case of AD, there is, in fact, no valid mammalian model for this uniquely human pathological form of aging—and as such, we must regard the title of this chapter with some caution. On the other hand, senescent forgetfulness represents a nonpathological entity—a normal form of cerebral aging not unique to human beings. This normal process of cerebral aging has also been referred to as "benign senescence" (1). Although there is no valid nonhuman pathologic model for AD, nevertheless there are some widely accepted mammalian models for normal senescent forgetfulness. In this chapter, the neuropathologic criteria that help determine the validity of the morphological model will be emphasized.

The major reason there are useful animal models for senescent forgetfulness is that all mammalian species that have been behaviorally tested show some degree of memory loss in the course of normal aging (for a review see ref. 2). This is in agreement with most studies showing similar memory deficits during normal aging in man (2). The behavioral change is typically observed as an age-related decline in performance on tests of learning and memory capabilities. The literature supplies numerous examples of such behavioral differences with aging in mice (3–6) and rats (7–12). Moreover, in view of the far more highly sophisticated behavioral repertoire of nonhuman primates, these animals, too, have gained importance as models to use in studying mental processes associated with age-related memory deficits (4, 13–17). Thus, viewed in conjunction with the behavioral literature on human aging (2) there seems to be convincing evidence that some nonhuman mammalian species clearly exhibit deficits in memory loss characteristic to nonpathological aging in humans, that is, normal senescent forgetfulness. Unfortunately, data concerning other common laboratory mammals such as dogs, cats, guinea pigs, and rabbits are absent from the behavioral literature with respect to age-related differences across the life span of these species. Accordingly, this remains an important area for future research. However, morphological characteristics of brain aging also contribute toward the validity of a particular species as a model for human senescence. Therefore, it is the pathoanatomical features of potential mammalian models which will now be considered.

Gross Morphologic Changes with Aging

The gross atrophic structural alterations in the human brain in the course of both normal aging and AD are well documented and are discussed elsewhere in this volume.

Studies of aging mammals also generally document similar atrophy. Thus, Ordy (18) has reported loss of brain weight in monkeys during senescence. In aging rats, brain shrinkage, cortical atrophy, and ventricular dilation have been found (19–24). However, other studies are not in agreement with these findings. Donaldson (25) has asserted that the rat brain maintains brain growth throughout life. Roberts and Goldberg (26) were unable to find age-related brain weight changes in several rat strains. In the C57BL/6J mouse, Curcio (27) reported that neither the height of the primary somatosensory cortex nor the height of layer IV changed with age (up to 33 months). It is interesting that a seemingly basic parameter of brain aging—well documented in humans—may not be characteristic for all mammalian species.

NEURONAL LOSS IN AGING

The brain has been referred to as a "multi-organ organ" (28) since the brain is highly heterogeneous; this is clearly reflected in the selective neuronal loss found in response to aging in both animals and humans. The topic has recently been extensively reviewed by several authors (2, 20, 29, 30). In humans, neuronal loss—either widespread or selective with respect to specific nuclei—has been linked to general age-related intellectual decline as well as contributing to dementia (31–33). Indeed, in the human neocortex age-related neuronal dropout has been well documented (34–39). Moreover, Terry and associates (40) have recently indicated that in AD there is significant loss of large ($90\mu m^2$) cortical neurons in comparison to normal age-matched controls.

Studies of subhuman primates have also shown an age-related loss of cortical neurons as reflected by a decline in cell density (41–44).

Contradictory evidence is found, however, in the literature pertaining to the rodent brain. Some reports have been in favor of age-related neuronal dropout (11, 22, 41, 45, 46). Alternatively, in other studies no age-related differences in rat cortical neuronal densities were found (42, 47). Peters and Vaughan (20) have suggested that this disparity may be attributed to differences in the rat strains being investigated. Moreover, in a study of the primary somatosensory cortex of C57BL mice, Curcio (27) was unable to find age-related cell loss in animals up to 33 months old.

In view of the presumed role of the hippocampus in memory function, this is an area of considerable importance for animal models of senescent forgetfulness; moreover, in AD the hippocampus is a region expressing considerable pathological alterations. Several studies on humans have demonstrated age-related neuronal loss in this region (48, 49). Similarly, neuronal loss has been found by Brizzee and colleagues (44) in the aging monkey hippocampus as well as in the rat hippocampus (11, 50). There have also, however, been reports of no apparent loss of granule cells or pyramidal cells in the hippocampus of aged rats (51, 52).

Purkinje cells of the cerebellum are easily identified neurons, which have made this anatomical region a valuable area in which to quantify age-related changes in humans, as well as in parallel studies of potential animal models. The Purkinje cell population has shown an age-related decrease in every mammalian species investigated: humans (53–55), monkeys (56), and rodents (57–59).

There are two additional areas deserving of special mention with regard to neuronal population, in view of their potential significance to AD. The first of these is the nucleus basalis of Meynert, a peripallidal nucleus of the basal forebrain. The neurons of this nucleus appear to be the principal source of extrinsic cholinergic input to the mammaliam neocortex

(33, 60, 61). As described elsewhere in this volume, dysfunction of the cholinergic system appears to play a major role in memory impairment in old age and, in particular, in AD (for an extensive evaluation of this issue see ref. 62). Studies have indicated that in the frontal-parietal cortex of the rat, 70% of the cholinergic innervation is extrinsic, derived from the nucleus basalis. Cholinergic neurons intrinsic to the neocortex provide the remaining 30%. Whitehouse and co-workers (33) have demonstrated that in humans there is a significant selective loss of cholinergic neurons from the nucleus basalis associated with AD. It is not yet known whether there is a correlation between memory loss and cell loss in the nucleus basalis of the aging rat.

The second nucleus of particular interest is the locus ceruleus. This brain stem nucleus is the source of noradrenergic projections to the cortex; and diminished monoamines may also play a role in memory impairments and/or dementia of the Alzheimer type. During normal human aging, it was shown that there is a 40% decrease in neurons of the locus ceruleus (62). In AD, Bondareff and associates (31) demonstrated a population subgroup showing a high (80%) loss of neurons in this nucleus. Coleman and Goldman (64), however, were unable to find any evidence of neuronal loss in the locus ceruleus of the aging rat.

AGE-RELATED CYTOPATHOLOGICAL CHANGES IN NEURONS AND NEUROPIL

LIPOFUSCIN

In mammalian pathological models of senescence, the accumulation of lipofuscin is probably the most conspicuous histological manifestation of aging. Lipofuscin is generally regarded as a byproduct of cellular metabolism, and is found in neurons and glia throughout the CNS. Lipofuscin is ubiquitous in mammals and has been studied in dogs (65), rats (66–68), mice (69, 70), subhuman primates (43, 71, 72), and humans (73). The degree of lipofuscin accumulation within the neuron appears to be dependent on the location of the cell (71, 74). Also, at least in neocortex and hippocampus of aged monkeys and dogs, there appears to be a greater accumulation of lipofuscin in glia than in neurons. Furthermore, lipofuscin differs in its appearance in these cell types (30) (Fig. 51–1). Although excessive lipofuscin deposition in humans has been associated with neuronal pathology (75, 76), since this is a widespread mammalian age-related phenomenon, it is still not known whether the presence and accumulation of lipofuscin is beneficial, detrimental, or harmless to the cell (77, 78).

NEURITIC (SENILE) PLAQUES

The nature of neuritic (senile) plaques is well described and reviewed in the literature (79–83). In humans, senile plaques (SPs) are found in both normal elderly and senile aged, although they are more prominent in the latter (84). SPs are one of the characteristic morphological hallmarks of dementia of the Alzheimer type. They are also referred to as neuritic plaques because typically, the lesion is characterized by altered or degenerating (predominantly axonal) neuronal processes (i.e., neurites), reactive neuroglial cells, and amyloid filaments (81).

In nonhuman mammalian models of aging, the neuritic plaques have also been described at the light and electron microscopic levels in monkeys (30, 79, 82). In dogs, several investiga-

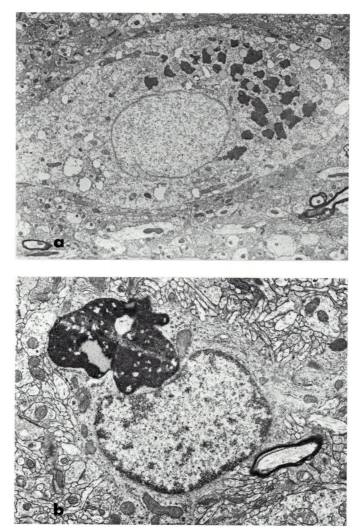

Figure 51–1. (a) Electron micrograph of a pyramidal cell soma from aged dog neocortex. There is a moderate accumulation of lipofuscin, with a polar distribution. × 2,800. (b) Glial cell (astrocyte) in the frontal cortex of an aged (20-year-old) monkey. This micrograph illustrates the large accumulation of pigment in this cell type and how its appearance differs from that in the neuron. × 6,300.

tors have described the light microscopic appearance of the senile plaques (SPs) (85–88). Ultrastructural features of canine neuritic plaques have also been evaluated (89).

The pathogenesis of SPs is unknown, but it has been suggested that aggregates of altered neurites may serve as a nidus for subsequent development of the neuritic lesion (80). In the monkey and the dog, where plaques may be found at the light microscopic level but are not abundant, ultrastructural studies of the parenchema have been shown to be a valuable adjunct in detecting these initial changes in the neuropil—some of which, in time, may subsequently develop into more definitive plaques (30, 80) (Fig. 51–2).

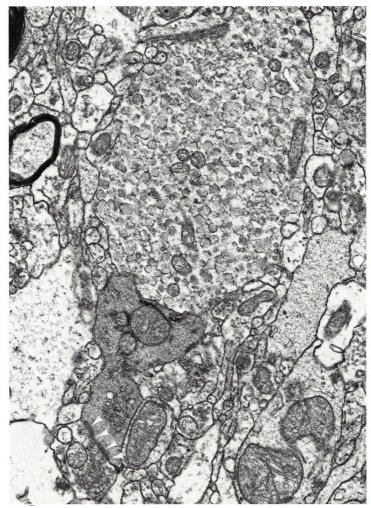

Figure 51–2. Large dystrophic neurite filled with vesicular profiles. The subadjacent dark structure is a degenerating dendrite. Arrows indicate synaptic zone of the dendrite with an apparently normal axonal terminal. Hippocampus, adult (10-year-old) monkey. × 13,000.

Recently, it has also been shown that neuritic plaques containing amyloid may be experimentally induced in mice infected with the scrapie virus (83, 89, 90).

Although plaques had not previously been shown to be a concomitant of normal aging in rodents, Vaughan and Peters (91) have now reported finding neuritic plaques containing amyloid in aged rats. The etiology is unknown but could reflect a true age-related change, or perhaps the expression of a viral infection.

NEUROFIBRILLARY CHANGES

As described elsewhere in this volume, neurons undergoing neurofibrillary degeneration are commonly found in the normally senescent human brain. Indeed the presence of this neurofibrillary change (along with SPs) is pathognomic for AD (92, 93).

The fibrillary change is of a very specific nature. Due to their light microscopic appearance in silver-stained tissue sections the neuronal changes are also called neurofibrillary tangles (NFTs). Electron microscopy has shown that NFTs are actually composed of paired helical 10-nm filaments (PHFs). This particular morphological finding, of PHFs, has been seen only in humans. Consequently, there cannot be a bona fide animal model for AD.

In aged monkeys, paired helical filaments (PHFs)—but of a different periodicity than those seen in humans—have been reported (82). This finding is, however, quite rare.

In experimental studies, neurofibrillary changes have been induced by various pharmacological agents such as mitotic spindle inhibitors (94) or maytansine (95). This topic has been recently reviewed by Wisniewski and associates (28). Typical neurofibrillary changes of this type are composed of aggregates of straight 10-nm neurofilaments and, hence, are not the same as the PHFs associated with NFTs in humans.

In the majority of experimental studies dealing with neurofibrillary degeneration, the inducing agent has been aluminum or aluminum salts. It is typically used to produce an acute model (rabbits go into status epilepticus within 1 to 3 weeks) (96–99). However, chronic animal models for producing neurofibrillary changes in both developing and mature rabbits by aluminum agents have recently been developed (100, 101). In the latter models, neurological signs and seizures have been minimized, particularly in the developing rabbit. Some of the aluminum models have also been shown to produce deficits in learning and memory (102, 103). However, as a potential model for AD there is currently contradictory evidence both in favor of (104) and against (105) changes in central cholinergic activity in aluminum-induced neurofibrillary degeneration. Thus, it might be stated that this model of neurofibrillary degeneration could be used to study the effects of neurofibrillary changes on neuronal function; however, it would not be appropriate to assume that these examples of neurofibrillary changes necessarily constitute an acceptable model for the pathogenesis of dementia of the Alzheimer type.

THE DENDRITIC FIELD AND SPINE CHANGES IN MAMMALIAN PATHOLOGIC MODELS

The Golgi impregnation method is an invaluable tool in evaluating both normal and pathological neuronal alterations in the senescent mammalian brain. This technique—through deposition of a silver-chrome precipitate—permits the investigator to visualize the entire soma-dendritic complex of the neuron (Fig. 51–3a).

THE DENDRITIC ARBOR AND DENDRITE SPINES

In a Golgi preparation, the dendritic field represents approximately 90% of the surface area of the average neuron (106). This arbor thereby constitutes the major source of afferent input to the neuron. It logically follows that any process which results in loss of dendritic integrity would also interfere with neuronal processing and—assuming that a sufficient number of neurons are involved—such loss would ultimately be reflected in behavioral or cognitive deficits in the organism.

Dendritic spines are small protrusions or excrescences found along the dendritic branches. They are postsynaptic specializations of the dendritic membrane which—in the case of cortical pyramidal neurons—mediate almost all input to that cell (Fig. 51–3b). Given this functional role, it is apparent that spine loss—like loss of the dendrites themselves—would have a major impact on the ability of a neuron to process information adequately. For example,

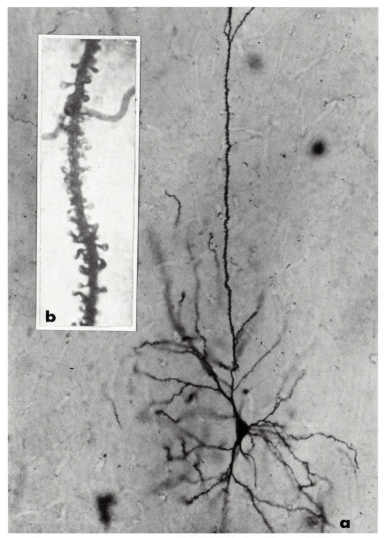

Figure 51–3. (a) Typical appearance of a Golgi-impregnated mammalian neocortical pyramidal cell. This is from canine frontal cortex. × 380. (b) At higher magnification, insert shows appearance of dendritic spines which embellish the dendritic branches; they serve as the primary loci for synaptic input to this cell type. × 1060. *Figure 51–3(a) is reproduced by permission of Academic Press.*

spine dysgenesis and/or loss of branches have been found in neurologic developmental disorders associated with diminished cognitive capacity (107–111).

ATROPHIC DENDRITIC CHANGES ACCOMPANYING SENESCENCE IN HUMANS

Studies by Scheibel and collaborators (112–120) have indicated that various neuronal cell types of the cortex, hippocampus, and spinal cord in the aging and senile human brain pass through a histopathological sequence of progressively atrophic structural changes which include a shrinking dendritic arbor and loss of dendritic spines. Some aspects of these atrophic changes in cortical neurons from senescent and senile human brain have also been described by others (30, 121–123). However, as will be discussed, it is possible that such atrophy may depict changes occurring in only a subpopulation of cortical neurons and may not necessarily be representative of the neuronal population as a whole.

In the cerebellum, atrophy of Purkinje cells accompanying senescence in humans has also been described (122).

ATROPHIC DENDRITIC CHANGES ACCOMPANYING SENESCENCE IN ANIMALS

Descriptions of dendritic atrophy accompanied by spine loss have also been ascribed to Golgi-impregnated cortical neurons in aged monkeys (30, 124–126) and aged dogs (30, 127).

Golgi studies of rodent brains have also depicted age-related regression of dendritic

Figure 51–4. (a) Golgi-impregnated Purkinje cell from the cerebellum of a young adult dog. × 212. (b) Higher magnification shows a dendritic arbor densely branched and heavily spined. × 1,060. *Reproduced by permission of the Plenum Press.*

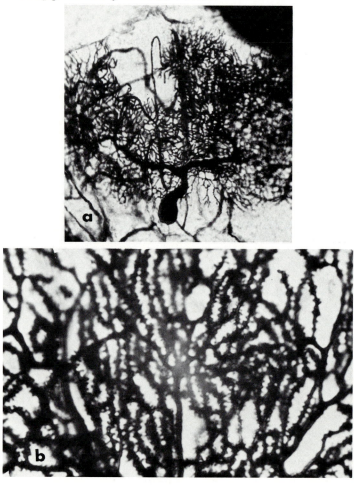

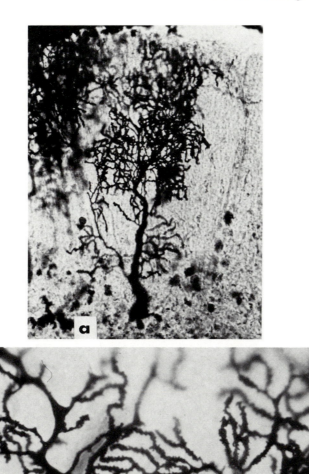

Figure 51–5. (a) Purkinje cell from an aged dog cerebellum. Golgi preparation shows reduction of the dendritic arbor. × 212. (b) Higher magnification reveals patchy areas of spine loss on thorny branchlets. × 1,060. *Reproduced by permission of the Plenum Press.*

fields and processes in cortical neuron branching or spine density (128–131). In a quantitative electron microscopic (EM) study in the hippocampus of aged rats, Geinesman and associates (132) reported dendritic atrophy in the dentate gyrus.

Apparent neuronal degeneration has also been described in Golgi studies of the aging mouse limbic system, spinal cord, lower brain stem, and hypothalamus (133–135).

In the cerebellum, age-related atrophy of the Purkinje cell dendritic field has been described in dogs (30) and rats (59, 136) (Figs. 51–4 and 51–5). However, Pysh and Benson (137) were unable to discern any atrophic alterations of these cells in their aged rats.

Synaptic Pathology in Mammalian Models of Aging

Synaptic Degeneration in the Aging Brain

Since light microscopy of Golgi preparations shows atrophic dendritic changes accompanying senescence, it is not surprising that there might well be concomitant evidence of synaptic alterations at the ultrastructural level. Certainly, synaptic loss has been described

Figure 51–6. (a) Electron micrograph of neuropil from adult (10-year-old) monkey frontal cortex. Note the dendritic spine (sp) projecting from the shaft (den) and synapsing (*arrow*) with axon terminal (at). × 8,750. (b) Electron-dense form of dendritic degeneration. Two apparently normal axon terminals seen synapsing with the dendrite (*arrows*). Adult monkey frontal cortex. × 22,900.

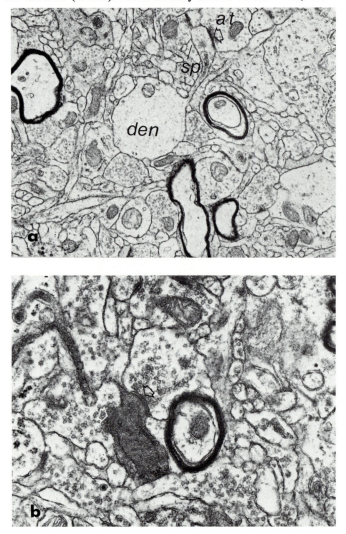

or quantified in a number of EM studies in the aging rat cortex (129, 138), hippocampus (51, 139–143), and cerebellum (59, 144, 145). In the monkey (*M. mulatta*), Uemura (125) has documented an age-related decline in synaptic density. Interestingly, studies of synaptic loss in the human cortex have not demonstrated comparable age-related changes (146, 147), but this may well be attributed to methodological and sampling difficulties inherent in such human studies.

Synaptic alterations may affect pre- and/or postsynaptic components. The appearance of presynaptic degeneration infers axonal loss and would thereby suggest extrinsic deafferentiation. Alternatively, loss of the postsynaptic element, the dendrite or its spine, would be indicative of age-related intrinsic neuronal deterioration. Both of these processes would most likely involve, to various degrees, affected synapses throughout the neuropil. Specific evidence of synaptic degeneration has, for example, been described in the cortex of aged monkeys (30, 82) and in the lateral vestibular nucleus of aging rats (148). Typically, degeneration takes the appearance of either an electron dense phase or of neurofilamentous hypertrophy (149) (Fig. 51–6). However, despite quantitative evidence of synaptic loss, it is perplexing that electron microscopy has not always been able to discern signs of synaptic degeneration in the neuropil (51, 129, 139, 140, 143, 144).

Evidence of synaptic degeneration may also be regarded as a normal process reflecting ongoing synaptic turnover which continues throughout the life span of the individual (150–152).

Dystrophic Neuritic Terminals

Synaptic pathology in both animals and humans may appear as more than just degeneration *per se*. Altered or dystrophic synapses and neuritic processes are found in AD, as well as in other forms of dementia or retardation (28, 153–157). Membraneous inclusions or whorls have been described in the cerebral cortex of aging monkeys (30) (Fig. 51–7a) and rats (129, 158). Membrane-bound degenerative and dense osmophilic products have been reported in aged dogs (87) and monkeys (30, 79, 82) (Fig. 51–7b). Tubulovesicular neuritic profiles filled with accumulations of tubular or cisternlike structures have also been described in the adult and aging monkey cortex (30) (Fig. 51–8a).

Axonal deterioration has also received attention and has been described in aging animals (20, 30, 82, 148, 159, 160) (Fig. 51–8b).

It is important to reiterate that some of these altered and dystrophic-appearing changes may also be found in normal adult brains of both animals and humans (30, 148, 152, 161). Their appearance, however atypical, may really only reflect a remodelling process, and thus suggests a continuing capacity for plasticity in the aging brains.

Plasticity in Mammalian Pathologic Models

It may be misleading and simplistic to paint a picture of the mammalian nervous system in senescence as one of atrophying dendritic fields and degenerating synapses. There is a growing body of evidence which clearly implies that the capacity of neurons to maintain plastic properties of growth and synapse renewal extends not only into adulthood but also into old age. This evidence has been described and evaluated in several recent reviews (27, 30, 150, 162, 163).

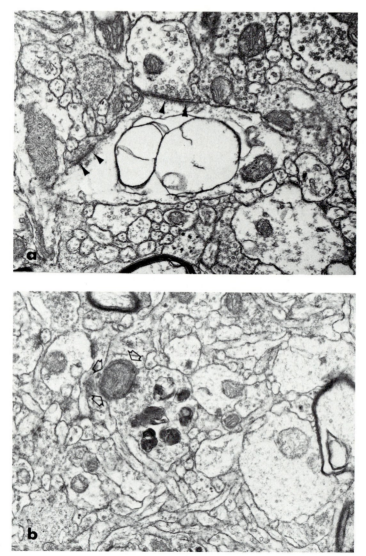

Figure 51–7. (a) Membranous inclusion in a dendritic process. Adult monkey neocortex. Two axons synapse on this dendrite (*arrows*). × 15,540. (b) Dystrophic synaptic complex in the frontal cortex of another adult monkey. Dense osmophilic products are located in axon terminal. Postsynaptically, there is extensive dendritic degeneration (*arrows*). × 11,350.

DENDRITIC FIELDS

In a computer-assisted study of the dendritic arbor of randomly selected Golgi-impregnated pyramidal cells from the human parahippocampal gyrus, Buell and Coleman (123, 164, 165) reported that during normal aging there was continued (and statistically significant) expansion of the dendritic tree and, particularly, of terminal dendritic segments. In neurons from these autopsied brains of Alzheimer patients, however, such continued dendritic plastic-

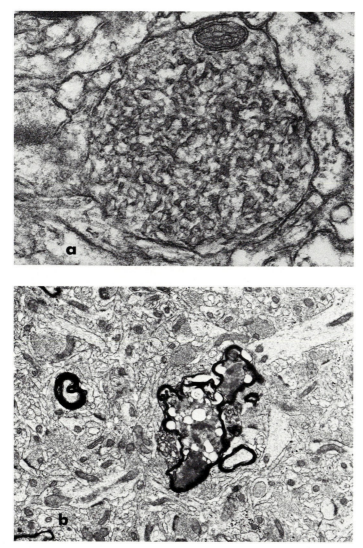

Figure 51–8. (a) A tubulovesicular filled neuritic profile in the frontal cortex of an aged (20-year-old) monkey. × 33,250. (b) An example of degeneration in a myelinated axon. Aged monkey neocortex. × 6,400.

ity ceased. Buell and Coleman observed that most senescent and AD brains contained neurons with both atrophic and normal-appearing dendritic arbors. This suggested that there may be, perhaps, two subpopulations of pyramidal cells; one regressing, and the other continuing to express plasticity. Findings of continued dendritic branching are also reported by Conner and associates (166, 167) and by Diamond and Connor (168) in aging rats. A shift in the balance between these two populations might explain the description of dendritic regression in other aged rats (128, 130, 169). A pattern of dendritic expansion into old age, followed by regression has also been seen in monkeys (126).

Dendritic Spines and Synapses

Dendritic spines are considered the major loci for information transfer to pyramidal cells, therefore, these structures are critical in determinating the functional capacity of neurons. Dendritic plasticity, to be functionally relevant, should also extend to spines. Descriptions of aging human neurons have noted that dendritic regression is typically accompanied by spine loss (115). Similar accounts are given for neocortical pyramidal cells from aging dogs (127) and rats (131). In the neocortex of the aging C57B1/6J mouse, spine loss in pyramidal cells also seems concomitant with normal aging (170). On the other hand, Conner and associates (171) described increased spine densities in rats which appear to correlate with enhanced dendritic growth. These descriptions of plasticity are not similar to the aberrant type of dendritic sprouting ("lawless") as seen by Scheibel and Tomiyasu (172) in two familial cases of AD. Occasionally, apparently abnormal dendritic spine growth was also observed in the aged dog brain (127), but these were not the same kind of changes described for AD.

Mervis has demonstrated that normal age-related loss of spines in the neocortex of C57B1/6J mice, which correlated with reduced retention of learning (173) could be repressed by chronic dietary choline enrichment (170). A similar change was found in synapses in the cerebellum (174). This implies that extrinsic influences such as diet or environment may also manipulate dendritic and synaptic integrity in the aging brain (166–168, 171, 175).

Cotman and Scheff (52, 176) have investigated synapse turnover and reactive synaptogenesis in the hippocampus of aged rats, i.e., the capacity of neurons to grow new synapses following partial denervation. Older animals have reduced plasticity as shown by a reduced growth rate as well as final magnitude of response.

Concluding Remarks

It is apparent from this review that there are valid mammalian models for the neuropathological findings seen during normal human aging. In rodents, dogs, and humans, Golgi and ultrastructural studies have shown there to be many similar alterations in neurons and neuropil (for additional reviews and discussion see refs. 20, 30, 177).

Additional quantitative studies are necessary both to further define age-related changes as well as to appreciate the widespread appearance of atypical structures in young are well as aging brains. Quantitative studies are especially needed to characterize the potential limits for continued neuronal plasticity in senescence.

A valid nonhuman mammalian model, per se, does not exist for AD or SDAT. Psychopharmacological models are available (Chap. 53). From a morphological perspective, however, the absence of typical neurofibrillary changes (composed of PHFs) in aging and senescent nonhuman mammals is a serious drawback to ultimately equating any senile behavioral changes in animals with AD. Animal models of neurofibrillary changes—such as aluminum-induced degeneration (101)—will, however, be helpful in understanding how such filamentous accumulation can modify neuronal function.

The greatest advantage of using animal models of senescence is not having to deal with the changes found in human brains which are a consequence of terminal therapeutic measures and/or prolonged agonal hypoxia, or postmortem fixation artifacts (178). Typically, these artifacts may well mask or distort the neuronal alterations which could lead to additional understanding of disease mechanisms.

Given these restrictions and limitations, however, animal models can be utilized and are valuable tools in the search for clues leading to greater understanding of the neuropathology of senescence.

REFERENCES

1. Kral VA: Benign senescent forgetfulness. *Aging NY* 1978; 7:47–51.
2. Kubanis P, Zornetzer SF: Age-related behavioral and neurobiological changes: a review with emphasis on memory. *Behav Neurol Biol* 1981: 31:115–172.
3. Dean RT, Scozzafava J, Goas JA, et al: Age-related differences in behavior across the life span of the C57BL/6J mouse. *Exp Aging Res* 1981; 7:427–451.
4. Bartus RT, Dean RL, Beer B: Memory deficits in aged cebus monkeys and facilitation with central cholinomimetics. *Neurobiol Aging* 1980; 1:145–152.
5. Fraley SM, Springer AD: Memory of simple learning in young, middle-aged, and aged C57/BL6 mice. *Behav Neurol Biol* 1981; 31:1–7.
6. Strong R, Hibkj P, Hsu L, et al: Age-related alterations in the rodent brain cholinergic system and behavior. *Neurobiol Aging* 1980; 1:59–63.
7. Goodrick C: Error goal-gradients of mature young and aged rats during training in a 14-unit spatial maze. *Psychol Rep* 1973; 32:359–362.
8. Ingram DK, London ED, Goodrick CL: Age and neurochemical correlates of radial maze performance in rats. *Neurobiol Aging* 1981; 2:41–47.
9. Lippa AS, Pelham RW, Beer B, et al: Brain cholinergic dysfunction and memory in aged rats. *Neurobiol Aging* 1980; 1:13–21.
10. Klein AW: A rat model for the neuroanatomical basis of performance decline with aging, in Stein D (ed): *The Psychobiology of Aging: Problems and Perspectives.* New York, Elsevier North-Holland, 1980, pp 81–97.
11. Brizzee KR, Ordy JM: Age pigments, cell loss, and hippocampal function. *Mech Ageing Dev* 1979; 9:143–162.
12. Gold PE, McGaugh JL: Changes in learning and memory during aging, in Ordy JM, Brizzee KR (eds): *Neurobiology of Aging.* New York, Plenum, 1975, pp 145–158.
13. Bartus RT, Fleming D, Johnson HR: Aging in the rhesus monkey: debilitating effects on short-term memory. *J Gerontol* 1978; 33:858–871.
14. Bartus RT: Physostigmine and recent memory: effects in young and aged non-human primates. *Science* 1979; 206:1087–1089.
15. Bartus RT: Effects of aging on visual memory, sensory processing and discrimination learning in the non-human primate. *Aging NY* 1979; 10:85–114.
16. Davis RT: Old monkey behavior. *Exp Geront* 1978; 13:237–250.
17. Medin DL: Form perception and pattern reproduction in monkeys. *J Comp Physiol Psychol* 1969; 68:412.
18. Ordy JM: Neurobiology and aging in non-human primates, in Ordy JM, Brizzee KR (eds): *Neurobiology of Aging.* New York, Plenum, 1975, pp 575–597.
19. Sabel BA, Stein DG: Extensive loss of subcortical neurons in the aging rat brain. *Exp Neurol* 1981; 73:507–516.
20. Peters A, Vaughan DW: Central nervous system, in Johnson TE Jr (ed): *Aging and Cell Structure.* New York, Plenum, 1981, vol 1, pp 1–34.

21. Diamond MC, Johnson RE, Gold MW: Changes in neuron number and size and glia number in the young, adult, and aging medial occipital cortex. *Behav Biol* 1977; 20:409–418.

22. Ordy JM, Brizzee KR, Kaack B, et al: Age differences in short-term memory and cell loss in the cortex of the rat. *Gerontology* 1978; 24:276–285.

23. Vaughan DW, Vincent JM: Ultrastructure of neurons in the auditory cortex of aging rats: a morphometric study. *J Neuropathol* 1979; 8:215–228.

24. Knox CA, Oliveira A: Brain aging in normotensive and hypertensive strains of rats: III. A quantitative study of cerebrovasculature. *Acta Neuropathol* 1980; 52:17–26.

25. Donaldson HH: *The Rat.* Philadelphia, Wistar Institute, 1924.

26. Roberts J, Goldberg PB: Some aspects of the central nervous system of the rat during aging, in Gibson DC, Adelman AC, Finch C (eds): *Development of the Rodent as a Model System of Aging,* US Dept of Health, Education, and Welfare publication no. (NIH) 79–161. Government Printing Office, 1979, pp 155–164.

27. Curcio CA: *A Computer-Assisted Morphometric Analysis of a Single Cortical Barrel in Aging Mice,* thesis. University of Rochester, Rochester, 1981.

28. Wisniewski HM, Sinatra RS, Iqbal K, et al: Neurofibrillary and synaptic pathology in the aged brain, in Johnson JE Jr (ed): *Aging and Cell Structure.* New York, Plenum, 1981, vol 1, pp 105–142.

29. Curcio CA, Buell SJ, Coleman PD: Morphology of the aging central nervous system. *Adv Neurogerontol* 1982.

30. Mervis RF: Cytomorphological alterations in the aging brain, with emphasis on Golgi studies, in Johnson J Jr (ed): *Aging and Cell Structure.* New York, Plenum, 1981, vol 1, pp 143–186.

31. Bowen DM, Spillane JA, Curzon G, et al: Accelerated aging or selective neuronal loss as an important cause of dementia. *Lancet* 1979; i:11–14.

32. Bondareff W, Mountjoy CQ, Roth M: Loss of neurons of origin of the adrenergic projection to cerebral cortex (nucleus locus ceruleus) in senile dementia. *Neurology* 1982; 32:164–168.

33. Whitehouse PJ, Price DL, Clark AW, et al: Alzheimer disease: evidence for selective loss of cholinergic neurons in the nucleus basalis. *Ann Neurol* 1981; 10:122–126.

34. Brody H: Organization of cerebral cortex: III. A study of aging in the human cerebral cortex. *J Comp Neurol* 1955; 102:511–556.

35. Brody H: An examination of cerebral cortex and brainstem aging. *Aging NY* 1976; 3:177–182.

36. Colon EJ: The elderly brain: a quantitative analysis in the cerebral cortex of two cases. *Psychiatr Neurol Neurochir* 1972; 75:261–270.

37. Henderson C, Tomlinson BE, Weightman D: Cell counts in the human cerebral cortex using a traditional and an automatic method. *J Neurol Sci* 1975; 25:129–144.

38. Henderson G, Tomlinson BE, Gibson PH: Cell counts in human cerebral cortex in normal adults throughout life using an image analyzing computer. *J Neurol Sci* 1980; 46:113–136.

39. Shefer VF: Absolute numbers of neurons and thickness of cerebral cortex during aging, senile and vascular dementia and Pick's and Alzheimer's disease. *Neurosci Behav Physiol* 1973; 6:319–324.

40. Terry RD, Peck A, deTeresa R, et al: Some morphometric aspects of the brain in senile dementia of the Alzheimer type. *Ann Neurol* 1981; 10:184–192.

41. Brizzee KR: Quantitative histological studies on aging changes in cerebral cortex of rhesus monkey and albino rat with notes on effects of prolonged low-dose ionizing irradiation in the rat. *Prog Brain Res* 1973; 40:141–160.

42. Brizzee KR: Gross morphometric analyses and quantitative histology of the aging brain. *Adv Behav Biol* 1975; 16:401–424.

43. Brizzee KR, Ordy JM, Hansche J, et al: Quantitative assessment of changes in neurons and glia cell packing density and lipofuscin accumulation with age in the cerebral cortex of a nonhuman primate (*Macaca mulatta*). *Aging NY* 1976; 3:229–244.

44. Brizzee KR, Ordy JM, Bartus RT: Localization of cellular changes within multimodal sensory regions in aged monkey brain: possible implications for age-related cognitive loss. *Neurobiol Aging* 1980; 1:45–52.

45. Landfield PW, Rose G, Sandles L, et al: Patterns of astroglial hypertrophy and neuronal degeneration in the hippocampus of aged memory-deficient rats. *J Gerontol* 1977; 32:3–12.

46. Mufson EJ, Stein DG: Behavioral and morphological aspects of aging: an analysis of rat frontal cortex, in Stein D (ed): *The Psychobiology of Aging: Problems and Perspectives.* New York, Elsevier North-Holland, 1980, pp 99–125.

47. Klein AW, Michael ME: A morphometric study of the neocortex of young adult and old maze-differentiated rats. *Mech Ageing Dev* 1977; 6:441–452.

48. Ball MJ: Neuronal loss, neurofibrillary tangles and granulovacuolar degeneration in the hippocampus with aging and dementia. *Acta Neuropathol* 1977; 37:111–118.

49. Mouritzen A: The density of neurons in the human hippocampus. *Neuropathol Appl Neurobiol* 1979; 5:249–264.

50. Landfield PW, Braun LD, Pitler TA, et al: Hippocampal aging in rats: a morphometric study of multiple variables in semi-thin sections. *Neurobiol Aging* 1981; 2:265–275.

51. Bondareff W: Synaptic atrophy in the senescent hippocampus. *Mech Ageing Dev* 1979; 9:163–171.

52. Cotman CW, Scheff SW: Compensatory synapse growth in aged animals after neuronal death. *Mech Ageing Dev* 1979; 9:103–118.

53. Ellis RS: Norms for some structural changes in the human cerebellum from birth to old age. *J Comp Neurol* 1920; 32:1–33.

54. Hall TC, Miller AKH, Corsellis JAN: Variations in the human Purkinje cell population according to age and sex. *Neuropathol Appl Neurobiol* 1975; 1:267–292.

55. Corsellis JAN: Some observations on the Purkinje cell population and on brain volume in human aging. *Aging NY* 1976; 3:205–209.

56. Nandy K: Morphological changes in the cerebellar cortex of aging *Macaca nemistrina. Neurobiol Aging* 1981; 2:61–64.

57. Inukai T: On the loss of Purkinje cells, with advancing age, from the cerebellar cortex of the albino rat. *J Comp Neurol* 1928; 45:1–31.

58. Rogers J, Silver MA, Shoemaker WJ, et al: Senescent changes in a neurobiological model system: cerebellar Purkinje cell electrophysiology and correlative anatomy. *Neurobiol Aging* 1980; 1:3–12.

59. Rogers J, Zornetzer SF, Bloom FE, et al: Senescent microstructural changes in rat cerebellum. Submitted for publication, 1982.

60. Coyle JT, McKinney M, Johnston MV: Cholinergic innervation of the cerebral cortex: implications for the pathophysiology of senile dementia of the Alzheimer's type. *Aging NY* 1981; 17:149–161.

61. Johnston MV, McKinney M, Coyle JT: Evidence for a cholinergic projection to neocortex from neurons in basal forebrain. *Proc Natl Acad Sci USA* 1979; 76:5392–5396.

62. Crook T, Gershon S (eds): *Strategies for the Development of an Effective Treatment for Senile Dementia.* New Canaan, Powley, 1981.

63. Vijayashankar N, Brody H: A quantitative study of the pigmented neurons in the nuclei locus coeruleus and subcoeruleus in man as related to aging. *J Neuropathol Exp Neurol* 1979; 38:490–497.

64. Coleman PD, Goldman G: Neuron counts in locus coeruleus of aging rat. *Aging NY* 1981:23–30.

65. Few A, Getty R: Occurrence of lipofuscin as related to aging in the canine and porcine nervous system. *J Gerontol* 1967; 22:357–368.

66. Heinsen H: Lipofuscin in the cerebellar cortex of albino rats: an electron microscopic study. *Anat Embryol* 1979; 155:333–345.

67. Brizzee KR, Johnson FA: Depth distribution of lipofuscin pigment in cerebral cortex of rat. *Acta Neuropathol* 1970; 16:205–219.

68. Reichel W, Hollander J, Clark JH, et al: Lipofuscin pigment accumulation as a function of age and distribution in rodent brain. *J Gerontol* 1968; 23:71–78.

69. Samorajski T, Ordy JM, Rady-Reimer P: Lipofuscin pigment accumulation in the nervous system of aging mice. *Anat Rec* 1968; 160:55–574.

70. Sekhon SS, Andrew JM, Maxwell DS: Accumulation and development of lipofuscin pigment in the aging central nervous system of the mouse. *J Cell Biol* 1966; 43:127A.

71. Brizzee KR, Ordy JM, Kaack B: Early appearance and regional differences in intraneuronal and extraneuronal lipofuscin accumulation with age in the brain of a non-human primate. *J Gerontol* 1974; 29:366–381.

72. Gless P, Spoerri PE, El-Ghazzawi E: An ultrastructural study of hypothalamic neurons in monkeys of different ages with special reference to age-related lipofuscin. *J Hirnforsh* 1975; 16:379–394.

73. Mann DMA, Yates PO, Stamp JE: The relationship between lipofuscin and aging in the human nervous system. *J Neurol Sci* 1978; 37:83–93.

74. Brizzee KR, Kaack B, Klara P: Lipofuscin: intra- and extra-neuronal accumulation and regional distribution. *Adv Behav Biol* 1975; 16:463–484.

75. Kornfeld M: Generalized lipofuscinosis (generalized Kuf's disease). *J Neuropathol Exp Neurol* 1972; 31:668–682.

76. Zeman W, Dyken P: Neuronal ceroid-lipofuscinosis (Batten's disease): relationship to amaurotic family idiocy? *Pediatrics* 1969; 44:570.

77. Mann DMA, Yates PO: Lipoprotein pigments: their relationship to aging in the human nervous system. *Brain* 1974; 97:481–488.

78. Mann DMA, Sinclair KGA: The quantitative assessment of lipofuscin pigment, cytoplasmic RNA, and nucleolar volume in senile dementia. *Neuropathol Appl Neurobiol* 1978; 4:129–135.

79. Wisniewski HM, Terry RD: Morphology of the aging brain, human and animal. *Brain Res* 1973; 40:167–186.

80. Wisniewski HM, Terry RD: Re-examination of the pathogenesis of the senile plaque. *Prog Neuropathol* 1973; 2:1–26.

81. Wisniewski HM, Terry RD: Neuropathology of the aging brain. *Aging NY* 1976; 3:265–280.

82. Wisniewski HM, Ghetti B, Terry RD: Neuritic (senile) plaques and filamentous changes in aged rhesus monkeys. *J Neuropathol Exp Neurol* 1973; 32:566–584.

83. Wisniewski HM, Moretz, Lossinsky AS: Evidence for induction of localized amyloid deposits and neuritic plaques by an infectious agent. *Ann Neurol* 1981; 10:517–522.

84. Tomlinson BE, Blessed G, Roth M: Observations on the brains of nondemented old people. *J Neurol Sci* 1968; 7:331–356.

85. von Braunmuhl A: Kongophile Angiopathie und "senile Plaques" bei greisen Hunden. *Arch Psychiatr Nervenkr* 1956; 194:396–414.

86. Dahme E: Altersveränderunges im Gehirn bei Tiern. *Bull Schweiz Akad Med Wiss* 1968; 24:133–142.

87. Wisniewski H, Johnson AB, Raine CS, et al: Senile plaques and amyloidosis in aged dogs. *Lab Invest* 1970; 23:287–296.

88. Pauli B, Luginbuhl H: Fluorescenzmikroskopische Untersuchungen der cerebralen Amyloidose bei alten Hunden und senilen Menschen. *Acta Neuropathol* 1971; 19:121–128.

89. Bruce ME, Fraser H: Amyloid plaques in the brains of mice infected with scrapie: morphological variation and staining properties. *Neuropathol Appl Neurobiol* 1975; 1:189–202.

90. Wisniewski HM, Bruce ME, Fraser H: Infectious etiology of neuritic (senile) plaques in mice. *Science* 1975; 190:1108–1110.

91. Vaughan DW, Peters A: The structure of neuritic plaques in the cerebral cortex of aged rats. *J Neuropathol Exp Neurol* 1981; 40:472–487.

92. Corsellis JAN: Aging and the dementias in Blackwood W, Corsellis JAN (eds): *Greenfield's Neuropathology,* ed 3. Chicago, Year Book, 1976, pp 796–848.

93. Hirano A: *A Guide to Neuropathology.* Tokyo, Igaku-Shoin, 1981.

94. Dahl D, Bignami A, Bich NT, et al: Immunohistochemical characterization of neurofibrillary tangles induced by mitotic spindle inhibitors. *Acta Neuropathol* 1980; 51:165–168.

95. Ghetti B: Induction of neurofibrillary degeneration following treatment with maytansine *in vivo. Brain Res* 1979; 163:9–19.

96. Klatzo I, Wisniewski HM, Streicher E: Experimental production of neurofibrillary degeneration: I. Light microscopic observation. *J Neuropathol Exp Neurol* 1965; 24:187–199.

97. de Boni U, Otvos A, Scot JW, et al: Neurofibrillary degeneration induced by systemic aluminum. *Acta Neuropathol* 1976; 35:285–294.

98. Wisniewski HM, Narkiewicz O, Wisniewski K: Topography and dynamics of neurofibrillary degeneration in aluminum encephalopathy. *Acta Neuropathol* 1967; 9:127–133.

99. Yates CM, Gordon A, Wilson H: Neurofibrillary degeneration induced in the rabbit by aluminum chloride: aluminum neurofibrillary tangles. *J Neuropathol Appl Neurobiol* 1976; 2:131–144.

100. Wisniewski HM, Sturman JA, Shek JW: Aluminum chloride induced neurofibrillary changes in the developing rabbit: a chronic animal model. *Ann Neurol* 1980; 8:479–490.

101. Wisniewski HM, Sterman, Shek JW: Chronic model of neurofibrillary changes induced in mature rabbits by metallic aluminum. *Neurobiol Aging* 1982; 3:11–22.

102. Petit TL, Biederman GB, McMullen PA: Neurofibrillary degeneration, dendritic dying back, and learning—memory deficits after aluminum administration: implications for brain aging. *Exp Neurol* 1980; 67:152–162.

103. Crapper DR, Krishnan, SS, Dalton AJ: Brain aluminum distribution in Alzheimer's disease and experimental neurofibrillary degenerating. *Science* 1973; 180:511–513.

104. Yates CM, Simpson J, Russell D, et al: Cholinergic enzymes in neurofibrillary degeneration produced by aluminum. *Brain Res* 1980; 197:269–274.

105. Hetnarski B, Wisniewski H, Iqbal K, et al: General cholinergic activity in aluminum-induced neurofibrillary degeneration. *Ann Neurol* 1980; 7:489–490.

106. Aiken JT, Bridges JE: Neuron size and neuron population density in the lumbosacral region of the cat's spinal cord. *J Anat* 1961; 95:38–53.

107. Purpura DP: Dendritic spine "dysgenesis" and mental retardation. *Science* 1974; 186:1126–1128.

108. Purpura DP: Normal and aberrant neuronal development in the cerebral cortex of human fetus and young infant, in Buckwald NA, Brazier MAB (eds): *Brain Mechanisms in Mental Retardations.* New York, Academic, 1975, pp 141–169.

109. Marin-Padilla M: Structural abnormalities of the cerebral cortex in human chromosomal aberrations: a Golgi study. *Brain Res* 1972; 44:625–629.

110. Marin-Padilla M: Structural organization of the cerebral cortex (motor area) in human chromosomal aberrations: a Golgi study. I. D_1 (13–15) Trisomy, Patau syndrome. *Brain Res* 1974; 66:375–391.

111. Marin-Padilla M: Pyramidal cell abnormalities in the motor cortex of a child with Down's syndrome: a Golgi study. *J Comp Neurol* 1976; 167:63–82.

112. Scheibel AB: Structural aspects of the aging brain: spine systems and the dendritic arbor. *Aging NY* 1978; 7:353–373.

113. Scheibel AB: The hippocampus: organizational patterns in health and senescence. *Mech Ageing Dev* 1979; 9:89–102.

114. Scheibel AB: Aging and senescence in selected motor systems of man, in Stein D (ed): *The Psychobiology of Aging: Problems and Perspectives.* New York, Elsevier North-Holland, 1980, pp 273–282.

115. Scheibel AB: The gerohistology of the aging human forebrain: some structural-functional considerations. *Aging NY* 1981; 17:31–41.

116. Scheibel ME, Scheibel AB: Structural changes in the aging brain. *Aging NY* 1975; 1:11–37.

117. Scheibel ME, Scheibel AB: Differential changes with aging in old and new cortices, in Nandy K, Sherwin I (eds): *The Aging Brain and Senile Dementia.* New York, Plenum, 1976, pp 39–58.

118. Scheibel ME, Lindsay RD, Tomiyasu U, et al: Progressive dendritic changes in the aging human cortex. *Exp Neurol* 1975; 47:392–403.

119. Scheibel ME, Lindsay RD, Tomiyasu U, et al: Progressive dendritic changes in the aging human limbic system. *Exp Neurol* 1976; 53:420–430.

120. Scheibel ME, Tomiyasu U, Scheibel AB: The aging human Betz cell. *Exp Neurol* 1977; 56:598–609.

121. Yamada M: Zahlemassige Verteilung der Dendritendorne am Apikalen Dendriten der Pyramidenzellen beim Morbus Alzheimer und seniler Demenz. *Bull Yamaguchi Med School* 1976; 23:229–235.

122. Mehraein P, Yamada M, Tarnowska E, et al: Quantitative study on dendrites and dendritic spines in Alzheimer's disease and senile dementia. *Adv Neurol* 1975; 12:453–458.

123. Buell SJ, Coleman PD: Dendritic growth in the aged human brain and failure of growth in senile dementia. *Science* 1979; 206:854–856.

124. Mervis R, Terry RD, Bowden D: Morphological correlates of aging in the monkey brain: a light and electron microscopic study. *Soc Neurosci* 1979; 5:8.

125. Uemura E: Age-related changes in prefrontal cortex of *Macaca mulatta:* synaptic density. *Exp Neurol* 1980; 69:164–172.

126. Cupp CJ, Uemura E: Age-related changes in prefrontal cortex of *Macacca mulatta:* quantitative analysis of dendritic branching patterns. *Exp Neurol* 1980; 69:143–163.

127. Mervis R: Structural alterations in neurons of aged canine neocortex: Golgi study. *Exp Neurol* 1978; 62:417–432.

128. Vaughan DW: Age-related deterioration of pyramidal cell basal dendrites in rat auditory cortex. *J Comp Neurol* 1977; 171:501–516.

129. Feldman ML: Aging changes in the morphology of cortical dendrites. *Aging NY* 1976; 3:211–227.

130. Feldman ML: Dendritic changes in aging rat brain: pyramidal cell dendrite length and ultrastructure, in Nandy K, Sherwin I (eds): *The Aging Brain and Senile Dementia.* New York, Plenum, 1977, pp 23–37.

131. Feldman MO, Dowd C: Loss of dendritic spines in aging cerebral cortex. *Anat Embryol* 1975; 148:279–301.

132. Geinisman Y, Bondareff W, Dodge JT: Dendritic atrophy in the dentate gyrus of the senescent rat. *Am J Anat* 1978; 152:311–330.

133. Machado-Salas JP, Scheibel AB: Limbic system of the aged mouse. *Exp Neurol* 1979; 63:347–355.

134. Machado-Salas J, Scheibel ME, Scheibel AB: Neuronal changes in the aging mouse: spinal cord and lower brain stem. *Exp Neurol* 1977; 54:504–512.

135. Machado-Salas J, Scheibel ME, Scheibel AB: Morphologic changes in the hypothalamus of the old mouse. *Exp Neurol* 1977: 57:102–111.

136. Mervis R, Cruce WLR, Rogers J, et al: Cerebellar senescence in the rat: Golgi studies of Purkinje cell alterations. *Neuroscience* 1982; 7(suppl):146.

137. Pysh JJ, Benson MD: Purkinje cell dendrites in aged rats: morphometric Golgi analysis. *Soc Neurosci* 1980; 6:281.

138. Artjukhina NI: An electron microscope study of aging changes of synapses of the cerebral cortex of rats. *Tsitologia* 1968; 10:1505–1513.

139. Bondareff W, Geinisman Y: Loss of synapses in the dentate gyrus of the senescent rat. *Am J Anat* 1976; 145:129–136.

140. Geinisman Y: Loss of axosomatic synapses in the dentate gyrus of aged rats. *Brain Res* 1979; 168:485–492.

141. Geinisman Y: Loss of axon terminals contacting neuronal somata in the dentate gyrus of aged rats. *Brain Res* 1981; 212:136–139.

142. Geinisman Y, Bondareff W, Dodge JT: Partial deafferentiation of neurons in the dentate gyrus of the senescent rat. *Brain Res* 1977; 134:541–545.

143. Hasan M, Glees P: Ultrastructural age changes in hippocampal neurons, synapses, and neuroglia. *Exp Gerontol* 1973; 8:75–83.

144. Glick R, Bondareff W: Loss of synapses in the cerebellar cortex of the senescent rat. *J Gerontol* 1979; 34:818–822.

145. Bertoni C, Guili C: A quantitative morphometric study on synapses of rat cerebellar glomeruli during aging. *Mech Ageing Dev* 1980; 12:127–136.

146. Cragg BG: The density of synapses and neurons in normal, mentally defective and aging human brains. *Brain* 1975; 98:81–90.

147. Huttenlocher PR: Synaptic density in human frontal cortex: development changes and effects of aging. *Brain Res* 1979; 163:195–205.

148. Johnson JE Jr, Miguel J: Fine structural changes in the lateral vestibular nucleus of aging rats. *Mech Ageing Dev* 1974; 3:203–224.

149. Sandbank U, Bubis JJ: The pathology of synapses. Available Brain Information Service/Brain Research Institute, University of California, Los Angeles, 1974.

150. Cotman CW, Scheff SW: Synaptic growth in aged animals. *Aging NY* 1979; 8:109–120.

151. Rees S: A quantitative electron microscopic study of the aging human cerebral cortex. *Acta Neuropathol* 1976; 36:347–362.

152. Sotelo C, Palay SL: Altered axon and axon terminals in the lateral vestibular nucleus of the rat: possible example of axonal remodeling. *Lab Invest* 1971; 25:653–671.

153. Terry RD, Gonatas NK, Weiss M: Ultrastructural studies in Alzheimer's presenile dementia. *Am J Pathol* 1964; 44:269–297.

154. Gonatas NK, Moss A: Pathologic axons and synapses in human neuropsychiatric disorders. *Hum Pathol* 1975; 6:571–582.

155. Gonatas NK, Gambetti P: The pathology of the synapse in Alzheimer's disease, in Wastenholme GEW, O'Connor M (eds): *Ciba Foundation Symposium on Alzheimer's Disease and Related Conditions.* Summit, NJ, Ciba, 1970, pp 169–183.

156. Gonatas NK, Goldensohn ES: Unusual neocortical presynaptic terminals in a patient with convul-

sions, mental retardation, and cortical blindness: an electron microscopic study. *J Neuropathol Exp Neurol* 1965; 26:179–199.

157. Gonatas NK, Terry RD, Weiss M: Electron microscopic study in two cases of Jakob–Creutzfeldt disease. *J Neuropathol Exp Neurol* 1965; 24:575–598.

158. Vaughan DW: Membranous bodies in the cerebral cortex of aging rats: an electron microscope study. *J Neuropathol Exp Neurol* 1976; 35:152–166.

159. Fujisawa K, Shiraki H: Study of axonal dystrophy: I. Pathology of the neuropil of the gracile and cureate nuclei in aging and old rats: a stereological study. *Neuropathol Appl Neurobiol* 1978; 4:1–20.

160. Fujisawa K, Shiraki H: Study of axonal dystrophy: II. Dystrophy and atrophy of the presynaptic boutons: a dual pathology. *Neuropathol Appl Neurobiol* 1980; 6:387–398.

161. Rees S: A quantitative electron microscopic study of atypical structures in normal human cerebral cortex. *Anat Embryol* 1975; 148:303–331.

162. Buell SJ, McNeill TH: New thoughts on old neurons. *Semin Neurol* 1981; 1:31–35.

163. Cotman CW, Nieto-Sampedro M: Brain function, synapse renewal, and plasticity. *Annu Rev Psychol* 1982; 33:371–401.

164. Buell SJ, Coleman PD: Individual differences in dendritic growth in human aging and senile dementia, in Stein D (ed): *The Psychobiology of Aging: Problems and Perspectives.* New York, Elsevier North-Holland, 1980; pp 283–296.

165. Buell SJ, Coleman PD: Quantitative evidence for selective dendritic growth in normal human aging but not in senile dementia. *Brain Res* 1981; 214:23–41.

166. Connor JR Jr, Diamond MC, Johnson RE: Occipital cortical morphology of the rat: alterations with age and environment. *Exp Neurol* 1980; 68:158–170.

167. Connor JR, Diamond MC, Connor JA, et al: A Golgi study of dendritic morphology in the occipital cortex of socially reared aged rats. *Exp Neurol* 1981; 73:525–533.

168. Diamond MC, Connor JR Jr: A search for the potential of the aging brain. *Aging NY* 1981; 17:43–58.

169. Hinds JW, McNelly NA: Aging of the rat olfactory bulb: growth and atrophy of constituent layers and changes in size and number of mitral cells. *J Comp Neurol* 1977; 171:345–367.

170. Mervis RF: Chronic dietary choline represses age-related loss of dendritic spines in mouse neocortical pyramidal cells. *J Neuropathol Exp Neurol* 1982; 41:363.

171. Connor JR Jr, Diamond MC, Johnson RE: Aging and environmental influences on two types of dendritic spines in the rat occipital cortex. *Exp Neurol* 1980; 70:371–379.

172. Scheibel AB, Tomiyasu U: Dendritic sprouting in Alzheimer's presenile dementia. *Exp Neurol* 1978; 60:1–8.

173. Mervis RF, Bartus RT: Modulation of pyramidal cell population in aging mouse neocortex: role of dietary choline. *J Neuropathol Exp Neurol* 1981; 40:313.

174. Bertoni-Freddari C, Mervis RF: Chronic dietary choline modulates synaptic plasticity in the cerebellum of aging mice. Submitted for publication, 1982.

175. Connor JR, Melone JH, Yuen AR, et al: Dendritic length in aged rat's occipital cortex: an environmentally induced response. *Exp Neurol* 1981; 73:827–830.

176. Cotman CW, Scheff SW: Synaptic growth in aged animals. *Aging NY* 1979; 8:109–120.

177. Brizzee KR, Ordy JM, Hofer H et al: Animal models for the study of senile brain disease and aging changes in the brain. *Aging NY* 1978; 7:515–553.

178. Williams RS, Ferrante RJ, Caviness VS: The Golgi rapid method in clinical neuropathology: the morphological consequences of suboptimal fixation. *J Neuropathol Exp Neurol* 1978; 37:13–33.

52 Neurochemical Lesion Models

Barbara Lerer
Eitan Friedman

THE MEMORY IMPAIRMENTS and reduced cognitive functioning characteristic of Alzheimer's disease (AD) have been correlated with deficits in central cholinergic neurotransmission (1). The most profound neurochemical deficits in AD involve choline acetyltransferase [CAT] (1–6) and acetylcholinesterase [ACh-E] (1, 3), the synthetic and catabolic enzymes for acetylcholine. Cholinergic dysfunction, which is pronounced in although not restricted to the hippocampus and frontoparietal areas of cortex, is correlated with the severity of cognitive impairment and also with the extent of neuritic plaques and neurofibrillary tangles (NFTs), the prominent morphological symptoms of AD (1).

Deficits in CAT, the presynaptic marker for central cholinergic neural pathways, have been reported as high as 90% in cortical tissue of patients with diagnosed AD as compared to tissue from age-matched controls. This presynaptic deficit is not accompanied by changes in the postsynaptic cholinergic receptors (4, 6, 7). It has been suggested that these CAT deficits are produced by loss of cholinergic afferents rather than by loss of intrinsic cortical cholinergic neurons (8, 9).

Several lines of converging evidence suggest that cholinergic activity may be involved in cognition and that memory impairment results from disruption of cholinergic neurotransmission (10, 11). First, in aged rodents, memory deficits in the retention of a single-trial passive avoidance task have been correlated with pre- and postsynaptic deficits in cholinergic functioning (12–14). In both young animals and normal adult humans, disrupting cholinergic activity produces memory retention deficits similar to those seen in aged subjects. For example, central cholinergic blockade with the muscarinic antagonists atropine and scopolamine produces memory deficits (15–21), as does inhibition of acetylcholine synthesis with pyrrolcholine and hemicholinium-3 (22, 23). Conversely, drugs that facilitate cholinergic transmission, such as physostigmine and arecoline, produce significant temporary improvements in memory and cognitive performance (24–27). The cholinomimetic drugs, when administered to young normal subjects, produced improved scores on verbal learning and cognitive tasks, and reversed the memory deficits induced by scopolamine (28–30). Finally, evidence suggests that acute and chronic administration of choline can alleviate deficits in passive avoidance learning in aged rats and mice (31, 32).

An afferent cholinergic pathway arises in the nucleus basalis of Meynert (nBM), a basal forebrain structure ventrolateral to the globus pallidus, and projects diffusely to frontal and parietal cortex (33–40). Data obtained through lesion studies with laboratory rats suggest that 70% of the cholinergic innervation of frontoparietal cortex may come from this nBM-cortex pathway, while the remaining 30% is derived from cholinergic neurons intrinsic to the cortex (41, 42). With the discovery that damage to nBM cell bodies reduces cortical CAT in rat brain, researchers have begun to look at the nBM of AD patients and to obtain data linking nBM damage to AD. A recent study of middle-aged and aged rhesus monkeys demonstrated that cortical neuritic plaques consist, in part, of presynaptic cholinergic axons. The data, obtained with ACh-E staining techniques, further indicate that many of these axons had origins within the nBM (43). Moreover, a recent series of studies has shown sharp morphological degeneration and neuronal loss in the nBM of an AD patient (44, 45). These studies report losses as high as 90% in the large neurons of AD nBM as compared to age-matched control tissue. The remaining nBM cells suffered granulovacuolar degeneration (GVD) and NFTs, the basic histopathological hallmarks of AD.

The neurochemical correlates of AD and its related memory deficits have not as yet been fully and systematically investigated. With this in mind, developing an animal model to facilitate an understanding of the etiology of AD through direct and chronic intervention into the central cholinergic system was pursued by Lerer and Friedman. Specifically, Lerer and Friedman examined the neurochemical and behavioral consequences of the destruction of the nBM-cortical cholinergic pathway.

To be useful in this respect, an animal model must fulfill two criteria: there must be a specific and significant deficit in cortical CAT, and there must be a concomitant memory impairment attributable to the CAT deficit.

Aged rodents show behavioral and memory impairments that parallel cognitive decline in human elderly (12, 13, 46–49) along with age-related pre- and postsynaptic impairments in cholinergic transmission (8, 50); for example, acetylcholine synthesis and choline uptake are decreased (14, 51). The most striking neurochemical aspect of AD, however, the profound reduction in cortical CAT, has not yet been observed in aged rodents; normal, aged rodents cannot therefore be said to have fulfilled the criteria as a good model for AD.

The nBM in the rat is a diffusely distributed group of large neurons with cell bodies located ventral to the globus pallidus. Destruction of cell bodies in the ventrolateral globus pallidus produces a specific and substantial CAT depletion in the frontoparietal cortex (41, 42). We have induced a cortical cholinergic deficit in young, male Sprague-Dawley rats via lesion of the nBM-cortex pathway in order to reproduce in the rat the cholinergic deficit of AD. Lesioned animals were tested for behavioral and cognitive impairments to examine the relationship between presynaptic cholinergic dysfunction and cognitive function. Research by Lerer and Friedman shows that destruction of the nBM-cortex pathway, with its resulting depletion of cortical CAT, produces behavioral deficits in the rat suggestive of memory impairment.

Bilateral microinjections of the neurotoxin kainic acid were placed stereotactically in the area of the nucleus basalis of Meynert in young, male Sprague-Dawley rats. The lesion coordinates were 0.7 mm posterior to the bregma landmark, 2.7 mm either side of the mid-sagittal suture, and 7.0 mm below the dura, with the skull in a horizontal position. Kainic acid (1.0 $\mu g/\mu l$, pH 7.2), which preferentially destroys cell bodies, was used to lesion nBM neurons. The resulting lesions reduced CAT levels in the frontoparietal cortex by 30–70% in the lesioned group, as compared to a sham-operated control group. In striatum and hippocampus, CAT levels remained unaffected.

For several days following surgery, lesioned rats were aphasic and adipsic, displaying motor and reflex abnormalities. During this recovery period, animals were maintained via intubation of liquid infant formula. Behavioral testing was conducted 10–14 days postoperatively, after normal ingestion, grooming, and locomotion had resumed.

The feeding deficits produced by the nBM lesions pose certain problems for designing a test battery to assess cognition and memory. The typical cognitive tasks used with animals involve appetitively motivated behavior, yet one could not assume that the lesioned rats would be motivated to earn a food reward; performance deficits on such tasks could reflect poor motivation rather than a memory deficit. Consequently, we chose an inhibitory learning task (passive avoidance) to measure learning (acquisition) and memory (retention) deficits. While severe cholinergic deficits had previously resulted in a high mortality rate, we discovered that CAT deficits of 15–25% were sufficient to produce reliable and replicable deficits in 24-hour retention of a step-through passive avoidance task.

Subjects were individually placed in the lighted front compartment of a two-compartment shuttle box. The latency to enter the second dark compartment was under 15 seconds for both lesioned and control subjects. After a 5-second stay in the dark compartment, a 1.5-mA scrambled shock was applied to the floor grids until the subject escaped to the lighted front compartment. After 60 seconds in this "safe" zone, subjects were returned to their home cages. If a rat returned to the dark compartment, it was given a second escapable foot shock and the 60-second timer was restarted. Lesioned and control subjects did not show any difference in the number of shocks to criterion. The maximum number of shocks given to any rat was 3; the mean number of shocks received was 1.84 for the lesioned group, and 1.5 for the control group. Twenty-four hours later, a subject was replaced in the lighted front compartment and the latency to enter the dark compartment was measured. The retention test was terminated after the subject entered the dark compartment or after 600 seconds. The latency to enter the dark chamber presumably reflected retention of the memory of the prior training trial; the rat was never shocked during the retention test. Control subjects did not generally reenter the dark side within 600 seconds; rats with nBM lesions had short reentry latencies, which suggests impaired memory for the shock of the previous day. The initial latency to enter the dark compartment was $8.44 + 2.96$ seconds for the lesioned group and $9.02 + 4.77$ seconds for the control group (Student's t-test, degrees of freedom = 10, $P > .10$, nonsignificant). The retention test latencies were $176.06 + 88.23$ seconds for the lesioned group and $503.89 + 96.10$ seconds for the control group ($P < .05$). During retention testing, five of six lesioned subjects entered the dark compartment in under 200 seconds, whereas five of six control subjects avoided the dark compartment for over 600 seconds. Motor activity rates and shock sensitivity were not significantly different in lesioned animals as compared to controls, and therefore do not account for the impaired performance.

In another experiment, Lerer and Friedman examined spontaneous alternation behavior. In the spontaneous alternation task, a rat placed in a two-armed Y maze, when allowed to freely choose between the arms (without receiving reward in either), will alternate in its choices, first choosing one arm and then the other on the next trial. Alternation occurs even though no food reward is involved and even when a delay as long as an hour is interposed between the first and second trial (52). The phenomenon is intriguing because it is not clear why the animals do not choose at random as there is no obvious reward influencing their choices. It has been suggested that the alternation results from "boredom" or satiation with the side just chosen and a curiosity which produces an active approach to the novel side (53). From an evolutionary standpoint, animals must explore their environments if they are to gain maximum information about available resources; if behavior is solely based on past experience with reward, animals will never learn about other potential resources in the area (54).

Because spontaneous alternation is not influenced by appetitive motivation, it is a good task to use with our experimental paradigm. Also, aged mice show decreased habituation of the exploratory drive (55–57) and preliminary evidence suggests that aged mice perseverate in their arm choices in a spontaneous alternation task in a T maze (M. Brennan, personal communication, 1982). Aged rats are slower to learn a complex maze than are mature young rats, and their failure to learn seems due to perseverative nonrandom sequences of errors (47, 48).

Experimentally naive, unoperated rats were individually placed in the lighted "start" alley of an unbaited Y maze with dark left and right side-arms. After 15 seconds in the start box, a guillotine door was raised and subjects were free to explore the maze. When a subject entered an arm, a door closed, preventing exit from the arm. The subject was then replaced in the start box for 15 seconds, the door was raised, and the subject was given the opportunity to make a second choice. Subjects were tested daily for 2 weeks, and the data showed that the rats alternated in arm choices on about 70% of the trials. After surgery and a recovery period, subjects were retested daily for an additional 2-week period. Subjects with sham operations showed the pre-operative alternation pattern. Lesioned subjects, however, alternated on only 25% of trials, and on the remainder of the trials they perseverated in their choice of the same arm on both the initial and reentry choice. The data were analyzed with a chi-square test, and the differences between the groups found significant at the $P < .005$ level.

Spontaneous alternation is not a learned behavior; however, the alternation from trial to trial reflects an underlying memory process which allows the animal to remember what it did before, so it can try something new. The perseveration of the lesioned rats suggests a deficit in this memory process analogous to the perseveration in the elderly who, for example, repeatedly tell their grandchildren the same story or keep checking the stove to make sure they turned off the gas.

It may be argued that if the lesioned animals were really unable to remember which arm they had previously chosen, then their postoperative rate of alternation should have been at the 50% chance level. A 25% rate of alternation (or 75% rate of perseveration) suggests a nonrandom sequence of responding, and the existence of some memory capacity. Similarly, while a senile person may not remember having shut off the gas burner, it is apparent that he or she does remember it was previously lit. The deficit may be interpreted either as a difficulty in adequate memory retrieval or as an inability to generate a new behavior pattern; more experimentation is necessary for an adequate understanding of the perseveration phenomenon.

Many animal and human studies point to the role of the cholinergic system in learning and memory. Indeed, the memory impairments and reduced cognitive functioning characteristic of AD have been correlated with reduced cortical CAT in postmortem human tissue. Data show that when this neurochemical aspect of AD is induced in young rats, behavioral impairments suggesting memory dysfunction result. This paradigm should prove useful as an animal model for studying the pathophysiology of AD, and to develop new treatment strategies for Alzheimer's disease.

REFERENCES

1. Perry EK, Tomlinson BE, Blessed G, et al: Correlation of cholinergic abnormalities with senile plaques and mental test scores in senile dementia. *Br Med J* 1978; 52:1457–1459.

2. Bowen DM, Smith CB, White P, et al: Neurotransmitter-related enzymes and indices of hypoxia in senile dementia and other abiotrophies. *Brain* 1976; 99:459–496.

3. Davies P, Maloney AJF: Selective loss of central cholinergic neurons in Alzheimer's disease. *Lancet* 1976; ii:1403.

4. Davies P, Verth AH: Regional distributions of muscarinic acetylcholine receptor in normal and Alzheimer's type dementia brains. *Brain Res* 1977; 158:385–392.

5. Spillane JA, White P, Goodhardt MJ, et al: Selective vulnerability of neurons in organic dementia. *Nature* 1977; 266:558–559.

6. White P, Goodhardt MT, Keet JP, et al: Neocortical neurons in elderly people. *Lancet* 1977; i:668–674.

7. Reisine T, Yamamura HI, Bird ED, et al: Pre- and post-synaptic neurochemical alteration in Alzheimer's disease. *Brain Res* 1978; 159:477–481.

8. Perry EK: The cholinergic system in old age and Alzheimer's disease. *Age Ageing* 1980; 9:1–8.

9. Rossor M, Fahrenkrug J, Emson P, et al: Reduced cortical choline acetyltransferase activity in senile dementia of Alzheimer type is not accompanied by changes in vasoactive intestinal polypeptide. *Brain Res* 1980; 201:209–253.

10. Deutsch JA: The cholinergic synapse in the site of memory. *Science* 1971; 174:788–794.

11. Glick SD, Mittag TW, Green JP: Central cholinergic correlates of impaired learning. *Neuropharmacol* 1973; 12:291–296.

12. Bartus RT, Dean RL, Beer B, et al: The cholinergic hypothesis of geriatric memory dysfunction. *Science* 1982; 217:408–417.

13. Lippa AS, Pelham RW, Beer B, et al: Brain cholinergic dysfunction and memory in aged rats. *Neurobiol Aging* 1980; 1:13–19.

14. Sherman KA, Kuster JE, Dean RL, et al: Presynaptic cholinergic mechanisms in brain of aged rats with memory impairments. *Neurobiol Aging* 1981; 2:99–104.

15. Bartus RT, Johnson HR: Short-term memory in the rhesus monkey: disruption from the anticholinergic scopolamine. *Pharmacol Biochem Behav* 1976; 5:39–40.

16. Bohdanechy Z, Jarvik ME: Impairment of one trial passive avoidance learning in mice by scopolamine, methylbromide, and physostigmine. *Int J Neuropharmacol* 1967; 6:217–222.

17. Buresova O, Bures J, Bohdanecky Z, et al: Effect of atropine on learning, extinction, retention and retrieval in rats. *Psychopharmacol* 1964; 5:255–263.

18. Carlton PL, Markiewicz B: Behavioral effects of atropine and scopolamine, in Furchtgott E (ed): *Pharmacological and biophysical Agents and Behavior*. New York, Academic, 1973, pp 345–373.

19. Crow T, Grove-White I: An analysis of the learning deficit following hyoscine administration to man. *Br J Pharmacol* 1973; 49:322–327.

20. Meyers B: Some effects of scopolamine on passive avoidance response in rats. *Psychopharmacol* 1965; 8:111–119.

21. Ostfeld AM, Araguete A: Central nervous system effects of hyoscine in man. *J Pharmacol Exp Ther* 1962; 137:133–139.

22. Caulfield MP, Fortune DH, Roberts PM, et al: Intracerebroventricular hemicholinium-3 (HC-3) impairs learning of a passive avoidance task in mice. *Br J Pharmacol* 1981; 74:865.

23. Glick SD, Crane AM, Barker LA, et al: Effects of N-hydroxyethylpyrrolidinium methiodide, a choline analogue, on passive avoidance behavior in mice. *Neuropharmacology* 1975; 14:561–564.

24. Bartus RT: Evidence for a direct cholinergic involvement in scopolamine-induced amnesia in monkeys: effects of concurrent administration of physostigmine and methylphenidate with scopolamine. *Pharmacol Biochem Behav* 1978; 9:833–836.

25. Bartus RT: Physostigmine and recent memory: effects in young and aged non-human primates. *Science* 1979; 206:1087–1089.

26. Sitaram N, Weingartner H, Gillin JC: Choline chloride and arecoline: effects on memory and sleep in man, in Barbeau A, Growdon JH, Wurtman RJ (eds): *Nutrition and the Brain.* New York, Raven, 1979, pp 367–375.

27. Whitehouse JM: The effects of physostigmine on discrimination learning. *Psychopharmacology* 1966; 9:183–188.

28. Drachman DA: Memory and cognitive function in man: does the cholinergic system have a specific role? *Neurology* 1977; 27:783–790.

29. Drachman DA, Leavitt J: Human memory and the cholinergic system: a relationship to aging? *Arch Neurol* 1974; 30:113–121.

30. Hington JN, Aprison MH: Behavioral and environmental aspects of the cholinergic system, in Goldberg AM, Hanin I (eds): *Biology of Cholinergic Function.* New York, Raven, 1976, pp 515–566.

31. Bartus RT, Dean RL, Goas JA, et al: Age-related changes in passive avoidance retention and modulation with chronic dietary choline. *Science* 1980; 209:301–303.

32. Bartus RT, Dean RL, Sherman KA, et al: Profound effects of combining choline and piracetam on memory enhancement and cholinergic function in aged rats. *Neurobiol Aging* 1981; 2:105–111.

33. Shute CCD, Lewis PR: The ascending cholinergic reticular system: neocortical, olfactory and subcortical projections. *Brain* 1967; 90:497–520.

34. Lewis PR, Shute CCD: The cholinergic limbic system: projections to hippocampal formation, medial cortex, nuclei of the ascending cholinergic reticular system, and the subfornical organ and supraoptic crest. *Brain* 1967; 90:521–540.

35. Kievit J, Kuypers HGJ: Basal forebrain and hypothalamic connections to the frontal and parietal cortex in the rhesus monkey. *Science* 1978; 187:660–662.

36. Gorry JD: Studies on the comparative anatomy of the ganglion basale of Meynert. *Acta Anat* 1963; 55:51–104.

37. Parent A, Gravel S, Olivier A: The extrapyramidal and limbic systems' relationship at the globus pallidus level: a comparative histochemical study in the rat, cat and monkey. *Adv Neurol* 1979; 24:1–11.

38. Divac I: Magnocellular nuclei of the basal forebrain project to neocortex, brainstem and olfactory bulb: review of some functional correlates. *Brain Res* 1975; 93:385–398.

39. Divac I, Kosmal A, Bjorklund A, et al: Subcortical projections to the prefrontal cortex in the rat as revealed by the horseradish peroxidase technique. *Neuroscience* 1978; 3:785–796.

40. Jones EB, Burton H, Saper CB, et al: Midbrain, diencephalic and cortical relationships of the basal nucleus of Meynert and associated structures in primates. *J Comp Neurol* 1976; 167:385–420.

41. Johnston MV, McKinney M, Coyle JT: Evidence for a cholinergic projection to neocortex from neurons in basal forebrain. *Proc Natl Acad Sci* 1979; 76:5392–5396.

42. Johnston MV, McKinney M, Coyle JT: Neocortical cholinergic innervation: a description of extrinsic and intrinsic components in the rat. *Exp Brain Res* 1981; 43:159–172.

43. Struble RG, Cork LC, Whitehouse PJ, et al: Cholinergic innervation in neuritic plaques. *Science* 1982; 216:413–414.

44. Whitehouse PJ, Price DL, Clark AW, et al: Alzheimer's disease and senile dementia: loss of neurons in the basal forebrain. *Science* 1982; 215:1237–1239.

45. Whitehouse PJ, Price DL, Clark AW, et al: Alzheimer disease: evidence for selective loss of cholinergic neurons in the nucleus basalis. *Ann Neurol* 1981; 10:122–126.

46. Barnes CA: Memory deficits associated with senescence: a neurophysiological and behavioral study in the rat. *J Comp Physiol Psychol* 1979; 93:74–104.

47. Goodrick CL: Learning, retention and extinction of a complex maze habit for mature-young and senescent Wistar albino rats. *J Gerontol* 1968; 23:298–304.

48. Goodrick CL: Learning by mature-young and aged Wistar albino rats as a function of test complexity. *J Gerontol* 1972; 27:353–357.

49. Wallace JE, Krauter EE, Campbell BA: Animal models of declining memory in the aged: short-term and spatial memory in aged rat. *J Gerontol* 1980; 35:355–363.

50. McGeer EG, McGeer PL: Neurotransmitter metabolism in the aging brain. *Aging NY* 1976; 3:389–403.

51. Gibson GE, Peterson C, Jenden DJ: Brain acetylcholine synthesis declines with senescence. *Science* 1981; 213:674–676.

52. Still AW: Memory and spontaneous alternation in the rat. *Nature* 1966; 210:401–402.

53. Dember WN, Fowler H: Spontaneous alternation behavior. *Psychol Bull* 1958; 55:412–428.

54. Staddon JER, Simmelhag VL: The superstition experiment: a reexamination of its implications for the principles of adaptive behavior. *Psychol Rev* 1971; 78:3–43.

55. Brennan MJ, Dallob A, Friedman E: Involvement of hippocampal serotonergic activity in age-related changes in exploratory behavior. *Neurobiol Aging* 1981; 2:199–203.

56. Brennan MJ, Quartermain D: Differential effects of aging on exploratory behavior. Read before the 51st Annual Meeting of the Eastern Psychological Association, Hartford, April 1980.

57. Brennan, MJ, Quartermain D, Aleman D: Stimulus complexity and exploratory behavior: age-related impairments of within-session habituation. Read before the Annual Meeting of the Gerontological Society, San Diego, Nov 1980.

53 Drug Evaluations in Aged Nonhuman Primates

RAYMOND T. BARTUS

REGINALD L. DEAN, III

BERNARD BEER

AMONG THE MANY BEHAVIORAL impairments that develop with old age (i.e., disturbances in cognition, affect, psychomotor function, sleep, and sexual function), loss of cognitive functions is generally recognized as the most debilitating (1). It has been particularly difficult, however, to accurately quantify the specific behavioral mechanisms impaired in the aged human subject, in part because of intertask differences, motivational factors, and other methodological problems which often plague gerontological research. Defining the etiology has also been difficult because of technical and moral restrictions which limit the type of neurological, biochemical, and pharmacological tests that may be conducted in humans.

Over the last several years, a nonhuman primate, behavioral test procedure which seems sensitive to many of the cognitive changes observed in aged humans has been developed (2). Early tests with this procedure, comparing performance between young and aged monkeys, revealed that one of the most severe and consistently observed deficits was decreased memory for recent (but not immediate) stimulus events. That is, a selective impairment was seen when information had to be remembered temporarily for a duration of several seconds to a few minutes, with no impairment under conditions allowing immediate recall. This age-related deficit in recent memory has been observed both in New World and Old World monkeys (3–5), as well as in mice and rats of different strains (for a review, see ref. 6).

Other behavioral studies demonstrated that (1) some degree of specificity for age-related behavioral deficits exist, since not all behaviors measured were impaired, nor to the same degree; and (2) reasonable similarity exists between the most serious age-related deficits in both human and nonhuman primates. On this basis it was suggested that the nonhuman primate may provide a valid and reliable means of assessing drugs ultimately intended to treat geriatric cognitive deficits.

Use of this primate model to study aging processes offers several important benefits. The usual advantages of using animal subjects in behavioral research (such as providing more specific test procedures and greater control and regimentation of the test and nontest environment) become particularly apparent when dealing with aged subjects who may confound accurate test measurements because of increased variability, decreased motivation, and so on. Another advantage of this model is that certain nonbiological changes (difficulties

428

in adjusting to the test environment; failure to completely understand test directions or procedures; various social or cultural influences) which might normally confound an accurate estimate of cognitive capacities in aged humans, are eliminated or greatly minimized by use of nonhuman primates who have been fully adapted to the laboratory and the routine of daily testing.

The use of this nonhuman primate model of aging has an additional advantage in that the behavioral repertoire of the nonhuman primate is sufficiently sophisticated to allow the study and measurement of many behaviors which are interesting and relevant to human aging (attention, reaction time, learning and memory, and so on). Thus, comparisons to human behavioral functions should be more meaningful and perhaps less hazardous than when alternative classes of animals are used.

Finally, recent evidence comparing brains from aged monkeys and humans has revealed certain similarities in age-related alterations in morphology, neurophysiology, and neurochemistry. The similarities suggest that the neurological and neurochemical changes observed may play common roles in similar behavioral deficits observed in aged humans and nonhuman primates. Thus, the possibility of obtaining valid and predictive information regarding the effects of drugs to reduce age-related memory loss by using nonhuman primates seemed well founded.

Systematic evaluations of several classes of drugs have been performed with this method. Some of these drugs, such as CNS stimulants, catecholaminergic enhancers, and anticoagulants, have failed to yield any encouraging data (7) and are not reviewed here. Other approaches have, however, produced interesting results, suggesting that some beneficial effects can be achieved. These classes include cholinomimetics, neuropeptides, and nootropics; the results obtained with these classes of drugs in this animal model constitute the remainder of this paper.

ENHANCEMENT OF CHOLINERGIC ACTIVITY

The idea that central cholinergic mechanisms are intimately involved with general learning and memory phenomena was first popularized by Deutsch (8). Drachman and Leavitt (9) later proposed that an age-related dysfunction in the cholinergic system might be responsible for the specific memory loss observed in elderly and senile dementia patients. In the last several years abundant pharmacological, neurochemical, and electrophysiological evidence has accumulated to support a plausible cholinergic involvement in age-related memory disorders (for a recent comprehensive review see ref. 10).

Three separate avenues have been used to enhance cholinergic activity in the elderly. The earliest attempt used was physostigmine, a drug that inhibits acetylcholinesterase activity. Inhibition of this enzyme results in a slower breakdown of acetylcholine in the synapse, thus allowing acetylcholine to remain active for longer periods of time, presumably increasing the degree of stimulation of cholinergic receptors.

Among aged subjects, relatively little improvement was observed with physostigmine, but only a single dose had been tested (11). More recently, the effect of physostigmine on recent memory in young (5–7 years) and memory-impaired, aged Rhesus monkeys (+ 18 years) was systematically evaluated over several doses on all subjects (12). The performance of the young monkeys treated with physostigmine was similar to that reported for young humans: no effect at low doses, some improvement at a restricted range of doses, and deficits at the highest dose. Although the aged monkeys also improved at the same general doses, their overall response as a group was much more variable than that of the younger subjects. That is, the performance of some aged monkeys was impaired at low doses which failed to affect young monkeys, and continued improvement was observed in a few aged monkeys at the highest dose, dosages which typically impaired young monkeys. Since this study, similar effects have been achieved in elderly humans (13, 14).

Another means of enhancing cholinergic activity may be through dietary manipulation of precursors to the cholinergic system. Numerous studies have demonstrated that dietary or systemic manipulation of choline, the precursor for synthesis of acetylcholine, or lecithin, the normal dietary source of choline, increases central cholinergic activity (for a review, see ref. 15). These studies suggest that geriatric cognition might therefore be improved by providing abundant amounts of choline or lecithin. Unfortunately, attempts to treat cognitively impaired elderly with cholinergic precursors have failed to demonstrate reliable or therapeutically relevant effects (10).

Consistent with these failures in elderly and demented humans, recent tests with the nonhuman primate model revealed that acute choline administration exerted no measurable effects on performance at any dose when tested (4). On the basis of several long-term clinical trials (for a review, see ref. 10) and the present monkey data involving a wide range of ineffective doses, it seems doubtful that any dose of choline could be expected to produce consistent effects in aged subjects on cognitive tests.

A third possible means of increasing cholinergic activity is through direct stimulation of the cholinergic receptors by muscarinic agonists (thereby mimicking acetylcholine at the receptor sites). One such potent muscarinic agonist is arecoline. When tested in the aged monkey model, arecoline produced significant improvement over baseline performance (4). Moreover, when compared directly to physostigmine, its effects were more impressive, in that consistent improvement across subjects and doses were observed. These results with aged monkeys have recently been independently corroborated in Alzheimer patients (13).

In summary, the results of cholinergic studies with aged nonhuman primates are generally similar to the limited data available from the geriatric clinic. That is, similar intrasubject variability in response to physostigmine and replicability using the best-dose paradigm have been observed in both aged humans and monkeys. Furthermore, choline has generally failed to improve geriatric memory in humans, and failed to enhance performance in the aged monkeys. Finally, the consistent improvement across subjects and doses with arecoline observed in aged monkeys has also been reported in Alzheimer patients. It is plausible that when longer-lasting cholinergics, with greater central to peripheral nervous system selectivity, are developed, greater therapeutic effects may be expected.

NEUROPEPTIDES

A wealth of evidence exists which implicates neuropeptides of mainly hypothalamic and pituitary origins in roles that influence behavior, independent of their neuroendocrine effects (for a review, see ref. 16). These extraendocrine effects appear to occur directly by influencing the central nervous system, and are long-lasting despite the short half-lives of neuropeptides (17).

Recently, measures of several neuropeptides have revealed reliable decreases in brain levels of aged and demented subjects (18–20). Of course, the implication is that factors normally controlled by these neuropeptides might therefore be impaired in aged subjects. In an effort to help establish the role that neuropeptides may play in modulating behavior, a number of studies have injected neuropeptides into the brains or bodies of animals and measured changes in behavior. From these studies it has been concluded that many neuropeptides, particularly vasopressin and $ACTH_{4-10}$, affect measures of attention, anxiety, and learning and memory in several mammalian species (for a thorough review see ref. 16). Interestingly, many of these same behaviors have been reported to be significantly altered in aged subjects and humans (1).

With regard to the age-related cognitive impairments in particular, the pioneering work of DeWeid first implicated vasopressin and $ACTH_{4-10}$ as playing important roles in modulating certain forms of learning and memory (21). Despite these findings, much controversy still exists over whether these behavioral effects represent improved learning or memory *per se,* or whether they have any relevance to cognitive problems that concern geriatric clinicians (22).

In the clinic, early case reports of improvement in posttrauma (23), as well as in Korsakoff's amnesia (24), created excitement, followed by additional success in controlled studies using cognitively elderly and demented patients (for a review, see ref. 25). However, clear improvement has not been universally achieved and some investigators conclude that little or no useful role for neuropeptides exists for the treatment of memory problems in the aged (25–27). Thus, the role that neuropeptides play in clinical problems involving learning and memory remains intriguing, but controversial.

In an effort to provide additional information regarding the role of neuropeptides in memory performance, as well as their potential usefulness in treating cognitive problems of the elderly, we evaluated and compared the effects of several neuropeptides (28).

Several doses of $ACTH_{4-10}$, lysine vasopressin, arginine vasopressin, oxytocin, and somatostatin were each tested in several aged monkeys. All of these neuropeptides apparently have multiple pharmacological effects and have recently been identified in the brains of mammals (29). $ACTH_{4-10}$, the behaviorally active amino acid sequence of the anterior pituitary adrenocorticotrophic hormone ($ACTH_{1-39}$), is devoid of endocrine effects and has been claimed to influence learning and memory. Vasopressin, traditionally known as the antidiuretic hormone, has two forms. One form, lysine vasopressin, is apparently unique to porcines but is the form used in several of the earlier clinical trials involving memory. The other form, arginine vasopressin, is common to most mammals, including human and nonhuman primates. Oxytocin, which like vasopressin is secreted from the posterior pituitary, has also been reported to impair memory in young rats and humans (30, 31). Finally, somatostatin is a hypothalamic hormone that inhibits the release of growth hormone. Recently, somatostatin has been reported as decreased in the brains of Alzheimer's patients (18, 19, 32) and aged rodents (33).

None of the neuropeptides produced sufficiently consistent effects across subjects to be reflected by changes in group means. Evaluations of each individual subject against his or her own baseline performance levels revealed that five neuropeptides produced some minimal improvement, but only three of the five did so with any consistency (both forms of vasopressin and $ACTH_{4-10}$) (12). In no case were clear, dose-response functions obtained, even within individual subjects (28).

Arginine vasopressin appeared to produce the best overall effects, with three of the five monkeys exhibiting significant improvement in performance. The same three monkeys who responded to arginine vasopressin also responded to the lysine form. Once again, the two monkeys who failed to improve with the arginine form of vasopressin also showed no improvement with the lysine form. Although not directly compared, the effects of the arginine form appeared to be somewhat more consistent and robust than those obtained under the lysine form. It may be relevant to these results that the arginine form, but not the lysine form of vasopressin, occurs naturally in human and nonhuman primates. Three of six aged monkeys also performed better under $ACTH_{4-10}$ compared to baseline. However, in two of these cases only a single dose was effective, while the third improved significantly on five of six tests (two tests for each of three doses). Very little improvement in performance was observed under any dose of somatostatin or oxytocin.

These data demonstrate that reliable changes in performance on a memory task with aged primates can be achieved, suggesting that certain neuropeptides may indeed play some role in the expression or mediation of memory for recent events. Additionally, the improvements observed in this study involve naturally impaired behavior by age and one which has many operational similarities and some empirical relevance to measures of recent memory in humans (34). At the same time, however, even the best effects obtained must be considered qualitatively subtle. In no case were consistent group effects obtained with any single dose of any neuropeptide tested. A question of certain importance, therefore, concerns what significance these data from aged monkeys may have. To the extent to which this animal model accurately predicts clinical reality, these limitations on overall improvement seriously question the therapeutic utility of the currently researched neuropeptides for treatment of age-related cognitive dysfunctions. A more optimistic viewpoint, however, might be that continued research and development of neuropeptides will ultimately lead to analogue structures that produce much more consistent or more robust effects.

NOOTROPICS

Nootropic compounds, a relatively new class of drugs which purportedly exert no sedative or stimulant effects, have been claimed to improve learning and memory in a number of behavioral paradigms. Four nootropiclike drugs which currently claim controversial efficacy for improving geriatric cognition are piracetam, vincamine, dihydroergotoxine, and centrophenoxine. While their chemical structures are quite different and their specific mechanism(s) of action still unknown, they share some common features, especially preservation of normal behavior and physiology under metabolically stressed states (i.e., hypoxia) (for reviews, see refs. 35–37).

Because the very efficacy of these drugs is still open to question, Bartus and associates evaluated representative nootropic drugs. Piracetam, vincamine, and dihydroergotoxine were administered to aged rhesus monkeys (+ 18 years) chronically in a counterbalanced manner for a minimum of nine consecutive days (p.o., BID) (37). A 1-week minimum washout period occurred between drugs. The results demonstrated that all three drugs produced some improvement in performance in the aged monkeys. Not all monkeys demonstrated the same qualitative response: some exhibited clear improvement, others showed no change, and a few isolated cases showed mild impairments in comparison to the nondrug control scores. These effects accord with the general findings of many clinical trials and help explain why some patients respond favorably to some of these agents, while others do not. One possibility is that the memory loss seen in aging is the result of a complex, multifaceted etiology and thus only a subpopulation of geriatric patients will respond to this type of treatment. Further characterization of this subpopulation to determine possible differences in the behavioral and neurochemical deficits should provide invaluable information to increase our understanding of this problem and develop effective therapy.

DISCUSSION

These studies suggest that it is indeed possible to develop procedures with animals to obtain valid information about drugs for treatment of geriatric-human-memory problems. Not only were certain classes of drugs found to induce modest but reliable improvement in memory in aged monkeys, but the similarity of the results obtained with this series of studies is strikingly similar to the consensus developed from recent clinical studies in humans. The similarity of these effects in aged monkeys and humans suggest that valid animal models may be used to facilitate the search for other, more therapeutically useful drugs.

One important advantage of using aged nonhuman primates, particularly in this test situation, is that the individual subject's response to a number of different drugs can be directly compared and individual differences objectively measured and accounted for. A consistent finding emerging from many of the studies in aged monkeys is that certain subpopulations of subjects exist which may respond favorably to several potentially useful therapeutic approaches. The current state of the art, however, is such that only subtle improvement can be expected with existing drugs and only in (as yet undefined) subpopulations of subjects. Whether the small improvement observed in certain aged monkeys is indicative of a pharmacological effect that can be related to meaningful clinical improvement in elderly or demented humans remains to be seen. However, because variations in individual responses to drugs can eventually be correlated with several neurochemical parameters as well as to the degree of memory impairment, information can be obtained to aid the search for more effective drugs. By systematically incorporating the information obtained from animal models into the search for new drugs and the design of clinical protocols in humans, the goal of achieving truly successful treatments would seem to be easier to achieve.

REFERENCES

1. Weinberg J: Geriatric psychiatry, in Kaplan HI, Freedman AM, Sadock BJ (eds): *Comprehensive Textbook of Psychiatry.* Baltimore, Williams & Wilkins, 1980, vol 3, pp 3024–3042.
2. Bartus RT: Effects of aging on visual memory, sensory processing and discrimination learning in the non-human primate. *Aging NY* 1979; 10:85–114.
3. Bartus RT, Fleming D, Johnson HR: Aging in the rhesus monkey: effects on short-term memory. *J Gerontol* 1978; 33:858–871.
4. Bartus RT, Dean RL, Beer B: Memory deficits in aged cebus monkeys and facilitation with central cholinomimetics. *Neurobiol Aging* 1980; 1:145–152.
5. Medin DL, O'Neil P, Smeltz E, et al; Age differences in retention of concurrent discrimination problems in monkeys. *J Gerontol* 1973; 28:63–67.
6. Dean RL, Scozzafava J, Goas JA, et al: Age-related differences in behavior across the life span of the C57B1/6j mouse. *Exp Aging Res* 1981; 7:427–451.
7. Dean RL, Loullis C, Bartus RT: Drug effects in an animal model of memory deficits in the aged: implications for future clinical trials, in Walker R, Cooper R (eds): *Experimental and Clinical Interventions in Aging.* New York, Dekker, 1983, 279–303.
8. Deutsch JA: The cholinergic synapse and the site of memory. *Science* 1971; 175:788–794.
9. Drachman D, Leavitt J: Human memory and the cholinergic system. *Arch Neurol* 1974; 30:113–121.

10. Bartus RT, Dean RL, Beer B, et al: The cholinergic hypothesis of geriatric memory dysfunction: a critical review. *Science* 1982; 217:408–417.

11. Drachman D: Central cholinergic system and memory, in Lipton M, DiMascio A, Killam K (eds): *Psychopharmacology: A Generation of Progress.* New York, Raven, 1978, pp 651–662.

12. Bartus RT: Physostigmine and recent memory: effects in young and aged non-human primates. *Science* 1979; 206:1087–1089.

13. Christie JF, Shering A, Ferguson J, et al: Physostigmine and arecoline: effects of intravenous infusions in Alzheimer presenile dementia. *Brit J Psychiatry* 1981; 138:46–50.

14. Davis KL, Mohs RC, Tinklenberg JR: Enhancement of memory by physostigmine. *N Eng J Med* 1979; 301:946.

15. Haubrich DR, Gerber NH, Pflueger AB: Choline availability and synthesis of acetylcholine, in Barbeau A, Growdon JH, Wurtman RJ (eds): *Nutrition and the Brain.* New York, Raven, 1979, vol 5 pp 57–71.

16. Rigter H, Crabbe JC: Modulation of memory by pituitary hormones and related peptides. *Vitam Horm* 1974; 37:153–241.

17. Kastin AJ, Olson RD, Schally AV, et al: CNS effects of peripherally administered brain peptides. *Life Sci* 1979; 25:401–414.

18. Davies P, Terry RD: Cortical somatostatin-like immunoreactivity in cases of Alzheimer's disease and senile dementia of the Alzheimer type. *Neurobiol Aging* 1981; 2:9–14.

19. Rossor NM, Emson PC, Mountjoy CQ: et al: Reduced amounts of immunoreactivite somatostatin in the temporal cortex in senile dementia of Alzheimer type. *Neurosci Lett* 1980; 20:373–377.

20. Rossor MN, Iversen LL, Mountjoy CQ, et al: Arginine vasopressin and choline acetyltransferase in brains of patients with Alzheimer type senile dementia. *Lancet* 1980; ii:1367.

21. de Wied D, Gispen WH: Behavioral effects of peptides, in Gainer H (ed): *Peptides in Neurobiology.* New York, Plenum, 1977, pp 391–442.

22. Sahgal A, Keith AB, Wright C, et al: Failure of vasopressin to enhance memory in a passive avoidance task in rats. *Neurosci Lett* 1982; 28:87–92.

23. Oliveros JC, Jandali MK, Timsit-Berthier M, et al: Vasopressin in amnesia. *Lancet* 1978; i:42.

24. leBoeuf A, Lodge J, Eames PG: Vasopressin and memory in Korsakoff syndrome. *Lancet* 1978; ii:1370.

25. Ferris SH, Reisberg B, Gershon S: Neuropeptide modulation of cognition and memory in humans, in Poon LW (ed): *Aging in the 1980s: Psychological Issues.* Washington DC, American Psychological Association, 1980, pp 212–220.

26. Branconnier RJ: The human behavioral pharmacology of the common core heptapeptides. *Pharmacol. Therapeutics* 1981; 14:161–175.

27. Prangle AJ, Loosen PT, Nemeroff CB: Peptides: application to research in nervous and mental disorders, in Fielding S, Effland RC (eds): *New Frontiers in Psychotropic Drug Research.* Mt. Kisco, Futura, 1979, pp 117–189.

28. Bartus RT, Dean RL, Beer B: Neuropeptide effects on memory in aged monkeys. *Neurobiol Aging* 1982; 3:61–68.

29. Gotto AM, Peck EJ, Boyd AE (eds): *Brain Peptides: A New Endocrinology.* New York, Elsevier North-Holland, 1979.

30. Bohus B, Urban I, van Wimersma Greidanus TB, et al: Opposite effects of oxytocin and vasopressin on avoidance behaviour and hippocampal theta rhythm in the rat. *Neuropharmacology* 1977; 12:239–247.

31. Ferrier BM, Kennett DJ, Devlin MC: Influence of oxytocin on human memory processes. *Life Sci* 1980; 27:2311–2317.

32. Davies P, Katzman R, Terry RD: Reduced somatostatin-like immunoreactivity in cerebral cortex from cases of Alzheimer disease and Alzheimer senile dementia. *Nature* 1980; 288:279–280.

33. Hoffman GE, Sladek JR: Age-related changes in dopamine, LHRH and somatostatin in the rat hypothalamus. *Neurobiol Aging* 1980; 1:27–38.

34. Bartus RT, Dean RL: Logical principles in the development of animal models of age-related memory loss, in Crook T, Ferris S, Bartus RT (eds): *Clinical and Preclinical Assessment in Geriatric Psychopharmacology.* New Canaan, Powley, 1983.

35. Loew DM: Pharmacologic approaches to the treatment of senile dementia. *Aging NY* 1980; 13:287–294.

36. Scott FL: A review of some current drugs used in the pharmacotherapy of organic brain syndrome. *Aging NY* 1979; 8:151–184.

37. Bartus RT, Dean RL: Age-related memory loss and drug therapy: possible directions based on animal models in aging. *Aging NY* 1981; 17:209–223.

SECTION XII

PSYCHOTHERAPEUTIC APPROACHES TO MANAGEMENT OF ALZHEIMER'S PATIENTS AND THEIR FAMILIES

54 Social Management

James A. Haycox

In 1950, an anonymous writer published "The Death of a Mind" in the *Lancet* (1). It was a touching account of the intellectual decline of the author's father, who had developed Alzheimer's disease, and of the helpless sorrow of his family. The father entered a nursing home, but when he died "it was as if we had already said goodbye." One can read of this account 30 years later and know that the pain of watching the progression of this disease still exists. Now one has a few more choices to ease the patient's suffering, and at least one alternative to nursing home placement or mental institutionalization, or keeping the patient confined at home in bed: dementia day care.

This chapter will describe

- The conditions for success in keeping a demented patient at home
- Choosing to place a patient in a nursing home
- The mental life of the demented
- A brief summary of pharmacology in dementia
- The important elements of a day care program
- What can be expected in the course of dementia day care

Correct diagnosis (2) is especially important in these cases since senile brain disease of the Alzheimer type (AD) generally tends to be overdiagnosed in up to 30% of cases (3, 4). Computerized tomographic x-ray scan (CT scan), new electroencephalographic knowledge, positron emission scanning, and cerebral blood flow measurement technology have lent vigor and increased accuracy in diagnostic evaluation, and have brought a larger public to diagnostic centers in search of help. Heretofore, the mental hospital has generally been the center for diagnosis, but 90% of patients can be evaluated less expensively and more safely as outpatients. There is an enormous economic advantage in an outpatient workup since the cost of very few days in a hospital or nursing home often exceeds the cost of an outpatient evaluation. One of the current aims of research in dementia is to find a clear biologic marker to use in diagnosis in order to increase diagnostic accuracy and reduce costs.

Keeping an Alzheimer Patient at Home Successfully

In keeping a demented patient at home one aims to

- Be alert to the patient's needs
- Capture wandering attention

- Communicate affection
- Provide assurance that all is well, the patient is safe

It is lonely labor for the caretaker, requiring tolerance of one's emotions and a capacity to suffer stoically. Friends help in time of crisis, but cannot be expected to endure over the long haul. They will depart; one learns to accept the leave-taking with minimal distress. The course of dementia is always downward and results in prolonged, repeated grieving.

When a patient is to live within the family confines, the family must first decide whether they can do what needs to be done and, second, whether it is too great a burden. The necessary social constrictions must be judged tolerable in order not to breed resentment.

Many will have already made a decision about what they'll want to do by the time the diagnosis is made. The physician need not consider the "correct" moral answer as to whether to keep a patient at home or in a nursing home. If a physician has misgivings about a family's intentions, the physician should say what they are and then collaborate as well as possible with what the family wants to do, realizing that human beings are willing to endure unimaginable hardships when there is no alternative. On the other hand, family members will often do what they wish in the face of all wisdom.

The following conditions will permit a demented patient to remain at home with a reasonable expectation of success:

1. When the family's wish to do it transcends all else and there is no other compelling task to accomplish. A person who must earn a living, for instance, cannot ignore economic necessity unless it is feasible to hire daytime helpers. Just as compelling is a demanding career. For these reasons an energetic, retired person may be in the best position to succeed.

2. When no one other than the demented patient has prior claim to the caretaker's time. A woman with a demented father may have to let go of him if her husband retires or when there are children.

3. It might be an asset to be female when caring for a demented person although there are many exceptions. A man who desires strongly to care for a demented female relative at home and who can arrange it will probably succeed as well as a woman, but it will be difficult. Women eventually care for demented males because they tend to be younger than their spouses and their life spans are longer. Put the other way around, demented women are statistically more likely to be cared for in nursing homes—unless they have daughters.

4. A childless woman is more strongly impelled to care for her demented husband than one who has children.

5. There are architectural constraints. Two people, one demented, in a small apartment aren't highly likely to succeed. One needs space, businesslike bathrooms, ways to thwart a wandering patient, and furnishings that accommodate to the patient's disabilities. Many spouses of patients report that they lock themselves in their bedrooms from time to time for much needed privacy.

6. An energetic and responsive family physician willing to help, make an occasional house call, and be accepting is a great asset. He or she will diagnose intercurrent illnesses, help with minor tranquilizing medication, and attend during terminal illness, usually pneumonia.

7. A day hospital or day care center may make the difference between managing and failing. It need not be attended every day; in fact, two or three times a week may be sufficient. Patients will improve in their orientation and enthusiastically recognize that there is a program for them to go to even though it does not occur every day.

8. Simple, repetitive, daily routine is necessary to give predictability to a patient's life, but some variety must be at hand to divert when the patient is restive and recalcitrant. It is almost always a mistake to take a demented patient on vacation: it will produce acute disorientation and decline, a severe disappointment to the person caring for the patient. When a vacation is necessary, leave the patient behind.

NURSING HOME PLACEMENT

The decision to place a patient in a nursing home ought to come from judgments as to which plan among alternatives will serve the patient and the family best. A disabled person who lives alone comes to the end of independence when it is impossible to feed and clean himself. Daily help if not constant care will be necessary. If the patient is disabled by dementia, needs assistance at night, wanders and gets lost, or makes dangerous mistakes in judgment and behavior, then a nursing home for adequate care and safety is probably best.

Each caretaker has unique capacities and tolerances; when they are exceeded, then a shift to institutional care should be made. When the time comes that the service needed is more crucial than the person who gives it, when it no longer matters who does it so long as it is done, then a nursing home is preferable. In the end, a patient may prefer to lie in bed undisturbed although someone must turn and bathe the patient. At this time physical needs and their satisfaction are nearly all that matter. A good nursing home offers someone in constant attendance day and night who is trained for the task and has relief after eight hours a day. It is a professional duty to see to the patient's needs in a cheerful, confident manner, without sorrow or anger. When the patient is no longer able to perceive others as individuals, then the patient is safer and more comfortable with professional service than in the care of family (5).

THE MIND OF DEMENTIA

What is in the mind of the person who becomes demented? Are faculties simply extirpated one by one, or is there a qualitative difference? The probable answer is yes to both questions (6), although those who know demented patients well agree that there is a real being at home behind the barriers of the disease. It sometimes seems that the patient is a quizzical spectator, a stranger in a strange land, trying to make sense both of that to which he or she is a witness and of the patient's own puzzling mental life. The patient's speculative gaze may indicate inability to find the word or the phrase with which to reply. Panic may indicate that all current circumstances have come out of context.

PRINCIPLES OF DAY CARE

REALITY ORIENTATION

Modern psychiatric treatment of demented patients can be traced back to Cameron's (7) groundbreaking report, published in 1941. He was able to reproduce nocturnal confusion in senile patients (often called sundowning) by placing them in a darkened room. Deprivation of visual cues for spatial orientation produced confusion and anxiety. He suggested, correctly, that maintaining visual orientation was good treatment and a prophylaxis for susceptible patients. This principle was used in the following years to treat mental confusion (8–10). In 1966, Folsom (11) and Taulbee (12) developed the specific concept of reality orientation, a method for presenting, repeating, and reinforcing the basic facts of time, place, and person. It is still the cornerstone of treatment efforts for the demented.

Reminiscence

Stimulating a patient's reminiscence is another way to bring back errant self-awareness. Reminiscence can be accomplished directly by encouraging it and by music, movement, and dance. When the mating instinct is transcended later in life and a search for meaning grows, reminiscence can occur. An older person's reminiscence has as its purpose the tendering of information more than a pushing of one's own self forward. As the older person recounts stories of the past, he tends to become again what he once was. For a demented patient reminiscence lights up the mind and illuminates the darkened threads and connections.

Music evokes the emotions and recaptures the past in another way we all recognize. The physical body has "memory" in it, too. Riding a bicycle is not remembered in any intellectual sense but once learned it is never forgotten. Dance (movement) therapists purposely evoke memory and reminiscence in their sessions. They also find that attitudes and emotions have bodily expression and that there is communication of ideas in body motions.

Social Expectations

Patients who are treated with dignity will respond in kind. Neat dress and good grooming tend to perpetuate themselves. Mealtimes can be arranged to be fairly normal socially. If the institution itself has the broad aim of rehabilitation, it fosters hopeful expectations in patients and receptivity to treatment efforts.

Psychotherapeutic Group Work

Group therapy is helpful for patients as well as families. Seeing patients in groups of seven or eight is difficult for the therapist and requires intense concentration, but it is worthwhile. Patients will articulate their frustrations and grief and strong bonds are often formed between patients. Many come to have an understanding and acceptance of their disabilities after interpretations and translations by the therapist and their peers. Group and individual work with families provides the information and techniques needed to carry on at home. It is also an important comfort in times of despair.

A Brief Pharmacology for Dementia

The old, the young, and those with damage to the nervous system often react in surprising ways to drugs. These surprises may be undesirable. Drugs interact with each other so one must be wary not only of the effect of single doses on the physiologically frail but also of potentiating a disaster with unfortunate drug combinations.

The mundane drugs of human life are tobacco, alcohol, and caffeine. A demented person should not smoke as a measure of fire safety, and because it is harmful to health. Alcohol tends to devastate the composure of the demented. Alcohol is not for them, nor do they even crave it. Geriatric units of hospitals sometimes make it a policy to serve decaffeinated coffee to avoid any interference with sleep, but it is not clear that caffeinism afflicts the demented more than usual.

Depression will worsen the symptoms of dementia and should be treated. An antidepressant which is also somewhat sedating if given at bedtime may help with sleep as well as elevate the mood. In dementia and in the elderly, smaller-than-usual doses may result in improved mood but because of this, overdosage is a greater danger. The side effects of tricyclic antidepressants are dangerous and include orthostatic hypotension leading to fainting, falling, and hip fracture. Arrhythmias may be produced from slowing of the conduction time (13).

Phenothiazines are used to calm agitation in the demented patient, and especially to mitigate intolerable behavior. Sometimes phenothiazines are useful but they can create misfortune by oversedating or overexciting a patient, or cause bizarre reactions (14). Sometimes one might better choose a benzodiazepine, which is often antipsychotic as well as tranquilizing in demented and elderly people. Diazepam endures up to 100 hours in the blood after a single dose, and if given even once or more each day may accumulate and overaffect a patient. Oxazepam is shorter acting and preferable. Flurazepam, chloral hydrate and diphenhydramine are three fairly safe hypnotic drugs, although the latter may be responsible for anticholinergic effects (15).

Difficulties in the brain in dementia with the neurotransmitter acetylcholine and with the enzyme choline acetyltransferase are described elsewhere in this book. Treatments for these problems have yet to be found. There is nothing at this time which has any lasting effect upon the memory or integrity of the mind in dementia.

EXPECTATIONS

Typically, a given patient's initial reaction to reality orientation and to day care in general is improvement. Memory will slightly revive and zest for life brighten. Initially patients will worry lest the day care center keep them overnight, and toward the end of the first several sessions they will worry about who is coming for them. The improvement will endure for three months or more and then the inexorable decline will proceed. Brief improvement is valuable but alone is not justification for day care. The longer aim is the production of as good an adaptation to the disabilities as possible—both in the patient and in the family. Patients respond better to discussion of memory problems than to avoidance of the topic. In some way they are aware of their mental derangements and many have come to feel they are insane. It is a relief when they can know that it is memory, not sanity, which has failed. This realization may be the beginning of a greater acceptance and a more efficient response to what is happening to them. Day care teaches how to accomplish the activities of daily life and to make the most of them in the face of loss of capacity. Families are less strained and more satisfied.

In the end, there is often a final, rapid decline. Somnolence, sharp loss of coordination, and dysphagia appear. The last development is often pneumonia, which has been called the old person's friend.

REFERENCES

1. Death of a mind. *Lancet* 1950; ii:1002–1015.
2. Roth M, Morrissy JD: Problems in the diagnosis and classification of mental disorders in old age. *Br J Psychiatry* 1952; 98:66–80.
3. Ron MA, Toone BK, Garralda ME, et al: Diagnostic accuracy in presenile dementia. *Br J Psychiatry* 1979; 134:161–168.
4. Nott PN, Fleminger JJ: Presenile dementia: the difficulties of early diagnosis. *Acta Psychiatr Scand* 1975; 51:210–217.
5. Haycox JA: Late care of the demented patient: the question of nursing home placement. *N Engl J Med* 1980; 303:165–166.
6. Miller E: Impaired recall and memory disturbance in presenile dementia. *Br J Soc Clin Psychol* 1975; 14:73–79.
7. Cameron DE: Studies in senile nocturnal delirium. *Psychiatr Q* 1941; 15:47–53.
8. Lindsley OR: Geriatric behavioral prosthetics, in Kastenbaum R (ed): *New Thoughts on Old Age.* New York, Springer, 1964.
9. Brody EM, Kleban MH, Lawton MP, et al: Longitudinal look at excess disabilities in the mentally impaired aged. *J Gerontol* 1974; 29:79–84.
10. Brook P, Degun G, Mather M: Reality orientation, a therapy for psychogeriatric patients: a controlled study. *Br J Psychiatry* 1975; 127:42–45.
11. Folsom JC: Reality orientation for the elderly patient. *J Geriatr Psychiatry* 1968; 1:291–307.
12. Taulbee LR, Folsom JC: Reality orientation for geriatric patients. *Hosp Community Psychiatry* 1966; 17:133–135.
13. Nies A, Robinson DS, Friedman MJ, et al: Relationship between age and tricyclic antidepressant plasma levels. *Am J Psychiatry* 1977; 134:790–793.
14. Davis JM: Antipsychotic drugs, in Crook T, Cohen G (eds): *Physicians' Handbook on Psychotropic Drugs Use in the Aged.* New Canaan, Powley, 1981.
15. Greenblatt DJ, Shader RT: The clinical choice of sedative hypnotics. *Ann Intern Med* 1972; 77:91–100.

55 Management of the Family

DONNA COHEN
DAVID COPPEL
CARL EISDORFER

FAMILIES ARE WILLING TO ENDURE considerable personal and economic sacrifices to care for relatives with dementia (1–4). While it is clear that the impaired aged rely more heavily upon the family for support than they do upon formalized clinical and community services (5–8), it is also clear that families are not receiving the support and training they need to effectively care for their relatives. It is important for health professionals to develop a strong partnership with family members. The health professional has an active role as clinician or service provider. Family members also have a formal role, not as lay therapists, but as knowledgeable caregivers (9).

Family members of dementia victims have an important responsibility to educate themselves and train the patient to cope with a range of physical, psychological, and social problems as the disease progresses. Families provide the motivational, emotional, and physical environments in which the patient must operate. Family members are not merely individuals related by blood. They have a profound personal influence upon each other. In this regard, families can be conceptualized as systems which operate to deal with crises and changes in the individual patient as well as within the entire family structure. In a family constellation where one member has a dementing disorder, the disease changes the roles of family members, including their various communication and behavioral patterns with one another (1, 10–12). Successful adjustment to these changes in the family constellation depends upon the ability of all family members to learn how to interact with the patient, cope with their own feelings, and maintain their health. If they do not learn how to cope with the dementia, they become vulnerable to physical and psychiatric disorders, and since the family is the first line of defense for the patient, if the family goes, the patient's survival in the community becomes unlikely.

The natural course of the dementing disorders is not known at this time (1). Some individuals decline rapidly, others more slowly. Some people cope successfully with their disabilities and progressive losses while others do not. Although it is clear that the rate of brain degeneration has a major impact on the patient's ability to function, several other factors affect the individual's level of performance. These include the patient's general health and the successful involvement of knowledgeable healthy family members as well as preventative social services in the community (1, 13). The level of responsiveness or tension within the family, as well as the family's financial status, determine what health care is affordable, and contribute to the functioning of the patient.

No amount of family love and attention can reverse or cure the effects of a progressive brain disease, but family members can influence the sense of control patients maintain throughout a major portion of the illness. Interactions that reinforce the patient's sense of dignity and control over the demands of daily life lead to increased independence and self-esteem rather than inducing dependency and helplessness (14, 15). In the earlier stages of the disease, when there appears to be a greater awareness of losses in abilities, the patient may be susceptible to secondary depression. At this time family support may be especially influential in maintaining the patient's motivation to function as long as possible.

Many patients report that they consciously invest a great deal of energy in "putting themselves together" each morning and in developing a sense of mastery over the stressful situations of the day. A number of patients have expressed their fears of awakening to ever declining functional capacities. One patient recited a quotation from Hammarskjöld's *Markings* each day upon awakening: "Tomorrow we shall meet, Death and I— And he shall thrust his sword into one who is wide awake." This man knew he could make it through the day if he remembered his lines.

Love does not restore a patient's memory, but love and the implementation of appropriate management strategies can reinforce whatever human skills, feelings, and abilities remain intact in the impaired person. The simple act of talking to a person stimulates feelings of being wanted. This may lead to enhanced mastery, more appropriate social actions, and a continued sense of participation. Families who talk less to their relative may inadvertently blunt intelligent behavior. Family members need to understand the necessity of pursuing an active role to strengthen the cognitive abilities and social skills of their relative. The challenge to the family and involved health care professionals is to have a realistic understanding not only of the patient's abilities but of their needs, desires, and preferences.

Families often experience their love for the patient in different ways than before. It may be difficult for families to apply "love" to an individual who is no longer responsive or communicative as they once were as a parent, spouse, companion, or lover. The positive supportive and emotional behaviors a family expresses does as much to help the patient as it does to help the family member adapt to the transitions they must make in relating to the patient. Another important issue is the understanding of the negative feelings which may arise in the course of caregiving which goes on "thirty-six hours a day" (Warren Easterly, in the film *The Thirty-Six-Hour Day,* August 1979). Family members report feelings of frustration and guilt concerning an angry thought or response to the irritating behavior of a demented spouse or parent. Denial of these negative reactions can create significant inner tensions in the caregiver.

There are a number of practical ways in which professionals and families can work together to maintain cognitively impaired patients at their maximum and enhance their dignity. It is important to understand that cultural and age-related attitudes concerning help seeking and/or seeing doctors for mental problems may surface within the family caregivers. Utilizing social, medical or psychological supports can be difficult for individuals who consider help-seeking (or receiving) as a weakness or a crack in their self-reliance. Often as the family's burden of love increases, the attitude of "wanting to do it all" becomes more and more entrenched.

The influence of family members on the patient with dementia can range from weak to strong, and from positive to negative. These influences can either foster feelings of dependence, isolation, rejection and hopelessness, or their positive counterparts: independence, involvement, intimacy, and thoughtfulness. Bringing families together to share their experiences and their range of feelings about the patient, and the disease in general, is useful for all involved. Programs with defined curricula can be designed and implemented to help the patient and the family cope successfully with the impact of the progressive, incurable dementing disease.

While mortality and the rate of cognitive decline are difficult to predict, it appears that anticipatory coping exercises may be quite useful, given the stage-related tasks and crises which are beginning to emerge from the current literature (1, 16). Group therapeutic programs provide families with opportunities to practice coping skills in preparation for sequelae of the disease, including the full range of potential problems that should be anticipated.

Structured behavioral programs guided by knowledgeable professionals should be implemented to teach groups of families how to deal successfully with disruptive and volatile behaviors and to reinforce appropriate social activities, exercise, dressing and eating behavior (17–19). Providing opportunities for cognitively impaired individuals to meet with one another is also rewarding, since these individuals can establish an unexpected communication and intimate rapport with one another. They can be friends with each other and support each other when their old friends reject them. They also report finding solace in their common destiny. Involving the family and patient jointly in some programs while separating them in others is also important. The key factor is early and direct intervention. The earlier these activities are begun and the longer they continue, the better the probability of success.

Obviously, a great deal needs to be done to meet the needs of struggling families while providing educational and clinical services in the community to foster a genuine partnership between families and health service professionals. This kind of therapeutic partnership implies a commitment of resources, time, energy, and a strong desire to learn from each other and to work together. However, a wide variety of effective clinical programs, such as geriatric family services (20), can emerge in the community only if there is strong government support and a social policy which recognize this as an area of high priority. We must begin to ask to what extent present government policies are helping or hurting families. The goal is at least threefold: to avoid such changes in current policy that place hardships on families with impaired relatives; to develop policies that provide alternative ways of strengthening families; and to determine how to provide the options that families need to do the best job.

There are some important issues to be addressed in this partnership between families and health professionals. How can professionals and families support each other and not undermine each other? How can they respect and learn from each other? What is the most effective way to share these expectations about each other's role in the care of the patient? What are the most effective paths of communication? What are the expectations and attitudes of each to the other? Where are health professionals supposed to learn how to understand and communicate with relatives and patients as well as how to learn from them? Where are families and caregivers supposed to learn how to communicate with the health care community? What priorities are lacking in federal, state, and local budgets to provide ways for each to relate to the other?

Many concrete changes can be implemented now, some will develop as research provides the empirical base, and others will require difficult choices. The clinician's role needs to be redefined to include the responsibility to build a partnership with demented older persons and their families. Medical schools and other professional schools need to reevaluate their curricula to prepare individuals for this responsibility. Professional schools must also experiment with innovative approaches to care. Such innovation should be carefully evaluated by both families and professionals. Families themselves can help say what is appropriate to ask from professionals in the way of support.

REFERENCES

1. Eisdorfer C, Cohen D: Management of the family and patient coping with dementing illness. *J Fam Pract* 1981; 12:831–837.
2. Fengler A, Goodrich N: Wives of elderly disabled men: the hidden patients. *Gerontologist* 1979; 19:175–183.
3. Isaacs B: Geriatric patients: do their families care? *Br Med J* 1971; 4:282–284.
4. Lowther CP, Williamson J: Old people and their relatives. *Lancet* 1966; ii:282–286.
5. Brody EM: Aging of the family personality: a developmental view. *Fam Process* 1974; 13:23–35.
6. Brody EM: *Long-term Care of Older People: A Practical Guide.* New York, Human Sciences, 1977.
7. Brody S, Poulshock W, Mascioschi F: The family caring unit: a major consideration in the long-term support system. *Gerontologist* 1978; 18:556–561.
8. Shanas E: The family as a social support system in old age. *Gerontologist* 1979; 19:169–174.
9. Cohen D, Eisdorfer C: Families as educators. Read before the Annual Association of Gerontologists for Higher Education Meeting, Washington, DC, Feb 1982.
10. Barnes RF, Raskind MA, Scott M, et al: Problems of family caring for Alzheimer patients: use of a support group. *J Am Geriatr Soc* 1981; 29:80–85.
11. Grossman L, London C, Berry C: Older women caring for disabled spouses. *Gerontologist* 1981; 21:464–470.
12. Lezak M: Living with the characterologically altered brain-injured patient. *J Clin Psychiatry* 1978; 39:592–598.
13. Tobin SS, Kulys R: The family and services. *Annu Rev Gerontol* 1980; 1:370–400.
14. Langer E, Rodin J: The effects of choice and enhanced personal responsibility for the aged: a field experiment in an institutional setting. *J Pers Soc Psychol* 1976; 34:191–198.
15. Rodin J, Langer E: Long-term effect of a control relevant intervention. *J Pers Soc Psychol* 1978; 35:897–902.
16. Moos RH (ed): *Coping with Physical Illness.* New York, Plenum, 1977.
17. Cohen D: Psychological issues in the diagnosis and treatment of the cognitively impaired aged, in Eisdorfer C, Fann E (eds): *Clinical Psychopharmacology of Aging.* New York, Springer, in press.
18. Eisdorfer C, Cohen D, Preston C: Behavioral and psychological therapies for the older patient with cognitive impairment. *Aging NY* 1981; 15:209–226.
19. Lawton, MP: Psychosocial and environmental approaches to the care of senile dementia patients, in Cole JO, Barrett, JE (eds): *Psychopathology in the Aged.* New York, Raven, 1978, pp 265–280.
20. Reifler BV, Eisdorfer C: A clinic for the impaired elderly and their families. *Am J Psychiatry* 1980; 137:1399–1403.

56 Reality Orientation

J. C. Folsom

REALITY ORIENTATION (R.O.) IS A GROUP-ORIENTED, psychotherapeutic technique for assisting confused, disoriented elderly individuals (frequently diagnosed as having Alzheimer's disease) to learn and practice techniques that help them cope with the problems caused by their confusion and disorientation. Reality orientation techniques have proven successful with three different groups of confused and disoriented patients.

GROUP ONE

The most severely confused, disoriented patients are frequently not responsive to any stimuli and require intensive 24-hour-a-day R.O. These patients are most frequently found in nursing homes and other long-term health-care facilities. Although they may be receiving excellent medical, nursing and physical care, as institutionalized persons, they have become progressively more debilitated, dehumanized, depersonalized, and socially disengaged. These patients are usually diagnosed as either senile or suffering from organic brain syndrome or Alzheimer's disease (AD).

In most cases these patients have been cared for by the institution for long periods. They have become "good" patients: they cause no trouble, do as they are told, and ask no questions. It is the norm of their existence that they have no opinions and simply accept their situation, gradually ceasing to make any meaningful input into their own lives and daily activities.

Much of the patients' confusion, disorientation, and disengagement results from their receiving such total physical care that they have no decision-making responsibility concerning their own life in the institution. Once they have been institutionalized and are receiving complete care, they have no need to be aware of the realities of their own existence or to question who they are, where they are and why they are there, the time of day or night, the season of the year or even the year.

The purpose of the R.O. program is to use *every* contact with the patient to help restore identity as to time, person, and place. The entire staff, and all volunteers and relatives who visit the patient, must be taught to use R.O. techniques every time they approach the patient—even though the patient may give no indication of noticing or understanding what is happening.

Every contact with the patient is used to reinforce the time, person, and place realities of the patient's existence. Furthermore, it is important to attempt constantly to let patients know why they are where they are and that they are expected to again become involved in their own self-care to the fullest extent possible.

A patient must always be addressed by his or her proper title and last name; for example, it is totally unacceptable for a staff person to address Mrs. Mary Smith as Sweetie, Grandma, Honey, or Mary. The proper form of address will be: Mrs. Smith. If a patient has an honorary title such as Doctor, Colonel, Governor, or the like, that will be used instead of Miss, Mrs., or Mr.

The patient must always be given an explanation of what is going to be done as well as reinforcement of the facts regarding time, person and place. For example, the following statements should accompany the actions being described:

> Good evening, Mrs. Smith. I am the ward nurse, Mrs. Johnson. Miss Brown, one of the nursing assistants, is with me. We are coming into your room to prepare you for bed. You seem to have dozed off already—the pillow I had placed behind your back has slipped out of your chair. I hope you haven't been too uncomfortable, Mrs. Smith. Ah, there now, you have opened your eyes. Do you remember Miss Brown? She works on the evening duty shift five times a week and you always seem happy to see her. It's 7:30 in the evening and time for you to go to bed. I see your TV set is turned to the Muppets' show. Do you like them? They are always on TV on Monday nights. Miss Brown will help you to the bathroom while I turn down your bed, Mrs. Smith.

Then, after Miss Brown has brought Mrs. Smith to the bedside, the conversation might continue as follows:

> I do hope you will have a good night's sleep. Remember, your daughter Suzanne will come to visit you tomorrow morning. She usually arrives shortly after she has dropped your grandson off at school—around 9 o'clock. Here is the nurse's call cord in case you need anything during the night. Good night, Mrs. Smith.

Each time a staff person contacts the patient for any reason, similar reinforcing conversation should follow. Family members are taught to reinforce reality by frequently calling the patient by name and by talking about what is going on in the family and the community, with specific dates and times being mentioned. This is continued even though the patient makes no response to any of the conversation.

GROUP TWO

These patients are still moderately to severely confused; however, they are capable of making some appropriate responses to interpersonal encounters with staff, volunteers and family members. For example, as soon as Mrs. Smith begins to respond to her own name, appropriately acknowledges the presence of those who speak to her, and indicates any knowledge of her current reality she is considered ready for a change in program. In addition to the 24-hour-a-day R.O. program she will now be taken to the R.O. Basic Classes.

These classes are 30-minute sessions held 5 days a week in a classroom setting. Class membership is limited to no more than five patients. The classroom instructor, usually a nursing assistant with special training in leading classroom sessions, will give individual attention to each of the moderately to severely confused and disoriented patients. Rigid adherence to scheduling and the assignment of the same nursing assistant/instructor throughout the program will ensure continuity.

The classroom approach should be direct, positive, and sufficiently flexible to meet the specific needs of the participants. Nursing assistants/instructors should remember the following: Introduce yourself to the patients. Repeat your name as necessary; ask patients to repeat it to you. Be sure they can pronounce it. Introduce patients to each other. Always call patients by their names, and encourage them to address each other by name.

Try to set a calm, friendly, and secure atmosphere. Confused patients will usually respond to a calm, friendly approach. Speak slowly and distinctly because older patients are frequently hard of hearing. Speak to them in a friendly manner, but do not talk to them as though they were children. Look directly at patients when addressing them.

Plan simple activities—things that the patients have probably done before. Use the reality board and the blackboard. Have all patients assemble a calendar notebook; be sure they write their names on them. Make a calendar each month, and mark off the day each morning. Move to more complex and gratifying activity only after patients have improved sufficiently—after they become more comfortable, and after they start showing interest in their surroundings.

Make minimal demands on the patients. Remember, they are already confused, upset, and possibly hostile. Give them one simple instruction at a time. Spend as much time with the patients as possible—do not get them started on their projects and leave them. Return to them often and give instruction.

Keep in mind that patients' social interaction with others, as much as their projects and activities, help them to return to reality as self-confidence and dignity are restored.

Ask all patients to sign in on a daily roster; encourage them to do so. Use spelling sessions and discussion; this may be done while in a group around a table. Keep words simple and close to reality. Ask the patients to spell the day, month, location of the hospital, next meal, and so forth; anagrams may be used. Reward patients immediately when they respond correctly; say "Good," "That's right," "Fine," and the like.

Many severely confused and disoriented patients are not able to respond appropriately when first placed in the R.O. classroom. The instructor must use much patience and emphasize by a consistent approach a genuine concern that the patient is expected to try to follow the instructions. Many days may pass before the patient gives his first positive response; however, when that breakthrough occurs, other appropriate responses usually follow very quickly.

As soon as patients show sufficient progress, they can be assigned to the R.O. Advanced Class. In the Advanced Class reinforcement of the basic facts of reality will continue to be emphasized through use of the reality board, the weekly calendar, the daily menu, and so on. In addition, discussion of current events, approaching holidays, preparations for visits from loved ones, and plans for parties and other activities become important parts of the classroom routines.

To ensure carryover of the relearning process from the classroom setting to the institution as a whole, large clocks, easily read calendars, and schedules of activities and of special events and upcoming holidays should be placed at key points. Reality boards are important and should be located in several strategic spots so that patients are encouraged to keep themselves oriented to the facts being reinforced by display on the boards. No hard-and-fast rules govern the style of make-up of the board. A typical one might display the following information:

The International Center for the Disabled (ICD)
Service Program for the Aging (SPA)
340 East 24th Street, New York, N.Y. 10010

Today is Monday, March 15, 1982
The next holiday is St. Patrick's Day
The weather is clear and cold
The next meal is lunch.

Some reality boards have slots for sliding letters and numbers in and out for updating information. Updating the board is not a very complicated task; it can be assigned to a patient who has demonstrated interest and is capable of the responsibility. Obviously, the line identifying the next meal must be changed three times a day. The weather line should be changed whenever the forecast or weather changes. It is important that the board be kept current.

Many reality boards are less stylized and are simply written on a chalkboard (Fig. 56–1). Some are made of cork or other material suitable for thumbtacking pieces of paper on which the necessary information is either printed or written in longhand. In every case, letters and figures should be of sufficient size so that even patients with diminished vision can read the information from several feet away. Proper lighting of the board is important.

Patients who have trouble remembering certain information of importance may be helped by being given 3″ × 5″ cards on which they write the pertinent facts, such as the names, addresses, and phone numbers of significant persons in their lives; important anniversaries, birthdays, and holidays. Many patients are helped by having with them a pocket-size calendar with important events noted against the appropriate dates. They should be encouraged to make a habit of marking off the current date at the same time each morning as the establishment of set routines and methods of coping with confusion and memory loss adds to their

Figure 56–1.

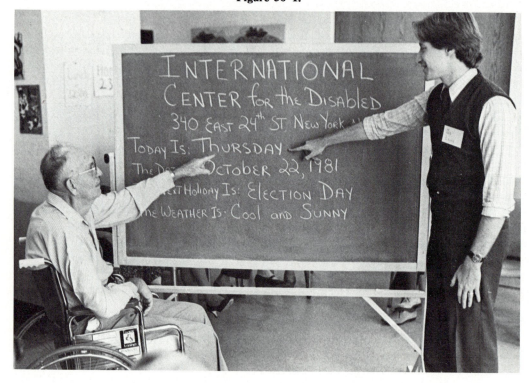

sense of self-confidence. Through continuing use of these memory aids, they become convinced that they can again cope with the responsibility of being decision-making individuals.

GROUP THREE

These patients have mild to moderate degrees of confusion and disorientation. They can be helped to live in relatively independent conditions with certain support services being provided. Use of R.O. techniques will help prevent further deterioration.

The International Center for the Disabled has published a pamphlet, *Help Begins at Home,* which discusses in detail simple and effective methods to be used in caring for confused and disoriented elderly persons. It is of utmost importance that those closest to the affected person—spouse, children, and others with a family relationship—become involved. Confusion and disorientation are not entirely and exclusively the problem of the elderly person exhibiting the symptoms; rather, they are a family responsibility. In describing how this responsibility can be met, the pamphlet stresses the importance of everybody understanding the problem and agreeing to treat the elderly person in a consistent manner. General guidelines list key do's and dont's.

Do:
- Recognize that the basic personality, hopes, and expectations of the person are still intact
- Treat the person as an adult with dignity—not as a child
- Expect the person to fulfill responsibilities as a member of the household
- Respond to confusion and disorientation with facts—no matter how painful this may seem to be for the person
- Reward accomplishment

Don't:
- Become overprotective and do everything for the person
- Focus on lost capacities and overlook those that remain
- Reinforce delusions and confusion by going along with them
- Give in to unreasonable demands
- Reward disability by being overly sympathetic

The importance of a careful assessment of the current medical status and diet is emphasized. It is particularly important that *all* medicines being taken—both those prescribed and those purchased over-the-counter—be thoroughly evaluated. Specific problems the affected person experiences should be listed, with the cooperation of and input from the affected person. Such a list might include

- Poor communication
- Memory loss
- Nonrecognition of people
- Overdependence
- Decreased participation in family life
- Falling off of recreation and leisure activities
- Difficulty in maintaining appropriate social behavior: hygiene, incontinence, table manners, attire

One simple way to combat confusion and disorientation in an elderly person is to set up a Reality Orientation center in the home. This should be done with the elderly person's participation and help—a cooperative project. The room selected should be central and accessible, not closed off, upstairs, or seldom used. The R.O. center should include

- A clock
- An easily read appointment calendar
- A chalkboard (or bulletin board) on which the elderly person can record the day's schedule
- A place for frequently used items such as keys and hearing aid
- Simple cues to jog memory; these can be flash cards or simple pictures. (It is much easier to recognize cues than it is to recall something out of the blue.)

The Reality Orientation center is the core of an organized system of clues and environmental aids that will enable the elderly person to function with more independence. In addition, he or she should always carry a pocket calendar when outside the home, containing the home address and phone number. If the person sometimes gets lost, an identification bracelet (with name, address, and phone number) will be helpful and will lower everyone's level of anxiety. If sent out to do errands, the elderly person should always take a note listing the errands to be done and any necessary bus or subway directions.

Help Begins at Home discusses in detail the approach to the specific problems listed above. It concludes with the following paragraph:

> No guidelines can cover all situations; no single situation can be generalized to cover all elderly persons or their families. But whatever the specific situation, certain principles remain valid. Above all, communication is important. In fact, very often open communication among all family members is the most important single ingredient to successful management of the situation. It is the *family* function that is to be managed, *not* simply the function of the confused member. This cannot be emphasized too strongly. The family does things with the person, not *to* the person.

REFERENCES

Folsom JC: Reality orientation for the elderly mental patient. *J Geriatr Psychiatry* 1968; 1.

International Center for the Disabled: *Help Begins at Home.* New York, International Center for the Disabled, 1981.

Keane EE: *Coping with Senility.* Pittsburgh, Chronic Organic Brain Syndrome Society, 1980.

Mitchel RA: Reality orientation for brain-damaged patients. *Staff Mag* 1966; 3:3–4.

57 Long-Term Continuous Support for Family Members of Alzheimer Patients

Gertrude Steinberg

Families of an Alzheimer's disease patient endure years of physical and emotional distress and strain. Additionally, they bear the frustration that results from knowing that no matter how much effort goes into caring for the patient, there is no hope of recovery. The family faces a harrowing future, caring for someone with whom communication eventually becomes impossible, whose personality changes, and one who will, if he/she lives long enough, become a human vegetable (1, 2).

The value of counseling for these family members, mainly through group participation, cannot be disputed (3–7). Furthermore, since Alzheimer's disease (AD) is a progressive, chronic process with gradual and inexorable decline, coping demands and emotional responses are also not static. They continuously manifest themselves in the family members as the illness evolves. Hence, truly effective supportive counseling and therapy for these caregivers must also continue over a period of months to years, depending on the individual case.

The theme of this chapter is to illustrate the need for long-term support and counseling. The more overt situations a family member may encounter during this traumatic period will be outlined and discussed.

CLINICAL OBSERVATIONS AND DISCUSSION

Although group participants become intellectually knowledgeable about the many possible behavioral and personality changes that may occur in the Alzheimer patient, when these changes actually do take place, family members experience major emotional trauma. Many of them may verbalize their acceptance of the patient's illness. But it is more and more apparent that rarely, if ever, does real acceptance come. Emotionally, it seems they are never prepared for each new occurrence.

The following case histories illustrate how emotionally unprepared the seemingly best adjusted family member is when further degenerative change develops in the Alzheimer patient. The individuals described had initially testified as to their "acceptance" of their spouses' illness, and as to their ability to cope with their home situation.

Mr. Smith, at the time he entered a counseling program, had previously been in individual therapy. Therefore, he felt he had overcome the denial universally experienced by family members. He was aware of the progressive nature of the disease, but since the deterioration in his wife was very slow, he was able to adjust to the slight changes in her behavior as they occurred, without significant emotional upheaval. His wife had been diagnosed as an Alzheimer patient approximately ten years before. He expressed skepticism about receiving much assistance from the group, but rather emphasized his potential contribution to other members because of his long experience. Initially, his attendance was irregular. However, after about six sessions, he was attending the meetings weekly. He began to express his feelings of depression about his wife's condition. He was disturbed with his friends for ignoring her in their conversations. This provided a rationale for his curtailment of their social life. However, this didn't pose too much of a problem for him since his wife was still able to accompany him to concerts, movies, and the theater.

Mr. Smith and his wife went on a vacation, from which he returned a very distressed and unhappy man. While they were away, his wife developed the delusion that her husband had died. Accordingly, she began to mourn him. Mr. Smith has become a stranger to her, and she treats him as such. She calls this stranger she is living with "stupid." She maintains he is not as smart as her deceased husband was. Also, she will not allow him to share her bed any longer.

Mr. Smith finds it very difficult to cope with this phase of his wife's illness. Understandably, considering her behavior, he feels rejected. With the help and support of the group, he is now undergoing the process of disengagement—emotionally divorcing himself from his wife.

Mr. Jones is a planner, very logical and organized. Since his wife's illness was not as advanced as the other group members' spouses, his initial upset was related to hearing about the others and their problems, not so much from his wife's condition. Intellectually, he was also aware of the progressive, debilitating nature of the illness. He stated he handled his emotions very well. For almost a year, from the time he joined a group, he planned his wife's day from the minute she awoke in the morning until she went to sleep at night. Since her major cognitive deficiency was in the area of recent memory, he arranged to visit and spend time with friends she had known for many years. Mrs. Jones could discuss the past with these old friends comfortably.

Currently, Mr. Jones is experiencing marked depression and overt emotional upset, not at hearing about the others in the group, but by what is happening to his planned life style. Due to the progressive nature of the disease, his wife is no longer able to participate in the social plans he previously made, and he can no longer control her day. Her condition prevents her cooperation. He is undergoing the anticipatory grief that often occurs in family members—facing the loss of his companion and partner. He is also mourning the plans he had for their retirement. Now that he is retired, and those plans are not materializing, he is very depressed. With the help of the group, he is now directing his organizational ability towards keeping his wife's environment as stable as possible.

Grief and bereavement are overtly expressed in the group setting. Even though the patient is still alive, for all intents and purposes, that individual is cognitively nonfunctioning. Therefore, the loss of what that person was is mourned. Additionally, the possibility of second marriages after the impaired spouse is deceased may be discussed. Outside relationships for sexual, as well as companionship gratification, is also spoken about.

When the patient ultimately becomes unmanageable at home, usually after a long period of deterioration, institutionalization is often seriously considered. The emotional impact on the family making this decision is devastating. Again, group participation helps the family member handle this guilt-provoking situation.

Incidents of verbal and physical abuse are progressively revealed. Abuse may occur in the form of violence on the part of the patient toward the caregiver. Conversely, the caregiver may frequently abuse the patient. It is quite evident that in spite of constant support, many caregivers still react violently to their long period of stress and frustration. These occurrences of abuse are not uncommon, but this information is usually revealed only after the deep, mutual trust formed in ongoing groups is established.

Handling of practical matters (finances, homemaking care, nursing home investigation, and so on) are usually discussed and acted upon in these groups. Alzheimer's disease is a very costly illness for which our social services do not provide. Many of the practical problems encountered are common to most of the members. Therefore, they are able to share and give each other the benefit of their mutual experiences.

Above are some of the more common situations that may arise within the family of an Alzheimer patient. The ongoing support groups provide an opportunity for the participant to ventilate feelings of anger, frustration, unhappiness, and guilt within the confines of an empathetic, understanding setting.

CONCLUSION

Moos (8), when speaking of family support, maintains families must endure years of siege with a chronically ill child, such as a leukemic. Hence, it is important to constantly help the family conserve their energies for a long, traumatic pull. We must apply this same concept to families with an Alzheimer's disease patient, for their energies, both physical and emotional, can also be expended very quickly. Thus, continuous support reinforcement for as long as the patient lives becomes necessary.

REFERENCES

1. Schneck M, Reisberg B, Ferris S: An overview of current concepts of Alzheimer's disease. *Am J Psychiatry* 1982; 139:165–173.

2. Angel RW: Understanding and diagnosing senile dementia. *Geriatrics* 1977 (Aug): 47–49.

3. Barnes RF, Raskind MA, Scott M, et al: Problems of families caring for Alzheimer patients: use of a support group. *J Am Geriatr Soc* 1981; 29:80–85.

4. Lezak MD: Living with the characterologically altered brain injured patient. *J Clin Psychiatry* 1978; 39:592–598.

5. Eisdorfer C, Cohen D: Management of the patient and family coping with dementing illness. *J Fam Pract* 1981; 12:831–837.

6. Zarit SM: The organic brain syndromes and family relationships, in Ragan PK (ed): *Aging Parents*. Los Angeles, University of Southern California Press, 1979, pp 237–257.

7. Zarit SM, Reever KE, Bach-Peterson J: Relatives of impaired elderly: correlates of feelings of burden. *Gerontologist* 1980; 20:649–655.

8. Moos RH (ed): *Coping with Physical Illness*. New York, Plenum, 1977.

SECTION XIII
FUTURE DIRECTIONS IN ALZHEIMER'S DISEASE RESEARCH

58 An American Perspective

Robert N. Butler
Marian Emr

In the summer of 1977, three United States federal organizations with interests in varying aspects of the aging brain—the National Institute on Aging (NIA), the National Institute of Neurological and Communicative Disorders and Stroke (NINCDS), and the National Institute of Mental Health (NIMH)—sponsored a conference to evaluate the status of research on senile dementia of the Alzheimer type (SDAT). The meeting brought to light the disturbing fact that a mere 12 significant research grants on dementia were being supported by the three institutes.

On a more positive note, the meeting served as a public forum for presenting research results of more than 15 years, including recognition of the fact that senile dementia is not an inevitable result of the aging process. In fact, one of the most important results of this meeting was to underline the relationship between senile brain disease and Alzheimer's disease: both involve progressive mental deterioration with increasing loss of memory and judgment, and pathological signs of brain atrophy, neurofibrillary tangles, neuritic plaques, and granulo-vacuolar bodies. A syndrome with these pathological findings was first classified in 1907 as "presenile dementia" by the German pathologist Alois Alzheimer. Clinical presentation, postmortem pathology, electron microscopy, and histochemical studies all seemed to support the concept that these syndromes are indistinguishable with one exception: Alzheimer's disease at that time was said to occur in the late forties and fifties, and senile dementia of the Alzheimer-type was said to occur only after the age of 65.

New knowledge was presented at the 1977 meeting regarding genetic and environmental factors, structural brain changes and abnormalities in structural proteins, chemical and metabolic changes, the role of slow viruses, and immunological factors associated with AD.

The discussion also recognized the importance of distinguishing between Alzheimer-type dementia, other irreversible forms of dementia, and the reversible dementias—a topic which was the focus of a later NIA-sponsored conference. A surprising number of confusional states are due to malnutrition, anemia, alcohol, and unrecognized physical ailments including congestive heart failure, infections, and even fecal impaction. If diagnosed correctly and treated promptly, these conditions are usually reversible.

Epidemiologists, citing the difficulties of dealing with a heterogeneous entity, noted the lack of baseline data necessary for scientific study of senile dementia and called for new studies of the incidence and prevalence of the dementias.

The meeting concluded with recommendations for future studies on the epidemiology and etiology of senile dementia of the Alzheimer's type.

Several years later, scientists are asking many of the same questions. Still, we have managed to set an action agenda for the ultimate cure and prevention of AD. Such an agenda embraces: (1) identifying the causes and mechanisms of development; (2) determining who is at greatest risk and why; (3) devising methods of early and accurate diagnosis as well as treatment and care of the dementias in their reversible and irreversible forms; and (4) applying this knowledge through well-trained and organized caregivers.

In 1981, the three institutes spent more than $15 million on dementia research—up from $3 million in 1976. The NIA has been particularly instrumental in stimulating interest in research on some of the very promising leads in dementia research:

1. GENETICS. Familiar clustering has been reported. Siblings of persons with Alzheimer-type dementia have a 3.8% risk of having the disease. The child of parents who had AD has a 10% risk. Researchers also find an elevated frequency of Down's syndrome and blood disorders such as leukemia and Hodgkin's disease among family members as compared with the general population. Conceivably, a gene or a group of genes may be identified as causing or promoting AD.

2. TRACE METAL STUDIES. As early as 1965, investigators working with experimental animals induced the development of neurofibrillary degeneration like that seen in postmortem study of the brains of AD patients by injecting aluminum salts. These studies stimulated other researchers who later reported an increase of 10 to 30 times the normal concentration of aluminum in the brains of individuals who had died having Alzheimer-type dementia. Still, the role of normal levels of aluminum and other metals in the brain, and aluminum's relation to AD have yet to be determined. Because of this, it is too early to say whether removal of aluminum from the body would be productive or practical.

3. IMMUNE REACTIONS. Some investigators believe that in old age, the immune system loses its ability to recognize elements of the host's body and that antibrain antibodies may be causes of neuronal degeneration. Other recent but very promising studies on AD involve tissue typing and the suggestion that people with certain tissue types may be more susceptible to specific diseases.

4. SLOW VIRUSES. AD may be among the nervous system diseases believed to be caused by slow viruses. In the late 1960s, material from several patients with rare familial cases of AD produced degenerative brain disease in chimpanzees and provided the first hint that the dementing disorders might be caused by slow-acting transmissible viruses. Numerous attempts to reproduce and corroborate these initial findings have been entirely unsuccessful. Still, the frequent similarity in symptoms and the demonstration of familial occurrence of AD is intriguing, as is the theory that a hidden virus is responsible for slowly progressive damage to the brain which produces symptoms of the disease only after a long period of time.

5. NEUROTRANSMITTERS. There are consistent findings that AD patients have a marked reduction in choline acetyltransferase (CAT), the enzyme instrumental in the production of the neurotransmitter acetylcholine. This change in neurochemical activity correlates with changes in memory and orientation, and also with the number of characteristic lesions seen in the brains of AD victims at autopsy. As this research began to unfold, some investigators attempted to supplement the brain's supply of choline. This approach would be comparable to the treatment of Parkinson's disease with L-dopa. Other investigators are attempting to increase cholinergic activity in the brain by preventing the fast breakdown of the neurotransmitter acetylcholine rather than overloading the system with choline. Still other investigators are administering choline in combination with a metabolic enhancer. The preliminary successes being reported in the literature are the most exciting findings in this area to date.

6. BASIC BRAIN STUDIES. Essential to understanding AD are studies of how the normal brain functions at various stages of life. At the NIA Laboratory of Neurosciences and at several other centers worldwide, scientists are applying a sophisticated research procedure, positron emission tomography (PET), to characterize regional brain metabolism in healthy individuals and AD patients. This procedure may eventually be useful in diagnosis and in developing a foundation for effective treatment of AD.

7. POPULATION STUDIES. NIA epidemiologists have outlined a strategy to study noninstitutionalized older adults who have early and mild dementia and who are generally overlooked in medical and statistical analysis of dementing disorders. In one community-based survey of mental illness, researchers will attempt to identify AD victims who have remained outside institutions. Meanwhile, small populations are being followed in an attempt to develop a more accurate picture of the natural progression of dementia and its relationship to certain risk factors.

Looking back at the research agenda shows that a fourth and vital step in the conquest of dementing illness is applying new knowledge through well-trained and organized caregivers. By 2030, the elderly population will have doubled such that nearly one in five Americans will be over the age of 65. Yet according to a 1983 report by the American Medical Association, only 697 physicians out of a total of 485,123 from 80 specialties cited care of the elderly as their primary specialty. Although interest in geriatric medicine is growing, some medical schools still do not offer courses in geriatrics. Even fewer offer clinical experience in the community, hospital, or nursing home with older patients who are generally healthy as well as those who are chronically ill. Given the success of medical science in prolonging life expectancy—and the effect that it is having on population trends—physicians will begin to see more and more cases of senile dementia. It is therefore essential that all health professions prepare students to handle the special needs and problems of AD victims and elderly patients in general.

Fortunately, in recent years, professional medical societies, medical students and faculty, private organizations, and a number of government agencies have recognized the need to promote geriatric medicine and clinical research on aging. From its inception, the NIA has spurred medical educators to incorporate geriatrics into their curricula and practical training programs. NIA's Geriatric Medicine Academic Awards have the dual purpose of improving the quality of curricula in geriatrics in medical and osteopathic schools and of fostering research and careers in the field of aging. A new mechanism, the NIA's Teaching Nursing Home award, would provide an organizational focus for geriatric research and training. As envisioned, these nursing homes would be affiliated with medical, nursing, and social service schools at major university centers and would serve as models for the 18,000 nursing homes around the country just as teaching hospitals are models for community hospitals. Teaching nursing homes could foster systematic basic and clinical investigations of disease in the elderly, train health care providers, and establish a research base for improving care, community services, and rehabilitative services.

If successful, teaching nursing homes would bring geriatrics into the mainstream of American medicine. Senile dementia provides evidence that this is needed. Because of exclusion at the hospital and the mass release of patients from mental hospitals, AD victims are concentrated in nursing homes, which have virtually no ties to academia. The AD patient is relatively unrepresented in clinical research but would be one of a number of high-priority subjects for research in the teaching nursing home.

In addition to the standard mechanisms offered by the National Institutes of Health, and the few special programs outlined above, the NIA now has or will soon initiate several funding mechanisms to enhance federal support for scientific research on the dementias. A Small Grant Award program, which is limited to four categories including AD, will, one hopes, encourage new investigators or seasoned investigators with new ideas to pursue this area of inquiry. NIA's Clinical Investigator Award, which also specifies dementia as an area of particular interest, is intended to encourage clinicians with some research experience to develop their ideas for biomedical research on clinical areas relevant to aging.

The NIA has done much in recent years to expand the scope of research on aging and training in geriatrics and to ensure that an aggressive program on AD is an integral part of this activity.

INDEX